Lelamour Herbal
(MS Sloane 5, ff. 13r–57r)
An Annotated Critical Edition

Late Middle English Texts 6

LMET

David Moreno Olalla

Lelamour Herbal
(MS Sloane 5, ff. 13r–57r)
An Annotated Critical Edition

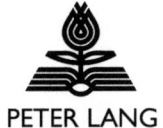

PETER LANG

Bern · Bruxelles · Frankfurt am Main · New York · Oxford · Warszawa · Wien

Bibliographic information published by die Deutsche Nationalbibliothek
Die Deutsche Nationalbibliothek lists this publication in the Deutsche National-
bibliografie; detailed bibliographic data is available on the Internet
at ‹http://dnb.d-nb.de›.

British Library Cataloguing-in-Publication Data: A catalogue record for this book
is available from The British Library, Great Britain

Library of Congress Control Number: 2017957170

Cover Image © The British Library.

ISSN 2235-0136 pb.
ISBN 978-3-0343-3155-5 pb.
ISBN 978-3-0343-3157-9 ePub

ISSN 2235-6401 eBook
ISBN 978-3-0343-3156-2 eBook
ISBN 978-3-0343-3158-6 Mobi

© Peter Lang AG, International Academic Publishers, Bern 2018
Wabernstrasse 40, CH-3007 Bern, Switzerland
bern@peterlang.com, www.peterlang.com

All rights reserved.
All parts of this publication are protected by copyright.
Any utilisation outside the strict limits of the copyright law, without the permission
of the publisher, is forbidden and liable to prosecution.
This applies in particular to reproductions, translations, microfilming, and storage
and processing in electronic retrieval systems.

Printed in Germany

of mylke ⁋ Also hit will make
pitte humours thynne ⁋ Also
stampe hit and hastyly hit
helyth wondys woundys worth
nc A man and his quo boy
shuld so y stamped y leyde
so to ⁋ Also ho amendyth byeth

Explicit mar

God grant of hyniche ha
byth y peny and y gra
uted Stipo in wordys stampe
and herbis of tho whiche erbis
a iust tho philizofur made a
boke in latyn ⁋ The whiche
boke Iohes Colinone pdena
ystor of hosfords est pey ho in
worthy vous in the yere of
oure lord. A. iij. cc lxxxny. tornyd
in to ynglio ⁋ And yff there be
any thynge myssaide in the tor
nynge of the langage the voso
reder and godely vndrestonde
he prayeth will all his herte
the faultes to amende ː⁓

A poldure ly satyffe

Take ny peny weyght
of Canonye tnch ij pe
ny weyrt of rubede ano xx
peny weyght of Sene. Ano ij.
peny weyrt of maltere. half a pe
ny weyrt of Redwale. & a peny
weyrt of spinage ⚬⚬⚬ & a peny
weyrt of floure of hanett Stā
oule of Spice And to all theso
endre & bare hem in A britein
water alt to pollere And lette
the patient vse hit fastynue eche
sawe a sponefull in swete & he
shatt be hole And hit purgeth
coteugre & dropesy in men and
woman

Contents

Acknowledgements 9
Introduction 11
   1. The text 11
      1.1. Authorship 13
      1.2. Sources 16
      1.3. The language of *LH* 28
   2. The manuscript 51
      2.1. Collation, quiring and foliation 51
      2.2. Materials, conditions and binding 54
      2.3. Watermarks 56
      2.4. Page layout and ruling 57
      2.5. Contents of the MS 58
      2.6. History of the MS 60
   3. The scribes 67
      3.1. The main scribe 68
      3.2. Other hands 76
   4. The edition 80
      4.1. Editorial criteria and typographic conventions 81
      4.2. Explanatory Notes 83
      4.3. Glossary 92
      4.4. Appendixes 93
   5. List of sources and abbreviations 95
   6. Works cited 97
Lelamour Herbal 115
Explanatory Notes 221
Glossary 467
Appendix A: Botanical names 497
Appendix B: Medical virtues 505

Acknowledgements

It is a pleasant duty to acknowledge here all the people who had some share in the making of this book. The edition had its origins in a dissertation for the degree of Ph.D. in the University of Málaga under the supervision of Dr Antonio Miranda García. To him I owe an enormous debt of personal and academic gratitude. I know that he will be particularly happy to see the book out after so many years waiting for it... but then, *nil sine magno vita labore dedit mortalibus.*

I would like to thank the British Library, not just for having waived the reproduction fees of the MS images used for the cover, frontispiece and p. 114, but also for all the help that I received from the staff at the desk of the Manuscripts Reading Room during my visits to London. My gratitude is especially directed towards Ms Claire Breay, who quickly and kindly provided expert answers to all my queries on the manuscript particulars. *Naviget Anticyram.*

Even though I do not always agree with his conclusions, my work also became so much easier and better after reading several papers on John Lelamour and his work written over the last twenty years by Professor George R. Keiser (Kansas State U.), who generously shared and discussed his ideas on the topic with a perfect stranger over several e-mails. For this and, in a less personal way, for being the author of the groundbreaking volume on *Fachliteratur* of the "Manual of the Writings in Middle English" as well, he deserves the highest praise. *Veluti pia mater, plus quam se sapere et virtutibus esse priorem vult.*

Closer home, I am particularly grateful to Mr Joaquín Garrido for his prompt and invaluable help in turning my lemmatized corpus into a proper Glossary, using his TexSEn application. Ms Jessica Carmona agreed to read large parts of the manuscript and her keen eye saved me from many infelicities. The general editors of the series read an early version of the book and provided many insightful comments that have raised the quality of the final volume. I regret to acknowledge that all remaining mistakes are unfortunately my own. *Sunt delicta tamen quibus ignovisse velimus.*

Publication expenses for this book were defrayed by a generous gift from the Department of English, French and German Philology of the University of Málaga. Thanks are particularly due to its Head, Dr. Rosario Arias, whose help was invaluable during the administrative process. *Rem facias, rem si possis, recte.*

This book is gratefully dedicated to my family: it would have never seen the light without their continuous support and forbearance. *Nunc est bibendum, nunc pede libero pulsanda tellus.*

Rincón de la Victoria (Málaga), St. Augustine's day 2017

Introduction

1. The text

This edition presents a medical herbal, a work of scientific *Fachliteratur* where the healing properties of a number of plants are collected together with several recipes where those species are used as ingredients. Some, but not all of them, include a broad physical description of the plant, its temperament according to the then current humoral theory, or practical advice on its proper harvesting, handling and usage as well. Medical herbals are therefore a derivation from treatises on *Materia Medica* or collections of *simples*, that is, lists of products frequently used in the confection of medicines, including not only vegetables but also minerals and animals, as well as their by-products (oils, distillates, chemical compounds, body fluids, and the like). As a rule, in herbals each of these simples was analysed in a chapter of its own, then arranged within the treatise in a number of ways: in alphabetical order (thus, Matthaeus Platearius's *Pandectae*), by temperament (as in the *Liber Serapionis*), by type of substance and/or perceived similarity to one another (so, Dioscorides's *Materia Medica*), or following no evident system (the case of *De Viribus Herbarum*, although here one could perhaps argue that longer entries appear at the beginning, shorter ones at the end). Although most of these works were written in prose, some of them, particularly the less technical and more popular-oriented ones, were composed in verse to benefit from the mnemonic power of rhythm and rhyme.

    Lelamour Herbal (henceforth *LH*) is a prose medical herbal written in late Middle English that contains the virtues of over two hundred species listed in a loose alphabetical arrangement using just the first letter of the plant name. *LH* survives in a single manuscript (London, British Library, Sloane MS 5, ff. 13ra–57ra, or S_1 for short). While some areas of Middle English utilitarian writing, such as historical chronicles or religious tracts, have traditionally enjoyed the continuous attention of editors, scientific prose has remained a textual Cinderella, so raising the awareness of this type of text among scholars by offering new published material is in itself reason enough for an edition of *LH*.[1] The main motive for an edition of this treatise is thus quite simple: although edited twice as parts of dissertations, the herbal has never been easily accessible in print, let alone as a commented critical edition. The lack of an edition is striking in itself, for the text contained in S_1 is one of the examples of herbals composed in Middle English that denotes some authorial desire to renovate the old formulas and even to create something new: the compiler of *LH* had evidently an encyclopaedic aim and drew his information from as many sources as he could lay his hands on, rather than offering a mere translation of a Latin poem (the cases of the Middle English versions of *De Viribus Herbarum*, *Circa Instans* and, perhaps, *Agnus Castus*). Its comprehensive spirit and the use of several sources in the compilation turn this treatise into a "designer herbal", as the text has been aptly dubbed (Keiser 2008b: 304), and makes an edition of this text a worthy addition to the library of any scholar interested in the development of science in England. Moreover, the critical use that the author of *LH* seems to have made of those sources, choosing not to reproduce a number of entries from *DVH* and *AC* dealing with plants such as ginger, zedoary or aloes probably because they were not indigenous to northern European climates but expensive Asian imports, adds to the interest of this particular ME herbal.

The present edition provides therefore the first widely available version of a very significant English medical work of the period, one which has attracted the attention of a substantial number of scholars

---

1 The reasons for the historical neglect of *Fachprosa* are manifold, see Pahta/Taavitsainen 2004; some of their remarks have been expanded and exemplified in the opening pages of Moreno Olalla 2013a.

since the late seventeenth century (not only among historians of science such as Eleanor Sinclair Rohde or Charles Talbot, but also among antiquarians and early literary historians such as Bishop Tanner or Thomas Warton and linguists such as the compilers of *OED* and *MED*) and been regarded by a contemporary scholar as one of the main herbals in ME that still awaited publication (Hunt 1989: ix–x, fn. 5).

1.1. Authorship

According to its *explicit* (reproduced in the frontispiece), *LH* is the English translation, executed by a certain ‹Joh*ann*es Lelamour›, of a treatise about the properties of plants that was originally composed in Latin by ‹Mac*er* the philizofur›, which obviously refers to Macer Floridus and his poem *De Viribus Herbarum* (*DVH* for short).² The inscription goes on to inform the reader that John Lelamour was a schoolmaster from Hereford and that he undertook the task of translating the Latin text into English in 1373. Nothing more is known about Lelamour and, since the

---

2 Ayscough 1782: 564 already read "Lelamour" and so did Halliwell-Phillipps 1889: i.xx, while Rohde 1922: 42 interpreted the final flourish as a brevigraph and thus renders the name as "John Lelamoure", but the author's name has been misspelt in a number of ways, such as "John Lelarmoner" (Bernard 1697: ii.251), "John Lelamar" (Tanner 1748: 477). Repetition of those versions in later authors is of course indicative of the ultimate source: Pulteney 1790: i.32 must have used Bernard; Albrecht von Haller must have used both Bernard's and Tanner's books, as he refers to the same volume using both designations (von Haller 1771–1772: i.215 and ii.657, respectively), while the name in Thomas Warton's widely influential *History of English Poetry* depends on the edition consulted (see Bravo Gozalo 1981: 119): the *editio princeps* mentions, under the old shelfmark "Sloane 29", both Bernard's and Tanner's versions ("John Lelarmoner, or Lelamar", Warton 1774–1781: ii.167, fn. h), while the 1824 and 1840 quarto editions, revised by Richard Price, spelt it "John Lelarmoure" (Warton 1840: ii.362, fn. h) and references the manuscript using Ayscough's shelfmark number. Hoffmann 1884: ii.765 plagiarized Warton's description, probably drawing the information from the 1871 edition (Warton 1871: iii.135), where the name is spelt Lelamar and Lelarmoner again and the pre-Ayscough shelfmark is repeated—even though that edition included "new notes and other additions" from such philological luminaries as Walter W. Skeat, R. Morris and Frederick Furnivall.

surname remains etymologically unexplained, a number of hypotheses have been put forward: it could be (faulty) French for an English name *John Love (so Talbot 1967: 187), or else it might be a copy mistake for an original *John Belamour (a conjecture hazarded in Moreno Olalla 2007: 123, fn. 28). As for Lelamour's trade, he could have been the master of Hereford Cathedral Grammar School (so Orme 1996: 55), because that was the sole establishment devoted to higher learning in that county and it was moreover known throughout medieval England as a school specialized in the teaching of Natural Sciences (Orme 1973: 172, 305). Unfortunately, no third-party record supporting any of the above ideas has been unearthed so far, in Hereford or elsewhere (see Moreno Olalla 2007: 123 and Keiser 2008b: 293). The use of different treatises in the creation of his work (→ Sources) does speak in any case for a well-stocked library such as those found in important learning centres such as a University or a Grammar School.

Generally speaking, all the statements in the *explicit* are hazy if not downright misleading: *LH* is in fact not a translation of Macer Floridus's treatise but a composite from several sources including *DVH*, and moreover S_1 was composed about ninety years later than the date provided in the inscription. It is therefore only natural, then, that the actual role of John Lelamour in the transmission of the text is called into question too. The traditional view was that all or most of the statements written in the *explicit* were trustworthy and therefore it was assumed that *LH* was indeed a translation of the Latin herbal completed in 1373 by John Lelamour. A few years ago, George Keiser demonstrated that *LH* did not stand in textual isolation, but other manuscripts must have shared a common ancestor with S_1; he hence hypothesized that John Lelamour's authorial rendering of *DVH* must have circulated around England and was reproduced in a number of copies. One is led to assume from here that the text copied in S_1, most entries of which do not derive from Macer's poem, is an amplification of John Lelamour's original translation with new matter borrowed from other textual traditions by later scribes (see Keiser 1996 for details).

Still, textual criticism and linguistic analysis indicate that the role of John Lelamour in the creation and transmission of *LH* must have been that of a compiler, not a mere translator. The common entries from *DVH* shared between S_1 and the other manuscripts, for example, cannot have been composed by a Herefordian, but by someone speaking a distinctively northern dialect. Textually as well, the composer of *LH* reproduced a collection of entries from *DVH* rather than the full translation of the Latin poem and, as fas as we can currently tell, neither one or the other was signed by John Lelamour: that name is indeed found in S_1 but missing from all other known copies of those treatises. Supporting evidence for all this is plentiful if a reconstruction of the original translation—in textual terms, the archetype Ω—is attempted from either a textological or a dialectal perspective (see Moreno Olalla 2013b and Moreno Olalla 2017, respectively).[3] The new picture suggests that in 1373 a speaker of a South-West Midland dialect, which in all likelihood was the Hereford-based John Lelamour, copied a selected Middle English translation of *DVH* that had been done somewhere in the North of England. Although this still needs further research, the presence of a few SWML words or spellings in entries taken from sources other than this translation of *DVH* suggests that Lelamour was responsible for the assemblage of the whole treatise, copying entries from different textual traditions. Several modifications of the original text (for example, a curious addition in the chapter Colombyne, → **344–346**,[4] or ⟨þe morfue⟩ → **319** substituting the more slavish rendition "black spots of the hide" that appears in the other MSS of the tradition) suggest that he was a person versed in Natural Sciences, and this certainly fits the image of a schoolmaster in Hereford Cathedral School.

Either the resulting autograph, which for all we know is now lost, or some copy thereof became the exemplar of S_1, which was composed in the London area *ca.* 1460 and remains the sole text that can be safely ascribed to John Lelamour's pen. The description of MS 497 (V.7.24) in the catalogue of the Hunterian Collection at Glasgow University Library (Young/Aitken 1908: 409) states that the sole treatise copied in this small quarto volume, dated in the early fifteenth century, is also a translation of *De Viribus Herbarum* into Middle English completed by

---

3 The textual transmission of *NM* is discussed in Moreno Olalla 2013b.
4 Bold numbers after a word/sentence refer to lines in the edition.

the same Hereford schoolmaster. Actually, the Secretary hand of the volume is better dated in the second half of the century and any cursory analysis demonstrates that the text contained there is yet another copy of the same ME herbal made in the south of England and edited in the late 1940s (Frisk 1949, → Sources). While the dating of the script and the general physical description of the book was corrected in the updated catalogue of the English MSS in that collection (Cross 2004: 33–34), the mistaken authorship attribution is unfortunately still maintained there (Moreno Olalla 2007: 121, fn. 17).

1.2. Sources

LH is a compilation of 215 entries taken from different textual families.[5] The usage of several sources can be demonstrated in a number of ways, one of them being the presence of a sizeable number of repeated species that were taken as separate plants since each of those traditions referred to the same vegetable under a different name (some of them misapplied already in the exemplar). This is different from the recopying of the same exemplary section due to some scribal mistake, as with wild chervil, spelt ‹kerwell› in **1061**, then ‹lerwell› in **1105**. Both are virtually the same entry (the first one offering additional materials borrowed from a second source) that got copied twice because the compiler misread the initial *κ in his exemplar when he was copying plant names beginning with letter L. The clearest case demonstrating Lelamour's use of several sources is that of the black hellebore (*Helleborus niger* L.), which is treated three times under different names: ‹Longwort› **1223**, ‹Pedelyon› **1851** and finally ‹Walworte› **2385**. Other instances include the following: black nightshade (*Solanum nigrum* L., **1371** and **1518**), bugle (*Ajuga reptans* L., **222** and **918**), common groundsel (*Senecio*

---

5   *LH* is generally described as containing 214 entries, but a very brief section on ‹Herba Plenius› **1045**, apparently a revisitation of the plant already treated in **656** as ‹erbe moyntayne›, was copied immediately at the end of ‹Jubarbe›, without starting a new paragraph, and was consequently skipped by Hand E in his reckoning.

vulgaris L., **794** and **824**), dill (*Anethum graveolens* L., **14** and **104**), dragons (*Dracunculus vulgaris* Schott, **37** and **538**), elecampane (*Inula elenium* L., **586** and **899**), hemlock (*Conium maculatum* L., **640** and **871**), houseleek (*Sempervivum tectorum* L., **708** and **1030**), lesser calamint (*Clinopodium nepeta* (L.) Kuntze, **1503** and **1525**), marshmallow (*Althaea officinalis* L., **848** and **2420**), onion (*Allium cepa* L., **188** and **1581**), purslane (*Portulaca oleracea* L., **975** and **1867**), rocket (*Eruca sativa* Mill., **313** and **2160**), soapwort (*Saponaria officinalis* L., **1570** and **2068**), sweet woodruff (*Galium odoratum* (L.) Scop., **629** and **2340**), thyme (*Thymum serpyllum* L., **1631** and **2313**), wild chervil (*Anthriscus sylvestris* (L.) Hoffm., **1061**, **1105**—see above—and **2136**), wild marjoram (*Origanum vulgare* L., **1552** and **1634**) and wood avens (*Geum urbanum* L., **29** and **843**). The cases of garden angelica (*Angelica archangelica* L., **655** and **1045**) and fleawort (*Plantago indica* L., **1880** and **1888**) are dubious as the identification of these plants is unsure.

Most of the treatises that Lelamour employed to create his herbal have been traced. As stated in the *explicit*, Macer Floridus's *De Viribus Herbarum* was one of these sources. Perhaps the most popular herbal in the Middle Ages (manuscript copies of the original text are literally counted by the hundreds, and translations were made into most of the major languages of Europe) and still well read until the end of the sixteenth century (Choulant 1841: 239–243 lists twenty printed editions, several of them pirated, from the 1477 Naples incunabulum to the 1590 Hamburg and Leipzig versions by Ranzovius, plus the French translation of Tremblay 1588), this poem in Latin hexameters describing the healing powers of 77 plants is thought to have been composed in France by a certain Odo de Meung-sur-Loire sometime during the late 11th or early 12th century. The original 2269 lines were supplemented in many manuscripts and early books by the *Spuria Macri*, a collection of extra simples—fixed into just 20 items in the two available modern editions—going from cheese and vinegar to manure, hartshorn and spider web (Jansen 2013).

The popularity and influence of *DVH* during the Middle Ages has made it the object of more scholarly attention than most texts of medical *Fachprosa*, including not only editions of the original Latin text (Choulant 1832, which is in sore need of revision) and long list of vernacular versions (Klemming 1883–1886, Hægstad 1906, Kålund 1907, Larsen 1931, Harpestræng 1936, Frisk 1949, Faraudo de Saint Germain 1955–1956, Bazzi 1959, Conerly/Ardemagni/Richards 1986, Capuano 1991, Corradini Bozzi 1997, Bos/Mensching 2000, Schnell/Crossgrove 2002, Hunt 2008), but a flurry of studies as well (Jansen 2013: 4–6 provides a brief yet complete and updated state of the art on the Latin text; literature on the High German rendering is thoroughly covered in Schnell/Crossgrove 2002: 53–58, while Pensado Figueiras 2012 cursorily mentions the most relevant works on the several translations into the Hispanic languages).

Notwithstanding the claims in the *explicit*, Macer Floridus's poem was the main source for just 68 entries, none of them from the *Spuria Macri*. All the chapters borrowed from *DVH* originated from translations other than the one edited in Frisk 1949, and appear to be divided into two groups. The following 23 sections are independent from any known Middle English version of the Latin text:[6] *Acedula* **2261**, *Allium* **758**, *Aristolochia* **66**, *Buglossa* **213**, *Caulis* **421**, *Cepa* **1581**, *Cicuta* **871**, *Colubrina* **37**, *Elleborus* **1223**, *Eruca* **2160**, *Galanga* **788**, *Gariofilus* **843**, *Iris* **834**, *Ligusticum* **498**, *Lolium* **1077**, *Nepeta* **1503**, *Origanum* **1552**, *Ostrutium* **1570**, *Pastinaca* **1719**, *Plantago* **1735**, *Portulaca* **1867**, *Senecio* **824**, and *Violae* **2517**. The lack of parallel manuscripts makes it very tempting to imagine that these sections were Lelamour's own work, which would give some grounds to the statement in the *explicit* that he had ‹tournyd [the original *DVH*] in-to Ynglis›, but positive evidence for this idea is yet to be found. Linguistic analysis is in fact against such notion (→ Dialect).

The other 45 sections derive ultimately from a translation done in the North of England, hence called *Northern Macer* (*NM*) to oppose it to the much better-known rendering of the same Latin text that was made

---

6   Since some of these sections either display no heading or were faultily spelt, reference to entries from this tradition is made using the plant names given in Choulant 1832 and crossreferenced with their opening line in the ME edition. The only exception is *Elleborus*, which corresponds to *Elleborus albus* (*DVH* 1774–1832) and *E. niger* (*DVH* 1833–1858): both chapters were copied as a continuous block of text in the translation.

in the Southern half of England and edited by Gösta Frisk.[7] Textually, this source can be easily spotted as most entries in *LH* without Latin heading belong here (only nine chapters from other sources miss their Latin titles), although the following ones were added by some later copyist: ⟨Anisum⟩ **14**, ⟨Apium risus⟩ **1060**, ⟨Beata⟩ **188**, ⟨Betania⟩ **149**, ⟨Bigula⟩ **204**, ⟨Camamilla⟩ **365**, ⟨Coriandrum⟩ **354**, ⟨Feniculum⟩ **693**, ⟨Genciana⟩ **803**, ⟨Lappa⟩ **560**, ⟨Papauer⟩ **1693**, ⟨Portulaca⟩ **975**, ⟨Rapa domestica⟩ **1525**, and ⟨Sacrefolium⟩ **708**.

Only one copy of *NM* is currently known (Oxford, Bodleian Library, Additional MS A.106, ff. 244r–259r, siglum *B* in the Explanatory Notes). This version contains 68 chapters out of the 77 of the Latin original, but there are good internal reasons to believe that at least two more entries (*Allium* and *Caulis*, corresponding to *DVH* 161–195 and 1201–1263, respectively) were included in its exemplar, which must have lost a sheet.[8] In two instances, moreover, the anonymous English translator decided to combine two Latin entries into a single chapter: the white and black hellebores (*DVH* 1774–1858) were presented as a continuous block ⟨Walworte⟩ **2385**, while the virtues of *Barrocus* (*DVH* 1641–1663) were copied immediately after those of *Aristolochia* (*DVH* 1395–1436) under ⟨Medewort⟩ **1355**. Therefore, besides the lost sections on cabbage and garlic, in fact only the following seven chapters are currently missing an equivalent in *NM*: *Lactuca* (*DVH* 765–775), *Ligusticum* (*DVH* 882–906), *Cyperus* (*DVH* 1585–1604), *Colubrina* (*DVH* 1728–1765), *Cicuta* (*DVH* 2030–2055), *Pyrethrum* (*DVH* 2086–2108) and *Cyminum* (*DVH* 2111–2124).

Textual analysis proves that Lelamour did not use a copy of *NM* as his exemplar, but an assortment from it, called *Rue Herbal* (*RH*)[9] since

---

7 A list of 43 entries from this source is given in Moreno Olalla 2013b: 932: note that ⟨Nepis⟩ **1526** and ⟨Papy⟩ **1694** were not included there as their origins had not been properly traced at the time.
8 Evidence in favour of this hypothesis is given in Moreno Olalla 2018 and mainly rests on the existence of a Renaissance edition of *DVH* that is textually very close to the one used as Latin exemplar by the anonymous translator of *NM*.
9 This abridgement from *NM* is alternatively referred as Branch β in the Explanatory Notes as it opposes Branch α (to which MS *B* belongs; see Moreno Olalla 2013b for details).

the virtues of rue (*Ruta graveolens* L.) probably opened the treatise. This compendium enjoyed some diffusion at the time: virtually the same selection of entries, copied in roughly the same order, is found in at least two other volumes (London, Wellcome Library, MS 5650, ff. 29r–39v and Cambridge, Magdalene College, Pepys MS 1661, pp. 266–284), and textual criticism strongly indicates that there were copies in other manuscripts which are now lost. These would include of course John Lelamour's autograph, called *Λ* in the stemma suggested in Moreno Olalla 2013b: 955. Parts of the fragmentary herbal kept in the so-called "Lincoln Thornton" (Lincoln Cathedral, Dean and Chapter Library MS 91, ff. 315r–321v; see Keiser 1996 for details) seem to belong here as well, and a very short text contained in London, British Library, Sloane MS 7, f. 105v must have derived from either *NM* or *RH*. The existence of these common entries both in S_1 and a number of manuscripts, all of which can be palaeographically dated after the third quarter of the 14th century, naturally led Prof. Keiser to assume that they were copies from the original 1373 version referred in the *explicit*, and hence he referred to *RH* as *Lelamour Herbal*, but textual and, above all, linguistic evidence are against this idea (as demonstrated in Moreno Olalla 2017).[10]

The most important source by number of entries in *LH*, yet, is not *DVH* but *Agnus Castus*. This anonymous herbal describes 248 plants alphabetically arranged under their Latin names, which turns it into one of the most important Middle English herbals even though this includes just letters A through S. (Some MSS offer entries beginning with the remaining letters, but the editor considered these to be later additions; see Brodin 1950: 11.) The author of *AC* kept a pattern in the confection of the entries: after the Latin name and a collection of vernacular synonyms comes a description of the morphology and known habitat(s) of the species. Then, except in a few short entries, a list of remedies

---

10 One would be at a loss, for instance, to find the "strong evidence of a Hereford dialect" that Keiser 2008a: 193 detects in the copy of *RH* contained in the Wellcome version. This text displays a strictly Northern dialect, as attested *inter alia* by verb endings or a collection of lexical choices. Only the alternation of *ā* and *ō* may cast some doubts about its origin, but this feature is regularly found in Northern dialects since the second half of the fourteenth century (Morsbach 1896: §§ 136–137) and is hence of little consequence.

follows, and frequently a simplified reference to the qualities of the species without mentioning its exact temperament.

AC outlived the Middle Ages and remained popular throughout the sixteenth century and was printed a number of times by Rycharde Banckes, Robert Redman, Anthony Askham, William Copland and Robert Wyer (Brodin 1950: 319–320; see also Arber 1953: 41–44), but its actual origins are disputed. It has been stated that "no known Latin source for this herbal exists" (Keiser 2008b: 294, fn. 1), although Gösta Brodin thought that the ME text was a translation of a Latin treatise akin to the one contained in London, British Library, Sloane MS 2948 (siglum *Sl*), and to prove his point he reproduced a number of entries (Brodin 1950: 20–25). Any cursory reading into this slim manuscript makes it impossible to escape the fact that the Latin and English versions are indeed very closely related not only in the choice of words and syntactic structures, but even in more minute details: Brodin is quick to point out the presence of common anacolutha and scribal mistakes in both versions. On the other hand, Sloane 2948 being written in a 15th-century Anglicana hand, there is always a chance that this manuscript is a translation *from* English *into* Latin. The presence of some English plant names interspersed in the Latin text, which Brodin quoted to demonstrate the insular origins of the Latin treatise, could then be re-interpreted as words in his exemplar for which the English translator did not know a Latin equivalent. The fact that, contrary to the ME version, the Latin text provides complete temperaments is also suspicious, for it quite unlikely that the English translator would have dropped such a piece of important information on purpose. As for the shared anacolutha and errors, they bear little to no weight in the argument as they can work both ways: from Latin to English, as Brodin wants them, but also vice versa. Unfortunately, the textual history of *AC* has been ignored since the 1950s and more research is needed before this matter can be settled.

The exact relationship between *LH* and *AC* is not completely transparent either. It is quite clear that no less than 101 sections of the former treatise derive from a copy of the latter. But, contrary to his usual policy with the other textual traditions used for his compilation,

Lelamour did not copy *literatim* from his exemplar in this case but in many cases he preferred to abridge the physical description of the species found there, sometimes heavily. Moreover, instead of copying all entries from *AC* beginning with the same letter continuously, as he did with *NM*, for most letters the group of sections from this source is split into two or more parts and spread over the whole letter block. To a lesser extent, the same happens to entries from the independent version of *DVH*, with which entries are frequently shuffled. See below about Lelamour's handling of his sources.

The third identifiable source in *LH* is the one used to compose a single entry, ‹Rose mary› **1985**. The longest section in the whole herbal (it contains almost 800 words), the chapter on the supposed medical powers of *Rosmarinus officinalis* L. is a copy of one of the several English translations of a Latin prose treatise known as *The Virtues of Rosemary*. This little piece became very popular in England, since it was copied several times during the Middle Ages and still printed as late as 1637 (Keiser 2008a: 198–204 provides a list of manuscripts and edits both a Latin version and a ME translation—that of *LH*, actually).[11]

Thirty-two entries stem from hitherto untraced sources. Most of these chapters share a number of structural traits, hence allowing their division into groups that might indicate a common origin. For convenience, these groups will be referred to here as *U*-sources (U_1, U_2, etc.). Needless to say, the groupings made here are largely hypothetical and hence bound to change—or indeed proved altogether wrong—as the matter is researched further. The first of these groups (U_1) is formed by ‹Basilica› **282**, ‹Fenigre[c]u*m*› **749**, ‹Spica celtica› **1048**, ‹Psiliu*m*› **1888** and ‹Apiu*m* siluaticu*m*› **2136**. These entries, in opposition to the other untraced chapters, offer a Latin heading and a full temperament, that is, indicating both qualities in their exact degrees, opening each section (whereas, for example, the temperament was given at the end in entries from *AC*). On the other hand, they offer neither Middle English synonyms nor botanical descriptions. ‹Psiliu*m*›, ‹Basilica›

---

11 The popularity of the text is shown as well in the number of translations into other European languages, including two Middle High German dialects (Zimmermann 1980: 368–370, Boot/Mayer 1990: 109–111) and Medieval Spanish (López 1987).

and ⟨Apium siluaticum⟩ present some small divergences from the rest but, all in all, they keep the same structure. In the first case, the Latin heading was used as headword, and thus the ME name (actually, the Latin borrowing ⟨policarya⟩) became a synonym. The chapter on basils does mention a very sketchy morphological description but simply because three different types were traditionally distinguished. ⟨Apium siluaticum⟩ also provides a physical description of the species, yet has been included into the same group as the above because the description looks like a later addition: the entry describes as a whole the virtues of chervil (*Anthriscus sylvestris* (L.) Hoffm.) but the described plant is surely a honeysuckle (*Lonicera periclymenum* L), so the mistake must be due to a scribal confusion between *CERFOIL(E) (whence ⟨Serfoyle⟩ **2137**) and *CHEVIRFOIL(E) < La. *caprifolium* during the transmission.

It is probable that ⟨Vrtica⟩ **1476**, ⟨Petrocillium⟩ **1798** and ⟨Epetimum⟩ **2313** belong to this group as well: they keep the same features as the above but their temperament consists of their relative heat only, while ⟨Diptanum⟩ **573**, ⟨Hastula regia⟩ **2340** and ⟨Salix⟩ **2510** similarly provide a faulty temperament that records one quality (either comparative heat or dryness), but this time without degrees. The sections ⟨Isopus⟩ **985** and ⟨Arthemesia⟩ **1384** agree with those characteristics but are slightly different as well: the second half of the former (**994–1004**) seems to have been a translation from *DVH* and a continuous block of lines from the latter (**1399–1405**) are strongly reminiscent of passages in *AC*, the final part being again similar to *DVH*. It is then possible that they are composite sections (see below). The adscription of these eight sections to U_1 is therefore unclear, but in any case the missing list of ME synonyms and descriptions makes them extremely close to the preceding group of chapters.[12]

Although there is a chance that they are just yet another subset within U_1, ⟨Euperatorium⟩ **132**, ⟨Sigilum Sancte Marie⟩ **2276**, ⟨Bursa pastoris⟩ **2306** and probably ⟨Caruium⟩ **406** should perhaps be segregated

---

12 One could perhaps argue that these three sections were copied from a herbal similar to the one printed in Wright/Wülcker 1968: I.553–554, where species were simply divided into "chaudes herbes", "freides herbes", "inter frigidum et calidum" and "inter frigidum et calidum temperatum", but I think it is improbable.

into a second group (U_2). These entries again offer a Latin heading and information on the temperament, but this time they are silent as to their exact degrees. As above, these sections do not record information on the morphology or usual habitat of the species treated but, in opposition to U_1, they do provide a list of ME synonyms. The only exception to this rule is ⟨Caruium⟩ as no synonyms are quoted there, but then this species had few, if any, synonyms in Middle English or Latin so this omission is only to be expected.[13]

A possible group (U_3) would be formed by a collection of entries that mention no temperament but do include some sort of botanical description (usually, but not always, covering both plant morphology and habitat). This group would be formed by ⟨Horeworte⟩ **884**, ⟨M[ir]tus⟩ **1097**, ⟨Lavandyr coton⟩ **1175**, ⟨Auricula muris⟩ **1467**, ⟨Ragworte⟩ **1930**, ⟨Crassula minor⟩ **2150** and ⟨Anabulla⟩ **2331**. Another common trait is their shortness: all these chapters are under a hundred words, noticeably shorter than the other U-sources. It is unclear whether the text displayed Latin headings in the exemplar since three of them miss it in S_1. About half the members of U_3 provide alternative Middle English plant names just after the headword but then, just like in the case of ⟨Caruium⟩ above, there seem to have been few synonyms in Middle English for those which offer none (⟨Lavandyr coton⟩, ⟨Mowsere⟩ or ⟨Stonecrop⟩),[14] so this feature probably carries little weight by itself.

---

13 Hunt 1989 includes *budthistil* (var. *bunthistil*) as a possible synonym under the headwords *bombix* and *cordimena*, but these derive from a scribal confusion between *CARDUUM and *CARU(I)UM, hence the intended ME word probably was *WUDTHISTEL (*MED*: s.v. wōde-thistel). The synonym *dominella* in the same source, glossed *carwi*, looks like a further deformation from *cordimena*. As for Latin synonyms, André 1985 only recorded *careum* and *caros*², both of which are of course the Latin and macaronic Greek versions of Classical Greek καρώ.

14 The same names are used for instance in *AC*, where only *stonore* is used to refer to the latter species. Hunt 1989 included the equivalents *lambes tounge* and *(h)er(t)swort(h)* in a few synonyma under the Latin name *Pilosella* which was also applied to mouse-ear, but note that all these plant names were copied together in the same gloss only once (in Cambridge, Gonville and Caius 200/106, pp. 196a–214, a synonyma described as "careless and inaccurate with frequent errors", Hunt 1989: xxx–xxxi). The evidence rather suggests that mouse-ear and lamb's-tongue/hartwort were taken to be separate species.

Lelamour Herbal 25

The mysterious ⟨H*erba* Plenius⟩ **1045** may also belong here as the entry succinctly provides both a morphological description and a habitat for the species, and the same goes for ⟨Tana[s]etu*m*⟩ **2323** which again provides a comparatively lengthy physical description in an otherwise brief chapter (just 76 words).

The last group of untraced sections (U_4) would be formed by the following chapters: ⟨Genes[t]ula⟩ **250**, ⟨Balsamu*m*⟩ **266**, ⟨Moleyne⟩ **1443**, ⟨Elactuericu*m*⟩ **2216**, ⟨Tanasetu*m*⟩ **2282**, ⟨Nasturciu*m* aquaticu*m*⟩ **2452**. These are extremely simple entries as they provide neither temperaments nor botanical descriptions and mention no synonyms either: they consist of just a list of medical virtues, which can be quite complete in some cases (three of the entries are well beyond the one-hundred-word length: 187 words in the case of ⟨Genes[t]ula⟩, 176 in ⟨Balsamu*m*⟩, and 172 in ⟨Nasturciu*m* aquaticu*m*⟩, and cf. also ⟨Elactuericu*m*⟩ with 99). All of them save ⟨Moleyne⟩ display Latin headings. It is possible that ⟨Sagge⟩ **2080** and ⟨Lolliu*m*⟩ **2537** belong to this group as well for they are also structurally very simple, although they do include some ME synonyms and, in the case of sage, the Latin headword is missing.

Next to the sections from untraced sources, a small but textually interesting group is formed by about a dozen entries which some scribe, perhaps Lelamour himself, must have created by merging information from several traditions into a single chapter. These conflations are demonstrated by the entry ⟨Kerwell⟩ **1061**, which offers virtually the same text copied from *NM* that will appear some few lines later as ⟨[K]erwell⟩ **1105** (including the misreading of an exemplary *MAUDEFLAUNKE as **maudeslamy(l)ke* **1063**, **1106**), but with the addition of several virtues taken from the entry *Apium risus* in *AC*, so that the first version more than doubles the length of the original chapter in *NM*: 167 vs. 72 words. The cases of ⟨Isope⟩ **986** and ⟨Mogwort⟩ **1385** are analysed above. ⟨Horehounde⟩ **935** similarly combines a translation of *Marrubium* in *DVH* with virtues of the parallel section from *AC* added at the end. But it is *AC* that served as basis for the larger number of these enhanced sections: ⟨Pelletir⟩ **1820** and ⟨Sowtheryne-wode⟩ **2111** were augmented with data taken from the chapters *Pyrethrum* and *Abrotanum* in *DVH*

(2086–2108 and 31–52, respectively), while ⟨Heyhofe⟩ **893**, ⟨Scabyeus⟩ **2206**, ⟨Synkefoly⟩ **2236**, ⟨Wodesoure⟩ **2469**, and ⟨Wodebynd⟩ **2484** offer in their second half a collection of virtues probably taken from one of the untraced groups outlined above. Like ⟨Mogwort⟩, ⟨Comyn⟩ **476** and ⟨Elenacampana⟩ **586** are particularly noteworthy as they combine fragments from three sources: first *AC*, then the appropriate sections from *DVH* and finally *U*.

Lelamour arranged his entries according to their ME plant names, using a loose alphabetical order that only attended to the first letter of the words and ignoring the rest. Plotting the entries of *LH* into a plectogram (Olmsted 1994) suggests that the compiler intended—quite logically—to reproduce his exemplars in batches, copying all entries beginning with a given letter in one of the books at his disposal, then consulting a second manuscript, then a third one, etc., and starting all over again once information under that particular letter was exhausted in all his sources. Still, the final result was messier than expected. Only the entries from *NM* were copied as continuous blocks, and even here the section for letter H is exceptional, since ⟨Helow⟩ **975** was not copied together with the other chapters from that source (⟨Horshele⟩ **899** and ⟨Henbane⟩ **905**) but added at the very end of the block. It is possible that the word was faultily spelt already in the exemplar and the copyist did not immediately identify the species (see Moreno Olalla 2013b: 946, fn. 27, where the reconstructed word is taken to have been *wowell).

Lelamour's handling of *DVH* and *AC* was not straightforward, because entries belonging to these traditions frequently appear scattered inside the letter-blocks. Although the sections from *AC* were copied continuously in blocks B, E, I and V/W, and there is a single entry from that tradition in blocks K and T, in the other blocks they appear split into two or more groups. For example, the six entries from *AC* are located thus within block F: first, lines **662–692** contain ⟨Filex campestris⟩, ⟨Filipendula⟩ and ⟨Fumus terre⟩, then come the two entries from *NM* (⟨Feniculum⟩ and ⟨Sacrefolium⟩), and finally three more entries from *AC* covering **712–748** (⟨Febrefuga⟩, ⟨Iris⟩ and ⟨Linum⟩). In the same vein, entries from *DVH* appear clustered together in block O only, and there is only one section from this tradition in blocks B, K, L, N and V/W, but they are distributed following no clear arrangement throughout blocks A, C, G, H, P and S (there are no entries from *DVH* under the rest of letters).

The reason behind Lelamour's different handling of his sources is not clear, although it must have something to do with the fact that the exemplar of *NM* was of course written in English, and hence gathering all the species beginning with the same letter presented no difficulty, while the other traditions at his disposal were either arranged by their Latin headings (certainly *AC* and probably the several *U*-sources) or else following no clear system (*DVH*), and therefore finding the English equivalents for the original plant names was not as immediate. Even so, it is hard to explain why ‹Anetum› **104**, which was to be glossed as ‹Annete› (hence posing little problems to the compiler in deciding its relative position within the herbal) and was placed in third position in his exemplar of *AC*, should appear after ‹Sana mu*n*da› **29** or ‹Agrimonia› **55**, which also begins with A but is positioned as the thirteenth entry in *AC*, unless Lelamour had some interest in having them at the beginning of the block, or else he used a copy of *AC* where the chapters were heavily shuffled.

Lelamour's handling of the untraced sources into batches while composing his herbal could give some support to the hypothesis that the four *U*-sources outlined above derived from as many exemplars: ‹Genes[t]ula› **250** and ‹Balsamu*m*› **266**, both associated to U_4, and ‹Tana[s]etu*m*› **2323** and ‹Anabulla› **2331**, both from U_3, form continuous blocks respectively under B and T. This could be taken as an indication that the compiler was maintaining the order kept in his exemplars for these sources. On the other hand, entries from U_1 are split, as shown by ‹Petrocilliu*m*› **1798** and ‹P[s]illiu*m*› **1888** in block P and ‹Hastula regia› **2340** and ‹Salix› **2510** in block V/W, so evidence is unconclusive.

Concerning the order used in selecting his sources, Lelamour did not follow a fixed system in the usage of the texts, but there is a marked preference for *AC* and *NM* to open the blocks: entries from *Agnus Castus* come first with letters D, E, F, H, M, O, P and R, while those from *Northern Macer* open blocks A, B, C, L and S. The untraced sources come next: U_1 provided the first chapter in blocks K, N, V/W, and (apparently with additional information copied from *DVH*) also I, while U_4 opened T. The independent translation from *DVH* was used first in block G only. Similarly, it seems that Lelamour used his exemplars from untraced sources, and U_3 in particular, at the very end of each letter-stint. There is be some tendency for entries from those families to appear in final positions: chapters from U_3 appear at the end of blocks I, K, M and T, while U_1 closes blocks B and F and U_2 closes blocks A and S.

1.3. The language of LH

The following is a description of the main linguistic features of *LH*, including an analysis of its dialect. The lists of words provided henceforward are as a rule not exhaustive but include illustrative examples only, but either exact figures or percentages are provided for those features that could be of interest to scholars. Some of the figures quoted here will also be found in Moreno Olalla 2007: 139–142, while the section on nouns and adjectives is for the most part an abridgement of Moreno Olalla 2011, which provides much more detailed information, including a larger collection of examples, and fuller discussion about the main features of those categories.

1.3.1. Phonetic and spelling overview

A. Vowels

The close front vowel is, as usual in ME texts, spelt through three allographs: ⟨i⟩, ⟨j⟩ and ⟨y⟩. The scribe largely avoided ⟨i⟩ in initial position if followed by a vowel, but there are some cases of ⟨j⟩ before consonants. As expected, ⟨y⟩ is frequently chosen in the vicinity of minims, being consistently chosen before and after ⟨m⟩, and most of the cases in the nearness of ⟨n⟩, but it alternates with ⟨i⟩ in writing environments where confusion is not likely to occur. Before ⟨u⟩ functioning as a vowel, the scribe preferred ⟨j⟩, the sole counterexample in the text being ⟨Plenyus⟩

2398. There is a single example of doubling of the vowel, ⟨myys⟩ **2128** (< La. *micae*). These graphs can stand for:

(1) OE, ON and Romance *i*: ⟨dym⟩ **1652** (< *dimm*), ⟨lyddis⟩ **2274** (< *hlid*); ⟨yl⟩ **1626** (< *illr*), ⟨skynne⟩ **2167** (< *skinn*); ⟨lycorys⟩ **1248** (< *licoris*), ⟨mylfoly⟩ **673** (< *milfoil*), etc. Cases of Anglian smoothing of *io*, simplification of initial *ġ-* before front vowels, and later shortenings also belong here, cf. ⟨mylk⟩ **1561** (< *mioluc*), ⟨siluer⟩ **632** (< *siolfor*); ⟨icching⟩ **1558** (< *ġiċċan*), ⟨iff⟩ **567** (< *ġif* and *ġiefan*); and ⟨lynsede⟩ **751** (< *līnsǣd*) or ⟨light⟩ (< *līht*), respectively. The corresponding long vowel is found in ⟨bliþe⟩ **212** (< *blīðe*) or ⟨swynes⟩ **774** (< *swīn*) and, with originally lengthened vowels, also in ⟨child⟩ **2072** (< *ċild*) or ⟨wilde⟩ **133** (< *wilde*), together with such OF words as ⟨frye⟩ **601** (< *frire*) or ⟨spicis⟩ **518** (< *espice*).

(2) OE *y* and OF *u*, both long and short: ⟨fill⟩ **738** (< *fyllan*), ⟨lyfte⟩ **2536** (< *lyft*); ⟨flix⟩ **2023** (< *flux*), ⟨hirt⟩ **2534** (< *hurter*), and maybe ⟨lymbrykys⟩ **1279** (< La. *lumbrīcus*). Examples of shortened vowels include ⟨filth⟩ **2059** (< *fylð*) and perhaps ⟨liþer⟩ **480** (< *lȳðre*), which is seldom found (see below). Some of these words alternate with ⟨u⟩-spellings, cf. ⟨flux⟩ **202**, which is much more common than ⟨flix⟩ (19× : 4×), or ⟨hurt⟩ **61**.[15] The vowel is long in ⟨fire⟩ **628** (< *fȳr*), or ⟨lyse⟩ **1178** (< *lȳs*) and, with lenthening, also ⟨kynde⟩ **142** (< *cynd*) or ⟨mynde⟩ **1184** (< *(ġe)mynd*).

(3) OE *īġ* and *ȳġ*: ⟨drye⟩ **1** (< *drȳġe*) or ⟨tyle⟩ **1294** (< *tiġule*); note also ⟨ly⟩ **1619** (< *licġan*, but reformulated from conjugated *liġest*, *liġeð*, cf. *-līð* already in eWS, Campbell 1959: § 267). Cases of Anglian smoothing of *ē(o)ġ*, such as ⟨flyes⟩ **1234** (< *flēoġe*) and ⟨dye⟩ **180** (< eME *dēʒen*, cf. ON *dø(y)ja*, *deyja*), belong here as well.

(4) eME *e* in a number of phonetic environments, mostly before nasal clusters, as in ⟨ynglis⟩ **2549** (< OE *englisċ*), ⟨quynche⟩ **2526** (< OE *cwenċan*) or ⟨swython⟩ **824** (< OF *sen(e)chion*, via **sinchon* > **suichon*). There are a few examples before other clusters, cf. ⟨dyrkyn⟩ **944**, ⟨dyrknes⟩ **1605** (< OE *deorcan, deorcnes*) or ⟨silfe-

---

15 It may worth mentioning that ⟨i⟩-spellings are recorded for both words from f. 40 onwards, and could hence be relics of exemplary readings vs. the ⟨u⟩-forms, which would represent the copyist's dialect.

‹hele› **223** (< OE *se(o)lf* + *hǣlan*). ‹e›-forms are also found alongside most of them, cf. ‹englishe› **709**, ‹quenchith› **1426**, ‹stenche› **1359** or ‹derknes› **160**. The case of ‹gris› **2367** must be included here too (→ Dialect).

Just like its front counterpart, the close back vowel is spelt in a variety of ways: ‹o›, ‹ou›, ‹ov›, ‹ow›, ‹u› and ‹v›. Of these, ‹ov› is very seldom used (just twice: ‹comovn› **663** and ‹movthe› **1603**), while ‹v› is generally found at the beginning of a word but extremely rare elsewhere (only ‹spvyng› **2050**).[16] Concerning ‹o›, see below. ‹u› stands for the short vowel, while ‹ou› and ‹ow› represent the long counterpart. In a few words of OF origin, ‹u› alternates with ‹eu›, ‹ew› (see below). Other than these cases, these letters stand for:

(1) OE, ON and OF *u*: ‹full› (< *full*), ‹lust› (< *lust*); ‹long› **1950** (< *lunga*); ‹jornaye› **1400** (< *journée*), ‹sodeyn› **1662** (< *sudain*), etc. The vowel is lengthened in ‹grounde› **238** (< *grund*), ‹hownde› **195** (< *hund*); ‹bowellis› **481** (< *bouel*), ‹powd*er*› **23** (< *poudre*), etc. and is etymologically long in ‹cowe› **81** (< *cū*), ‹mouþe› **27** (< *mūð*), etc. ‹i-drowid› **342** (< *drūgian*) belongs here as well.

(2) OE *y*, particularly if followed by tautosyllabic *r*: ‹borþen› **766** (< *byrðen*) and ‹wort› **253** (< *wyrt*). Probable examples of the same trend might be ‹woll› **310** (< *wil(l)e*), next to the much more frequent ‹wil-› (5× : 145×), and ‹woman› **48** (< *wīfmann*), via intermediate **wyl(l)e* and *wymman in lOE due to labialization of the original front vowel after *w*- (Hogg 1992: §§ 5.180–181). The sole example of the long vowel are the several instances of ‹brusid› **491** (< *brȳsan*), which is spelt ‹broyse› in **1603**.

‹e› represents both the short, the long close-mid and the long open-mid front vowels. The letter is seldom doubled for the last two cases (only nine instances in the whole treatise, including the apparently misspelt ‹holee› **950** and the otherwise unknown ‹diuee› **963**). ‹ea› is even less frequent since—besides *EARTHNOTE, miscopied as ‹carthnote›

---

16 In ‹bvgill› **205**, ‹cvlrage› **517**, ‹fvmyter› **681**, ‹lvnary› **1253**, ‹lvpyne› **1192** and ‹tvtymallys› **2332** the presence of ‹v› is due to a conscious scribal choice as he drew the second letter of the opening word of each section as a smaller capital.

458—it is recorded just twice in the whole treatise, ⟨beatis⟩ **189** and ⟨seall⟩ **2277**.[17] The graph represents:

(1) OE, ON and Romance *e*: ⟨helpe⟩ **225** (< *help*), ⟨rest⟩ **948** (< *restan*); ⟨egge⟩ **1214** (< *egg*), ⟨leggis⟩ **1804** (< *legr*); ⟨afferme⟩ **851** (< *affermer*), ⟨erbe⟩ **36** (< *herbe*), etc. These include as well ⟨smert⟩ **1199** (related to < **smiertu*, Gmc. **smart-iþō*) and ⟨yerde⟩ **113** (< *ġierd*, Gmc. **gazdī*), i.e. possible cases of Anglian *e* instead of WS *ie*, and instances of shortened vowels such as ⟨yett⟩ **873** (< OE *ġīet*) and perhaps ⟨chessboll⟩ **1696** (if from OE *cīese* "cheese"). OE and OF examples with a long vowel are frequently due to lengthening processes, as in ⟨breke⟩ **524** (< *brecan*), ⟨mete⟩ **63** (< *mete*); ⟨beste⟩ **948** (< *beste*), or ⟨spece⟩ **530** (< *espece*).[18] Cases of OF *e* from La. *a* (Nyrop 1899–1930: § I.170) also belong here, cf. ⟨degre⟩ **103** (< *degradus*) or ⟨grece⟩ **774** (< *crassus*), as are those of reduction of OF *ai*, as in ⟨entrellys⟩ **1166** (< *entrailles*) or ⟨esyle⟩ **2211** (< *aisil*), for which ⟨ai⟩-variants are recorded as well.

(2) OE *eo*: ⟨hert⟩ **924** (< *heorot*) and ⟨yellowe⟩ **1468** (< *ġeolu*), but also cases of earlier *io* like ⟨cleue⟩ **31** (< *cleofian*) or ⟨pese⟩ **1193** (< *peose*). The long vowel is found in ⟨be⟩ **15** (< *bēon*) or ⟨chese⟩ **1540** (< *ċēosan*). Lengthened cases such as ⟨smere-worte⟩ **1312** (< *smeoru-*) belong here as well, and do those of ON and OF *ø*, to which they were assimilated, cf. ⟨seme⟩ **632** (< *sǿma*); ⟨keuerchiff⟩ **2479** (< *cuevrechief*) or ⟨pepill⟩ **2437** (< *poeple*).

(3) OE *ē*: ⟨geese⟩ **973** (< *gēs*), ⟨teþe⟩ **332** (< *tēð*), etc. Anglian reflexes of Gmc. **ā*, i.e. the so-called *ǣ*₁, and of the i-mutation of *ēa* (Campbell 1959: §§ 128, 200) also belong here, cf. ⟨sede⟩ **26** (< *sǣd*), ⟨threde⟩ **1281** (< *ðrǣd*); ⟨herynge⟩ **546** (< *hīeran*). A number of ⟨a⟩-forms are found side to side with others displaying ⟨e⟩ for "let" (⟨lat⟩ **97**), the preferred vowel being unclear: *lat* 17× vs. *let* 18×.

---

17 Since ⟨ee⟩, rather than ⟨ea⟩, would be etymologically expected in ⟨beatis⟩ (< OE *bēte*, ultimately from La. *bēta*), it is likely that the spelling suffered influence from La. *beatus*.

18 The scribe made a careful distinction between "species" and "spices" (spelt ⟨spices⟩ **1225**), both of them ultimately from La. *speciēs*, in all instances except ⟨spice⟩ **666**.

(4) OE ǣ, i.e. the i-mutation of ā (Gmc. *ai*): ⟨clene⟩ **115** (< *clǣne*), ⟨hele⟩ **36** (< *hǣlan*), etc. In the case of OE ǣniġ, ⟨e⟩-forms are clearly hegemonic, but there are examples of ⟨a⟩- and ⟨o⟩-spellings too: ⟨eny⟩ 23×, ⟨any⟩ 9×, ⟨ony⟩ 3×. Note the ⟨a⟩-spelling of ⟨silfehale⟩ **919** in a text where Gmc. **xailjan* "to heal" and its derivations are always spelt ⟨hel-⟩.

(5) OE ēa: ⟨ere⟩ **696** (< *ēare*), ⟨lefe⟩ **607** (< *lēaf*), etc. This includes lengthened cases such as ⟨berde⟩ **1989** (< *beard*) and perhaps ⟨ferne⟩ **663** (< *fearn*).

(6) eME *i* if before a nasal, *r* and, most frequently, in the vicinity of a labial consonant (Luick 1964: §§ 379–380): ⟨senowys⟩ **339** (< OE *sionu*); ⟨þerd⟩ **1553** (< OE *ðridda*); ⟨medill⟩ **1256** (< OE *middel*), ⟨wekkyd⟩ **1314** (< OE *wicca*), ⟨wete⟩ **1089** and apparently ⟨bellyre⟩ **240** (< OIr *biolar*). These include instances of OE *y/ie* in the same environments, cf. ⟨dente⟩ **152** (< *dynt*), ⟨hemloke⟩ **533** (< *hymeliċe*), ⟨herdis⟩ **147** (< *hierde*) or ⟨kernyng⟩ **2320** (< **ciernung*); ⟨skemmyd⟩ **328** (< OF *escumer*) may also belong here. Alternative ⟨i⟩-spellings are much more frequent for "sinew" (18× out of 19×) or "third" (26× out of 31×) and are sometimes found for "wicked" (5× vs. 19×). It is not clear whether ⟨weth⟩ **1856** belongs here as this is a weakly stressed word, but it is the sole case in a text where ⟨i⟩-spellings are hegemonic (411×, plus 52× of compounds such as *within*, *without*, *withhold*, etc.). Note as well ⟨kyrnyng⟩ **108** and the unexpected ⟨þorst⟩ **2033**, which could be just a badly written **þerst*. Lengthened eME *i* from OE *y* is found in ⟨euyll⟩ **12** (< *ȳfel*) and perhaps ⟨leþer⟩ **127** (< *lȳðre*), which is much more frequent than ⟨liþer⟩ (12× vs. 2×).

⟨o⟩ can stand in *LH* for the short, the long close-mid and the long open-mid back vowels. Moreover, the letter frequently represents the short close back vowel, particularly when in the vicinity of minims. The vowel is geminated just twice to indicate the close-mid vowel of ⟨horshoo⟩ **984** and ⟨twoo⟩ **228** (Jordan 1974: § 45). The graph can stand for:

(1) OE, ON and Romance *o*: ⟨dokk⟩ **569** (< *docce*), ⟨stok⟩ **478** (< *stocc*); ⟨crosse⟩ **474** (< *kross*), ⟨skolle⟩ **2532** (< *skolt*); ⟨forse⟩ **1661** (< *force*),

⟨olife⟩ **270** (< *olive*), etc. Examples of lengthened vowel are ⟨hore⟩ **1203** (< *horu*), ⟨smoke⟩ **77** (< *smoca*); ⟨close⟩ **972** (< *clos-*) or ⟨sole⟩ **2536** (< *sole*). Etymologically long vowels are found in ⟨blode⟩ **148** (< *blōd*), ⟨toþe⟩ **332** (< *tōð*); ⟨crokid⟩ **542** (< *krók*), ⟨rote⟩ **4** (< *rót*), etc., and shortened in ⟨blossu*m*⟩ **499** (< *blōstm(a)*), ⟨softe⟩ **1786** (< *sōfte*) or ⟨yox⟩ **109** (< *ġeōcsa*).

(2) OE and ON *ā*: ⟨cloþe⟩ **101** (< *clāð*), ⟨go⟩ **337** (< *gān*); ⟨boþe⟩ **1027** (< *báðir*), etc. OE *a* by homorganic lengthening, in ⟨colde⟩ **119** (< *cald*) also belong here, as do Anglian forms displaying *a* instead of WS *ea* such as ⟨foldyng⟩ **2471** (< *fealdan*), ⟨olde⟩ **144** (< *eald*), etc.

(3) OE, ON and OF *u* by the so-called Open Syllable Lengthening, in ⟨dor⟩ **2008** (< *duru*) and ⟨wodis⟩ **459** (< *wudu*). In the vicinity of minims, including ⟨v⟩, ⟨r⟩ and ⟨t⟩, the letter is generally spelt ⟨o⟩, as in ⟨hony⟩ **45** (< *huniġ*), ⟨not⟩ **1543** (< *hnutu*); ⟨horting⟩ **528** (< *hurter*), ⟨norys⟩ **1210** (< *nurice*), etc. Cf. also ⟨clofe-tonge⟩ **1851** (< *clufðunge*), ⟨opon⟩ **110** (< *upon*); ⟨podyngs⟩ **1268** (< *boudin*), or ⟨soffyr⟩ **53** (< *suffrir*), without surrounding minims. Some of these words are also spelt with ⟨u⟩ or ⟨v⟩ in the treatise (⟨spurge⟩ **2217**, ⟨vpon⟩ **183**, etc.).

(4) eME *a* followed by a tautosyllabic nasal, as in ⟨bondis⟩ **296** (< ON *band*), ⟨cerelonge⟩ **923** (< OF *cer(f)langue*) or ⟨hond⟩ **1915** (< OE *hand*). A few of these display alternatives with ⟨a⟩, but ⟨o⟩-spellings are as a rule much more frequent, being the sole possibility for "among", "hand", "hang", "long", "stand" and "strong", and hegemonic with "handful" (2× : 1×). "Bond" and "cerelong" appear only once. ⟨mon⟩ is on the other hand found just once, in opposition to the virtually universal ⟨man-⟩ (113×).

⟨a⟩ represents both the short and long open vowel; there are no instances of doubled letters. In stressed position, the letter stands for:

(1) OE, ON and Romance *a*: ⟨kalketrap⟩ **1049** (< *calcatræppe*); ⟨call⟩ **646** (< *kalla*), ⟨stang⟩ **1138** (< *stǫng*); ⟨branche⟩ **474** (< *branche*), ⟨passe⟩ **179** (< *passer*), etc. These also include cases of Anglian *a* (instead of WS *ea*), as in ⟨ballok*is*⟩ **21** (< *beallucas*), or ⟨fall⟩ **103**

(< *feallan*). The letter can appear before a tautosyllabic nasal, as in ⟨handfull⟩ **485** (< *handful*) or ⟨land⟩ **884** (< *land*), although ⟨o⟩-spellings are usually much more frequent (see above). The vowel was lengthened in cases such as ⟨fare⟩ **529** (< *faran*), ⟨nakyd⟩ **1917** (< *nacod*); ⟨kake⟩ **1197** (< *kaka*), ⟨take⟩ **86** (< *taka*); ⟨face⟩ **302** (< *face*), ⟨place⟩ **100** (< *place*); ⟨ale⟩ **20** (< *ealu*), ⟨schappe⟩ **1143** (< *sċeap*), etc.

(2) OE *æ*, including shortened cases: ⟨bak⟩ **1470** (< *bæc*), ⟨small⟩ **973** (< *smæl*); ⟨fatte⟩ **973** (< *fætt*), ⟨adder⟩ **2009** (< *næddre*), and probably also ⟨drad⟩ **43** (< *drǣdan*; see Luick 1964: § 363.3). This includes also ⟨lady⟩ **1521** (< *hlǣfdīġe*), shortened and then lengthened after the simplification of the cluster. OE *tōgæder* is sometimes spelt ⟨to-gader⟩ but is more frequently found as ⟨togeder⟩ (20× : 54×).

(3) OF *au* before a labial consonant, a nasal cluster, or an affricate *g* (Luick 1964: § 427.1–2): ⟨chafe⟩ **2503** (< *chaufer*), ⟨chambur⟩ **65** (< *chaumbre*), and ⟨sage⟩ **2092** (< *sauge*), respectively. ⟨au⟩-forms can be also found alongside these (cf. ⟨jau*n*dys⟩ **612**, or ⟨sauge⟩ **927**), see below.

(4) eME *e* and *eo* before tautosyllabic *r*, alternating with etymological ⟨e⟩-spellings: ⟨cars⟩ **2454** (< OE *cerse*), ⟨marche⟩ **1809** (< OE *mereċe*); there seem to be a few cases of the same trend before tautosyllabic *r* as well, cf. ⟨newffratik⟩ **701** (< OF *nefretique*) or ⟨franticles⟩ **1667** (< ON *freknur*).

As for diphthongs, the scribe of *LH* used ⟨ai⟩/⟨ay⟩ and ⟨ei⟩/⟨ey⟩ interchangeably, as shown by pairs such as ⟨lay⟩ **115** /⟨ley⟩ **144**, ⟨raynes⟩ **129**/⟨reynes⟩ **117** and many others. ⟨a⟩-variants are by far the most frequent allographs (80.66%), including many lexemes where *ei* would be etymologically expected (cf. for instance ⟨way⟩ **2015** or ⟨payne⟩ **1778**, < OE *weġ*, OF *peine*). The diphthong has for the most part the usual origins (OE *aġ, æġ, ǣġ, eġ, ēġ*, ON *ei*, OF *ai, ei*), but it is also found before the cluster ⟨nth⟩ in words such as ⟨leynthe⟩ **541** or ⟨streynthe⟩ **407**, and in the words ⟨kayre⟩ **1046** and ⟨laiste⟩ **888**, about which, → Dialect. Concerning ⟨playntayn⟩ **167** and ⟨plaist*er*⟩ **11** (< OF *plantain, plastre*), see von Wartburg 1928–2002: *s.vv.* plantago, emplastrum. There are no clear instances of smoothing in the text: ⟨mygrane⟩ **1844** (< OF *migraine*) is the sole candidate, but the presence of minims immediately afterwards makes it more likely that this is just a scribal mistake, as is ⟨seide⟩ **543** "seed", perhaps through influence of "said".

Parallel to the merging of *ai* and *ei*, *LH* displays several examples suggesting that ⟨au⟩/⟨aw⟩[19] and ⟨ou⟩/⟨ow⟩ (when not used to indicate a close back vowel) could have represented the same sound sometimes, cf. ⟨clawynge⟩ **420**/⟨clowyng⟩ **1403**, ⟨lawe⟩ **2237**/⟨lowe⟩ **296** or ⟨strawe⟩ **110**/⟨strow⟩ **1394** and spellings such as ⟨blawiþ⟩ **609**, ⟨knawleche⟩ **1909** or ⟨jawys⟩ **73** (< OE *blāwan, cnāwan*, OF *joue*). But in opposition to *ai/ei*, though, in the case of *au/ou* for the most part the scribe kept their etymological spellings. Other than the instances noted above, which must include also ⟨lawe⟩/⟨lowe⟩ (< **hlēow*) and ⟨strawe⟩/⟨strowe⟩ (< *strēowan*)—about which, see below—the origin of the diphthongs are the usual: ⟨au⟩ comes either from OE *a* or *ēa* followed by *w* or *g* or from Romance *au* (including AN *a* before nasals instead of OF *a*), while ⟨ou⟩ derives from either OE *ā* or *o* followed by *w* or *g*, or else it represents the usual off-glides before ⟨gh⟩. Smoothing of this diphthong is frequently verified in OF borrowings before nasals, as in ⟨jandis⟩ **235** (< *jaunice*), but there are examples before other consonants as well, cf. ⟨chafe⟩ **2503** (< *chaufer*), ⟨sagge⟩ **2080** (< *sauge*).

⟨eu⟩ and ⟨ew⟩ derive regularly from either OE *ēow, ēaw* or OF *eu*. The words ⟨lowe⟩ **2050** "tepid" and ⟨strowe⟩ **64** "scatter" (also spelt ⟨law(e)⟩ **1130**, ⟨strawe⟩ **110**) should be included here as well, cf. OE **hlēow, strēowian* whence PDE *lew* (dialectal) and *strew*, but must have evolved from the rising diphthong (cf. ⟨foure⟩ **1079** or ⟨trowe⟩ **2440** < OE *fēower, trēow(i)an*); about ⟨euche⟩ **179**, → Dialect. In the following four words ⟨eu⟩/⟨ew⟩ alternated with ⟨u⟩/⟨v⟩/⟨w⟩: ⟨leuke-warme⟩ **830** /⟨luke-warme⟩ **17** (< OE *hlēow-*), ⟨rew⟩ **1955**/⟨rwe⟩ **599** (< OF *rue*), ⟨du⟩/⟨dew⟩ **1430** (< OF *deü*) and ⟨spewynge⟩ **2319**/⟨spvyng⟩ **2050** (< OE *spēowan*). In the first case ⟨u⟩-forms are hegemonic (5× vs. 1×), but with "rue" ⟨ew⟩-spellings are clearly the majority (15× vs. 2×); the last words only

---

19 The spelling ⟨av⟩ is recorded twice in the text, with the same word and in an interval of just a few lines: ⟨javndys⟩ **1382** and ⟨javndis⟩ **1392**. Hence the spelling probably answers to a passing scribal fancy.

appear once each in the text. Note as well ⟨grewell⟩ **778** and ⟨fedyrfewe⟩ **2284** to represent OF *grüel, fevrefue*.

The unstable ME diphthong *ui* is spelt as a monophthong in ⟨frute⟩ **1007**, ⟨jule⟩ **659** and ⟨june⟩ **633**, but note ⟨froite⟩ **1539** as well as the very frequent ⟨juis⟩ **1**, rather than the rare ⟨iuse⟩ **195** (277× vs. 8×). ⟨superfluyte⟩ is *de facto* a Latin borrowing. The rest of the diphthongs used in *LH* (⟨oi⟩ and ⟨io⟩) are of lesser interest as they appear in the expected places (i.e. a number of OF loanwords), except for ⟨voymett⟩ **161**, which looks like a scribal attempt to make sense of an exemplary reading which may have displayed four minims; ⟨stoyned⟩ **958**, probably from an exemplary *STONYED; and the pair ⟨broyse⟩ and ⟨hoyles⟩, about which, → Dialect. The case of ⟨voce⟩ **452** may be a Northernism but it appears in an entry with no evident Northern links, so it may be yet another scribal mistake.

Concerning unstressed vowels, and putting aside the case of words of Romance origin, where etymological and phonetic spellings coexisted (cf. ⟨autours⟩ **363**/⟨autor⟩ **2063**, ⟨playnteyn⟩ **167**/⟨playnton⟩ **1939**, ⟨sodeynly⟩ **196**/⟨sodenly⟩ **1846**, etc.), and a few examples such as ⟨blossu*m*⟩ **499**, where the following labial consonant must have helped to round the unstressed vowel, it seems clear that the scribe of *LH* had a marked preference to employ ⟨i⟩/⟨y⟩ rather than ⟨e⟩ except in absolute final position, where the letter was actually silent and was frequently added unetymologically (Moreno Olalla 2011: 56–58, 62–64). An analysis of the vowel used in the more usual grammatical endings (-*s*, -*þ*, -*d*) has demonstrated that ⟨i⟩/⟨y⟩ is used in about 80% of the total number of instances (79.53%, 83.92% and 83.27%, respectively). There is a sizeable number of instances where these endings were written without a vowel but, other than in cases such as ⟨ancles⟩ **1028** or ⟨brayd⟩ **389** which are caused by the peculiarity of their lexemes, the dropping is verified in very few nouns only (⟨addris⟩ **1591**, ⟨corners⟩ **652**, ⟨man*er*s⟩ **366**, ⟨naddirs⟩ **1610**, ⟨synews⟩ **1783**, ⟨vertus⟩ **2322**, or ⟨waters⟩ **241**).

B. CONSONANTS

The consonantal system of *LH* is fairly typical of a late ME text. Double consonants regularly indicate a preceding short vowel, even if the cluster is followed by ⟨e⟩, although there are a few counterexamples: ⟨gommys⟩

73, ⟨grette⟩ 880, ⟨mell⟩ 1202, ⟨nosse⟩ 547, ⟨oppyn⟩ 1272, ⟨rippe⟩ 1204, ⟨rosse⟩ 924, ⟨woddis⟩ 1099 and particularly ⟨shappe⟩ 799, which is spelt with a single ⟨p⟩ just twice (as opposed to 11× with gemination). ⟨deppir⟩ 1028 (< OE *dēop*) and probably ⟨rykkylles⟩ 795 (< OE *rīecels*) do not belong here as they had shortened vowels. On the other hand, a single consonant followed by final ⟨e⟩ does not necessarily mean a preceding long vowel, as seen for example in ⟨pute⟩ 881 next to ⟨put⟩ 33, ⟨putt⟩ 1925 and conjugated ⟨puttiþ⟩ 11, or ⟨sone⟩, which stands for "soon" in 248 but for "sun" in 1875. Even so, the coda "single consonant-plus-⟨e⟩" is comparatively so frequent in the treatise to mark a preceding long vowel that spellings such as ⟨doþ⟩ 424, ⟨mor⟩ 2481 or ⟨wyn⟩ 234 feel slightly alien—an impression that is reassured by data, cf. ⟨doþ⟩ 9× vs. ⟨doþe, dothe⟩ 59×, ⟨mor⟩ 1× vs. ⟨more⟩ 26× or ⟨wyn⟩ 12× vs. ⟨wyne⟩ 190×.

The alternation between the velar plosives and their palatalized counterparts is for the most part the one expected in a Southern dialect, except for a few exemplary forms in entries from *NM*, such as ⟨mekyll⟩ 2406 (1×), ⟨skap⟩ 2381 (2×) alternating with the usual ⟨myche⟩/⟨moche⟩ (40×), ⟨shappe⟩ (17×), or ⟨kerwell⟩ 1105 as opposed to ⟨cheruell⟩ 1061 (and also ⟨serfoyle⟩ 2137). Dialectal differences within the OF continuum explain ⟨skallyd⟩ 1853 vs. ⟨shaldid⟩ 111. The sole unexpected forms are ⟨kyrnyng⟩ 108, also spelt ⟨kerning⟩ 2320, and ⟨askys⟩ 446, ⟨askyn⟩ 2376. Concerning the other plosives, the final alveolar seems to have been voiced in ⟨appetide⟩ 402 (4× as opposed to ⟨appetite⟩ 1603, which only appears once), as well as in the noun and verb "comfort", spelt with ⟨d⟩ if in absolute final position (⟨conford⟩ 715) but with ⟨t⟩ elsewhere (⟨comfortiþ⟩ 78).

The situation of the fricatives and affricates is typical of a late Southern ME text. Both the voiced and the voiceless dental fricatives are indifferently represented by the graphs ⟨þ⟩ (3051×) and ⟨th⟩ (3150×). The voiced alveolar is spelt with ⟨s⟩ except in ⟨philozofur⟩ 2547, and the same graph, together with ⟨c⟩, serves to represent its voiceless counterpart. In a few cases ⟨sc⟩ was chosen for the task, mainly when followed by *l*: ⟨scleith⟩ 396; ⟨sclepe⟩ 187, 202, 1414; ⟨slcepy⟩ 1352 and ⟨resceyved⟩ 2350, but variants without ⟨c⟩ are more frequent by far.

The voiceless postalveolar is as a rule spelt ‹sh›, seldom ‹sch›: 283×
vs. 21×, while *sk-* (spelt ‹sc› and ‹sk›) is found mostly in borrowings
such as ‹skabbe› **565**, ‹scamony› **1281** or ‹scome› **1374** (< ON *skabbr*,
La. *scammōnia*, OF *escume*); see above about ‹skallyd› and ‹askys›.
The voiceless velar fricative is spelt ‹gh› (90×), less usually ‹ȝ› (20×),
without any clear instance of dropping of the phoneme other than in
the preposition ‹þrow› **428**. The voiced affricate is as a rule spelt ‹j›
and less frequently ‹i› in initial position, and ‹g› elsewhere: ‹jaundys›
612, ‹iuse› **195**, ‹magiron› **1265**, ‹age› **1057**, ‹rige› **1095**. ‹g› appears
in initial position as well in a few OF borrowings (‹gencyan› **804**,
‹genderith› **1621**, ‹gentill› **407**, ‹germandir› **812**, ‹gus› **2368**), and the
scribe used medial ‹gh› in ‹eghe› **1873** and ‹gg› in ‹sagge› **2080**. The
voiceless counterpart is always ‹ch›, which can be spelt ‹cch› after a
short vowel (‹bocchis› **941**, note yet ‹ychchyng› **1403**). The voiceless
labio-velar fricative is consistently spelt ‹wh›, except in ‹welkys› **1804**
and ‹s[t]andylwelkys› **2195** next to etymological ‹whelkys› **1578** (< OE
*hwelca) and where mutual influence with the mollusc *whelk* (< OE
weoloc) should perhaps not be ruled out. The glottal fricative is spelt
‹h› and always found whenever it is historically expected, including
weakly stressed words such as *he*, *him*, *hit*, etc. There are no cases of
excrescent *h-* other than ‹hache› **6–9**.

Voiceless fricatives in absolute initial position became voiced
sometimes, although the change is visible only in the case of the
labiodental and then rarely, as the sole noted examples are ‹verne› **1046**,
‹vylmyd› **599** and ‹vretyng› **1749**. As a rule ‹f›-forms clearly prevail in
LH even with the above examples, except in the case of "fern", where ‹v›-
forms outnumber those with ‹f-› (5× : 3×). The inverse spellings ‹fessell›
1982 and ‹fomyte› **1660** make it likely that the scribe emended other
cases of voiced *f-* in his exemplar, although here as well the expected
‹v›-spellings are hegemonic (3× for ‹vessell›, 7× for ‹vomyt(e)›). In
opposition to this, devoicing of *-v* in absolute final position is evinced
in cases such as ‹dryfe› **2532**, ‹hafe› **1861**, ‹yff› **1160** (whence also
‹yfith› **2359**) or ‹laxatife› **232**. ‹potache› **1297** and ‹sache› **11** may also
indicate devoicing or else influence from *ache*; ‹ch› in ‹pichon-is› **258** is
dialectally correct (Nyrop 1899–1930: § 472, von Wartburg 1928–2002:

s.v. pīpio). The form ⟨leue⟩ **1302** is a reverse spelling influenced by the plural form ⟨levis⟩.

Confusion between *ð* and *d* is infrequent yet verified not only in the vicinity of *r* (⟨oþer⟩ **576**, ⟨wedders⟩ **2456**) but also in final position, cf. ⟨wekiþ⟩ **80**, the past participles ⟨calliþ⟩ **373**, ⟨i-fryeþ⟩ **2173** and ⟨vsith⟩ **901**, and the 3rd sg. present ⟨castid⟩ **341**. Other confusions, equally rare in the treatise, include *w* and *v* in ⟨wyne⟩ **548** or ⟨sawyne⟩ **2058** on the one hand and ⟨vlake⟩ **33, 2228** or ⟨ureste⟩ **1918** on the other, and *ng* and *n* in ⟨stynkyn⟩ **809** and, oppositely, ⟨dronkyng(e)⟩ **567, 2382**, ⟨holdynge⟩ **2359**.

1.3.2. Accidence

A. Nouns

Analysis of the noun declension of *LH* strongly indicates a paradigm where the case system has been greatly weakened, as there is no morphemic distinction between nominative, accusative and dative. The several declensions that were possible in OE have been equally reduced to a heavily simplified version of a typical *a*-stem, albeit with a small collection of words which display the usual endings of *n*-stems and a few relics of some of the so-called minor declensions in the genitive and plural forms.

For the singular case, a distinction must be made between the core case and the genitive. The core case displays no ending, since final *-e* was no longer pronounced and had simply become part of the spelling of many words—often unetymologically. The study of this letter in combination with nouns suggests that the orthography of most nouns was becoming standardized: the scribe had marked spelling preferences for over 83% of the substantives. Other than the value of *-e*, the only point of any interest in connection with the core case is ⟨childire⟩ **1357**, backformed from the plural (cf. OE *ćildru*), next to the much more usual ⟨childe⟩ (35×).

Other than a few relics of minor declensions (about which, see below), cases of analytic constructions with *of* and noun premodification, the Saxon genitive is found everywhere in the herbal.

Several endings are used for the task, but there is an evident scribal preference for -*is/-ys* (79.31% of the total number of instances), followed from afar by -*es(s)* (15.86%), -*s* (4.14%) and -*ese* (0.69%). As a general rule, the synthetic genitive is used with animate beings, either humans or animals, while inanimate entities, including body parts, generally indicate the genitival relation syntactically as mere premodificators. Even so, there are a few examples of the Saxon genitive with plants, such as ‹annys-is sede› **2530**, ‹bornete-is leuys› **230** or ‹okys tre› **1462**, and with body parts ‹eyese re*n*nyng› **160**, and conversely there are several instances of premodification with animate beings, including humans: ‹nadder stynggynge› **395**, ‹addir stinge› **1531**, ‹shepe blode› **1268**; ‹mayden pappis› **642**, ‹woman flouris› **363** or ‹woman p*r*evy me*m*bris› **832**. Phrases such as ‹cowe mylke› **81–82, 148, 1216, 1561** are not necessarily instances of premodification but continuations of the OE genitive form *cū* (Campbell 1959: § 628). Other relics from the minor declensions include the athematic ‹gose gres› **310** (< OE *gōse*) and the *r*-stem ‹modir wombe› (< OE *mōdor*). The two instances of ‹woman› mentioned above could therefore answer to a shifting of that noun from the masculine athematic (OE -*es*) to the feminine athematic (OE -*e*). Note as well the old *n*-stems ‹lady day› **1521** (< OE *hlǣfdīgan*), ‹sparowe-tongue› **2156** (< OE *spearwan*) and ‹wesyll bitt› **1965** (< OE *wesulan*), where the original morpheme -*an* was reduced to -*e*, then dropped.

LH displays a couple of group genitives: ‹of man and of woman-is p*r*iuete› **442**, ‹in man and woman-is body› **2015**. The analysis of the treatise has yielded no instances of the so-called *his* genitive, but there are almost forty instances where the genitival ending is spelt as a separate word, which is likely to be at the root of this Renaissance feature, cf. the two examples just quoted, a couple of plant names such as ‹ram-ys-fote› **1907**, ‹wolfe-ys þistill› **2490** or phrases like ‹body-ys stomake› **2106** or ‹pichon-is geserys› **258**. The detached genitival ending is mostly used with animate beings, but there are two examples in conjunction with inanimate entities: ‹annys-is sede› **2530** and ‹bornete-is leuys› **230**. In nearly half the instances, the detached morpheme appears in connection with the word *one* (18×):

⟨one-is cloþes⟩ **31**, ⟨one-ys lyu*er*⟩ **1296**, etc., followed by *woman* (7×); *man*, on the other hand, seldom displays it: just ⟨man*n*-ys lyvir⟩ **233** and ⟨man-ys skynne⟩ **2167**. This feature is recorded in entries from different traditions and hence can be traced back to either Lelamour or the Sloane copyist.

As expected, the regular plural endings are virtually the same as those of the genitive case, and their percentages are strikingly similar: *-is/-ys* (79.75%), *-es* (17.85%), *-s* (1.92%), *-esse* (0.29%), *-isse* (0.19%). In opposition to genitival *-is*, yet, the morpheme is detached from its lexeme just once: ⟨dry scabbe-ys⟩ **2339**. There is a sizeable number of umlauted plurals, none of them having any particular interest, and slightly over seventy instances of weak forms, which frequently alternate with strong endings, as in ⟨askyn⟩ **2376**/⟨askys⟩ **446** (OE *æsce*) or ⟨eryn⟩ **697**/⟨erys⟩ **44**; only *child, eye, house* and *toe* always follow the weak declension. Most of them are original OE *n*-stems, but note ⟨childryn⟩ (< OE *ċild*, *s*-stem), ⟨housyn⟩ (< OE *hūs*, neuter *a*-stem) and ⟨flene⟩ as well, in case this was originally a masculine *a*-stem (< OE *flēah*, see Hogg/Fulk 2011: § 3.25). The pair ⟨eryn⟩ **1741**/⟨eggis⟩ **12** does not really belong here as each word derives from a different lexeme (OE *ǣġ* and ON *egg*). The doublets just quoted and a single instance of *that* determining a plural noun (→ Pronouns) could perhaps be used as evidence to suggest that *n*-plurals were part of the Sloane scribe's passive knowledge only and that most, if not all, weak forms in the treatise should be better regarded as relics from John Lelamour's exemplar.

The treatise offers a modicum of zero plurals too, which are diversely explained: a few are old OE long-stemmed neuters, where zero ending is in fact etymological, so ⟨lefe⟩ **607** (< OE *lēaf*), ⟨maiden⟩ **1120** (< OE *mǣġden*) or ⟨þinge⟩ **1232** (< OE *ðing*), but most instances of zero plural are nouns premodified by quantifiers, as in ⟨all man*er*⟩ **377**, ⟨diu*er*[se] akyng⟩ **748** or ⟨all þe in-warde sekenys⟩ **1567**. This is frequent of course with nouns expressing measures that are preceded by cardinal numbers, as in ⟨xx peny-wiȝt⟩ **162**, ⟨iij sponefull⟩ **17** or ⟨ij vnce⟩ **168**. Some of these words were also long-stemmed neuters in Old English, cf. ⟨viij wynt*er*⟩ **1679** < OE *winter*.

B. ADJECTIVES

As indicated in the preceding section, -*e* was demonstrably mute in *LH*, and therefore earlier distinctions between singular vs. plural or weak vs. strong declensions were erased from the adjectival paradigm: the presence or absence of the letter is as a rule dictated by its new use as a length diacritic, so that adjectives having a long stressed vowel usually display it (for instance, ‹clene› **115** or ‹gode› **35**), while those having a short stressed vowel do not (‹black› **398** or ‹fat› **777**), or else is written after a geminated consonant, as in ‹blacke› **334** or ‹fatte› **1901**. Consequently, adjectives in the treatise already function as an indeclinable grammatical category.

As regards gradation, the situation is equally predictable for a late ME text. Both synthetic and analytic formations were in use, applied indistinctively to Germanic and Romance items and, although there are no instances of synthetic gradation with polysyllabic roots, probably chosen irrespective of syllabic structure: cf. ‹more white› **512**, ‹more black› **2202** or ‹more large› **674** on the one hand and ‹more bustous› **581** or ‹more violent› **1227, 2387** on the other. In the case of synthetic comparisons, regular shortening of the root vowel is very plausible in ‹whitter› **936** (cf. also the adverb ‹deppir› **1028**), but apparently not in ‹greter› **582** and unclear in ‹febler› **1153**. The sole instance of umlauted comparative is ‹more strenger› **292–293**, which is the only example of double comparative as well. Irregular comparatives and superlatives include the following: ‹better› **777**/‹beste› **183**; ‹worste› **393**; ‹lasse› **125**/‹laste› **274**; ‹more› **323**/‹moste› **835**.

C. PRONOUNS

The paradigm of the personal pronouns is incomplete: there are no instances in the treatise of either the 1st pl. gen. or 2nd pl. obj.; moreover, the whole 1st sg. forms are missing. Concerning the 3rd person, the text belongs to the mixed type model, which combines Old English and Scandinavian forms for the 3rd plural. The paradigm for the 3rd m. is therefore *he* : *him* : *his*, that of the 3rd f. is *she* : *hir* : *hir*. The neuter paradigm uses both *hit* and *him* for the objective case, but the cases of *him* could easily be ascribed to the masculine paradigm as the scribe shifts from one gender to the other when the antecedent is a plant, cf.

⟨set hit [mustard] to þe hede and he brennyth him wiþ his hete⟩ **1328**. There seems to be some preference for *him* to appear in prepositional phrases and for *hit* to stand for the direct object, but this wants further research as counterexamples are not lacking, cf. ⟨Þe rote of hit⟩ **330**, ⟨a-noynte þe with hit⟩ **1160–1161**, or ⟨sit vpon hit⟩ **1445**. In keeping with the general ME usage, the genitive is unexceptionally *his*. As for the 3rd pl., the paradigm is as follows: *þei* (34×), *þai* (9×) : *ham(me)* (111×), *hem* (14×) : *her* (5×), *har* (1×), *hir* (1×).[20]

The deictic system consists of a proximal and a distal demonstrative pronouns, both of which frequently double as determiners.[21] The scribe has a marked preference for *this* over *thes* in the singular of the proximal pronoun (314× vs. 2×), while the reverse seems to happen for the plural (5× vs. 8×). The distal pronoun consists of a single member, *that*, which is as a rule employed as a singular form but once in the plural (⟨that askyn⟩ **2376**). Given such a small sample, it would be a moot question to decide whether this demonstrates that the same form was employed indifferently for the singular and the plural, or simply answer to a confusion by the scribe, who mistook *askyn* as a singular noun; cf. as well the few cases of verbal *-n* below.

D. VERBS

The conjugation table in *LH* is incomplete since there are no instances of the 1st person sg. either in the present or past tenses, and there are comparatively very few examples of the 2nd sg., but as far as the available evidence allows to tell, the situation is, all in all, a fairly typical one for a late ME Southern text. Even so, it is possible to detect influences from other dialects now and then. The subjunctive mood is still in use in the treatise, although it is poorly represented: just 66 noted instances, all of which are marked via either *-e* or no ending. The imperative is on the other hand very frequent (909×), but is equally unremarkable as regards the ending, which is again *-e/-Ø*; singular and plural forms are not distinguished.

---

20 ⟨hir⟩ **325** is missing from the filled *LALME* questionnaire in Moreno Olalla 2007: 139.
21 I borrow the convenient terms "proximal" and "distal", which are of general use in anatomical and psychological texts, from Lass 1992: 113.

The conjugation of the present indicative is as follows:[22]

    2nd sg.   -*st* (5×)
    3rd sg.   -*th* (1145×), -*s* (13×), -Ø (13×), -*n* (3×), -*d* (2×), -*t* (2×)
    Pl.   -*th* (103×), -Ø (19×), -*n* (1×)

It is evident from the table that -*th* is hegemonic both for the 3rd sg. (97.1%) and the plural (83.7%), but the appearance of some 3rd sg. endings is striking and deserves some comment (concerning -*d*, -*s* and -*t*, → Dialect). Most instances of zero endings in the singular (and perhaps also in the plural, but -Ø can be dialectally regular there) can be explained as examples of syncopated -*þ* after (post-)alveolar consonants, both plosives and sibilants, cf. ⟨put⟩ **271**, ⟨conford⟩ **715**, ⟨sese⟩ **1821** or ⟨staunche⟩ **1490** (Görlach 1991: 88); even so, with all these verbs alternative forms with -*þ* are hegemonic. Cases like ⟨lat hi*m* not be war*e* of the erbe and but he sclepe e *con*trario⟩ **1414** or ⟨this erbe y-ete make gode digestion⟩ **2547**, on the other hand, are perhaps best explained as instances of a missing future auxiliary *will* since they appear in clauses describing the effects of a medicine, while ⟨hit helpe the long⟩ **1950** could be a simple instance of haplography. The three cases of -*n* are not so clear. ⟨Also i*n* plaster-wise of caule, fenecrek and vynegir that helpyn to al sorys of synewys⟩ **443–445** could be actually a plural form agreeing *ad sensum* with a preceding *that* having a plural antecedent (unless the pronoun itself is plural or else indifferent to number, which is not completely impossible, see above); in ⟨The sede y-stampid and medlid wi*th* hony & etyn avoyden wormes oute of the wombe⟩ **1194–1195** and ⟨Þe juis y-dronkyn helpyn a-yene the colde cogh⟩ **1477–1478** the presence of strong past participles immediately preceding the verb may have played a paronomasiastic part, a a sort of verbal case attraction.

---

[22] The figures quoted here do not match those of Moreno Olalla 2007: 139–142 as they contain not only those for the items "3rd sg pres" or "pres pl" but also the data drawn from other items which were segregated in the questionnaire (DO, GIVE, GO, HAVE, etc.). The copula and the modals are on the other hand not included. The two plural instances of -*is* recorded in the questionnaire, on the other hand, were later found to be cases of zero ending. To make the table as compact as possible, both the preceding unstressed vowels and final ⟨-e⟩ have been dispensed with.

The present paradigm of the copula mixes *b*- and *s*-forms (< IE *b^hueH_2*- and *H_1es*-; Hogg/Fulk 2011: § 6.146; Rix/Kümmel 2001: 98, 241). The 3rd sg. is overwhelmingly marked with *is* (644×) together with a couple of instances of *be*-forms; oppositely, the plural forms generally display *beth* or *ben* (93×), seldom *ar* or *er* (5×). Concerning auxiliaries, HAVE combines syncopated *ha-* (65×) and full-stem *hav-* (48×), the ending *-th* being hegemonic both for the 3rd sg. (95×) and the plural (10×). *-s* is very infrequent (4×, always in the singular), and even rarer are zero endings and *-n* (once each, always in the plural). The 2nd sg. displays *-st*. As for the future auxiliaries, *LH* uses both SHALL (146×) and WILL (150×), the 2nd sg. ending in *-t* and the rest of persons displaying no ending; the usual vocalism for the latter is *i*, seldom *o*. MAY (26×), is always *may* for the 3rd sg. and *might* for the sole instance of the 2nd sg. (‹myght› **440**, although this could arguably be a preterite form); MUST is found only once, as a 2nd sg. form (‹moste› **2221**).

In opposition to the present tense, the preterite is seldom found in *LH*. Other than a few instances of the irregular *was* (5×), *woll* (4×), *were* (2×), *did* (1×) and *hadest* (1×), verbs in the past tense amount to just the following nine forms, most of them included in a passage of the entry "Peony": the old strong ‹fell› **1681**, ‹lett› **1680**, ‹rose› **1682**, ‹sawe› **1678** and ‹toke› **1681** and the weak ‹made› **2547**, ‹savid› **1680**, ‹taʒte› **1962** and ‹tournyd› **2549**.

Non-finite verb forms include infinitives and participles, both present and past ones. There is little to say about the infinitive other than there are five instances of *-n*, always with the verb *do*: ‹don› **1965**, ‹done› **733**, **982**, **1169**, **2009**. Other than in **1169** (‹shall done the sede›), the maintenance of the morpheme probably answers to phonotactical reasons: in **733** and **982** *-n* appears before a vowel, while in **1965** and **2009** *-n* precedes a word beginning with *n-* inside a medical phrase that was probably becoming fossilized: *shall don none harm*. (The variant without *-n* appears just once: ‹shall do no harme› **966**.) As for present participles, the ending is *-ing* as a rule (29×), rarely *-eng* (2×), but *-and* is found sometimes (about which, → Dialect).

In opposition to the other non-finite verbs, the past participle is extremely frequent (702×). About a third of them (233×) display the prefix *y-*, which is noticeably more frequent with old strong verbs than with weak ones (respectively, 149× out of 338 instances, i.e. 44.08%, vs. 101× out of 364 instances, i.e. 27.75%). Usage of *y-* was due either to Lelamour or the scribe of Sloane 5, since the prefix is regularly recorded in entries from all textual traditions, including those from *NM* where it would be unexpected. A substantial collection of strong verbs (119×) keeps the *-n* ending (a few times misspelt *-ng*, → Phonetic and spelling overview),²³ an even larger number maintains the marker *y-* (142×) and a sizeable quantity use just the bare participle (70×), but it is very seldom that both prefix and suffix are used together, just 7×. The figures for *drink* and *seethe*, the two more frequent strong verbs in the treatise, are revealing, cf. ‹y-dronke› 74× : ‹dronkyn› 25× : ‹dronke› 25× : ‹y-dronkyn› 3×, and ‹y-sod› 18× : ‹soden› 51× : ‹sodde› 17× : ‹y-soden› 3×, respectively. Alternations between the strong and the weak conjugations for the same root are not frequent in the text, but note ‹swell› **967** : ‹swellyd› **1968** (< OE *swelgan*) or ‹washen› **431** : ‹weshid› **1702** (< OE *wascan*). The case of ‹slyt› **658** : ‹slyttid› **2507** (< OE *slītan*) is dubious, as is ‹y-lok› **2274** : ‹lokkyd› **1079**, since they could derive from different verbs (OE weak **locan* and strong *lūcan*).

The most frequent past participle ending for weak verbs is *-id* (seldom *-iþ*, → Phonetic and spelling overview), which is frequently syncopated after an alveolar, as seen from ‹a-corde› **2519**, ‹y-hette› **1875**, ‹hurt› **61**, ‹y-put› **215**, ‹shred› **894** or ‹wette› **101** nexto to ‹a-noynted› **43**, ‹shaldid› **111**, ‹wastid› **254** or ‹y-grauntid› **2545**. Cf. as well pairs such as ‹brent› **766** next to ‹y-brende› **23**, ‹caste› **1267** next to ‹castid› **341** or ‹slyt› **658** next to ‹slyttid› **2507**. Just like the genitive and plural ending of the nouns, the weak past participle morpheme is detached sometimes and spelt *-it*, apparently due to confusion with the neuter pronoun. The trend is particularly frequent with *use* and *stamp* (4× each), but there are a few instances with old strong verbs, where the explanation is less obvious: ‹drinke it› **60** = *drunken*, ‹ete hit› **1600** = *eaten*. Oppositely, ‹gadryt› **342** is to be read as an imperative *gather it*. As with other features of the treatise mentioned above, this characteristic is found in

---

23 Again, the even distribution within the treatise strongly suggests that usage of *-n* was not carried over from a particular tradition but was a feature of a later scribe.

entries from different textual traditions and hence must derive either from Λ or the copyist of S_1.

1.3.3. Dialect

LH is a composite text from several sources originating from different parts of England, hence the task of describing its dialect is no straightforward matter. The *LALME* team analysed most of the texts contained in Sloane 5 (not just *LH*) and validated the information found in the *explicit* of *LH* by plotting Linguistic Profile 7361 inside Herefordshire, apparently in some location not too far from Hereford city (Grid 344 233; McIntosh/Samuels/Benskin 1986: I.199). The fitting suggested in the *Atlas* was later examined and its Hereford origin confirmed a few years later in a dissertation devoted to the re-assessment of the linguistic evidence from *LALME* associated with that county (Black 1997: 81–90).

Even so, the suitability of Sloane 5 as a reliable witness for *LALME* and the completeness of the evidence gathered and presented there remain questionable.[24] Therefore a fresh linguistic analysis of *LH*, combining information from the *Atlas* and a more traditional approach, has been attempted in a number of works (Moreno Olalla 2007, 2011, 2017). Those studies, the main ideas of which are condensed here, have

---

24 According to McIntosh 1963: 5, a manuscript such as Sloane 5, which is palaeographically dated in the 1460s would be outside the team's self-imposed time span, since Middle English texts "cease to have much value after about 1450 or 1460 [...] because they are by then becoming highly standardised". Although that statement would require some qualification as regards some types of *Fachliteratur*, particularly their most private forms, as in letter-writing, personal notes, and some receptaria, it is on the whole surely correct. On the perceived shortcomings of *LALME*, Burton 1991 makes several valid points on the selection and treatment of the manuscript evidence, although it is sometimes unnecessarily belligerent; the equally sharp retort by one of the members of the team (Benskin 1991) is a very able but ultimately unconvincing defence, as he fails to tackle the main criticisms levelled at the *Atlas*, one of them being the use of hand-filled questionnaires. Comparison of the computer-generated wordlist in Moreno Olalla 2007: 139–142 with the items presented in McIntosh *et al.* 1986: III.166–167 is certainly revealing.

revealed the presence of several dialects in *LH*, corresponding to as many scribal layers which mark, strata-like, the main episodes in the creation of the herbal. On the surface and as seen from the preceding two sections, *LH* displays a fairly typical South-Eastern dialect of the second part of the 15th century. Since there are good reasons to think that the volume was in that area from an early date, the best course is surely to assume that this must represent the speech of Hand A, that is the main scribe of the herbal, who clearly did not behave like a *literatim* scribe but chose instead to turn his exemplar into his own idiolect. Most forms and spellings in *LH* are on the whole similar to those known for London in that period, and applying *LALME*'s fit-technique to the items suggests a location around the London-Middlesex-Essex border.

Underneath the thick London fabric woven by the copyist of the Sloane text it is possible to detect at least two more layers, albeit quite faintly. The first of them has a South-Western colouring and points to some location around the Bristol Channel, which could well be somewhere in Hereford and hence represent a direct link to the elusive John Lelamour. Detectable—although arguably, as shown below—in a limited set of spelling choices (⟨o⟩, ⟨u⟩, ⟨eu⟩ and ⟨oy⟩ deriving from OE *y*, and ⟨eynth⟩ to represent OE *-engð*) and in some morphemes, this SW layer is best seen in a few lexical items. The clearest ones are ⟨kayre⟩ **1046**, the word used to refer to the rowan (*Sorbus aucuparia* L.), the group formed by ⟨kenynge⟩ **2108, 2182**, ⟨kennyng⟩ **2328** and the compound ⟨kennyng-worte⟩ **1859**, all of which derive from a word that designates an eye ailment, and the pair of synonyms ⟨s[t]andilgose⟩ and ⟨s[t]andylwelkys⟩ **2195** which refer to some plant, probably the early purple orchid (*Orchis mascula* (L.) L.).

The first two of these words evince influence from a Celtic, and particularly a Brittonic, language (cf. Gaelic *caor* "berry" or We *cerddinen* "rowan, mountain ash", and We *caenen/cen* "film"); this idea is reassured as well by word geography, for these words have been recorded as being in use in Devon and Cornwall. The third item has Germanic origins (cf. MLG *standelwort*, MHG *standelwurz*), and seems to have been a dialectal word employed in Somerset (Wright 1896–1905: *s.vv.* care *sb.*², kenning *sb.*³, standel *sb.*). All instances of these words are recorded in section drawn from *AC*, save ⟨kayre⟩ **1046** and ⟨kennyng⟩ **2328**, both of which are found in entries that belong, at least structurally, to U_3 (⟨H*erba* Plenius⟩ and ⟨Tana[s]etu*m*⟩, respectively).

Concerning the rest of the possible South-Western evidence, i.e. spellings such as ⟨borthen⟩ **71**, ⟨broyse⟩ **1603**, or ⟨euche⟩ **179** on the one hand, and ⟨le(y)nthe⟩, ⟨stre(y)nth(e)⟩ on the other, these dialectal forms are found in entries copied from several sources. For example, ⟨borþen⟩ is recorded in entries from *DVH*, U_1 and U_4, ⟨broys-⟩/⟨brus-⟩ in *DVH*, *NH* and *AC*, ⟨euche⟩ in *NM*, ⟨leynthe⟩/⟨lenthe⟩ in the *AC*, *Virtues of Rosemary*, and ⟨streynth⟩/⟨strenth⟩ in *DVH*, *NM*, *AC*, *Virtues of Rosemary* and U_2. That fact strongly suggests that these forms are not relics from the exemplar of a particular tradition used by the compiler of *LH*, but rather spellings that some scribe used as part of his active inventory for the creation of his copy. It is therefore tempting, and probably correct, to assume that these must correspond to John Lelamour's idiolect. Even so, it is fair to indicate that they could be due to the pen of the copyist of the Sloane version: *LALME* records these or similar spellings not only in areas of the SW Midlands but also in a number of locations in Essex (→ History of the MS).

Morphologically, 3rd sg. forms such as ⟨gendrit⟩ **1209**, ⟨helyt⟩ **1107**, ⟨castid⟩ **341** or ⟨helid⟩ **1976** may well be evidence of the SWML layer too. The missing **h* in the first two cases are probably to be accounted for as simple copy mistakes, but a change *-þ* > ⟨-d⟩ is harder to explain unless read as scribal hypercorrections from an earlier mistake *-þ* > **-t* in the exemplar, which would in turn mean that **-t* could be used as the past/past participle ending in the exemplar, which was emended by a later scribe who was aware of that feature. Devoicing of final *-d* is a feature found in Western dialects (Jordan 1974: § 200). Three of the four instances (all but the first of the list) appear in entries from *NM*, but the readings are unremarkable in the parallel MSS: ⟨helis⟩ *W*.36r/16, ⟨heleþ⟩ *P*.282/19 (the passage is missing in *B*); ⟨cast*is*⟩ *B*.252r/20, *W*.36r/28; ⟨helis⟩ *W*.35v/7, ⟨heleþ⟩ *P*.280/13 (the passage is again missing in the Bodley version). Hence the ending *-t* is unlikely to have derived from the exemplar used by Lelamour but rather from his own holograph, which later served as exemplar to S_1.

LH also evinces a collection of Northernisms, overwhelmingly detected in those entries copied from *NM*. Most of them were thickly daubed over with later scribes' dialects—no doubt including Lelamour's—but they can be reconstructed using the other versions of that herbal and a number of linguistic relics and copy mistakes in S_1. Phonetically and orthographically, spellings such as ⟨laiste⟩ **888** or ⟨hoyles⟩ **1157** (< OE *latost, hulu*) suggests an exemplar where long vowels could be indicated by the presence of a diacritic ⟨i⟩, while mistranslations such as ⟨colde⟩ **150** instead of *CALDE* "called" that must have rendered *DVH* 429 *soliti sunt... dicere* in the exemplar or ⟨Etyn ham colde⟩ **563** for *DVH* 1999 *sumptaque sicut olus* (which is to be explained as an exemplary *CALE translating *(h)olus* "broth"), are clear proofs of an original dialect where OE *ā* had not become *ǭ*. The spelling ⟨gris⟩ **2367** (< OE *græs*, early Scots *gres*), next to ⟨gresse⟩ **1855** and ⟨grasse⟩ **789** and which evinces raising of original *e* before an alveolar (Aitken 2002: § 14.15(8)), must be included as well in the list of phonetically Northern forms. Relics such as ⟨mekyll⟩ **2406** or ⟨skap⟩ **2381** (→ Phonetic and spelling overview) belong here as well.

From a morphological perspective, the scribe of *LH* used as a rule *-th* to mark the 3rd sg. and plural present indicative forms, but in both cases there are a small number of forms ending in the sibilant, meaning little more than 1.3% of the total number of instances. The number is comparatively so tiny that these endings cannot have been really active in the scribe's inventory, but are rather to be interpreted as remnants from his Northern exemplar that he forgot to iron out during the copying process, all the more so since there are good internal reasons to believe that either John Lelamour or the Sloane copyist altered some exemplary *-s into ⟨th⟩ (→ **1260**). Another morpheme in the text suggestive of a Northern layer in *LH* is *-and(e)* to mark the present participle (⟨rennand⟩ **1960**, ⟨stynkande⟩ **1961** and ⟨brennand⟩ **2057**), which is a very striking feature in a Southern text, where the rule is to find *-ing(e)*.

The scribes who worked on the development of *LH* (not only John Lelamour but probably the anonymous 1460s London copyist as well) were more careful in the task of turning the actual words of the exemplar into their own dialects, but even here one can find a few odd lexical choices, such as ⟨rennith⟩ **311** "it deoppilates", ⟨adeleth⟩ **372** "face" or ⟨host⟩ **1334** "cough", all of which are quite unexpected in a Southern text but would be not odd at all in a text written in a dialect with a strong Norse component (cf. ON *renna, andlit, hósti*). Cf. as well the case of ⟨beatys⟩ **189**, which ultimately derives from a misreading of an exemplary *LEC*IS* as shown by the fact that it translates *DVH* 1087 *cepis*. While OE *lēac* could stand for several alliaceous species having a pungent taste or smell, including not only onion (*Allium cepa* L.), but also garlic (*A. sativum* L.) or leek (*A. porrum* L.), during the Middle English period the sense of the word was narrowed so as to refer to leeks only except in areas having a strong Scandinavian element, where the same general meaning as the OE word was still kept or else had been especialized to mean only the onion due to ON influence (cf. Swedish *lök*, Danish *løg* or Icelandic *lauk*).

2. The manuscript

This section presents London, British Library, Sloane MS 5 as a physical artifact, both in itself and as an object in time. Therefore it contains not only a description of the present conditions of the materials which form the book (support, inks, binding, etc.) and some basic information on the book contents, but it also tries to trace the early history of the volume, from its creation in the mid-fifteenth century to its acquisition by Hans Sloane more than two hundred years later.

2.1. Collation, quiring and foliation

Sloane 5 is composed of 198 folios, collated into twenty quires as follows: $A^1 + B^2 + C^{12} + D-I^{12} + J^5 + K^{10} + L-M^{12} + N^{8+1} + O^{12} + P^{11+1+1} + Q-S^{12} + T^2$. Gatherings A, B and T once served as flyleaves to the original book, before it was modernly rebound (→ Materials, Conditions and

Binding), while the remaining quires can be divided into two groups, codicologically as well as palaeographically. On the one hand, Quire C looks like an old membrane quinternion that was later wrapped in an imperfect bifolium for protection. On the other, Quires D–S consist of a combination of two parchment folios sandwiching a paper quaternion, an arrangement that is neither random nor whimsical but answers to a frequent scribal design during the fifteenth century (De Hamel 1992: 16). Exceptions to this rule are signatures J, K and N and P. The last of these quires includes as f. 156 a small paper insert (about 180mm × 205mm) containing four recipes in a sixteenth-century Secretary; the rest were mutilated after the treatises were copied—as there is missing text in all cases. The missing folios were not carelessly torn off but painstakingly excised as close as possible to the hinge, but the thin stubs are still generally visible. For convenience, here the two main sections of the manuscript will be called Part I and Part II. Since *LH* belongs to the latter half, the information provided henceforward will refer to that section of the book unless stated otherwise, the particulars of Part I being attended to in less detail.

There are three different paginations in the manuscript, but none of them is completely accurate. The oldest one can be found in Part II only, was added by the main scribe, and follows the usual bifolium signature system. This consists of a capital letter—except for the first five bifolia of Quire H, which display lowercases—followed by an Arabic number written on the lower outer margin of the rectos of the bifolia before the cord, indicating hence the relative position of both gathering and bifolium within the volume (Muzerelle 1985: *s.v.* Signature par bifeuillets). Both the letter and the number are followed by a *punctus*, and in the first two bifolia of Quire Q (ff. 158r, 159r), they were moreover framed with the same system that serves to call the reader's attention to *lemmata* in the text. Since all those quires were originally sexternions, naturally the numbers range goes from 1 to 6, except naturally for mutilated gatherings: thus, Quire J begins on "C.5." but keeps folio "C.4." after the cord, K begins on "D.3." but keeps folios "D.1." and "D.2." after the cord, and N misses the whole bifolium "G.3." and folio "G.4." before the cord.

As a further assurance that the gatherings would be bound in the right order, the scribe added catchwords to most gatherings. Exceptions to this rule are Quires E and F, where a few missing words from the body text appear instead: ‹distroy› and ‹A-yene the son*n*e›, respectively. (Quires G and P display no catchword for reasons explained below.) The actual structure of the catchword depends on the first words of the new quire. When a quire ends mid-sentence, the scribe as a rule copied the two or—more frequently—three opening words of the next signature, always trying to end the catchword with a noun or pronoun. The sole counterexample to this rule is the single ‹Arabik› in Quire K, perhaps because the scribe felt it odd that the noun phrase did not end in a noun this time but in a Roman number (‹Arab*ik* ʒ.ij.›). When a new section begins a new gathering (as in Quires H and I), on the other hand, the full heading was repeated. For the most part, catchwords were open-boxed just like *lemmata*, the only exception being those of Quires M, O and Q, which were not underlined, and ‹Obtalmye› in Quire H, which was framed.

This early foliation is not continuous but was restarted twice, suggesting that the scribe must have completed his portion of the volume on three uneven stints, but probably during a comparatively short period of time as the paper remains the same (→ Watermarks). The first one begins on f. 13 (= D_1) and covers four quires that correspond to the whole text of *LH* and seven blank pages (= G.3.–G.6.) filled by a Tudor reader with a list of diseases and plant names. The second block is the largest, going from f. 61 (= H_1, although strictly speaking the first signature is found on the second folio as "a.2") until f. 157 (= P_{12}, signature "I.6"), hence consisting of nine quires. The third job was the shortest as it contains only three quires (ff. 158–193 = Q_1–S_{12}). Catchwords were not included in the last quire of each batch, which furthers the notion that the volume was created in batches.

The other two paginations are modern. The first of them was done by a firm hand using good-quality black ink on the upper right corner; folio numbers are usually followed by a thick dot. This is the one used for reference in the unpublished *Catalogus librorum manuscriptorum Bibliothecæ Sloanianæ* (no date, but *ca.* 1837–1840; Nickson 1998:

5). The first numbered page was the second folio of Quire C, i.e. the opening page of a short 14th century uroscopical treatise. This foliator skipped the Tudor insert, so the last folio in the MS bears number 191. A contemporary hand, who might have been the same scribe using a pen with a thinner nib, numbered each major treatise according to its relative position within the volume.

The last pagination seems to have been completed sometime during the late nineteenth or early twentieth century. Its author struck out both the treatise numbers and the previous pagination and added the new folio numbers under it, using a pen with a very thin nib. This is the foliation used by all scholars at least since Scott 1904, and hence it is the one used in this edition as well. Like the preceding two, this is also imperfect. Just like the previous librarian, the author of this one also chose to ignore the first and last folios of Quire C, although he did take into account both the single-page insert and the flyleaves that form Quire B. Quire A on the other hand remained unfoliated; it may be that the singleton was still functioning as the actual flyleaf of the volume at the time. Hence Sloane 5 is now officially composed of 194 folios.

2.2. Materials, conditions and binding

Sloane 5 is a hybrid manuscript, i.e. it was made up using both paper and parchment bifolia. Neither rodent or worm action, nor damp or fire damage has been detected, so the volume can be regarded as a finely preserved manuscript. The folios were evenly trimmed, especially as regards their width, which is roughly 205–206mm throughout the whole volume. There is a slight variation in length, though again an almost imperceptible one, the measure going from 270mm to 275mm.

All in all, parchment leaves are of middling quality. Folios of Part I are thin membranes, perhaps sheepskin to judge from its colour, while those in Part II are made of thicker vellum and sometimes keep remnants of the more keratinized extremities or else display traces of follicles in large areas of their hair side, evincing some carelessness during the pumicing process (for instance, f. 163). A sizeable number of bifolia were either unskilfully cut or severely flayed. Such manufacture holes were mended after the text was copied by gluing a piece of new parchment onto the old one, the new parchment overlapping parts of some letters in the process, as with ‹clansiþ› **348**. A scribal tendency appears to exist for those imperfect membranes to be selected as the six, i.e. central, bifolia (→ Collation, Quiring and Foliation), cf. ff. 18 (= D_6), 31 (= E_6), 42–43 (= F_{6-7}), 163 (= Q_6), and 175 (= R_6), although they functioned as the outside bifolium in ff. 73/84 (= I_{1-12}) and 111 (= L_{12}), and both as outside and central bifolia in ff. 124/127–128 (= $N_{1,\ 6-7}$), 138/144 (= $O_{6,\ 12}$), and 150–151/157 (= $P_{6-7,\ 12}$).

Paper folios, which were employed in Part II only, are quite thick and a bit rough to the touch. Their fibres run vertically. All of them—save naturally the Tudor insert in f. 156—exhibit the same watermark throughout the whole manuscript, which suggests that the reams were imported from somewhere in the Continent, probably Northern Italy (→ Watermarks). The paper being still quite crisp is a token of its good quality. The colour is matt white to clear ivory and virtually free from dirt or lint at the edges.

Several types of ink were in use in Sloane 5, but for the sake of brevity only those employed by the main scribe will be briefly dealt with here. As Hands A_1 and A_2, the main scribe used the same matt brownish iron-gall ink throughout the three stints. The ink flowed smoothly, and as a rule it is not easily possible now to spot when the scribe dipped the quill, as he was careful never to let it run dry. Hand A_3, because of the peculiar nature of his task, chose differently and used mainly a matt vermilion which has withstood the test of time remarkably well, together with matt dark blue ink to render the big initial capital letter of the main treatises of the volume (De Hamel 1992: 45).

As with so many items from the Sloane collection, the volume has not maintained its original boards but was rebound in 1971 according to a notice added at the very end of the volume. There is strong internal evidence suggesting that there was at least an earlier binding, probably done in the last quarter of the seventeenth century (→ Watermarks), and it stands to reason that there was at least an earlier one, which contained all of Part II issued as a single book *ca.* 1460. The book is now in the characteristic half-calf binding in red cloth with the oval bookpress of the Sloane family plate encircled by the legend "Bibliotheca Manuscript. Sloaneiana" gold-embossed in the middle of both the front and back panels. Since the current binding is contemporary, it is not possible to be absolutely certain now on which quires were originally assembled together and which are additions, but it is very likely that Quire C, containing the excerpt on urines and the synonyma, were sewn into an already complete MS during the late 1600s (Moreno Olalla 2004: 90). The rest of the MS must have been a single unit since the very beginning, because a Tudor hand compiled a list of diseases and plant names drawn, as a sort of index, from *LH* (a text copied in the first scribal batch, → Collation, Quiring and Foliation) and from the two medical treatises that follow and which were copied in the second stint.

2.3. Watermarks

Several watermarks can be detected in the paper folios of the volume. The one on f. 1 is a heavily decorated coat of arms depicting a horn, like those used in hunting or the post. The pattern is clearly post-medieval and quite similar to, but not exactly the same as, no. 318 in Churchill 1935: the name of the paper-maker found in that picture ("L. V. Gerrevink"), for example, is not found in the volume. This is dated 1724, but the hand of an ownership inscription on the verso side and the unmistakable fact that the volume was part of Hans Sloane's library more than 30 years before Gerrevink's paper was manufactured (→ History of the MS) strongly indicate that the paper must be older. The *ad quem* date seems to be 1668, where a similar watermark is detected for the first time in reams of paper made in Amsterdam (Heawood 1950: no. 2715). Given that both Churchill's and Heawood's watermarks had Dutch origins, we can perhaps hypothesize that this folio was manufactured in the Netherlands as well, and the bifolium used as flyleaves in the 17th-century binding.

The second post-medieval watermark in the volume is found on the Tudor insert that forms f. 156 (listed as item (12) in Contents of the

MS below). The motif is an open hand pointing upward with a five-petalled flower or some star-like object protruding from its forefinger and seems to be the same as no. 10719 in Briquet's collection, appearing in reams manufactured mostly in Italy during the first quarter of the sixteenth century (Genoa 1501–1503, 1507–1519, Rome 1515), but with variations in Spain (Toledo 1502) and France (Provence 1512–1527). The hand of the recipes, which probably dates from some of Henry VIII's early reigning years, agrees with that dating.

The third watermark is medieval and appears in virtually all paper bifolia of Part II (bar the insert, of course). The image is a griffin segreant, i.e. rampart and with extended wings, but the pattern cannot be seen at a glance as the image is in the center of the bifolium and hence each folio offers either the head, wings and forepaws or else the hind legs and the tail. The carefully drawn hairy tailtip and outline of the griffin's hind legs seems to be the same as Briquet no. 7464, a paper manufactured in Udine (1461) with contemporary variations in nearby Venice (same year) and Rome (1464).[25] The use of the same motif in the whole of Part II reinforces the idea that the book, although written in three batches, was probably commissioned as a single unit, and copied and assembled in a comparatively short timespan.

2.4. Page layout and ruling

The manuscript does not present any sign of pricking to the eye, although the noticeable evenness in the measures of the columns strongly suggests that this is simply due to the book having been trimmed prior to its binding. The folios themselves are frame-ruled in lead. The bounding area encompassed by this rectangle is 190mm × 145mm. This frame was, with a single exception, then divided into two columns, where the texts were accommodated and which are still visible (cf. for example the fully prepared yet blank f. 193v). The sizes of those two columns are strikingly even throughout the whole book:

---

[25] Images of Churchill's and Briquet's watermarks were reproduced in Moreno Olalla 2004: 91.

the outer column measures 190mm × 66mm, whereas the inner one is 190mm × 65mm. Those are the measures of the top line; the bottom lines are somewhat wider (67mm for the inner column and 70mm for the outer one). Each complete column houses 29 lines at an average. The only noted exception to the presence of two columns are ff. 61r–84v (i.e. Quires H and I), which were copied as a single column housing 35 lines to a complete page. Columns seem not to have been line-ruled so the copying task was completed freehanded—with remarkable skill as sloping is minimal. The lack of line-ruling is further strengthened by the fact that there is no correspondence between the number of lines on respective recto and verso, nor even between the two columns.

The main scribe regularly restricted himself within those self-imposed boundaries, although he always used the horizontal frame lines as rules on which to write section titles.[26] Although the final result of his work gives quite a square impression to the columns, the copyist made no real attempt to justify the lines other than by adding some wavy lines at the end of the final line in some sections (→ Decoration). In fact, he did not mind writing beyond the vertical framelines, sometimes well into the margins, as in lines 1 and 10 of f. 46rb, where ⟨ut sup*ra* de v*er*tutib*us* playnteyn⟩ **1939–1940** and ⟨vbi sup*ra*⟩ **1946** were added at the end of the entries *Rybwort* and *Rodewort,* or in 52rb, where ⟨*in* met*is*⟩ **2284** appears at the bottom line of the column after the sentence ⟨Also the juis is holsu*m*⟩.

2.5. Contents of the MS

The following list records all the texts in S_1, using the description in Scott 1904 as basis. Whenever they are included there, items are accompanied by the Voigts-Kurtz (VK) electronic catalogue number (Voigts/Kurtz 2000). Between (12) and (13) the Catalogue includes item VK 260.00 ("and in? the patient eke? measure? electuary to the restoring of the moisthood"), but these are actually the opening words of the final page

---

26 Word(s) written on the upper frame line will be referenced here using line number zero.

of VK 4072.00, which became physically separated by the Tudor insert. Note as well that VK 3527.00 is apparently Richard Dod's supplying a missing portion of the treatise that for some reason had been deleted: note that f. 157va begins with the words "[A]lma gestor*um* that yf..." written by Hand A, and they correspond to the final words in Dod's inscription. Both items have therefore been ignored here.

(1)   *De Urinis*, cum medicamentis nonnullis 3r
(2)   *Synonyma de herbis Latine, Gallice et Anglice*. 4r–12v
(3) VK 729.00. Lelamour, John. *Herbal*. *Incip*. "Ache is hote and dry" . 13ra–57ra
(4)   *Incip*. "A Powdre laskatyffe" 57rb
(5)   "Table of contents to the two treatises" 57va–60vb
(6) VK 765.00. *Incip*. "Age is moder of forretilhed". 61r–62
(7) VK 7115.00. Gordon, Bernard, *De pronosticis* (incomplete). *Incip*. "Thanne we may not pronstik maladies" 62r–63r
(8) VK 424.00. Gilbert of England, *Compendium Medicinae* (incomplete). *Incip*. "Scotomye is suche a sekenesse of the brayn" 63v–151v
(9) VK 1436.00. *Incip*. "Concepciou*n* i*d est* þe conceyvinge" 152ra–153ra
(10) VK 3339.00. *Incip*. "Lepra is a corruptiou*n* of the me*m*bris" 153ra–155ra
(11) VK 4072.00. *Incip*. "Raucedo i*d est* horshed" 155ra–155vb
(12) VK 4943.00. *Incip*. "Take an[e]ge & roste it herde" 156r
(13) VK 3527.00. *Incip*. "Mast*er* barnard wrote in a in a boke". 157rb–157va
(14) VK 4554.00. Gilbert of England, *Compendium Medicinae* (excerpt). *Incip*. "Sires we shull vnd*er*stonde" 158ra–172vb
(15) VK 2247.00. *Incip*. "Here begynneth the merueylous and sothefaste co*m*nynge of Astrologye" 173ra
(16) VK 8184.00. *Incip*. "Wete ye well in-dowtable" 173ra–179ra
(17) VK 3785.00. *Incip*. "Nowe þu man þa*t* desirest" 179ra
(18) VK 2251.00. Moon of Ptolemy. *Incip*. "Here begy*n*myth þe mone [P]tolome" 179rb–179vb
(19) VK 3817.00. *Incip*. "Nowe ye moste vnderstond that þ*ere* ben .7. planetis" 179vb–181ra
(20) VK 1539.00. *Incip*. "Evermore after oþ*er* regneþe þe .7. planetis" 181ra–182v
(21) VK 3086.00. *Incip*. "In vryne ben xviij contentis" 182vb–187rb
(22) VK 2575.00. *Incip*. "If a woman milke her right brest" 187rb

(23) VK 3287.00. *Incip.* "Carapos signifieth þe dropcye" 187va–190rb
(24) VK 1911.00. *Incip.* "For to knowe eviles that comen of postoumes" 191ra–193rb
(25) *Incip.* "no*ta* A pley att the Cardys" 194r

2.6. History of the MS

We know little about the history of Sloane 5 prior to its acquisition by Hans Sloane. The manuscript folios are still quite clean (for further details, → Materials, Conditions and Binding) while marginal inscriptions are comparatively few and, to judge from the hands, added within a short timespan, so it is possible that the volume was read only a few times. The number of people whose names are linked to this volume is similarly very reduced.

The earliest name attached to this MS appears on f. 157r, in an ownership inscription written in a textura script which reads ‹Iste liber constat Richardo/Dod. de London. Barbor/Sorior›. An Anglicana signature "Rc' dod" is scribbled immediately afterwards, and again at the bottom of ff. 164v and 165r as "Ryc' dod". We know several things about Richard Dod thanks to Keiser 2008b: 296–298; some additional information will be provided here.[27] His name appears in a number of documents dated between the 1440s and 1460s, some of which confirm that Richard Dod was indeed a citizen of London and a barber (‹Sorior› is obviously a mistake for *Sorion, i.e. "surgeon" as seen from such 15th-century spellings as *surion* and *serion*). Comparison of his Anglicana hand with the several scribblings in S_1 makes it evident that he was one of the annotators of the herbal, albeit not a very prolific one (for a brief palaeographical analysis, → Hand B). As expected in a barber-surgeon, his marginal annotations on the herbal are of a strictly practical nature, consisting for the most part of names of illnesses added in the margins next to the sentences in the treatise where they are mentioned for quick reference.

---

27 I have drawn the new information from the excellent repository *British History Online* (www.british-history.ac.uk).

The same documents disclose some information about Richard's family as well: his parents' names were William (*a*. †1445) and Alice, and he had at least one brother called William, who may have been older than him and a haberdasher by trade. (Richard's father was a haberdasher too according to Keiser's account, but I have found no document confirming this.) It is possible that a Richard Dod, tailor, who was pilloried for three hours on December 1406 for having acted as pander between his own wife Margaret and a chaplain called William Langford (Riley 1868: 566) was some relation of his, maybe his uncle. The contented cuckold and his wife lived in Bishopsgate Without, roughly the same area where the namesake barber would operate forty years later, and it seems clear that Richard Dod had close ties with the sartorial community of London. His own brother was a haberdasher, and Richard is frequently accompanied by tailors, mercers and drapers in his suits (about which, see next): such were John Asshe, Roger Moyne, John Sabyn or John Wolsale. A Richard Little in particular must have been a close associate of Richard Dod's as their names were recorded together several times. A memorandum dated 1 July 1484 (Ledward 1954: 430) mentions a Thomas and a Richard Dod, citizens and chandlers of London, and a William Dod, husbandman in Blackmore (Essex), all of whom may have belonged to the next generation of the same family.

Richard Dod appeared before the Court of Common Pleas several times during his life. From February 1441 to November 1444, a carpenter called Thomas Coventre felled a substantial number of trees in a Chigwell close once owned by William Dod, which his son Richard had enfeoffed a third party but which Thomas claimed Alice had enfeoffed him. Coventre was found guilty and committed to the Fleet as a consequence in 1446 (CP 40/739, rot.611d and 40/740, rot. 321; Michaelmas 1445 and Hilary 1446, respectively). In February 1444 Richard, who was living in Barking, made a bond with the same Coventre in £40, which he never paid as the arbitrators they had chosen to settle their differences on the Chigwell Close suit had not yet reached an agreement (CP 40/740, rot. 302; Hilary 1446). Dod later claimed that the bond was obtained under duress, because Coventre and some associates had forcefully retained him in the parish of St

Mildred Poultry (CP 40/745, rot. 408d; Easter 1447). A dispute over the actual enfeoffment of a tenement near St Mary Fenchurch back in 1447 sent Dod to the Fleet for some time during 1449 as he was unable to pay the fine and costs, which amounted to £11 13s 4d (CP 40/748, rot. 405; Hilary 1448). Curiously, Dod pleaded that when the original writ was composed (16 October 1447) "he was a yeoman, and was not, and never was afterwards a barber" as the writ supposed (maybe some legal ploy: the ownership autograph makes clear that he was a barber-surgeon in the 1460s). In September 1458 he assaulted William Dod, which probably meant his brother, and carried off a box containing a number of documents and charters related to several messuages in or near Barking (CP 40/800, rot. 122; Hilary 1461). Richard was probably trying to obtain the legal documents that would have entitled him to these messuages; the dispute must have lagged for years as Dod was granted licence to imparl to octave of Michaelmas 1465. In 1461 Dod was still operating in St Mary Fenchurch, since on March that year he trespassed on one of John Garter's properties there, which Dod claimed to have been legally enfeoffed (CP 40/802, rot. 215, Michaelmas 1461). In May 1465 he quitclaimed all the lands and chattels in Barking that a John Boder had earlier granted him, except those which had been once owned by Richard's grandfather, John (Bird/Ledward 1949: I.303). The last record we have about him is dated 1468 when, together with other three London citizens, he was a plaintiff against a Thomas Chopyn, who had disseised them of a messuage in Warwickshire (CP 40/829, rot. 407, tried at Michaelmas that same year). It is evident that Chopyn was an old acquaintance of Richard's: both had been executioners of William Dod Jr.'s gift of all his goods and chattels in June 1448 (Flower 1933–1947: V.61).

The most revealing thing about Richard Dod's legal battles, including his assault on William, is that they all revolved around real estate, and this naturally suggests that he must have been a person of some wealth. His insistence on being a yeoman during his 1447 dispute could also be construed as an indication that he was a proud landowner. Further support for this status as a well-off person is found in his having built up a modest library: an inscription on its first folio

(‹Hic incipit p*ro*logus in libr*um* vricrisiar*um* Ricardi Dodd› by the main scribe in red ink) teaches us that Richard Dod was not only the first known possessor of Sloane 5 but that he also commissioned a copy of the *Dome of Urines*, a ME version of Isaac Judaeus's *De Urinis* generally ascribed to Henry Daniel and now housed in San Marino, Huntington Library MS HM 505. Comparison of the hand of the main scribe of the Huntington MS with that of *LH* and most treatises of Sloane 5 makes it evident moreover that the same person executed both jobs: the ductus, most elements of decoration (capitals slashed with a red line, occasional bottom-line flourishes, framing of side notes and catchwords in red, etc.) and even the inks used in the creation of both volumes are obviously the same scribe's.[28] The gathering of the folios into sexternions and the pagination system is again the same and, while the watermark in Huntington is a crown (similar if not the same as Briquet 4846, dated Genoa 1465 with variations the following year; Briquet 1958: II.293, Dutschke/Rouse 1989: 242) and hence different from the griffin used in Sloane 5, they are exact contemporaries and share a North Italian origin.

The similarities between both MSS make it more than likely that Richard Dod was not only the earliest known reader of *LH* but could have commissioned the copying of both books to one and the same person over a relatively short period of time in the 1460s, Sloane 5 being older than HM 505 by a few years if we are to trust the watermarks. This idea cannot be cogently proved using hard evidence but a tantalizing hypothesis on the genesis of the manuscript can be built on a number of striking coincidences. The legal documentation strongly suggests that Richard Dod's closest family was not London-based but originated

---

28 A (very cursory) analysis over a few images of the Huntington MS has revealed some minor divergences. While HM 505 is a paper MS, Sloane 5 combines parchment and paper. Palaeographically, the form of ‹w› is as a rule Secretary in *LH* but Anglicana in the *Liber*, while final ‹s› is sigma-shaped in *LH* but alternates with diamond-shaped ones in the *Liber* (at least in the Latin prologue). The decoration of the initials is different as well: the scribe used simple geometric patterns—if anything—in S_1 but went for free-hand flourishes in HM 505. Some linguistic choices seem different in the two texts as well, but a more detailed research is needed before a conclusion on this point can be reached.

from the South Western tip of Essex, probably Barking where Richard seems to have lived until the mid-1440s before he moved to St Mary Fenchurch in NE London,[29] and this is relevant for the argument: *LH* has been linguistically fitted in the area comprising NE London-SW Essex-SE Middlesex (→ Dialect), and Barking would be an ideally central location. It is also evident, just by checking the hands, that Richard Dod could not have been the main scribe of the MS, but we know that Richard was acquainted and apparently on excellent terms with a Peter Vynt and his son John, both of which worked as clerks in Barking. Peter Vynt was dead by 1456, before either of the two volumes could have been copied (→ Watermarks), but two legal documents inform us that in January 1457 Richard had agreed to maintain John for life with "mete and drynk and also bed" in exchange for his estates in Barking (Flower 1933–1947: VI.184–185), since the previous month John had granted Dod all his possessions, which were substantial: it consisted of a large messuage with several houses, gardens and barns, a number of tenements and 2 acres of land (Flower 1933–1947: VI.196). Note moreover that Richard's 1458 assault on William Dod was over several charters by which Edith, John Vynt's widowed mother, had granted certain messuages in Barking and Leigh-on-Sea to several third parties. It stands to reason, therefore, that Dod would have resorted to the Essex-born John Vynt for the job of copying both the Sloane and the Huntington volumes in the 1460s as it would have been a more logical step than commissioning a third party. It would have been surely cheaper as well, since Vynt had been dependent on Dod *de jure* since 1457.

After Richard Dod, the marginalia demonstrate that several anonymous people read and annotated the MS during the late 15th century. Of those who read or owned the book previously to Hans Sloane, the quantity of text recorded by Hand C (over a thousand

---

29 Keiser mentions in his account that he could have been a parishioner of St Andrew in Holborn, which would explain Dod's marginal inscriptions ‹Seynt G› and ‹Gilys› appearing respectively over the two columns of f. 157r and which must refer to St Giles Hospital in that borough, but so far I have not been able to confirm this.

words) allows a succinct linguistic analysis that may help pinpoint him geographically. The results obtained fit the image of a late 15th century South East or London dialect. In opposition to the main scribe, long vowels are frequently doubled in this hand: ⟨leeke⟩ **93**,[30] ⟨seed⟩ **22**, ⟨good⟩ **22**, ⟨soo⟩ **1471**, etc., although -*e* serves the same purpose in cases like ⟨dede⟩ **576** or ⟨brode⟩ **568**. Doubling of consonants as a rule indicates a preceding short vowel: ⟨putt⟩ **22**. The scribe used ⟨o(o)⟩ to represent the sound derived from OE $\bar{a}$ (⟨colde⟩ **1841**, ⟨hoot⟩ **2378**; ⟨nat⟩ **1851** is unstressed). ME $\bar{e}$, both open and close, is as a rule spelt ⟨e⟩, but it is yotized once (cf. *ear*, spelt ⟨yere⟩ **2358** next to ⟨erys⟩ **547**); in the same vein, ME $\bar{\imath}$ is regularly spelt ⟨i, y⟩ but note ⟨e⟩ in the word *like* ⟨leke⟩ (< *ġelīc*) **80** (10× vs. just once ⟨lyke⟩ **74**). ME *a* before a nasal is spelt with ⟨a⟩ (⟨man⟩ **6**), but note ⟨eny⟩ **576** and ⟨meny⟩ **80** (twice). ME *i* is sometimes lowered to ⟨e⟩, as in ⟨spete⟩ **866**, ⟨chekwede⟩ **1861**, ⟨wekid⟩ **647**, ⟨yeven⟩ **6** as opposed to ⟨birde⟩ **533**, ⟨children⟩ **6** or ⟨spiret⟩ **647**; ⟨hem⟩ **870** is unclear as it could arguably be a plural form. Unstressed vowels are generally spelt with ⟨e⟩, sometimes ⟨i⟩, and it is clear that final -*e* has no grammatical value but is used rather as a length diacritic. OE $\dot{g}$ is ⟨y⟩ in ⟨yeven⟩ **6** but ⟨gh⟩ in ⟨ighen⟩ **1718**. The spellings ⟨sch⟩ and ⟨ssh⟩ alternate for the voiceless prepalatal fricative, the former in initial and the latter in final position: ⟨sche*r*des⟩ **1263**, ⟨florissheth⟩ **125**, ⟨wassh⟩ **514**. Morphologically, the scribe used a dialect that did not differentiate the 3rd sg. and plural ending in the present, using -*th* for both (cf. sg. ⟨brekyth⟩ **368** vs. pl. ⟨comyth⟩ **125**), although the plural form -(*n*) is used with the verbs *be* and *have* (⟨be⟩ **61**, ⟨ben⟩ **1851**, ⟨haue⟩ **6**). Present participles are created using -*ing*, while past participles do not display *y*-; infinitives bear no -*n*. Noun plural forms almost unexceptionally end in -*es*, just twice in -*is* (⟨erys⟩ **547** and ⟨nyttis⟩ **197**) and once in -*s* (⟨medicyns⟩ **22**). As for personal pronouns, the scribe used subject ⟨they⟩ **61** and genitive ⟨theire⟩ **1471** next to object ⟨hem⟩ **1471**. The 3rd sg. neuter forms seldom display *h*- (5× : 25×); *(h)it* is used as the object form. The demonstrative plural form is ⟨þoo⟩ **6**.

---

[30] For convenience, I use the line of the corresponding lemmas in the apparatus criticus to reference marginalia both here and in the description of the hands in the MS other than the main scribe's.

Whoever the person behind Hand C may have been, he was perhaps older than both the scribe and Richard Dod, if we are to judge from his script (which looks rather like a 1450s hand), and he seems to have had access to the volume around the 1470s (→ Hand C for the reasons). He must have been a person of some culture, able to jot down a couple of sentences in decent Latin: ⟨Et di*citur* nepta fac*it* dente*m* cadertu tactu*m* ips*a*⟩ **1509**, ⟨Et dic*itur* q*uo*d fac*it* ve*r*a responsa h*a*b*er*i portanti ad interrogationes sue⟩ **1866**. During his annotation of *LH* he also supplied a number of correct Latin headwords (⟨Nasturciu*m*⟩ **300**, ⟨Menta⟩ **1318**, etc.) and temperaments (for instance, those of henbane or gromwell) that were originally missing, emended a few others which in the treatise were wrong, for example betony (⟨Betayn is by som bok*es* hot & drie⟩ **150**) or camomile, which was correctly described as a hot species instead of the nonsensical original ⟨dry and wete⟩ **367**. He expanded the information given by Lelamour by adding more detailed descriptions, some new medical virtues or better ways to receive a medicine, like the indication that hart's-tongue fern (*Asplenium scolopendrium* L.) has neither seed nor stalk in **923**, the powers of leeks against inebriation in **1116**, or washing the forehead, instead of the eyes, with crushed cranesbill (*Geranium columbinum* L.) in **514**.

After several anonymous hands, the next positive identification is found on the verso of the second front flyleaf, where a Latin ownership inscription written in a Humanistic script reads ⟨Robartus Sandis est possessor istius Libri⟩. Rossell H. Robbins suggested that Robert Sandys might have been Dod's apprentice (Robbins 1970: 410); while indemonstrable today and maybe inaccurate, the idea is not completely misguided either as there is every chance that the Dods and the Sandys were connected, for both families demonstrably had dealings together since the mid-1450s. A "William Sandys gentilman" is mentioned in a Memorandum of acknowledgement dated 18 November 1456 (Flower 1933–1947: VI.176) as one of the executors and assigns of John Vynt. (Another of these was Richard Little, citizen and tailor of London who was mentioned above as one of Richard Dod's associates.) Both Little and Dod appear in the Memorandum dated 10 December 1456 through which Vynt granted his messuages to Dod and where a "William Sondes gentilman" is also mentioned in connection with the enfeoffment of one of Vynt's tenements. As his hand can be dated in the first half of the 16th century, Robert Sandys may have been William's (great-)grandson, but unfortunately the information provided in the MS is so scarce that it is very difficult to be more precise concerning identification. It seems probable in any case that the volume must have been either sold or bequeathed by the Dods into the Sandys, and hence there is a good chance that Hand C as well belonged to one of these two families.

The history of the MS after Robert Sandys is a blank until the time when it was bought by Hans Sloane (1660–1753), i.e. the last private owner of the volume. Thanks to his meticulous nature, we now know not only the time when he bought the book but also how much he paid for it. On f. 1r a scribbling in light brown crayon reads ⟨∩⟩2|o.∩*.*⟩. This type of cabbalistic inscriptions is not exceptional among items from the Sloane collection; quite the contrary, they appear in many volumes from his cabinet, particularly printed books, making it sure that the handwriting is the Baronet's (Pearson 1998: 19). The table of equivalences provided in Nickson 1979: 16–17, where the code was cracked, shows that the mysterious inscription indicates that Sloane bought the book in 1693, having paid 10s.0d for it. No acquisition place is provided (this was written in his usual Italic script), but it is quite safe to suggest London as all known previous owners of the book lived in or near London and Sloane himself had been living in Great Russell Street and settled in practice at Bloomsbury Square since 1689 (Davenport 1909: 342).

3. The scribes

Several hands can be found in Sloane 5, but only those used in *LH* will be studied in detail here. To ease locating the analysed passages, and since references will be made to treatises outside *LH*, references will be made using the folio, column and line system rather than the line in this edition. As mentioned in previous sections and just like the rest of the treatises included in Part II, the herbal was the work of a single scribe and hence most features described here apply to most texts of the volume. Besides the work of the main scribe, the writings and scribblings of a number of people who read the volume can be distinguished in the margins; a description of these hands' main traits will be briefly given here as well.

3.1. *The main scribe*

The person who copied *LH* used three separate hands, distinguished here as Hand A_1, A_2, and A_3 since either the scripts or their textual functions within the manuscript are different. Subscripts indicate the order in which the scribe must have selected each of these hands. We can be certain that the main scribe did not switch between two scripts (i.e. between Hand A_1 and Hand A_2) while copying the text but that Hand A_2 acted after the treatises were virtually complete because some of the words written using Hand A_2 were crammed or awkwardly spelt (for instance ‹Astrologi› 45rb/27 instead of the expected **Astrologie*, which is in keeping with his usual spelling customs). This suggests that the scribe, working as Hand A_1, had left gaps to be filled later but sometimes made some miscalculation in the layout, which he then tried to fix as Hand A_2. Hand A_2 must in turn precede Hand A_3 because the latter underlined the work already completed by the former. Moreover, there are a few mistaken inclusions of red pilcrows in unexpected places suggesting that, while acting as Hand A_3, the main scribe was again simply looking for the blanks that the previous hands had left in an otherwise complete text. Cf. for example ‹Drinke þe juis of þe rote of ¶ for brokyn bonys› 30ra/27–28, where Hand A_1 intended Hand A_2 to include a plant name (either jubarbe or a synonym) that he forgot to add, hence triggering Hand A_3 to write the paragraph marker—probably as a matter of course and without paying any real attention, as the inclusion of the pilcrow in the middle of a sentence would have stricken any scribe as nonsensical.

With all three Hands the main scribe used quills cut at an Anglicana angle and a fairy thin nib, ≅ 0.8mm for its heaviest stroke. The palaeographical analysis suggests that he was an able scribe, but probably not a particularly skilled one. He wrote in two different scripts, but displayed some competence in just the most cursive of them. Concerning his ductus, his pen flowed naturally over the support and the lettering itself is continuous and fairly regular, without noticeable variations neither in shape nor size.

3.1.1. Hand A_1

Hand A_1 was used to write the body of text, except for some minor details (*lemmata* and *auctoritates*, section titles, etc.), and a lot of marginal annotations that served as index to the reader. For the task, he used a Bastard Anglicana script that can be dated in the 1460s (a date which reinforces the information provided by the paper folios, → Watermarks). As frequent with cursive scripts, the scribe made no effort to differentiate minims, although **i** is marked by means of an arc in a few words where the position of the letter within the word might render it confusable (‹in›, ‹juis›, ‹virginis›, etc.; Johnson/Jenkinson 1915: i.25), and the Rules of Meyer were disregarded, except in the biting of geminate **pp** (Derolez 2003: 77–79). Letterforms are small (x-height ≅ 2.3–2.5mm),[31] rounded and well proportioned, as ascenders and descenders are not too long (*ca.* 2.5mm above x-height and *ca.* 2.8mm below it). This creates a sensation of compactness; yet the script always remains legible. Letterforms in the margins are sometimes much smaller (x-height about *ca.* 1.5mm in the long list at the bottom of 39va, for example).

The study of the different allographs indicates a marked preference for the Anglicana 8-shaped **g** and for round lobes and loops in **b**, **d**, **h**, **k** and **l**, although the lower lobe of **d** was frequently drawn with a cusp instead of an arc, which is suggestive of Secretary influence. This influence is visible as well in **a**, which has one compartment and

---

[31] To describe letter anatomy, I use the terminology in Petti 1977 with some additions from Gaskell 1976.

is sometimes drawn with a single bold stroke that makes it look like a capital letter (for example ⟨jau*n*dyce⟩ 39rb/a), and the simpler **w** rather than the more exuberant Anglicana graph. Even so, counterexamples are frequent. The open-tailed Secretary form for **g**, for example, can be spotted with some frequency (⟨degre⟩ 15ra/2, ⟨gode⟩ 23va/6, etc.),[32] and in the case of geminate **gg** the rule is to find first the Anglicana and then the Secretary forms combined (⟨egge⟩ 25rb/6, ⟨mandragge⟩ 37ra/12, ⟨leggis⟩ 43vb/8). There are also a few instances of Anglicana **w** (⟨browne⟩ 16va/19, ⟨newffratik⟩ 24va/17, ⟨warance⟩ 34ra/16, etc.) and one instance of two-compartment **a** (⟨smalache⟩ 52va/16). In the case of **v**, both the Anglicana and the Secretary forms are used interchangeably, although there is a tendency for the Secretary form to appear in the word ⟨v*er*tue⟩ as it is easier to draw the abbreviation sign over that variant than over the looped Anglicana version.

e is written using two graphs. The first one is written with two strokes, is similar to the modern letterform, and can be found anywhere but it is very infrequent in final position beyond the first folios, as the scribe became more comfortable with his text. The second graph is the reversed **e**, written in a single stroke and which can also appear at any place but it is most common in final position and comparatively rare at the beginning of a word. The same happens to **r**, but in this case they stand in complementary distribution: the long Anglicana version is used in the beginning of a word while the shorter Secretary counterpart is found at the end of the word, except when the abbreviation *-re* follows, as in ⟨ber*e*⟩ 48va/22, ⟨flour*e*⟩ 25ra/26 or ⟨purpur*e*⟩ 24rb/7. In middle position a very low shouldered long **r** is more frequent than the Secretary type, although the latter allograph is normally used after **o** (instead of the expected 2-shaped form, which this hand never uses). Geminated **r** is usually written with the long Anglicana form, with the exception of ⟨lorrey⟩ 46va/24 and ⟨ȝekesterris⟩ 50vb/5, where the first graph is Secretary. As for **s**, the long and sigma-shaped close versions alternate

---

32 The upper stroke closing the head-bowl of Secretary **g** was sometimes not drawn (cf. ⟨to-ged*er*⟩ 15va/8, ⟨gode⟩ 17rb/14 and 29), which made Whytlaw-Gray misread them as ⟨y⟩ in her edition; those readings have unfortunately crept as ghost spellings into the MED (s.vv. *tǒgeder, gǒd*).

but in final position, where only the latter is possible (in keeping with the usual Anglicana custom) except when the **s** is doubled, as in ‹less› 32ra/17, ‹Swiness› 34va/9 or ‹gress› 54rb/3, where long **s** is employed. Long **s** is also more frequent in initial position and particularly with clusters, although sigmas can be seen with some frequency as well, mainly before vowels and **p**—but never before **t**.

A number of graphs in final position frequently display a final stroke which could be interpreted as a brevigraph. In the case of **m, n, r**, the stroke is an upward prolongation of the final arm or shoulder that curls over the letter, while with **c, d, f, g, k**, sigma-shaped **s** and **t** it takes the form of a thin oblique line from the head-stroke, terminal, bar, ear or tongue. A more detailed analysis of these letterforms suggests that these are in fact otiose and meant as a modest flourish. Such final strokes were also used in the middle of the word when this is split over two lines, as **r** in ‹por|cion› 13rb/25–26, **c** in ‹sc|hall› 21ra/23–24 or **t** in ‹st|ampe› 56ra/7–8, and in places when -*e* would be unexpected, as **n** in ‹womans› 25vb/2. The slant line in **g** or **s** is less pronounced and could just be an unintended serif due to the scribal ductus. The crossbar added to the ascenders of digraphs such as **ch, gh, th** or **sh** and **ll** is a mere ligature answering to the same decorative purpose, as demonstrated by its appearance in words already ending in **e**, such as ‹coghe› 13vb/9, ‹brethe› 21ra/8, ‹freshe› 27ra/5, ‹wolle› 21vb/29, etc.; note as well ‹sight› 25va/10, with crossbar across **gh** *and* final slant line in **t**, or cases like ‹fleshis› 44va/24 or ‹myghty› 51rb/5, which display the stroke over clusters in non-final position.

3.1.2. Hand A_2

Whenever some keyword or medical authority was mentioned in the text, Hand A_1 left blanks that could house the estimated letters and further enclosed them with *virgulae* which can be seen sometimes (for example ‹/ypocras/› 31rb/22). The scribe was not fully consistent and the names of some of the *auctoritates* were copied without making any difference with the rest of the sentence but, for the most part, these, *lemmata*, and the headings of the sections were written in a different script from the one used in the body. To distinguish this scribal role, his job in filling in those gaps will be designated Hand A_2. Letterforms here are slightly taller (about 1.2mm than the regular letterforms in the text) and, as a whole, more carefully drawn than those of Hand A_1. It seems to be an attempt to write in a Textura semiquadrata script, but the scribe was largely unsuccessful. The first problem was the absence of line ruling, so that x-height varies noticeably even within a single heading, as clearly seen in ‹Caulus domestic*us*› 19vb/23. The minims are poorly executed and frequently slant rather than keep vertical as expected in a professional job and, even though the scribe tried to add the right elbows or feet, his use of exaggerated serifs flawed his intention sometimes, as in ‹Sana› 13rb/28 or ‹Plenius› 15vb/24. More importantly, interferences from more cursive scripts are everywhere to be seen, and some headings are in virtually undistinguishable from Hand A_1, as in ‹Morsus diaboli› 34vb/6.

In opposition to Hand A_1, for example, the scribe used three graphs to render **r** when as Hand A_2. The two Textura forms are by far the most frequent: the short one, similar to those of modern typefaces (for example, ‹Aristologia› 14ra/11), and the 2-shaped allograph after a bowl (‹Portulaca› 29ra/10). But the Rules of Meyer are broken most times and the short Textura form is generally used also in those cases: ‹Borago› 16rb/29, ‹Coriandrum› 18vb/1, ‹Maior› 21ra/9, or ‹Mandragora› 36ra/19. The long Anglicana type also pops in now and then, as in ‹Birula› 16vb/18, including one example after round letters: ‹Morella› 38va/6. Similar confusions between Textura and Anglicana are regularly found with other letters, particularly **a**, **g** and **s**.

3.1.3. Hand A_3

Being a book designed with an eminently practical purpose, Sloane 5 contains neither miniatures or drawings (other than the outline of some urine vials on ff. 187v–190r, where the liquid never got actually painted), but some colours can be seen other than the usual brown of the ink used to copy the main text. Hand A_3 is the main scribe setting aside his regular writing ink and taking up colour pigments to lure the reader's eyes into some portion of the text. In keeping with the general unexpensive features of the work, the palette was modest in

Lelamour Herbal 73

range and hardly original, as only red and blue—the loudest and most usual colours, De Hamel 1992: 62—were selected for the task. Blue was used just to draw the *littera notabilior* that opens the major treatises of the manuscript, whereas the scribe dipped his pen in vermilion in the following instances:

(1) To draw the Lombardic letter at the beginning of each section. Hand A_1 had written the intended minuscule inside a blank which A_3 would later fill with a capital—incidentally making an error once, since the scribe misread the original ‹k› in ‹Kerwell› 31rb/7, which is still clearly visible, as an **l*. Lombardic letters are crude but confidently drawn. The columns of some of these letters were sometimes not filled with solid red but with a middle vertical line, several horizontal lines—usually five—or else a simple zigzag pattern, although the scribe seems to have got tired of that from Quire F onwards. (The scribe will add a surrounding dot pattern to many letters in Quires H–J at the beginning of the second stint.) Other than that, the style of the letters is homogenous except for the peculiar initials of ‹Fethirfoy› 24vb/10 and ‹Wedebynd› 55vb/27, which where drawn following a markedly different design. Letter size is uneven: two lines (*ca.* 11mm) is the usual measure, but the range goes from the five lines of ‹Ache› 13ra/1 to just one whenever the new section begins in the last line of a column, as in ‹Calamynte› 19ra/28, ‹Endiue› 22vb/28, ‹Ivbarbe› 29vb/28, ‹Lauandyr coton› 32rb/28, ‹Rose mary› 46vb/29, ‹Vervey*n*› 54vb/27 and ‹Wedebynd› 55vb/27.

(2) To indicate Latin headwords, which were not only underscored, but enclosed in inverted brackets as well: ‹)Aristologia(› 14ra/11. The following three headwords were not underlined: ‹Crenta› 27rb/19 (a copy mistake for *CICUTA), ‹H*erba* Plenius› 30rb/1–2 and ‹Auricula muris› 37va/17.

(3) To highlight the beginning of a new recipe or chapter subsection. In order to do this, the scribe combined two devices. On the one hand, the opening letter was added a vertical red line, hence distinguishing proper capitalization from any other use of majuscules within a sentence. Moreover, Hand A_1 had placed middle dots, similar to

a *punctus elevatus*, in between recipes/subsections, and Hand A₃ then proceeded to cover them with a paragraph sign. Although there are a few examples where he missed the mark (for example 13rb/15 or 31ra/3), all in all the scribe scanned the text very carefully, even ignoring several instances where the function of *punctus* was different, as in ⟨The ve*r*tu · he is a gode heler⟩ 23va/6. Even so, he added the sign mistakenly sometimes, cf. ⟨the evill y-callid scietica passio ¶ And also þe narthe of þe brest⟩ 32va/24–26 or ⟨The juis þ*e*re-of stanchis þe flux ¶ Of women⟩ 35vb/21–22. In these and a few other similar cases the copyist must have been misled by the presence of the capital letter, which usually marked the beginning of a new recipe (→ Punctuation).

(4) To call the reader's attention towards *lemmata, auctoritates* and some plant names. A number of these had already been emphasized by writing them using a different script (→ Hand A₂). Just like the Latin headwords, these were open-boxed rather than just underlined, the inverted brackets being drawn over the initial *virgulae* that Hand A₁ wrote. The scribe was not particularly consistent and he skipped the *auctoritas* about half of the time, while once he may have mistaken an illness as a medical authority (⟨ypocandria⟩ 19ra/9, surely interpreting that this meant the same as *ypocras, i.e. Hippocrates).³³ A few plant names were also lemmatized (⟨Elebure⟩ 33rb/28, ⟨Pyretu*m*⟩ 44rb/8, ⟨Astrologi⟩ 45rb/27), as was the Latin phrase ⟨medici*n*a vt sup*ra*⟩ in 43rb/26.

(5) For marginal annotations by the main scribe, including the repetition of Latin headwords in the upper or lower margins, a few page references and most catchwords (→ Collation, Quiring and Foliation). One of the few exceptions to this rule is ⟨Cankyr hede ache⟩ on the outer margin of 31r, which was not framed.

---

33 Pliny, by far the most frequently quoted authority in the treatise, was underlined 9 out of 16 instances. Only one of the five references to Galen passed without red marking, while the name Hippocrates was highlighted one out of four times. Platearius appears twice, being underlined just once. Mithridates, Palladius, Discorides and Macer appear once in the treatise: the first two names were marked, while the last two were not. ⟨An autor⟩, which probably meant Oribasius, was lemmatized in 48rb/25–26 but not ⟨Autours⟩ in 18vb/18 (meaning Xenocrates).

3.1.4. Punctuation

The main scribe made little use of punctuation marks. The *punctus* is found only very sparsely and then only immediately before or—more generally—after Roman numbers, and at the end of a few entries (for example ⟨Fabaria⟩ or ⟨Granum solis⟩), being very infrequent elsewhere (just a few instances in the first folios, for example after ⟨derknes⟩ 15va/19, ⟨longg*is*⟩ 16rb/23 or ⟨sonne⟩ 17ra/25). There is a possible virgula after ⟨cogh⟩ 13ra/12 (but this could also be a slant line used as flourish, see above), and what seems to be a *punctus elevatus* after ⟨vertu⟩ 23va/6. Breaking of words at the end of a line, which all in all is an uncommon trait in the treatise, is not indicated by hyphens. The only symbol worth mentioning is the *paragraphus*, a reading device to locate the beginning of a new virtue/subsection within the entry. These pilcrows are slashed in red and were obviously made by the main scribe as Hand A_3 once the text was completed, by drawing the paraphs in the middle of a blank—usually over a thickish middle dot—that Hand A_1 had left for the purpose while copying the text. The original dot can still be seen under the red paint in many cases. He missed a few of these gaps (for instance in 14rb/10, 15ra/9, 17ra/25, 19rb/13, 22va/12, 44vb/19, 50ra/18 or 56ra/5) and conversely added the sign in blanks where a *paragraphus* was not expected, cf. ⟨drinke hit ¶ wyne⟩ 40vb/16 or ⟨swelling ¶ drynke⟩ 51va/22. Note the minuscules in these instances, as opposed to the capital letters that were used to begin a new subsection.[34]

3.1.5. Decoration

Sloane 5 was surely designed as a utilitarian volume, and it is hence sparsely decorated. Very simple geometrical patterns fill the last line of several sections in the first folios of the treatise and then randomly in a

---

34 There are a number of instances in *LH* where a recipe does not begin with a capital. Most of them are not mistakes but answer to shortcomings in the script: such is the case of sentences starting with **h, u, v, w** or **y**, since there were no capital counterparts for these minuscules in the scribal inventory. Only three instances qualify as mistakes in the whole herbal: ⟨harr witt ¶ but yett⟩ 27rb/22–23, ⟨saynte mary sede ¶ the juis⟩ 50va/27–28 and ⟨oþer swelling ¶ drinke þe juis⟩ 51va/22, which is remarkable if we take into account that there are 867 pilcrows in the text.

few entries throughout the treatise, so as to create the illusion of a fully justified block of text. This was normally done by drawing a number of wavy lines in red ink (so after the last word of the entries ‹Ache› (also in 13ra/13 as the entry was mistakenly split into two halves), ‹Annete›, ‹Ambrose›, ‹Betayne›, ‹Beatis›, ‹Bvgill›, ‹Bellyre›, ‹Brome› and ‹erbe moyntayne›), once as an array of figures of 2 (at the end of ‹Rose›). A very stylized red trefoil that marks the end of the *explicit* serves the same purpose. Such modest decoration was added once the copying task of the text was completed, as it was the cursory vision of a gap, rather than the end of an entry, what attracted the eye of Hand A_3. This is evident because the scribe added this type of decoration mistakenly on one occasion: in the middle of the section *Astrologie* (after ‹mowthe› 14ra/28), one can find the same simple scrolls drawn in red ink, just because Hand A_1 left some blank space there and passed on to write in the following column. Hand A_3 then mistook this as the end of the section and filled the space as a matter of course.

Other than this, the text of some folios was modestly decorated by the simple procedure of elongating the descenders of a few **f** and **s** in the bottom line, then letting the quill run free into as many hasty flourishes. In the case of *LH*, this device is found only in the final line of folios 13r, 15v and 36v, but in the medical treatises that follow the herbal he added them more frequently, usually every two or three folios. In the three final treatises, on the other hand, such embellishments are absent. It stands to reason that the main scribe would be willing to add some decoration of the opening pages, but it is unclear why he exaggerated the descenders on the other folios better than by suggesting that it was largely a question of fancy. He may have found it amusing to do it sometime and another, to spice up this slightly unsavoury text.

3.2. Other hands

A number of people read Sloane 5 prior to its acquisition by Hans Sloane, some of whom left their mark in form of marginal annotations, cross-references or corrections. Some of them scribbled long and learned passages in the margins, discussing the data and affirmations given in Lelamour's account, whereas others simply left one or more brief annotations or emended some minor mistakes. Such divergences make it impossible to offer a full description of all these hands, so a short coverage of each script will be provided. Hands are arranged here in chronological order according to their estimated palaeographical dates; line references are those of the appropriate entries in the apparatus criticus.

3.2.1. Hand B

Hand B is a typical example of Anglicana script, written with a pen cut into a nib slightly larger than that of the main scribe ($\cong$ 0.9mm for its heaviest stroke) and dipped in a brown ink. Letterforms are slightly larger (x-height $\cong$ 2.5mm) and more splayed (n-breadth $\cong$ 2.5–3mm) than those of Hand A, which gives the script a compressed look. Letterforms are carelessly drawn, sometime slope, and generally display a more open-rounded style that other hands in the MS. Minims are, as expected in a *media-currens* version of Anglicana, not distinguished but **þ** and **y** are, since the shaft of the first is straight whereas the second shows a tail finished with a quick upward stroke to the right. The script is roughly contemporary to the main scribe, as it can be safely dated in the 1460s–1470s.

Comparison with a cursive inscription by the same hand on ff. 157rb–157va makes it evident that Hand B belongs to Richard Dod, the earliest known owner of the volume and likely to be the person who had *LH* copied ($\rightarrow$ History of the MS). Note in both cases the custom of using the *punctus* to separate some words, the same broken strokes to form the two compartments of **a**, the very low and round shaft of **d**, the inverted **e**, which is closed when carefully written but open and rather splayed in its most *currens* version so that it is reminiscent of a laid down open Greek theta (ϑ), the peculiar **g** with the lower bowl standing almost on the baseline, so that the upper compartment becomes an ascender or else it is so compressed that the letter seems to be linear, or the hastily-drawn **w**, resembling two consecutive C's.

3.2.2. Hand C

Hand C is the most prolific writer in the treatise, second only to the main scribe, not only as regards the number of marginal inscription but also with respect to their length. He used a quill cut into quite a thin nib, ≅ 0.5mm for its heaviest stroke and using for the most part a greyish brown ink not too different from the one used by the main scribe. The script is a hasty but proficient version of Anglicana: two-compartment **a** with an exaggerated upper lobe written over the mean line, which makes the graph reminiscent of a capital letter, reversed close **e** in all positions, long **r**, elaborate **w** and the usual distribution of long and sigma **s** (initial and medial vs. final position). The ductus of **g** is peculiar as it curls counter-clockwise, as does **y**, the last stroke being prolonged so as to link both letters to the following one. **y** and **þ** remain distinguished, but no effort was made to differentiate minims. Loops in ascenders and lobes are, as usual in Anglicana, very round. In compliance with the Rules of Meyer, 2-shaped **r** is in general use after **o**, and it is used sometimes also before that vowel (cf. ‹dronken› **74**).

Hands A and C are palaeographically quite close in time and in fact the marginal annotations by Hand C look as if they had been written some years *before* the main text itself, *ca.* 1450. Still, the person behind Hand C is likely to have added those notes much later since he added a brief Latin recipe against drunkenness on f. 157rb immediately after a Secretary inscription which can be palaeographically dated in the 1470s, and hence Hand C must follow Hand B chronologically. Perhaps Hand C was already an elderly person by the time he made the inscriptions.

3.2.3. *Hand D*

Hand D is found only once (‹Cepe› **1581**). The scribe used a Textura script of middling quality using a quill cut to ≅ 1mm dipped in black ink. With such a limited sample, the hand is quite difficult to date, but the general style is reminiscent of scribes working in the last quarter of the 15th century. Richard Dod used a Textura script in his ownership inscription of f. 157rb/20–22, but whereas his script was an attempt at a Quadrata version of that script, that of Hand D is clearly Rotunda. The ink used in each case seems to be different as well. The ductus of ⟨e⟩ also suggests a different person: Hand D drew the thick stroke forming the eye with a concave line but this is perfectly straight in Dod's hand.[35] Moreover, there is no letter biting in **pe** in opposition to Dod's ⟨Ricardo⟩ 157rb/20, ⟨de⟩ or ⟨london⟩ 157rb/21 (but note that the Rules of Meyer were followed in the case of **d**-plus-round vowel but not in other possible cases, as there is no biting in ⟨liber⟩ 157rb/20, ⟨Dod⟩ or ⟨Barbor⟩ 157rb/21).

3.2.4. Hand E

Hand E was the person who numbered the entries, writing the appropriate figure as a rule to the right of the Latin headword whenever there is one, or roughly in the centre of the blank space between two entries when there was none. For the task the scribe cut his quill into a nib of $\cong$ 0.7mm for its heaviest stroke, which he dipped in pitch-black ink. The figures were drawn in their modern shapes, barring neither **0** nor **7**, and are not very peculiar with the exception of **5**, which is slightly rotated clockwise. The x-height for linear numbers (0, 1 and 2) is $\cong$ 3mm, while the rest measure $\cong$ 6mm.

Dating a hand using only figures is quite difficult but the form of **5** points towards a late fifteenth- or early sixteenth century hand. In any case, it has to be later than Hand C, since he wrote the number to the right of the additions and emendations done by that scribe (cf. for instance ⟨Nastucium⟩ **300**, ⟨Jusquiamus⟩ **905**, ⟨Lauriola⟩ **1149**, ⟨Menta⟩ **1318** or ⟨Absinthium⟩ **2350**; concerning emendations, cf. ⟨vel Cicuta i. herba benedicta⟩ **871**, ⟨Albus⟩ **1223** or ⟨vel Asterion⟩ **1252**). An earlier addition ⟨niger⟩ **1850** by Hand C explains that, contrary to his custom, the number of ⟨Eleborus⟩ was written to its left rather than to its right. The numerator must be also younger than Hand B as the number ⟨164⟩ was added to the right of a brief ⟨nota⟩ **1930** which Dod wrote in the middle of the blank between the entries *Radich* and *Ragworte*.

---

35 The person who wrote the recipe for a laxative also drew **e** with a concave stroke sometimes, but the writing angle, the colour of the ink and the form of **C** seem to point to two different people.

Hand E made at least two mistakes during the job. The five entries on f. 23v were misnumbered, but the scribe realized his mistake in time and managed to emend it: the sections ⟨Herba Roberti⟩ to ⟨Filex campestris⟩ first bore numbers ⟨47⟩–⟨51⟩, but those were washed off (probably because the ink was still wet, although the smudges make the old figures quite visible). The correct numbers (⟨53⟩–⟨57⟩) were then added next to them except for the last two entries, where the scribe only deleted the last figure and wrote the correct ones over them. He also wrote ⟨55⟩ instead of expected *45 in the entry ⟨Lappa⟩ but here he seems not to have realized his lapsus.

3.2.5. Hand F

Hand F is a Tudor script written in black ink using a quill cut to a thin nib of ≅ 0.6mm. Comparison with the plates offered in Petti 1977, Hector 1980 and Brown 1990 matches the script of this hand with one typical of the first decades of the second quarter of the 16th century, as seen by the handwriting of Thomas More (letter to Cardinal Wolsey dated 30/10/1523; Petti 1977: 17) or Henry Gold (letter, *ca.* 1534; Hector 1980: xvii (a)). As with those, letterforms are broad, open and firm, although Hand F presents a hastier ductus than either of them, which gives the hand a sprawled look: x-height varies from 1.5 to 2mm, and n-breadth ranges from 1.6 to 2.2mm. It seems quite safe to date it sometime *ca.* 1525–1530.

4. The edition

The present edition of *Lelamour Herbal* is critical and based on the sole known witness (S_1). The text is accompanied by two apparatus critici at the bottom of each page. The first of these records all editorial changes from the original readings of the manuscript; since this treatise is a collection of entries copied from several sources, a number of emendations is based on parallel readings taken from other MSS.

Lelamour Herbal

The rationale for such decisions is further discussed and—whenever possible—textually supported in the corresponding entries of the Explanatory Notes section that immediately follows the edition. Since a single-copy tradition makes this feasible, a second apparatus is included that records the marginalia by the several readers and owners of the book.

4.1. Editorial criteria and typographic conventions

Capitalization, punctuation, and word-division are modern. Contractions and abbreviations are expanded and italicized, with the exception of the ampersand, which is left unaltered. Thorn and yogh are retained, as is the scribal distinction between **u** and **v**. On the other hand, **i** and **j** are spelt according to the modern usage. The horizontal line over digraphs such as **ch**, **gh**, **sh** or **th** at final position is taken to be a mere ligature mark, or else a modest flourish, just like the upward prolongation of the final stroke that frequently curls over final **m**, **n**, **r** and the thin oblique line of **c**, **d**, **f**, **g**, **k**, sigma-shaped **s** and **t**. They have therefore been ignored as otiose in the edition. On the other hand, **n** with a clear tilde hovering over it has been regularly transcribed as ⟨n*n*⟩ except in absolute final position where it is rendered as ⟨ne⟩, a policy which makes sense in ⟨bene⟩ **1968** or ⟨done⟩ **794**, but not really in ⟨mane⟩ **692** or ⟨pane⟩ **328**, where ⟨n*n*⟩ is surely preferable. With non-monosyllabic stems, the choice is less obvious, but pairs like ⟨cotidiane⟩ **362** vs. ⟨cotidiane⟩ **8**, ⟨molayne⟩ **891** vs. ⟨moleyne⟩ **1443** or ⟨planteyne⟩ **899** vs. ⟨plantoyne⟩ **1775** suggest the convenience of transcribing as ⟨-ne⟩ here too.

Editorial emendations are enclosed within square brackets. Generally speaking, I have taken a conservative stance, emending only when the word/passage is clearly garbled or nonsensical, as in ⟨ferntiklys⟩ **11**, or can be put down as a spoonerism, as in "dotovs" **341**. On the other hand, I have kept such cases as ⟨ete þe levis⟩ **2038**, which derives from an original Latin *ethicus* but manages yet to make some sense in the passage (the reading was emended to ⟨etik⟩ in Keiser 2008a: 203), or ⟨woll oylle⟩ **2117**. In the same vein, the reading MS ⟨est⟩

has been kept over the possible emendation "eft", even though a cursory research on the topic suggests that the expression "Hereford East" dates from the second half of the fifteenth century and was prevalent in the South West of England, where the name was likely to be confused with Haverfordwest in Pembrokeshire. Therefore, John Lelamour could hardly have added the tag when referring to his home town, since he lived in the second half of the fourteenth century according to the information provided in the *explicit*, while, from another perspective, it is unclear that the London scribe of S_1 would have added the tag *motu proprio* (Moreno Olalla 2007: 122, fn. 23). Such cases are as a rule teamed with an accompanying note in the Explanatory Notes section.

As most MSS, S_1 is sometimes faulty, so missing fragments were added whenever a homoioteleuton was detected that rendered the passage nonsensical (see for instance ‹bvgill› **205**), but for the most part I have preferred to make the best of what is actually in the MS, which has meant that the sense of a number of obscure passages does not necessarily correspond to the one originally intended in the source text (the case of the *ethicus* : ‹ete þe levis› opposition that was mentioned above). Readings from *NM* are taken from the Pepys version whenever this is available and correct, because this MS is linguistically closest to the dialect used in S_1. If not, the reading from Wellcome is preferred, because it is genetically related to the Sloane 5 version via Subarchetype γ. Perhaps paradoxically, MS *B*, which is the best known version of *NM* so far, has been sparingly used for the purpose, since it stands furthest from S_1 as regards both dialect and textual pedigree.

Besides its use with botanical binomina, where it is standard practice, italics are used to quote words or lines from *De Viribus Herbarum* and also to mark lexemes generally, without reference to any particular context (for example, in etymologies). Bold letters are used to indicate letterforms in a palaeographical context, while chevrons (‹ ›) enclose readings from the edition and are therefore followed by a line reference: hence, ‹Iris› **724** as opposed to *Iris* which, depending on the context, may refer to the entry under that name in *DVH*, in *AC*, etc. or else to the botanical genus of flowering plants.

An asterisk before a spaced word indicates that this reading was expected in the text but not actually found there (they are used, for example, to provide the correct form of a mistranslated word, or missing fragments in the text due to homoioteleuta). Starred small capitals indicate reconstructed forms from Q, Ω or any of its proposed subarchetypes. Starred italics mark reconstructed scribal readings (be they correct or wrong): *LŌSIS > *lāsis ‹layses›.

4.2. Explanatory Notes

Explanatory notes come in three main forms: linguistic, textual and medical. Notes of linguistic nature do not include all the perceived dialectal modifications done by the scribes of the ΛS_1 branch, but only those that are helpful for the reconstruction of the archetype or are significant in any other way. Some attention is paid to lexical matters as well, particularly to explain obscure words and *hapax legomena*; see for example the note on ‹strechillis› **449**. Textual notes serve a triple purpose. First and foremost, they comment or provide evidence to support editorial emendations. Secondarily, these notes demonstrate that a given entry was borrowed from this or that tradition and therefore they support the ideas presented in the Sources section by tracing back the original Latin or Greek passages. Tracing the ultimate source(s) of any given entry is naturally beyond the scope of this edition, so I only indicate the immediate textual tradition from which the entry in *LH* seems likelier to have derived, although some commentary, mostly of historical or metatextual interest, is added sometimes. See for example the endnote to **385** on the assumed anaphrodisiac powers of calamint, or the one to lines **374–375**, where Choulant's claimed source for *DVH* 580–584 is disputed. Finally, these notes show how the text has evolved in time and how the initial meaning has become sometimes corrupt. Although some of them are devoted to the description and medieval etiology of diseases, comment on technical matters such as weights or succinctly inform about the *auctoritas* mentioned in the fragment, medical notes will for the most part attend to the much-vexed question of species identification, i.e. pairing the medieval name with a modern phytonym.

4.2.1. Species identification

It is unnecessary to insist on the idea that identification of the species hidden under the ME phytonym is as a rule problematic because plant names are not univocal: the same vernacular name can, and normally will, refer to more than one species. In order to provide an educated guess, a discussion is required that will include close reading of the entry, and above all of the morphological description whenever available. This should prevail over any general *consensus doctorum* not matter how universal (see Moreno Olalla 2015), since the procedure has shown that in *LH*, and probably in many other herbals, textual transmission and subsequent scribal emendations—*lectiones faciliores* in particular—have distorted parts of the original text almost beyond recognition, to the sad result that plant names were used in entries which demonstrably described the medical properties of very different species. The clearest case of this trend in *LH* is surely ‹beatis› **189**. This suggested the convenience of including a note attached to each headword in *LH* where all that matter is considered in some length. The species ‹dodyr› **745** and ‹herba Plenius› **1045** are also attended in similar depth, because textually they function as sections even though in the first case the virtues are subjoined to the chapter on flax and in the second case the poor performance of the main scribe misled later readers into perceiving it as a part of the chapter on houseleek which precedes it. There is a description of the medical virtues attached to them and, in the latter case, even a brief physical description. Other plants mentioned in the herbal, like ‹forse› **1057**, on the other hand, have not received such attention because they are just mentioned as ingredients of a recipe, or used for morphological comparisons of leaves, roots and the like.

While of course desirable in itself, the ultimate purpose of botanical notes, which can be quite lengthy and even discursive, is not be necessarily the correct identification of the species. Rather, editors of texts on medieval materia medica should strive to provide as complete an image as possible of the evidence, textual or otherwise, that we have on the topic, and arrive to a well-supported conclusion even if that means that the traditional or more obvious identification cannot be correct and the editor's botanical ingenuity falls short to provide a plausible alternative, as with ‹bornete-is› **230**.

It is obvious that, in order to achieve this, the editor must attend first and foremost to the physical description provided by the author of the herbal himself. In the particular case of *LH*, the amount and quality of the botanical data depends on the tradition whence Lelamour drew his information for the entry, ranging from the relatively good physical descriptions provided by *AC* to no information at all, as is usually the case of *NM*, which naturally mirrors its source text *DVH*. The frequent lack of an accurate physical description means that in many cases we must extract the information elsewhere. In the case of medical herbals such as *LH*, using the assumed pharmacographical properties of the plant is an evident scholarly choice: if they can be shown to be roughly the same as those mentioned by Dioscorides, Galen or Pliny in their works, then we can assimilate the ME plant name with the species suggested by Classical scholars. See for example how medical considerations demonstrate the convenience of preferring *Lavandula angustifolia* Mill. over *L. stoechas* L. as the species intended in the chapter ‹Lauandyr› **1172**.

Equating Latin/Greek and Middle English phytonyms is, strictly speaking, as far as an editor can get when it comes to plant identification, unless some good description is given. Going any further than this has something of an editorial leap of faith since the editor will be building on a syllogism: since plant A in, say, Dioscorides's *Materia Medica* is generally assumed to be species B, and the Middle English entry C is ultimately based on the information provided by A, therefore the species in entry C must also be B. This is admittedly not be the wisest procedure, since the species growing in the Mediterranean basin that were described in the Latin and Greek books are not necessarily the same as those that we must assume that Lelamour and other medical herbalists from England or Germany had seen. Even so, I think that trying to provide a corresponding Atlantic species (a sort of a *Quid pro quo*) is a futile enterprise since it is very likely that the medieval English physician was convinced that he was describing the medical virtues of the same species already mentioned in the Classical literature. Contrary to Renaissance scholars such as Matthioli, Fuchs or Gerarde (who frequently expressed doubts concerning what Dioscorides described and what they saw in their countries), the medieval herbalists do not normally provide any extra information that may be of help in this matter.

Plant names are given using their scientific binomina, according to *The Plant List* website (www.theplantlist.org), together with a Present-day English name, which for most entries will be the one used in *PNME*, unless the description of the species provided in *LH* is contradictory. Whenever the information given in the entry does not grant an accurate species identification (as in the case of ‹astrologie› **67** or ‹basilicon› **283**) I have refrained from identifying the plant through the type species (*species typica*) but mentioned only the genus (in these cases, *Aristolochia* L. ssp. and *Ocimum* L. ssp.). In some cases (for example, ‹dent de lion› **556**) even reference to a single genus (*Taraxacum* F.H.Wigg. ssp.) has meant a certain degree of editorial imposition on the text, as the ME name might have possibly been used to refer to a number of species not well distinguished in medieval times but now taken to belong to different genera (among other possibilities, *Leontodon* L. ssp. or *Crepis* L. ssp.).

4.2.2. On the Literature *section*

As indicated above, each chapter of the herbal has an opening endnote discussing the possible candidate species for every plant name. Such notes also include a list of the more relevant literature on that particular plant. While strictly speaking not a *Quellenforschung* apparatus, it may serve to present a general—if incomplete—overview of the possible names by which the plant has been known, many of which were also used in *LH*, since Theophrastus's time. The sources are arranged chronologically so that the evolution of certain plant names becomes as obvious as possible; to mark the relative position of *LH* in that development the symbol ⚜ is used. Renaissance botanical literature is wide so only a few treatises were selected, mainly those composed or translated into English; the only exception is Leonhart Fuchs's seminal *Historia Stirpium*. The catalogue of abbreviated titles, edition used and the reference system used for each of them will be found in the List of sources and abbreviations below.

To make the apparatus as compact as possible, only the first name of the several synonyms provided by the Classical authors, which normally serves as headword of the entry, is recorded. The entries merely indicate the chapter(s) where the same species as the one in the ME text seem to be treated. Medieval and Renaissance synonyms, on the other hand, are quoted in full as one of them may serve to explain a name used in *LH*, which in turn may have also been used by a later author, Gerard being of particular interest here.

Although in fact the list does not aim for comprehensiveness, one could wonder why some very important sources are missing. Apuleius Platonicus's *De Herbarum virtutibus* (*HAP*) has been sparsely used in the Explanatory Notes but was dropped in favour of the *Old English Herbarium* as it is a translation of that work and has the benefit of including the Old English synonym. Similar considerations made the Middle English version of *Alphita* (Mowat 1887) preferable to the otherwise more solid Latin version (García González 2007). Oppositely, the 1512 Latin edition of Matthaeus Platearius's *Circa instans* was chosen over its ME translation (Garrido Anes 2005) as the text of the latter is defective and misses several important items (for example, the entry on onions); for completeness' sake the ME plant names have yet been added whenever the entry is included in the translation.

Due to well-known reasons (see Moreno Olalla 2013a: 398–399), the plant names given there are illustrative and not necessarily correspond to the same species suggested for the ME text. This is particularly true with those plant names quoted from synonyma, but to a certain degree also happens with the Classical sources. The guiding force in the selection of the information has been historical rather than botanical, and thus in the section one will find references to Greek or Latin plant names that are known to be species other than the one meant in *LH*: they are included nonetheless because they were thought to be one and the same during the Middle Ages and the Renaissance. For instance, ⟨mowsere⟩ **1468**, the plant thought to be the same as the one called *auricula muris* in Latin and μυὸς ὦτα or μυὸς ὠτίς in Greek, probably refers to some hawkweed, generally identified with *Pilosella officinarum* Vaill., even though the Latin name is as a rule taken to be either *Theligonum cynocambre* L. or some subspecies of *Anagallis arvensis* L. (André 1985: *s.v.* auricula), and the Greek plant has been traditionally identified with *Asperugo procumbens* L. or *Myosotis scorpioides* L. = *M. palustris* (L.) Nathh. (Berendes 1902: 258). On the other hand, when the species has been identified with some degree of security, the other candidates have been dropped: ⟨pympirnell⟩ **1859** refers to *Anagallis arvensis* L., not to *Pimpinella saxifraga* L., hence the entries in Fuchs's or Dodoens-Lyte's treatises on that species (Fu$_{231}$, DL$_{97}$) are missing.

The names are spelt as given in the source, maintaining the heterogeneous use of diacritics of Greek words in Renaissance treatises (cf. for example the missing asper and accent in Tu's ⟨ραφονις [...] ραφανος⟩ or Fu's ⟨ραφανίς⟩, vs. the more correct ⟨ῥαφανὶς⟩ in DL and Ge), although the original capitalization has been ignored and abbreviations have been silently expanded. The only exception to this are the plant names in Tu, a few of which have been emended as the modern editors regularly mistransliterated **x** in the blackletter original book as ⟨r⟩ (for example, ⟨Iros⟩ on p. 599 instead of **Ixos** on f. 164v of the second part of the original, reprinted as p. 352 in that edition).[36]

A present-day English name (as a rule, the one used by Hunt in *PNME*) and its scientific binomen are also provided for the reader's convenience. In those entries where the several species identified in the text are now taken to belong to different families or genera, the basionyms have been used instead whenever one is suitable; for example ⟨camamyll⟩ **366**, an umbrella term probably covering either *Chamaemelum nobile* (L.) All. or *Anthemis arvensis* L., *Cota tinctoria* (L.) J. Gay, and *Anthemis rosea* Sm., is referred to simply as *Anthemis*

---

36 The transcription of Tu is not to be trusted as regards the distribution of **i** and **y**, **u** and **v** in the original edition, but the editorial spellings have been kept unaltered nonetheless for quotation purposes as this is naturally a very minor point.

L. ssp., (cf. the old Linnaean names *Anthemis nobilis* L. and *Anthemis tinctoria* L. for the former two species). The accepted binomina will be found in the Explanatory Notes and the Glossary. Starred names before a vulgar name indicate that the proposed identification is tentative, perhaps even probable, but unwarranted by known textual or pharmacographical evidence. The interested reader is strongly advised to read the full note for further details and discussion.

Alph. and *Sin.Bart.* frequently include entries where information already given under a previous headword is rearranged or abridged, being thus virtual duplicates. In the apparatus, only that entry offering the largest number of synonyms is quoted, while the other(s) are simply referenced through the appropriate page(s). If two or more references to the same species are given in the same page, these will be separated with a double vertical bar as in "*Alph.* 202 (*ammi, cyminella, pe perdium* || *vmurcula, redi domum*)". While *Sin.Bart.* generally offers English synonyms only (the same is true with other sources, such as *OEH*), *Alph.* includes French ones as well. To distinguish both groups, in this source French and English plant names are preceded by the subscript tags GA and/or AN, respectively. For example, the plant called *auens* is treated at least four times in *Alph.* (first on page 17, then on 70, 141, and 162), in all cases offering the same Latin synonyms: the reference is therefore "*Alph.* 17, 70, 141, 162 (*avencia, pes leporis, gariofilata, sanamunda, zimis.* $_{\text{GA,AN}}$*auense*)". In case that some entry adds fresh synonyms, only the new pieces of information will be consigned. Alternative spellings will be normally ignored unless identification is not obvious. Thus, the several references to *apium* in *Alphita* will be indicated as "*Alph.* 11–12, 202 (*apium domesticum sive ortolanum.* $_{\text{A}}$*smalache*), 194, 235 (*xilenum*), 211 (*charasis*), 212 (*elimon*), 216 (*gaxit*)". Note that *xilinon* on p. 235 is taken as a mere variant of *xilenum* whereas *elimon* on p. 212, which is in fact yet another faulty rendering of the same synonym (< Gk σέλινον), is kept as a separate reference.

In several sources, and most noticeably in Serapion's work, several different—if akin—species are described under one and the same heading. For example, the plants called ‹ditander›, ‹origanum› and ‹pulyoll monten› in *LH* appear under the same heading *fandenigi* in

De simplici medicina, cap. 300 together with several other Lamiaceae, even though inside the entry they are given different names (which are not clearly distinguished: *mescatremephir* [مشكطرامشير *maškaṭrāmašīr*] seems to refer to *Origanum dictamnus* L., while both *alnam* and *alnegem* [spelling variants of النيجل *al-nīǧl*] are probably *Thymum serpillum* L.). The same happens to *luf* (*LS* 43), which refers both to ‹addyrworte› and ‹dragancia femall›. In *MM* iii.35 καλαμίνθη seems to refer to both ‹calamynte› (*Calamintha* L. spp.) and ‹nepte ryall› (*Clinopodium nepeta* (L.) Kuntze). Occasionally, the heading of a parallel entry may indicate a different species, as is the case of *kauroch* (*LS* 296), which describes the celandines (*Chelidonium majus* L. and *Ranunculus ficaria* L.) even though the Arabic and Latin names refer to turmeric (*Curcuma longa* L.).

The structure of Matthaeus Sylvaticus's *Opus* (or *Liber*) *Pandectarum* combines, in a strict alphabetical order, both numbered chapters devoted to individual species and a sort of *synonyma*, which are unnumbered. Only those species that were warranted a numbered chapter have made it into the list, but this has meant that a few important species, such as *origanum* or *pullegium*, do not appear in the Literature section because Sylvaticus included these species in the *synonyma* section only. Spellings have been kept unaltered even in cases of obvious typos (‹coriamium› < Gk κορίαννον, ‹dasnoides› < Gk δαφνοιδές, ‹herbena› < La *berbena*), but some synonyms, particularly Arabic ones, have been discarded when they are evident spelling variants (the cases of ‹lisen alhamel› and ‹lisemalhamel›, cf. لسان الحمل *lisān al-ḥamal*, or ‹bebonig›, ‹bebonigi›, cf. بابونج *bābūniǧ*)[37] or are repeated (‹serpillum› is said to be both a Greek and a Latin synonym). The subscript tags AR, GR and LA are respectively added to the first Arabic, Greek and Latin synonym provided in that work; I have maintained the information as given in the text even when that it is demonstrably wrong (for instance, ‹calib› and ‹calebum› are tagged GR although they are in fact aberrant variants of Arabic قلب *qulb*). Arabic forms in Serapion (many of which were also repeated by Sylvaticus) have been taken from Guigues 1905a–b.

---

37 Other spellings such as ‹bebonici›, ‹beborugi› or ‹bebunegiemara›, on the other hand, have been kept even though they stem from the same Arabic word.

4.2.3. Temperaments

As indicated, there is a sizeable number of entries where the Latin name, the ME synonym(s) or the suggested identification do not match. When the rest fails, checking the species temperament stated in *LH* against the one offered in the usual literature may be used to advantage to support or discard possible candidates. For example, identification of ‹pelletir› **1820** as pellitory of Spain (*Anacyclus pyrethrum* (L.) Lag.) rather than pellitory-of-the-wall (*Parietaria judaica* L.) mainly rests on its temperament, since *Anaclysus* was taken to be ‹hote & drye› while, according to medical *auctoritates*, *Parietaria* was cold and humid.

This made information on temperaments in those treatises included in the Literature section a convenient addition to those notes discussing plant identification. To reduce the space devoted to this matter to a minimum, I include only the Latin initial of the four possible states (*Frigidus/Calidus* and *Humidus/Siccus*), followed by a superscript number indicating the exact degree whenever this is stated. Letter Æ (standing for *aequalis*, cf. *LS* 1–12) is used for those few species where the preponderance of one of the two opposing states over the other is uncertain (for instance, ‹maydenhere› **1301**). As with the Literature section, if identification is unclear or the entry demonstrably combines information from two or more species, the temperament of the several candidates is recorded, as in ‹comyn› **477**, which seems to be a blending of cumin (*Cuminum cyminum* L.) and anise (*Pimpinella anisum* L.).

The temperament has not been consigned in a reduced number of species. In cases like ‹savygill› **2068**, for instance, the temperament was never recorded in the medical literature consulted, while for those cases of repeated species (for example, ‹dragancia femall› **539**), or where the species was thought to be narrowly related to another one which is also treated in the text (‹lasse sper-wort› **1180**, identified as *Ranunculus flammula* L. and traditionally taken to be the *minor* counterpart of *R. lingua* L., i.e. ‹spereworte› **2175**), that particular information is recorded elsewhere in the treatise and cross-referenced to the appropriate chapter. Similarly, ‹longwort› **1224** provides full information on the white hellebore (*Veratrum album* L.) even though both the white and the black hellebores are treated there, because the back hellebore (*Helleborus niger* L.) has its own chapter later in the treatise (‹pedelyon› **1851**). To cross-reference an entry the sign "→" is used.

Additional information on sources and temperaments is also cross-referenced using the same sign: for example, information provided in the general chapter on ferns ‹ferne› **663**, can be supplemented with the information given under ‹polipody› **1899** on a particular species of ferns (common polypody, *Polypodium vulgare* L.). The same with ‹lawreoll› **1149** (*Daphne laureola* L.) and ‹spurge› **2217** (*Euphorbia lathyris* L.), or ‹coluyr-fote› **511**, ‹erbe Robert› **636**, and ‹maworte› **1286**, all of which refer to similar *Geranium* L. spp., ‹mynte› **1454** (*Mentha longifolia* (L.) L.) and ‹horsmynte› **863** (*Mentha aquatica* L.), black and white mustard (**1327** and **2506**), etc.

4.3. Glossary

The glossary is complete, except from obvious Latin words and phrases (‹virginis› **1261**, ‹Cap*ri*cornis› **2492**, ‹e *con*trario›, **1414**, ‹vt sup*ra*› **1787**, etc.) and section headings, while an Index of proper nouns is included at the end as an addendum. The letters ‹k› and ‹y› are taken as mere spelling variants of ‹c› and ‹i› and arranged accordingly, while ‹þ›/‹th› are segregated from **T** and ‹ȝ›/‹gh› follows **G** as a separate section. ‹u› and ‹v› remain distinct according to their value in the word: hence ‹vryne› or ‹vndir› will be found under **U** (there are no examples of word-initial ‹u› as a consonant, ‹ureste› being under **W**). A few words which are spelt both with and without initial ‹h› in the treatise (‹(h)ache›, ‹(h)erbe› or ‹(h)it›) are arranged under the latter variant; ‹addyr› and ‹quynacy› will be on the other hand found under **N** and **S**.

The headword represents the most frequent spelling, but is frequently modified so that it includes optional letters, which are bracketed. When none of the variants of a word is clearly hegemonic (for instance, ‹yryn› **801** and ‹iren› **61**), that one which separates the most from the current British English spelling has been chosen for the benefit of the readers (hence **yryn**). Spellings are crossreferenced to their headwords in the Glossary whenever identification is not immediately evident, but the following minor variants are ignored for the purpose: final -⟨er⟩ vs. -⟨re⟩ (stretched to include akin cases like ⟨coryandry⟩ or ⟨Februare⟩), soft ⟨c⟩ vs. ⟨s⟩, the alternations between tautosyllabic ⟨ar⟩ and ⟨er⟩, ⟨con-⟩ and ⟨com-⟩, ⟨ay⟩ and ⟨ey⟩, ⟨au⟩ and ⟨ou⟩, ⟨o⟩ and ⟨u⟩ to indicate the close vowel, or ⟨sch⟩/⟨sh⟩. Unstressed vowels (generally ⟨e⟩ and ⟨i⟩) are similarly not distinguished. But even comprehensive headwords such as **ab(o)ute** or **gres(se** make spellings such as ⟨a-bote⟩ or ⟨gris⟩, ⟨grasse⟩ invisible.

Headwords are spelt without hyphens, unless it is a compound (including cases like **an-oþer** or **in-to**), or the scribe always split the word. The different meanings of a word are separated by semicolons, collocations and idioms by a pilcrow. Plant names and those Middle English words of dubious meaning which are analysed in the Explanatory Notes are crossreferenced to the appropriate line (for example, **kyrning** → **108**). The Index of proper nouns similarly crossreferences those entries in the Explanatory Notes that include a biographical sketch of the *auctoritas* mentioned in the passage.

Verbs not recorded in the infinitive or imperative are reconstructed and followed by an asterisk, as are nouns not found in the singular and pronouns not in the subject case. Homographs have separate headwords and are distinguished by a raised number after the grammatical category whenever they belong to the same grammatical category (e.g. **more** $n.^1$ "root" vs. **more** $n.^2$ "moor, wasteland" as opposed to **mor)e** *a.* "larger" or **more** *adv.* "more").

4.4. Appendixes

Two appendixes follow the glossary. For the benefit of the interested botanists, plant names have been recorded separately according to their modern binomina as Appendix A. To make it as comprehensive as possible and particularly since a number of entries are botanically unclear, this appendix includes all the identifications discussed in the appropriate note. To make the list as compact as possible, the abbreviated authorities have been dropped; only the genus and epithet(s) are included. The full binomina, crossreferenced to the edition lines, will be found in the respective glossary entries under their ME plant names. Latin names between slants indicate that the same species was treated at least once in a headless section: for example, the healing properties of *Alium cepa* L. are described in **189–203** under the heading ⟨beata⟩, but with no heading in **1581–1606**. Words in parentheses indicate variations in the heading, as with *Dracunculus vulgaris* Schott, described in the sections ⟨dragancia⟩ **37** and later as ⟨dragancia fe*mina*⟩ **538**.

A large number of words of a very technical nature were used in the Explanatory Notes as a quick way to refer to the assumed healing properties of a given plant (called *vires* or *virtutes* in Latin). Aware that many of these terms will prove mystifying to the lay reader (and even to the specialists, as many of them are no longer part of the usual medical vocabulary) and because many are not recorded in general dictionaries (not even in OED), a second appendix has been included that will serve as a glossary to those remedies. The term "remedy" is stretched here to cover also such things as exorcisms, avoidance of pests or the health of domestic animals, which strictly speaking do not belong to medicine but to theology, husbandry or veterinary.

A few of these words have been created for the purpose from already existing words, generally by adding the *anti-* prefix to an illness (for example, "antipleurodynic" or "antitonsillitic" cf. pleurodynia, tonsillitic), while others have been used etymologically ("antigonorrheic" or "hysteric"), or else in the broadest sense possible *faut de mieux* (for example, "eloquent"). Most of the words, however, were drawn from medical dictionaries such as the erstwhile very popular by Robley Dunglison (I use the 1893 edition, revised and enlarged by Robley's son, Richard). Hoping to make the appendix more useful, terms are indexed to the lines in the edition where these remedies appear. This might prove helpful to scholars interested in *Quellenforschung* and in tracing the origins and dissemination of medieval medical recipes.

5. List of sources and abbreviations

Abbreviations of the grammatical categories follow those of the second edition of the OED, except for deverbative nouns and adjectives (*vbl. n.* and *ppl. a.* in OED), which are tagged *n.* and *a.*, respectively. Raised numbers after the tag separate homographs within the same category.

A. PRIMARY SOURCES

AC	Page,Line (Brodin 1950)
Alph.	Page (Mowat 1887)
Chir.(ME)	Page (Ogden 1971)
Cl	Letter.Chapter (Platearius 1512)
CM	Page (de Capella 1510)
CMR	Book.Chapter.Section.Sentence (Raeder 1928–1933)
DL	Page (Dodoens 1619)
Dur.Glos.	Page (Cockayne 1864–1866: iii.298–305)
DVH	Line (Choulant 1832)
DVH(NME)	Folio.Line (MS *B*, unless stated otherwise)
DVH(SME)	Folio.Line (Frisk 1949)
EPN	Chapter (Earle 1880)
Fu	Chapter (Fuchs 1542)
Ge	Page (Gerard 1597)
GH	Chapter (*Great Herball* 1539)
Grad.	Page (Constantinus Africanus 1536: 343–387)
HAP	Page (de Vries 1984)
HP	Book.Chapter.Section (Hort 1916)
LS	Chapter (Alpagus 1550)
MM	Book.Chapter (Wellman 1906–1914)
NH	Book.Section (Rackham/Jones 1938–1963)
OEH	Chapter (de Vries 1984)
Pand.	Chapter (Silvaticus 1521)
Ps.Dios.	Book.Chapter (Wellman 1906–1914)
RM	Page (Heiberg 1924)
Sin.Bart.	Page (Mowat 1882)

SM	Volume.Page (Kühn 1821–1833: xi.789–xii.158)
SpMa	Line (Jansen 2013)
Συν	Page (Langkavel 1868)
TH	Chapter (Ventura 2009)
Tu	Volume.Page (Chapman *et al.* 1995)
Viat.	Book.Chapter (Constantinus Africanus 1536: 1–167)

B. SECONDARY SOURCES

AND *Anglo-Norman Dictionary* online [www.anglo-norman.net/gate])
DEPN *Dictionary of English Plant Names* (Britten/Holland 1886)
DMF *Dictionnaire du Moyen Français* online [www.atilf.fr/dmf])
DSL *Dictionary of the Scots Language* online [www.dsl.ac.uk])
EDD *English Dialect Dictionary* (Wright 1896–1905)
FEW *Französiches Etymologisches Wörterbuch* (von Wartburg 1928–2002)
LSJ *Greek-English Lexicon* (Liddell/Scott/Jones *et al.* 1996)
MED *Middle English Dictionary* online [quod.lib.umich.edu/m/med]
OED *Oxford English Dictionary* (Simpson/Weiner 1989)
OLD *Oxford Latin Dictionary* (Glare 1997)
WG   Whytlaw-Gray 1938

C. MANUSCRIPTS

B	Oxford, Bodleian Library, Additional MS A.106, ff. 244r–259r
H	London, British Library, Harley MS 3840, ff. 139r–178v
L	Oxford, Bodleian Library, Laud Misc. MS 553, ff. 7v–21r
P	Cambridge, Magdalene College, Pepys MS 1661, pp. 266–284
R	London, British Library, Royal MS 18.A.6, ff. 64r–87v, 89r–101v
S_1	London, British Library, Sloane MS 5, ff. 13ra–57ra
S_2	London, British Library, Sloane MS 7, f. 105v
Sl	London, British Library, Sloane MS 2948, ff. 1r–19v
W	London, Wellcome Library, MS 5650, ff. 29r–39v
X	Stockholm, Kungliga Biblioteket, MS X 90, pp. 156–216

6. Works cited

Alpagus, Andreas (ed.) 1550. Johannes Serapion: *Serapionis medici arabis celeberrimi Practica.* Venetiis: Apud Iuntas.

André, Jacques 1956. *Lexique de termes de botanique en latin.* Paris: Klincksieck.

André, Jacques 1985. *Les noms de plants dans la Rome antique.* Paris: Les Belles Lettres.

Andrews, Alfred C. 1958. The mints of the Greeks and Romans and their condimentary uses. *Osiris* 13, 127–149.

Appendino, Giovanni / Pollastro, Federica / Verotta, Luisella *et al.* 2009. Polyacetylenes from Sardinian *Oenanthe fistulosa*: A molecular clue to *risus sardonicus*. *Journal of Natural Products* 72.5, 962–965.

Arber, Agnes [1912] ²1953. *Herbals. Their origin and evolution. A chapter in the history of Botany 1470–1670.* Cambridge: Cambridge University Press.

Aufmesser, Max 2000. *Etymologische und wortgeschichtliche Erläuterungen zu De materia medica des Pedanius Dioscurides Anazarbeus.* (Altertumswissenschaftliche Texte und Studien 34). Hildesheim: Olms-Weidmann.

Austin, Thomas (ed.) 1888. *Two fifteenth-century cookery-books: Harleian MS. 279 (ab. 1430), & Harl. MS. 4016 (ab. 1450), with extracts from Ashmole MS. 1429 Laud MS. 553, & Douce MS. 55.* (EETS Original series 91). London: N. Trübner.

Ayscough, Samuel 1782. *A catalogue of the manuscripts preserved in the British Museum hitherto undescribed consisting of five thousand volumes.* 2 vols. London: John Rivington.

Banckes, Rycharde (ed.) 1526. *Here begynneth a newe marer* [sic]/ *þe whiche sheweth and treateth of the vertues & propertes of herbes/the whiche is callyd an Herball.* London: Rycharde Banckes.

Bauhin, Caspar 1623. *ΠΙΝΑΞ. Theatri botanici.* Basileae Helvet[iae]: Sumptibus et typis Ludovici Regis.

Bazzi, Franco 1959. Un inedito erbario del secolo XV. Presentazione e commento (Prima traduzione in volgare nota del Macer Floridus). In *Atti del III Bienale della Marca per la storia dell'arte medica*. Fermo, 233–245.

Beck, Lily Y. (ed., trans.) 2005. Pedanius Dioscorides of Anazarbus: *De materia medica*. (Altertumswissenschaftliche Texte und Studien 38). Hildesheim / New York: Olms-Weidmann.

Benskin, Michael 1991. In reply to Dr Burton. *Leeds Studies in English, New Series* 22, 209–262.

Berendes, Julius Dominikus (ed., trans.) 1902. Pedanius Dioscorides of Anazarbus: *Arzneimittellehre in fünf Büchern*. Stuttgart: Enke.

Bernard, Edward 1697. *Catalogi librorum manuscriptorum Angliæ et Hiberniæ in unum collecti, cum indice alphabetico*. 2 vols. Oxoniæ: e Theatro Sheldoniano.

Bierbaumer, Peter 1975–1979. *Der botanische Wortschatz des Altenglischen*. (Grazer Beiträge zur englischen Philologie 1–3). Bern / Frankfurt am Main: Peter Lang.

Bird, W. H. B. / Ledward, K. H. (eds.) 1949. *Calendar of the close rolls preserved in the Public Record Office. Edward IV.* 2 vols. London: HMSO

Björkman, Erik 1900–1902. *Scandinavian loan-words in Middle English*. 2 vols. Halle: Max Niemeyer.

Black, Merja Riita 1997. *Studies in the dialect materials of medieval Herefordshire* (Ph.D. Dissertation). Glasgow: Glasgow University.

Boot, Christine / Mayer, Johannes 1990. Zwei Neufunde zur altdeutschen Überlieferung des Rosmarintraktats. *Sudhoffs Archiv* 74.1, 104–111.

Bos, Gerrit / Mensching, Guido 2000. The Hebrew translation of Macer Floridus: A fragment with Romance elements. *Jewish Quarterly Review* 91, 17–51.

Bravo Gozalo, José María 1981. *Problemática e historia de la historiografía literaria inglesa*. Valladolid: Secretariado de Publicaciones de la Universidad de Valladolid.

Briquet, Charles Moÿse [1907] 1958. *Les filigranes. Dictionnaire historique des marques du papier dès leur apparition vers 1282 jusqu'en 1600.* Amsterdam: The Paper Publications Society.

Britten, James / Holland, Robert 1886. *A dictionary of English plant-names.* (English Dialect Society 22, 26, 45). London: Trübner.

Brodin, Gösta (ed.) 1950. *Agnus Castus. A Middle English herbal, reconstructed from various manuscripts.* (Essays and Studies on English Language and Literature 6). Upsala / Copenhagen / Cambridge (Mass.): A.-B. Lundequistska Bokhandeln / Ejnar Munksgaard / Harvard University Press.

Brown, Michelle P. 1990. *A guide to Western historical scripts from antiquity to 1600.* London: British Library.

Burgess, Edward Sandford 1902. *History of pre-Clusian botany in its relation to Aster.* (Memoirs of the Torrey Botanical Club 10). New York: Published by the Club.

Burton, Tom L. 1991. On the current state of Middle English dialectology. *Leeds Studies in English, New Series* 22, 167–208.

Butler, Alban 2003. *Butler's Lives of the saints.* 12 vols. London: Burns & Oates.

Campbell, Alistair 1959. *Old English grammar.* Oxford: Clarendon Press.

Cappelli, Adriano [1912] ⁶1990. *Lexicon abbreviaturarum.* Milano: Ulrico Hoepli.

Capuano, Thomas M. (ed.) 1991. *Texto y concordancias del Libro de Medicina llamado Macer: Granada, 1518 y 1519.* Madison: L.E.A. Publishing House.

Chantraine, Pierre [1968–1980] ²1999. *Dictionnaire étymologique de la langue grecque. Histoire des mots.* Paris: Klinksieck.

Chapman, George T. L. / Tweedle, Marilyn N. / McCombie, Frank / Wesencraft, Anne (eds.) 1995. *William Turner: A New Herball.* 2 vols. Cambridge: Cambridge University Press.

Choulant, Ludwig (ed.) 1832. *De viribus herbarum.* Lipsiae: sumptibus Leopoldi Vossii.

Choulant, Ludwig [1828] ²1841. *Handbuch der Bücherkunde für die ältere Medizin.* Leipzig: Leopold Voss.

Churchill, William Algernon 1935. *Watermarks in paper in Holland, England, France, etc. in the XVII and XVIII centuries and their connection.* Amsterdam: Menno Hertzberger.

Cleasby, Richard / Vígfusson, Gudbrand [1874] ²1957. *An Icelandic-English dictionary.* Oxford: Clarendon Press.

Cocco, Vicenzo 1955. D'un'antichissima designazione mediterranea della 'malva': preell. μῶλυ *pianta magica, malva. Archivio glottologico italiano* 40.1, 10–28.

Cockayne, Oswald (ed.) 1864–1866. *Leechdoms, wortcunning, and starcraft of early England.* 3 vols. (Rolls Series 35). London: Longman.

Conerly, Peter / Ardemagni, Enrica J. / Richards, Ruth M. (eds.) 1986. *The text and concordances of Seville Colombina manuscript 7-6-27: Macer herbolario.* (Medieval Spanish Medical Text Series 7). Madison: Hispanic Seminary of Medieval Studies.

Constantinus Africanus 1536. *Constantini Africani post Hippocratem et Galenum, quorum, Grœcę linguœ doctus, sedulus fuit lector, medicorum nulli prorsus, multis doctissimis testibus, posthabendi opera.* Basileae: Apud Henricum Petrum.

Corradini Bozzi, Maria Sofia 1997. *Ricettari medico-farmaceutici medievali nella Francia meridionale.* (Studi / Accademia toscana di scienze e lettere "La Colombaria" 159). Firenze: L.S. Olschki.

Cramer, John Anthony (ed.) 1835–1837. *Anecdota Graeca e codd. manuscriptis bibliothecarum Oxoniensium.* 4 vols. Oxonii: e Typographeo academico.

Cross, Rowin 2004. *A handlist of manuscripts containing English in the Hunterian Collection.* Glasgow: Glasgow University Library.

Culpeper, Nicholas 1652. *The English physitian, or an astrologo-physical discourse of the vulgar herbs of this nation.* London: Peter Cole.

Daems, Willem Frans 1993. *Nomina simplicium medicinarum ex synonymariis medii aevi collecta. Semantische Untersuchungen zum Fachwortschatz hoch- und spätmittelalterlicher Drogenkunde.* (Studies in ancient Medicine 6). Leiden: Brill.

Davenport, Cyril 1909. *English heraldic book-stamps.* London: Constable & Co.

de Capella, Michael (ed.) 1510. *Compendium medicine Gilberti anglici.* Lugduni: per Jacobum Saccon expensis Uincentij de Portonarijs.

De Hamel, Christopher 1992. *Scribes and illuminators.* London: British Museum Press.

de Vere, Gaston du C. (trad.) 1912–1915. *Lives of the most eminent painters, sculptors & architects by Girogio Vasari* (10 vols.). London: Philip Lee Warner/The Medici Society.

de Vriend, Hubert Jan (ed.) 1984. *The Old English Herbarium and Medicina de quadrupedibus.* (EETS Original Series 286). London: Oxford University Press.

de Vries, Jan Pieter Marie Laurens [1957–1961] ^{2}1962. *Altnordisches etymologisches Wörterbuch.* Leiden: Brill.

Demaitre, Luke E. 2013. *Medieval medicine: the art of healing, from head to toe.* Santa Barbara / Denver / Oxford: Praeger.

Derolez, Albert 2003. *The palaeography of Gothic manuscript books: from the twelfth to the early sixteenth century.* Cambridge: Cambridge University Press.

Dodoens, Rembert 1619. *An Newe Herball, or historie of plants.* (Trans. Henry Lyte.) London: Edward Griffin.

du Fresne, Charles 1938. *Glossarium mediae et infirmae latinitatis.* 10 vols. Paris: Librairie des Sciences et des Arts.

Dunglison, Robley [1874] ^{21}1893. *A dictionary of medical science.* Philadelphia: Lea Brothers.

Dutschke, Consuelo W. / Rouse, Richard H. 1989. *Guide to medieval and Renaissance manuscripts in the Huntington Library.* 2 vols. San Marino: Huntington Library.

Dyce, Keith M. / Sack, Wolfgang O. / Wensing, Cornelius Johannes Gerardus [1987] ^{4}2010. *Textbook of veterinary anatomy.* Philadelphia / London: Saunders.

Earle, John 1880. *English plant names from the tenth to the fifteenth century.* London / Oxford: Henry Frowde / Oxford University Press.

Faraudo de Saint Germain, Lluís 1955–1956. Una versió catalana del *libre de les herbes de Macer*. *Estudis romànics* 5, 1–54.

Fischer, Hermann 1929. *Mittelalterliche Pflanzenkunde*. München: Münchner Drucke.

Flower, Cyril Thomas 1933–1947. *Calendar of the close rolls preserved in the Public Record Office. Henry VI.* 6 vols. London: HMSO

Font Quer, Pío [1961] [10]1987. *Plantas medicinales. El Dioscórides renovado*. Barcelona: Labor.

Frisk, Gösta (ed.) 1949. *A Middle English translation of Macer Floridus De Viribus Herbarum*. Uppsala: Almqvist & Wiksells Boktryckeri AB.

Frisk, Hjalmar 1960. *Griechisches etymologisches Wörterbuch*. 3 vols. (Indogermanische Bibliothek. II. Reihe, Wörterbücher). Heidelberg: Winter.

Fuchs, Leonhart 1542. *De historia stirpium*. Basileæ: In officina Isingriniana.

García González, Alejandro 2007 (ed.). *Alphita*. (Edizione nazionale «la scuola medica salernitana» 2). Firenze: SISMEL edizioni del Galluzzo.

García Valdés, Manuela (ed., trans.) 1998. Pedanius Dioscorides of Anazarbus: *Plantas y remedios medicinales (De materia medica)*. 2 vols. (Biblioteca Clásica Gredos 253–254). Madrid: Gredos.

Garrido Anes, Edurne 2005. *De simplici medicina (Circa instans) en inglés medio: vernacularización del tratado salernitano de Mateo Plateario* (Ph.D. Dissertation). Universidad de Huelva.

Gaskell, Philip 1976. A nomenclature for the letterforms of roman type. *Visible Language* 10.1, 41–51.

Gerard, John 1597. *The herball or Generall historie of plantes*. London: John Norton.

Glare, Peter Geoffrey William 1997. *Oxford Latin dictionary*. Oxford: Clarendon Press.

Görlach, Manfred 1991. *Introduction to Early Modern English*. Cambridge: Cambridge University Press.

The great herball, newly corrected. 1539. Londini: in edibus Thome Gybson.

Grimal, Pierre [1951] ⁷1982. *Dictionnaire de la mythologie grecque et romaine*. Paris: Presses Universitaires de France.
Groom, Nigel St John 1992. *The perfume handbook*. London: Chapman & Hall.
Guigues, Pierre 1905a. Les noms arabes dans Sérapion, «Liber de simplici medicina». Essai de restitution et d'identification de noms arabes de médicaments usités au Moyen Âge. *Journal asiatique* 10.5, 473–546.
Guigues, Pierre 1905b. Les noms arabes dans Sérapion, «Liber de simplici medicina». Essai de restitution et d'identification de noms arabes de médicaments usités au Moyen Âge (suite et fin). *Journal asiatique* 10.6, 49–112.
Hægstad, Kristofer Marius 1906. *Gamalnorsk fragment av Henrik Harpestreng*. (Videnskabsselsk. Skrifter ii: Historisk-filolosofisk Klasse 2). Christiania: Dybwad.
Halliwell-Phillipps, James Orchard [1847] ¹¹1889. *A dictionary of archaic and provincial words, obsolete phrases, proverbs and ancient customs from the fourteenth century*. 2 vols. London: Reeves and Turner.
Hamilton, George L. 1906. Trotula. *Modern Philology* 4.2, 377–380.
Harvey, John H. 1987. The Square Garden of Henry the Poet. *Garden History* 15.1, 1–11.
Hauberg, Poul (ed.) 1936. Henrik Harpestræng: *Liber herbarum*. København: Carl Kretzschmer.
Heawood, Edward 1950. *Watermarks mainly of the 17th and 18th centuries*. (Monumenta Chartæ Papyraceæ Historiae Illustrantia 1). Hilversum: Paper Publication Society.
Hector, Leonard Charles 1980. *The handwriting of English documents*. Dorking: Kohler and Coombes.
Hepper, Peter / Wells, Deborah 2015. Olfaction in the order Carnivora: family Canidae. In Doty, Richard L. (ed.) *Handbook of olfaction and gustation*. Chichester: Wiley-Blackwell, 591–603.
Herrtage, Sydney John Hervon (ed.) 1881. *Catholicon Anglicum, an English-Latin wordbook, dated 1483*. (EETS Original Series 75). London: Trübner.

Hoffmann, Frederick August 1884. *Poetry, its origin, nature, and history. To which is added a compendium of the works of the poets of all times and countries.* 2 vols. London: Thurgate & Sons.

Hofmann, Konrad / Auracher, Theodor M. 1883. Der Longobardische Dioskorides des Marcellus Virgilius. *Romanische Forschungen* 1.3, 49–105.

Hogg, Richard M. 1992. *A Grammar of Old English. Volume I: Phonology.* Oxford / Cambridge (Mass.): Blackwell.

Hogg, Richard M. / Fulk, Robert Dennis 2011. *A grammar of Old English. Volume II: Morphology.* Oxford: Wiley Blackwell.

Holthausen, Ferdinand [1933] ³1974. *Altenglisches etymologisches Wörterbuch.* (Germanische Bibliothek. II. Reihe, Wörterbücher). Heidelberg: Carl Winter.

Hort, Arthur (ed., trans.) 1916. Theophrastus: *Enquiry into plants and minor works on odours and weather signs.* 2 vols. (Loeb Classical Library 70, 79). London / Cambridge (Mass.): W. Heinemann / Harvard University Press.

Hunt, Tony 1986–1987. The botanical glossaries in MS London, B.L. Add. 15236. *Pluteus* 4–5, 101–150.

Hunt, Tony 1989. *Plant names of medieval England.* Cambridge: D. S. Brewer.

Hunt, Tony 2008. *An Old French herbal (MS Princeton U.L. Garrett 131).* (Textes vernaculaires du Moyen Âge 4). Turnhout: Brepols.

Jansen, Ulrike 2013. *»Spuria Macri«: ein Anhang zu »Macer Floridus, De viribus herbarum«.* (Beiträge zur Altertumskunde 314). Berlin / Boston: De Gruyter.

Johnson, Charles / Jenkinson, Hilary 1915. *English court hand A.D. 1066 to 1500.* 2 vols. Oxford: Clarendon Press.

Jordan, Richard 1974. *Handbook of Middle English grammar: Phonology.* (Janua linguarum. Series practica 218). The Hague / Paris: Mouton.

Kålund, Peder Erasmus Kristian 1907. *Den islandske laegebog: Codex Arnamagnaeanus 434 a, 12mo.* (Kgl. danske videnskabsselk.

skrifter, 6. raekke: historisk og filosofisk 4). København: B. Luno.

Keiser, George R. 1996. Reconstructing Robert Thornton's herbal. *Medium Ævum* 65.1, 35–53.

Keiser, George R. 1998. *Works of science and information.* (A manual of the writings in Middle English 1050–1500 10). New Haven: The Connecticut Academy of Arts and Sciences.

Keiser, George R. 2005. A Middle English rosemary treatise in verse and prose. *American Notes and Queries* 18.3, 7–17.

Keiser, George R. 2008a. Rosemary: not just for remembrance. In Dendle, Peter / Touwaide, Alain (eds.) *Health and healing from the medieval garden.* Cambridge: Boydell & Brewer, 180–204.

Keiser, George R. 2008b. Vernacular herbals: a growth industry in late medieval England. In Connolly, Margaret / Mooney, Linne R. (eds.) *Design and distribution of late medieval manuscripts in England.* Cambridge: Boydell & Brewer, 292–307.

Klein, Ernest David 1987. *A comprehensive etymological dictionary of the Hebrew language for readers of English.* Jerusalem: Carta.

Klemming, Gustaf Edvard (ed.) 1883–1886. *Läke- och örte-böcker från Sveriges medeltid.* (Samlingar utgivna av Svenska fornskriftsällskapet 26). Stockholm: Kongl. boktryckeriet / P. A. Norstedt & söner.

Kühn, Karl Gottlob (ed., trans.) 1821–1833. Claudius Galenus: Ἅπαντα. *Opera omnia.* 20 vols. Lipsiae: officina libraria Car. Cnoblochii.

Künkele, Siegfried 1987. Beiträge zur Geschichte der europäischen Orchideen. I. Leonhart Fuchs, der Vater der Väter der Botanik. *Mitteilungsblatt Arbeitskreis Heimische Orchideen Baden-Württemberg* 19.2, 197–383.

Langkavel, Bernhard August (ed.) 1868. Simeon Seth: *Syntagma de alimentorum facultatibus.* Lipsiae: in aedibus B. G. Teubneri.

Larsen, Henning 1931. *An old Icelandic medical miscellany: MS Royal Irish Academy 23 D 43, with supplement from MS Trinity College (Dublin) L-2-27.* Oslo: Jacob Dybwad.

Lass, Roger 1992. Phonology and morphology. In Blake, Norman (ed.) *The Cambridge History of the English Language. Volume II: 1066–1476.* Cambridge: Cambridge University Press, 23–155.

Ledward, K. H. (ed.) 1954. *Calendar of the close rolls preserved in the Public Record Office. Edward IV, Edward V and Richard III, A.D. 1476–1485.* London: HMSO

Legré, Ludovic 1899. *La botanique en Provence au XVIe siècle. Pierre Pena et Mathias de Lobel.* Marseille: H. Aubertin & G. Rolle.

Liddell, Henry George / Scott, Robert / Jones, Henry Stuart et al. (eds.) 1996. *A Greek-English lexicon. With a revised supplement.* Oxford / New York: Clarendon Press.

Lodge, Barton (ed.) [1873] 2000. Rutilius Taurus Aemilianus Palladius: *Palladius on husbandrie from the unique MS. of about 1420 in Colchester Castle, with a ryme index by J. H. Herrtage.* 2 vols. (EETS Original Series 52, 72). London / New York / Toronto: Oxford University Press.

López, Marcela (ed.) 1987. *The text and concordance of Biblioteca Universitaria, Salamanca, MS 2262, Propiedades del romero.* (Medieval Spanish Medical Text Series 21). Madison: Hispanic Seminary of Medieval Studies.

Luick, Karl [1914–1940] ²1964. *Historische Grammatik der englischen Sprache.* 2 vols. Oxford / Stuttgart: Blackwell / Bernhard Tauchnitz.

Macafee, Caroline I. (ed.) 2002. Adam Jack Aitken: *The older Scots vowels: a history of the stressed vowels of older Scots from the beginnings to the eighteenth century.* (Scottish Text Society fifth series, 1). Edinburgh: Scottish Text Society.

Martin, Charles Trice 1892. *The record interpreter: a collection of abbreviations, Latin words and names used in English historical manuscripts and records.* London: Reeves and Turner.

McIntosh, Angus / Samuels, Michael L. / Benskin, Michael 1986. *A linguistic atlas of late mediaeval English.* 4 vols. Aberdeen: Aberdeen University Press.

McIntosh, Angus 1963. A new approach to Middle English dialectology. *English Studies* 44, 1–11.

Miranda García, Antonio / González Fernández-Corugedo, Santiago (eds.) 2011. *Benvenutus Grassus' On the well-proven art of the eye. Practica oculorum & De probatissima arte oculorum. synoptic edition and philological studies*. (Late Middle English texts 1). Bern: Peter Lang.

Morales, Ramón *et al.* (ed.) 1996. *Nombres vulgares*. (Archivos de Flora Ibérica 7). Madrid: Consejo Superior de Investigaciones Científicas.

Moreno Olalla, David 2004. A manuscript life. BL, Sloane 5 from a physical perspective. In Rodríguez Álvarez, Alicia / Alonso Almeida, Francisco J. (eds.) *Voices of the past. Studies in Old and Middle English language and literature*. A Coruña: Netbiblo, 89–98.

Moreno Olalla, David 2007. *The fautys to amende*. On the interpretation of the *explicit* of Sloane 5, ff. 13–57, and related matters. *English Studies* 88.2, 119–142.

Moreno Olalla, David 2011. Nominal morphemes in *Lelamour's Herbal*. In Thaisen, Jacob / Rutkowska, Hanna (eds.) *Scribes, printers and the accidentals of their texts*. (Studies in English medieval language and literature 33). Frankfurt: Peter Lang, 53–71.

Moreno Olalla, David 2013a. A plea for ME botanical synonyma. In Gillespie, Vincent / Hudson, Anne (eds.) *Probable truth. Editing medieval texts from Britain in the twenty-first century*. (Texts and Transitions 5). Brussels: Brepols, 387–404.

Moreno Olalla, David 2013b. The textual transmission of the *Northern Macer* tradition. *English Studies* 94.8, 931–957.

Moreno Olalla, David 2015. Is plant species identification possible in Middle English herbals? In Shaw, Philip / Erman, Britt / Melchers, Gunnel *et al.* (eds.) *From clerks to corpora: essays on the English language yesterday and today*. (Stockholm English Studies 2). Stockholm: Stockholm University Press, 53–70.

Moreno Olalla, David 2017. Reconstructing 'John Lelamour's' herbal: the linguistic evidence. *Anglia* 135.4, 669–699.

Moreno Olalla, David 2018. Notes on the Latin original of the Middle English *Northern Macer* herbal. *Manuscripta* 62.1.

Morris, Richard 1865. Liber cure cocorum. In *The Philological Society's Early English volume, 1862–4: containing: I. Liber cure cocorum, ab. 1440 A.D. II. Hampole's Pricke of conscience, ab. 1340 A.D. III. The castel off loue, ab. 1320 A.D.* 3 vols. London / Berlin: Published for the Philological Society by A. Asher & Co., 1–61.

Morsbach, Lorenz 1896. *Mittelenglische Grammatik.* (Sammlung kurzer Grammatiken germanischer Dialekte 8). Halle: Max Niemeyer.

Mossé, Fernand [1952] 1968. *A handbook of Middle English.* Baltimore: Johns Hopkins Press.

Mowat, John Lancaster Gough (ed.) 1882. *Sinonoma Bartholomei. A glossary from a fourteenth-century manuscript in the Library of Pembroke College, Oxford.* (Anecdota Oxoniensia. Mediaeval and modern series 1.i). London / Oxford: Henry Frowde / Oxford University Press.

Mowat, John Lancaster Gough (ed.) 1887. *Alphita. A medico-botanical glossary from the Bodleian Manuscript, Selden B.35.* (Anecdota Oxoniensia. Mediaeval and modern series 1.ii). London / Oxford: Henry Frowde / Oxford University Press.

Muzerelle, Denis 1985. *Vocabulaire codicologique: répertoire méthodique des termes français relatifs aux manuscrits.* (Rubricae 1). Paris: CEMI.

Nickson, Margaret Annie Eugenie 1979. Sloane's codes: the solution to a mystery. *Factotum. Newsletter of the XVIIIth Century* 7, 13–18.

Nickson, Margaret Annie Eugenie 1998. *The British Library: guide to the catalogues and indexes of the Department of Manuscripts.* London: British Library Board.

Norri, Juhani 1992. *Names of sicknesses in English, 1400–1550: an exploration of the lexical field.* (Annales Academiae Scientiarum Fennica. Dissertationes Humanarum Litterarum 6). Helsinki: Suomalainen Tiedeakatemia.

Nyrop, Kristoffer 1899–1930. *Grammaire historique de la langue française.* 6 vols. Copenhague: Gyldendalske Boghandel Nordisk Forlag.

Ogden, Margaret Sinclair (ed.) 1971. *The Cyrurgie of Guy de Chauliac*. (EETS Original Series 265). London / New York / Toronto: Oxford University Press.

Olmsted, Hugh 1994. Modeling the genealogy of Maksim Grek's collection types: the 'plectogram' as visual aid in reconstruction. In Flier, Michael S. / Rowland, Daniel B. (eds.) *Medieval Russian culture, Volume II*. (California Slavic studies 19). Berkeley: University of California Press, 107–133.

Orme, Nicholas 1973. *English schools in the Middle Ages*. London: Methuen & Co.

Orme, Nicholas 1996. Medieval schools of Herefordshire. *Nottingham Medieval Studies* 40, 47–62.

Ortoleva, Vincenzo 2014. The meaning and etymology of the adjective *apiosus*. In Maire, Brigitte (ed.) *'Greek' and 'Roman' in Latin medical texts: studies in cultural change and exchange in ancient medicine*. (Studies in ancient medicine 42). Leiden: Brill, 259–288.

Pahta, Päivi / Taavitsainen, Irma 2004. Vernacularisation of scientific and medical writing. In Taavitsainen, Irma / Pahta, Päivi (eds.) *Medical and scientific writing in late medieval English*. Cambridge: Cambridge University Press, 1–22.

Pearson, David [1994] ²1998. *Provenance research in book history. A handbook.*. London: The British Library / Oak Knoll Press.

Pensado Figueiras, Jesús 2012. Pasajes del *Macer Floridus* castellano en el ms. II-3063 de la Real Biblioteca. *Revista de Filología Española* 92.2, 341–362.

Petti, Anthony Gaetano 1977. *English literary hands from Chaucer to Dryden*. Cambridge (Mass.): Harvard University Press.

Platearius, Matthaeus 1512. *Liber de simplici medicina*. Lugdunum: Constantin Fradin.

Polito, Roberto 1999. On the life of Asclepiades of Bithynia. *The Journal of Hellenic Studies* 119, 48–66.

Potter, Paul (ed., trans., comm.) 1980. *Hippocratis De Morbis III* (Corpus Medicorum Graecorum I 2,3). Berlin: Academia Scientiarum.

Prior, Richard Chandler Alexander 1863. *On the popular names of British plants.* London: Williams and Norgate.

Pulteney, Richard 1790. *Historical and biographical sketches of the progress of botany in England, from its origin to the introduction of the Linnæan system.* 2 vols. London: printed for T. Cadell.

Quincy, John [1721] ²1727. *The dispensatory of the Royal College of Physicians in London.* London: Printed by J. Bettenham, for R. Knaplock, D. Midwinter, W. and J. Innys, J. Osborn and T. Longman, B. Motte, and J. Clarke.

Rackham, Harris / Jones, William Henry Samuel (eds., trans.) 1938–1963. Pliny: *Natural History.* 10 vols. (Loeb Classical Library 330, 352, 353, 370, 371, 392, 393, 394, 418, 419). Cambridge (Mass.): Harvard University Press.

Raeder, Hans (ed.) 1928–1933. Oribasius: *Collectionum medicarum reliquiae.* 4 vols. Lipsiae: B. G. Teubneri.

Rawson, Elizabeth 1982. The life and death of Asclepiades of Bithynia. *The Classical Quarterly* 32.2, 358–370.

Redwood, Theophilus [1821] ²1848. *Gray's supplement to the pharmacopœia.* London: Longman and Co.

Ribichini, Sergio 2003. *Il riso sardonico: storia di un proverbio antico.* Sassari: Carlo Delfino.

Riddle, John M. 1984. Byzantine commentaries on Dioscorides. *Dumbarton Oaks Papers* 38, 95–102.

Riley, Henry Thomas 1868. *Memorials of London and London life, in the XIIIth, XIVth, and XVth centuries, being a series of extracts, local, social, and political, from the early archives of the City of London, A.D. 1276–1419.* London: Longmans, Green and Co.

Rix, Helmut / Kümmel, Martin (eds.) 2001. *LIV. Lexikon der indogermanischen Verben. Die Wurzeln und ihre Primärstammbildungen.* Wiesbaden: Dr. Ludwig Reichert.

Robbins, Rossell Hope 1970. Medical manuscripts in Middle English. *Speculum* 45.3, 393–415.

Rodgers, Robert H. (ed.) 1975. Rutilius Taurus Aemilianus Palladius: *Opus agriculturae. De veterinaria medicina. De insitione.*

(Bibliotheca scriptorum Graecorum et Romanorum Teubneriana). Leipzig: Teubner.

Rohde, Eleanor Sinclair 1922. *The Old English herbals*. London: Longmans, Green and Co.

Rolland, Eugène 1896–1914. *Flore populaire, ou, Histoire naturelle des plantes dans leurs rapports avec la linguistique et le folklore*. 11 vols. Paris: Librairie Rolland.

Schnell, Berhard / Crossgrove, William C. (eds.) 2002. *Der deutsche »Macer« (Vulgatfassung). Mit einem Abdruck des lateinischen Macer Floridus »De Viribus Herbarum«*. (Texte und Textgeschichte 50). Tübingen: Niemeyer.

Scott, Edward John Long 1904. *Catalogus librorum manuscriptorum Bibliothecæ Sloanianæ*. London.

Seymour, Michael C. et al. (ed.) 1975–1988. *On the Properties of Things. John Trevisa's translation of Bartholomeus Anglicus' De Proprietatibus Rerum*. 3 vols. Oxford: Clarendon.

Silvaticus, Matthaeus 1521. *Opus pandectarum medicine Matthaei Siluatici*. Papie: Bernadinum de Garaldis.

Simpson, J. A. / Weiner, E. S. C. (eds.) 1989. *The Oxford English dictionary*. Oxford: Oxford University Press.

Sprengel, Kurt Polycarp Joachim (ed.) 1829–1830. Pedanius Dioscorides of Anazarbus: *De materia medica libri quinque*. 2 vols. (Medicorum Graecorum Opera 25–26). Lipsiae: Officina libraria Car. Cnoblochii.

Stadler, Hermann 1897a. Dioscorides Longobardus. (Cod. Lat. Monacensis 337.). *Romanische Forschungen* 10.2, 181–247.

Stadler, Hermann 1897b. Dioscorides Longobardus. (Cod. Lat. Monacensis 337.). *Romanische Forschungen* 10.2, 369–446.

Stadler, Hermann 1899. Dioscorides Longobardus. (Cod. Lat. Monacensis 337.). *Romanische Forschungen* 11.1, 1–121.

Stadler, Hermann 1901. Dioscorides Longobardus. (Cod. Lat. Monacensis 337.). *Romanische Forschungen* 13.1, 161–243.

Stein, Gabriele 2006. The English Edition of Hadrianus Junius' *Nomenclator* (1585). *Lexicographica* 21, 35–46.

Stearn, William Thomas (ed.) 1965. William Turner: *Libellus de Re Herbaria 1538. The Name of Herbes 1548* (The Ray Society Series 145). London: The Ray Society.

Stirling, János 1995–1998. *Lexicon nominum herbarum, arborum fruticumque linguae Latinae: ex fontibus Latinitatis ante saeculum XVII scriptis collegit et descriptionibus botanicis illustravit.* 4 vols. Budapest: Encyclopaedia.

Talbot, Charles H. 1967. *Medicine in medieval England.* London: Olbourne.

Tanner, Thomas 1748. *Bibliotheca Britannico-Hibernica: sive, De scriptoribus, qui in Anglia, Scotia, et Hibernia ad saeculi XVII initium floruerunt, literarum ordine juxta familiarum nomina dispositis commentarius.* Londini: Excudit Gulielmus Bowyer, impensis Societatis ad Literas Promovendas institutae.

Tremblay, Lucas 1588. *Les fleurs du livre des vertus des herbes.* Rouen: chez Martin et Honoré Mallard.

Turner, William 1551–1568. *The first and seconde partes of the Herbal.* London-Collen: Stephen Mierdman-Arnold Birckman.

Vázquez de Benito, María Concepción / Herrera, María Teresa 1989. *Los arabismos de los textos médicos latinos y castellanos de la Edad Media y de la Modernidad.* Madrid: Consejo Superior de Investigaciones Científicas.

Ventura, Iolanda (ed.) 2009. Ps. Bartholomaeus Mini de Senis: *Tractatus de herbis (Ms London, British Library, Egerton 747).* (Edizione nazionale «la scuola medica salernitana» 5). Firenze: SISMEL edizioni del Galluzzo.

Voigts, Linda Ehrsam / Kurtz, Patricia Deery 2000. *Scientific and medical writings in Old and Middle English: An electronic reference.* (ver. 1.0). Ann Arbor: University of Michigan Press.

von Fleischhacker, Robert (ed.) 1894. *Lanfrank's "Science of cirurgie".* (EETS Original series 102). London: K. Paul, Trench, Trübner & Co.

von Haller, Albrecht 1771–1772. *Bibliotheca botanica. Qua scripta ad rem herbariam facientia a rerum initiis recensentur.* 2 vols. Tiguri: apud Orell, Gessner, Fuessli, et socc.

von Wartburg, Walther 1928–2002. *Französisches etymologisches Wörterbuch: eine Darstellung des galloromanischen Sprachschatzes.* 25 vols. Bonn: F. Klopp.

Warton, Thomas 1774–1781. *The history of English poetry from the close of the eleventh to the commencement of the eighteenth century.* 3 vols. London: J. Dodsley.

Warton, Thomas 1840. *The history of English poetry from the close of the eleventh century to the commencement of the eighteenth century.* 3 vols. London: Thomas Tegg.

Warton, Thomas 1871. *History of English poetry from the twelfth to the close of the sixteenth century.* 4 vols. London: Reeves and Turner.

Wellmann, Max (ed.) 1906–1914. *Pedanius Dioscorides of Anazarbus: De materia medica libri quinque.* 3 vols. Berolini: apud Weidmannos.

Whytlaw-Gray, Alianore 1938. *John Lelamour's translation of Macer's Herbal* (M.A. Dissertation). Leeds: University of Leeds.

Wilson, William James Erasmus 1864. On the nature, the varieties, and the treatment of eczema. *The British Medical Journal* 2.203, 567–573.

Wright, Joseph (ed.) 1896–1905. *The English dialect dictionary.* 6 vols. London / New York: Henry Frowde / G. P. Putnam's Sons.

Wright, Thomas / Wülcker, Richard Paul [1884] ³1968. *Anglo-Saxon and Old English vocabularies.* 2 vols. Darmstadt: Wissenschaftliche Buchgesellschaft.

Young, John P. / Aitken, Henderson 1908. *A catalogue of the manuscripts in the Library of the Hunterian Museum in the University of Glasgow.* 2 vols. Glasgow: James MacLehose & Son.

Zimmermann, Volker 1980. Der Rosmarin als Heilpflanze und Wunderdroge: Ein Beitrag zu den mittelalterlichen Drogenmonographien. *Sudhoffs Archiv* 64.4, 351–370.

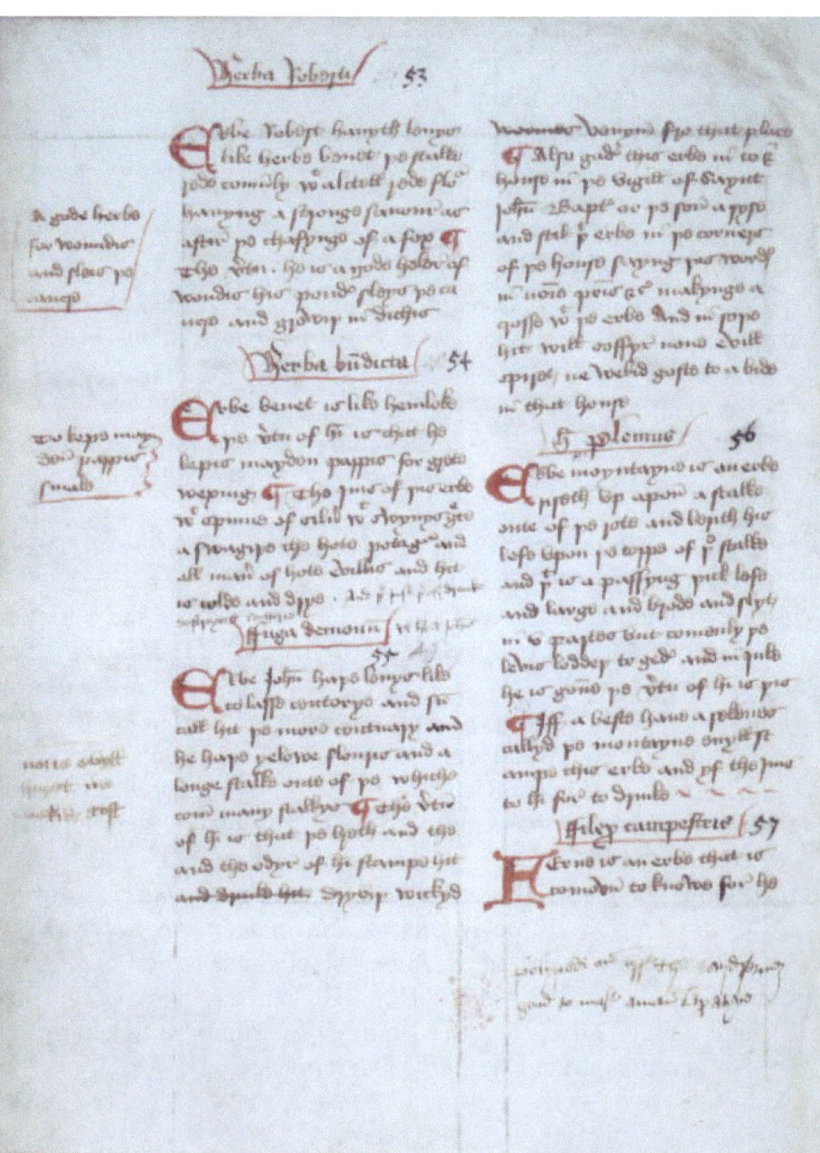

Fig. I. Sloane 5, f. 23v (reproduced with permission from the British Library)

Lelamour Herbal

Ache is hote and drye. The juis of ache and cro*m*es of brede
y-made of whete, made in a plastyr, swagiþ swellinge and
akynge of þe eyne, & swagiþ akynge of the pappis, and doþe
a-way the brenynge of þe stom*a*ke. The rote, sodyn and
dronkyn, abatith venym, and helpiþ for the cogh. For to haue
mylke. [Hache, sodyn in watyr, sesith þe wombe of castynge.
Vse hache rawe all fastynge, and hit shall make þe well
colouryd. And he that haþe feu*er* cotidiane by-for þe accesse
ete hache, and hit a-batiþ þe accesse. Drynke ache and fenell,
and hit helpiþ for þe dropsy, and for þe splene, and for þe
geser, and puttiþ a-way [ferntiklys]. A plaist*er* of sache &
doust of [myll] and eggis by even porcion helpith to euyll helid
wou*n*des and sursano*ur*is].

Anisum

Annys is hote and dry. Yf hit be customable reseyvid, hit yevith
to þe noryshe largely of mylke, and puttiþ a-waye evillis of þe

---

1 ache¹] [Marc]he *.id est.* Apy. Apiu*m* [for brenyng of the stomake] *written, perhaps by Hand A, on the upper margin but now almost completely erased.* and¹] and and *MS.*   **6** hache...13 sursanouris] *This fragment was copied immediately after the entry* Anisum.   sesith] .a. *written on the outer margin.*   **11** ferntiklys] serutiklys *MS.*   **12** myll] milk *MS.*   **15** annys] .b. *written on the inner margin.*

---

1 ache¹] 1 *added by Hand E immediately after the word* Apiu*m that was written by Hand A on the upper margin* || vel smaleach or marche *written by Hand C over the line.*   **6** sodyn] *id est.* ache & smaleach dic*itur* wyll make a man to make water & openeth the [sro *deleted after this word*] stoppyng of the lyu*er*. But it is not to be yeven to women þat been wi*th* child neþer to þoo that haue sokyng children for it draweth evyl humo*re*s to the wombe *written by Hand C on the outer margin.*   **14** anisum] 2 *written by Hand E after this word.*

stomake. Resayue iij sponefull of þe juis luke-warme, and yf þu haue evil stomake, hit opynneþ hit, & castiþ oute þe evil wynde þere-of and vomyte, and helpiþ to make vryn, and helpiþ þat is in womanys schappe. And yf hit be [washen] in ale and drounkyn, hit helpiþ all sore ballokis, and makiþe þe wombe solabill. But he so etyth hit ofte, | hit perith þe sight, and stoppyth þe yate of the engendir. The rote y-brende and y-made pouder fretiþ a-way the fleshe in the wonde. Grynde him and he heliþ bilys, and clensyþ foule wondis, and namely in manns membres. The oudoure þer-of reneyth the brenyng of þe eyne. Sede of annys heliþ knottys that stoppith þe mouþe of þe stomake, & that evill comyþe of colde, and hit castiþ a-way þe hede-ake.

Sana munda

Avance is an herbe that som men calliþ hare-fote. He beriþ a yelowe floure, and sede of him ‖ will cleue in one-is cloþes ȝiff one tuche him. The vertue of hym is þis: make pouder of him, and put a litell þere-off in vlake wyne oþer water, and yf that to him that haþe þe feuerys, and hit shall saue hym. Also hit comfortith þe stomake, and makeþ gode digestion. Also he is a worthi erbe for þe cankyr, and for to hele wondis y-drank.

Dragancia

Addyrworte ys an erbe þat som manne callith dragans, oþer serpentary. Þis erbe is like to þe colour of an nadder, all spraklyd. Hit is hote and drye in the thirde de-gre. The vertue of

---

20 washen] wethe *MS.* **30** som] .c. *written on the outer margin.*

18 stomake] þe juis off annys ys good for evill winds pwrgit vomyte *written by Hand F on the inner margin.* **22** perith] The seed of annys made in pouder is good to putt in all medicyns *written by Hand C on the outer margin.* **29** sana munda] 3 *written by Hand E after this word.* **33** vlake] v *deleted and* u *added over the line with a caret before the letter* a *by Hand C.* **37** dragancia] 4 *written by Hand E after this word.*

him is, braye him and drinke þe juis wiþ wyne, and hit will hele him þat is stonngid with a naddir oþere eny oþer venyme. Also yf one be a-noynted with juis of þat erbe, he thar not drad no venyme worme. Also put þe juis in-to sore erys, and hit will hele ham. Also þe juis, y-medlid with hony, is a worþi þinge for al sore eyne. Also þis erbe is | gode for to distroy þe cankyr, and the goute, and þe festeryng of a wonde. Also þe savir of his flouris makiþ a woman to ber hir childe hastely. Also poudir made of his more and medlid with hony and ete hit: that is souerayne for þe coghe. And þe same medicyne helpiþ a-yeyne humouris of a manys brest. And yff ye seþe the rote, hit will do þe same. Also seþe the rote in watir well, and he that haþe gibbis on his helis washe him þere-in as hote as he may soffyr hit, and he shall be hole.

Agrimonia

Agrymony is an erbe that hauythe sede that will honge in one-is cloþes. This erbe is hote and drye. The vertue of him is this: who that etiþe him all grene wiþ the rote, he helpiþ þe akynge of the wombe. Also yf þis erbe be dried, and made to pouder, and drinke hit with hote water, that is a nobill medicyne for þe same evill. Also yf ‖ eny body be hurt with eny iren tole, mell þe juis wiþ aysell and drinke hit, oþer so y-stampid and layde to he shall be hole. Also yf þu vse him in potage oþer in mete, that heliþe akynge of sorys of þe mylte. Also strowe him in a chambur and in bedis and hit killyth flene.

---

61 eny body] Agrimonia *written on the upper margin.*

55 agrimonia] 5 *written by Hand E after this word.*   **61** yf] Agrimonie hath leves leke to tansie but they be grener then tansie & haþe a yelow flour and after þe flour the sede hongeth on mennes clothes and it groweth in diches hegges & vales *written by Hand C on the lower margin.*

Aristologia

Astrologie beth of iij specys: the longe is callid rede mader. All þei beþ hote in þe secound de-gre and drye in the first de-gre and haviþ one vertue. The vertue of ham is þis: yf one drinke þe juis in wyne, hit distroyeth all maner of venym, and heliþ all poyson, and bryngeþ oute the hastier borthen of a womane, and heliþ nature of þe brest. Also with hony and gladeyne hit clensiþ wondis and þe filþe of þe teþe, yf the gommys and þe jawys be a-noynted ther-with in the mowthe. | Also drynke hit with warme water and that helpeth þe splene, and þe sidis, and þe feuerys, and þe crampe, and the potager, and the fallyng evill, and þe sore of þe wombe, and þe paralitik hit lettiþ. Also þe smoke þere-of dryvith a-wey evill spiritis and comfortiþ chilryn, and hit helpiþ for þe youske. And this þe longe may done as well as the rounde. Also he vnbyndiþ þe stopping of þe lyuer and castiþ oute wekiþ wyndis of manys body. Also sethe the rotis of þe rounde in cowe mylke till hit wax rede: vse that mylke and that will stanche þe blody menysoun, for þis sayþe Ipocras.

Alexandrum

Alixsandir is an erbe that som men calliþ him stammarche. He beryth grete black sede. Þe vertu of him is for to take his levis and vse hame a-monge wortis, and that potage shall distroy all

---

66 aristologia] 6 *written by Hand E after this word.* **73** wondis] with-in or with-oute *written by Hand C over the line.* **74** also] Aristologia rotunda hath leves lyke burre leves or clotte leves & hath but oon branche & grene leves a-bove & it is cleped ganygale. And it dronken with warme water is good for the stoppyng of the brest, and it is good for the fallyng evyll for the potager & for the the crampe & it wold be gadered in hervest *written by Hand C on the outer margin.* **80** also] Aristologia longa hath leves leke to mader & hath branches a cubite of lenght & meny branches comyth of hym hauyng meny knottes as mader & som-what a white flour and it woll be gadered in hervest. *written by Hand C on the outer margin.* **84** alexandrum] 7 *written by Hand E after this word.*

man*er* of postome. Also ete the sede eu*ery* day: that distroyeth tre*m*lyng hondis. ‖

Centu*m* cap[i]ta

Affodill is an herbe þ*at* beriþe a faire yolewe floure, and at þe toppe he haþe ronde coddys in þe whiche he berith sede, and his levis beth smale and longe. The vertu of hi*m* is that þe branchis of this erbe ben gode to hele þe dropesy. Also drynke þe juis of þe flourys of the͜s͵ erbe in wyne and that will sle byti*ng* of venymo*us* wormys. Also take þe more of this erbe and þe juis of his leuys and a litell safar, lat this boyle to-gadrys w*ith* swete wyne streyned fayr: hit is gode for renynge eyen. Also þe more, i-brent and made to poud*er*, temp*er* þ*at* w*ith* a litell oyle, a-noynte that place wher that lackyth here, and hit shall make hit to growe a-yene. Also and a harde sharpe cloþe be wette in þe juis of this erbe, let rubbe the morfue w*ith* that cloþe and hit shall fall a-way, for this erbe is hote and drye in the secund deg*re*.

Anetum |

Annete is an erbe that som men callethe dyll. This herbe ys like to fynell. The v*er*tu of hym is this: who-so drynkiþ þe juis of hi*m* w*ith* stale ale, he will make hi*m* well to pisse. Also þe same drynke will swage the kyrnyng and wikkyd wyndys in þe wombe, and hit puttiþ a-way the yox. Also take þe sede of this erbe and bren hit, and make poudir þ*ere*-of, and strawe hit opon

---

89 hondis] *written on the outer margin.* **90** centum capita] *written on the upper margin;* capta MS. **95** thes] s *written over the line.* **105** annete] Anetum *written on the upper margin.*

---

90 centum capita] 8 *written by Hand E after this word.* **91** affodill] or senichief *written by Hand C over the line.* **93** longe] leke to leeke *written by Hand C over the line.* **96** wormys] or bestes *written by Hand C over the line.* þe juis] or put mirre to þ*is* medicyn *written by Hand C on the outer margin.* **105** annete] 9 *written by Hand E after the word* Anetum *that Hand A had repeated on the upper margin.*

a wou*n*de, and hit heliþe hi*m*, and namely yf a man ben shaldid on his pyntill, oþ*er* in ony oþ*er* me*m*bre, and whate harme arysiþe in onys yerde, w*ith* that medicyne he schall be hole. Also make a plaster of þe sede y-brent, oþ*er* stampe þe rote, and lay to þe emerodys: hit heliþ ham clene. Also þe juis i-dronke makiþ norshys haue plente of mylke and is gode for þe stom*a*ke. Also that drynke clensiþ menstrue and also þe reynes, makeþ gode digestyou*n*. Also þe flo*ur* of hi*m* i-sodd in oyle is a worþi þinge a-yene all colde þingis, and to þe hede, and to þe synowys, ‖ for he is hote and drye in the secounde de-gre. But [who-]so vsiþe hi*m* myche in drynke, he periþe þ*e* sight and lettiþ the gettyng of childryn*e*.

Ameos

Ameos ys an erbe well y-like to elryn*e* in levis, but thei ben lasse. Þe v*er*tu of þ*i*s erbe is þis: yf he be dronke w*ith* hony, he sleyth wormys in þe wo*m*be. And that vnbyndiþ þe grete stoppyng of leþ*er* wyndis in one-is body, and hit brekiþ þe stone. Hit comfortiþ a manys stom*a*ke yf he be colde, and hit [clansiþ] a man*n*s lyu*er* and his raynes. Also he helith wond*is* and þe styng oþ*er* bitynge of venymys best*is* oþ*er* wormes, for þ*i*s erbe is dry and hote.

Euperatoriu*m*

Ambrose ys an erbe that som men calleþ wilde sauge, oþ*er* wode-merche, oþ*er*e hyndale. He is hote and drye. The v*er*tu of him is this: who-so drynkeþ þe juis of þ*i*s erbe, that laskiþ as myche in | quantite as he drynkeþ þ*er*e-of. Also yf ye bray hit

---

121 who-so] so *MS.*   129 clansiþ] causiþ *MS.*

---

123 ameos[1]] 10 *written by Hand E after this word.*   124 ameos] called amye *written by Hand C over the line.*   125 lasse] And amye hath a longe brau*n*che & florissheth & sedeth as p*er*lys *written by Hand C on the inner margin.*   132 euperatorium] 11 *written by Hand E after this word.*

w*ith* egrymony and botyr, þ*at* helpiþ hastely newe wondis. Also
take ambros, and daysye y-called brysewort, and hare-fote
y-like myche, seþ ham in wat*er*, put þ*er*-to pyp[er] and hony
largely, and þis is sou*er*ayn for to be dronke to hele wondis and 140
strayne ha*m* to-gader. Also that drynke will knytt and hele
brokyn ribbis, for he is hote and drye of kynde. Also yf þ*u*
drynke hi*m*, he vnbyndiþ þe stoppyng of þe lyu*er*. Also stampe
this erbe w*ith* olde wyne and ley to wou*n*dis: hit helpiþ ham.
Also ete þe erbe oþ*er*e drinke þe juis or the axces com, and hit 145
shall not greue the. Also take an hondfull of þis erbe and a
hondfull of herdis purse, bray ham and drynke þ*at* juse w*ith*
gotis mylke oþ*er* cowe mylke to saue ham þ*at* pissiþ blode.

Betania

Betayne is colde, and makiþ to pisse, and brekiþ þe stone. ‖ 150
Betayne, hony, and wyne drowith þe dropesye and helpiþe þe 15va
empetik. Stampe þe leuys and make a plastre, hit heliþ þe dente
of þe eye. The juis þ*er*e-of and oyle of rose in [erys] a-batiþ
akynge. Þe poud*er* of betayne and hony sod to-ged*er* is gode for þe
cogh and a-batith þ*e* [ʒis]kyng*e* and diu*er*se akyng of þe stomake. 155
And drinke hit in wyne, hit helpiþ for feu*er*. The levis w*ith* salt,
in man*er* of a plaster, hit helpiþ newe wou*n*dis and brokyn
hedis. The levis, soden in man*er* of a plastre laide to þe eyen, is
gode for many evillis of þe eyne. Ete hit oþ*er* drinke hit, hit

---

139 pyper] pyp *MS.*   **150** betayne] Betayny *before the emendation.*
151 betayne hony] Betayne *written on the upper margin.*   **153** erys] erye *MS.*
155 ʒiskynge] kyng*e* *MS.*   **157** and brokyn] for newe mou*n*dis and brokyn
hedis *written on the outer margin.*

---

149 betania] 12 *written by Hand E after this word.*   **150** betayne is] Betayn is
by som bok*es* hot & drie *written by Hand C on the outer margin.*
151 betayne hony] Betayn brused w*ith* salt & put in the nostrelles stancheth þe
bledyng þ*er*-of. Also sta*m*ped w*ith* wyn & playstered to a manes yerd þ*at* is
swolle & sor*e* it helpeth *written by Hand C on the outer margin.*

160 stoppiþe þe eyese rennyng and doþe a-way derknes. Drynke him in wyne, hit addys voymett and doþe a-way evill of þe breste. Take an vnce of betayne and þryse xx peny-wiȝt of olde wyne and xxvij cornes of peper, stampe hit to-geder, and hit heliþ þe splene, þe geser, and the reynes, and doþe a-way akynge of þe
165 reynes, and of þe eyen, & of þe wombe. The juis of him and |
15vb hony, i-vsid to-geder, a-batith the cough and nescheith þe wombe þat is harde, with an vnce of the juis of playntayn put þere-to. For þe feuer cotidian drinke ij vnce of the juis of betayn and hit helpiþ. drynke x peny-wiȝte with olde wyne, hit
170 helpiþ þe dropsie. Drinke þu most [&] þe rote estampit, he castiþ oute evill humours of þe body. Plenius commaundith to take xx peny-wiȝte of þe rote of betony and drinke hit with juis of grapis, and hit spurgith flewme þrowe vomyte. Þe sede, soden in wyne, is gode for venyme. An vnce of betaynne,
175 sodyne in wyne, helpiþ þe jandys, and drinke hit with muste, hit brekiþe þe flour. Take pouder of betayn, as myche as a bene, and hony and ete hit after soper, and hit helpiþe þe stomake for to defie. Plenius saiþe: "make a sercle a-boute nadderes of grete venym with betony, and þei shall not passe oute but euche bete
180 oþer with her taylles till þei dye." The maister of medecynes
16ra biddiþ vs to take betony to all || maner of medicynesse, for þere nys none herbe so gode to þe stomake. Plenius saiþe: "who-so euer beriþ hit vpon him þer may none evill beste do him disses." Drinke þe juis in wyne, hit amendiþ a manys colour. Take
185 betony, egrymoyne and camamyll sodyn in watir, and weshe þe seke hede ther-with and ley the erbis as a plaster to, and hit dothe a-waye evill akyng and makiþ hym to haue sclepe.

161 þe breste] for þe eyne and þe feuer & þe stone þe dropesye *written on the outer margin.* **170** &] *om. MS.* **181** all] Betany *written on the upper margin.*

Beata

Beatis some lechis seiþ that hit swelliþ þe hede. Also Galyen saythe that hit is not gode to him that haþe myche of gall, but he saiþ þat hit is gode and holsome to þe flewmatike, and he affirmeth that hit is holsome to þe stomake and makiþ faire colour. Also he saiþ: "who-so vsiþ hit wiþ vynegre hit makeþ him to haue sauor & nescheith þe wombe." Þe levys, hony, and eysell i-mengid to-geder [heliþ] hownde bitte. Þe iuse and water dronkyn helpith him that has sodeynly loste his speche. | Þe juis þere-of, done in þe nose-holles, doþe a-waye evill vmeris of þe hede. Ete hit or drinke hit, and lay ham to bilys, and he heliþ hit. Take þe juis, aysell, and hony to-gederis, hit cleriþ þe siȝte and puttiþ a-way frenteklys. Who-so etiþ hit a-batith swelling of ouer-myche hete. Þe juis, y-dronkyn wiþ wyne, makiþ a man to sclepe and þe noryce to haue mylke, and hit helpiþe þe flux, and who-so etith þere-of hit helpiþe þe sighte.

Bigula

Bvgill is hote and drye in that oþer de-gre. Drinke him wiþ wyne i-stampid hit clensiþ rede colour and purgith brenynge of þe hert þat þer comiþ of blacke colour, þat is callid cardiaca yn [grewe] and helpiþ evill humers of þe longgis. Þe juis mengid with water and vse hit [helpeþ mennys memorye in þe hete ȝif it be ofte vsed]. Þe wyne that hit is soden inne oþer the watir, yf hit be caste a-monge men at a feste, hit shall make hem be bliþe and gladd.

---

195 heliþ] *om. MS.*   **196** þe juis] Beta *written on the upper margin.*
208 grewe] gowe *MS.*   **209** helpeþ...vsed] *om. MS.*

---

188 beata] vel Beta *written by Hand C after this word, then* 13 *written by Hand E immediately after.*   **189** beatis] or bete *written by Hand C over the line.*   **197** nose-holles] Also it clensith þe hede from nyttis & oþer vermyn *written by Hand C on the outer margin.*   **204** bigula] 14 *written by Hand E after this word.*

Borago ||

16va
215
Borage is a worþi erbe after þe wordis of Macer. Þe vertu of him is that he will clense þe rede coloure. Also þis erbe y-put þe levis in wyne, who that drynkiþ þere-of hit shall make ham mery and glade. And also poyson shall not do ham harme. Also he is gode to distroye þe cardiacle and postemys that comyþ of black colour, for he is hote & drye. Also braye þe rote of borage
220 and drinke hit with ale and a litell safur, and soupe þre soppis iij tymes, first and laste, for þe jandys.

Bigula

Browne bugill som calliþ him silfe-hele and sum calliþ him hart-worte. The vertue of this erbe is þis: þat he will hele a wonde in
225 whate place so þat hit be with ony oþere helpe. Also þis erbe brekiþ and distroyeth þe rewme in a manys hede and þe leþer stopping of the hede and þe akynge, for he is hote and drye, & þere beþe twoo spicis of him. |

16vb
230
Burneta

Bornete-is leuys beþ like almoste to tansey, but þey beþ not so grete and a blewe flour like to heyhofe. Þe vertu of him is þis: that he will distroye grete humouris and laxatife with-in a man. Also þis herbe openyþ the stoppinge of a mann-ys lyvir, and he makiþ a man well to pisse. Also drinke him wiþ wyn and þat

---

214 borage] Borago *written on the upper margin.* **216** in wyne] in wyne in wyne *MS.* **221** for þe] d *deleted after this word.* **229** burneta] *written on the upper margin.* **233** lyvir] *apparently,* lever *before the emendation.*

---

214 borage] 15 *written by Hand E after the word* Borago *that Hand A had repeated on the upper margin.* **222** bigula] 16 *written by Hand E after this word.* **223** browne bugill] Thys bugyll [or selfhele *over the line*] hath leves somdel ronde & blak & haþe a blew flour sumdel softe. *written by Hand C on the outer margin.* **225** erbe] dronke *written by Hand C over the line.* **227** the hede] And heleth broke bones in hit *written by Hand C over the line.* **229** burneta] 17 *written by Hand E after this word.*

sauyþ one of þe jandis. Also þe juis of þis erbe wiþ hony 235
y-dronke vnbyndiþ þe sore vndir þe ribbis and of sore pappis,
for þere be ij specis of this erbe: one growith in þe medis,
an-oþer in harde grounde.

Birula

Bellyre is an herbe that þe levis be like to skyrwhite, and he 240
growith in waters, and he hauyþ a longe stalke. Þe vertu of þis
erbe is þis: that he is myche worthe for to ripe bylis and bochis.
He is hote and drye.

Fabaria

Brokleuys is an erbe þat þe levis beþe like well to mynte. The 245
vertue of þis erbe is þat, yf he be pouwnyd and medlid || with 17ra
schepis tallowe and made hote in water in maner of a plaster
and y-leide to eny maner of swellyng, he shall swage hit sone.
Þis herbe growith in smale brokys, and namely a-monge bellyry.

Genes[t]ula

Brome is a worþi erbe. Þe vertu of him is þis: take þe grene 250
croppe of his levis and choppe hem smale, þan take a galon of
gode stronge worte i-made of otyn malt, and boyle ham well þe
brome and þe worte till halfe oþer more be wastid. Let hit kele
and strayne hit, and yf to sponefull to him that is seke in þe 255
dropsye, first at morowe. Mylke ham and strayne hame, kepe
þat in a box for þe colde gowte. Also take þe sede of brome,
and grommyll sede, and þe ynny[r]er pithe of pichon-is geserys,

---

246 with schepis] Fabaria *written on the upper margin.* **250** genestula] Genescula *MS.* **258** ynnyrer] ynnyter *MS.*

---

239 birula] 18 *written by Hand E after this word.* **243** drye] & þer be ij spices ther of *written by Hand C over the line.* **244** fabaria] 19 *written by Hand E after this word.* **250** genestula] 20 *written by Hand E after this word.*

of euery like moche, dry þis in þe sonne, þen take centorye as myche as one of ham in pouder. Medill all þes to-gadrys and drinke hit in stale ale, first and laste, for the stone. Also drinke þe juis of | hym, and he is gode to knytte bonys and synewys to-gedir. Also take grene branchis of him and þe þirde parte of alyme i-brent, melle þis to-gadrys wiþ water, and frett with that þe teþe, and hit will make ham clene and put a-way blacknes.

Balsamum

Balme is gode and dilicius of sauour. Þe vertu of him is, stampe him and drynke hit for þe feuerys. Also drinke him wiþ wyne, and þat makiþ gode digestion and puttiþ a-way þe sore of þe bladder. Also stampe þe juis of him and oile olyfe to-gader, and þere-wiþ a-noynte þe for-hede & wasche þe hede, and þat put a-wey þe hede-ache and oþer soris þer-of. Also stampe him and drinke him, and þat lettith him þat caste myche, and helpiþ for þe yox, and hit bryngiþ oute þe laste burþen of a woman when she haþe borne childe. Also medill him with hony and oyle, and þat heliþe þe potagir that he swell noȝte. Also hit is gode but, yf þe seke be in feuerys, | drinke þe juis wiþ water oþer with wyne. Also braye him and the juis of nepe, and toun hit in a gotis horne, and yf him to drinke that haþe þe fallinge evill, for þe sauor is gode. Also seþe him and washe lymes þere-wiþ for grete travaill.

Basilica

Basilicon is an erbe that is hote in þe firste degre and in [drye] that oþere degre. He hathe dyuerse kyndis, for his levis beþe

---

262 hym and] Genestula *written on the upper margin.*   **273** þat²] to *deleted after this word.*   **277** be] *written over the line.*   drinke þe] Balsamum *written on the upper margin.*   **283** drye] *om. MS.*

---

266 balsamum] 21 *written by Hand E after this word.*   **282** basilica] 22 *written by Hand E after this word.*

like rewe and with flouris and savyr of franke-incense. That oþer haþe a blewe flour, and þe third is calliþ garifilatum. The vertues of ham is þis: ete him wiþ þe blewe flour to-for oþere metis fastyng, and he shall make a gladde hart, and put a-way quakynge and suspecion, and comfortith in defautis, and heliþ þe brannyd colour. Also he helpiþ a colde stomake, and confortith þe brayne, and makeþ one for to slepe esily. Also to swellyng and to sore eyne þe gare[f]ill helpiþe—þat is more strenger in medicyne. And he comfortith þe stomake and makeþ | him to defye all grete metis. Also he is gode for þe cardiacle and for black colour. Also for f[l]ewmatik y-put to þe nose-þrillis hit vnbyndiþ þe lowe bondis of þe brayne and confortith þe brayne. Also yf an arme swell for blode lettynge, braye him and put þer-to: hit swagiþ sone and hit helpiþ well to a-mend the siȝte of þe eyne.

Crasse is hote and drye, for hit hansith lecherye. Stampe þe sede and menge hit with bere mele: hit heliþe þe antracas þat men clepiþ þe vncomes in þe face þat men riseth wiþ quitter, and a-batith all akynge. The iuse þere-of a-batiþe þe toþe-ake yf hit be don in þe halfe side that akiþe. Þe juis of carse holdith her that will away. Drinke þe sede þere-of and hit castiþ þe dede childe from his modir wombe, and hit is gode for venym. Þe smell þere-of makeþ naddres fle. Drinke the juis with aysell: hit helpiþ the splene. Take þe sede and aysell and baryes gres y-made a plaster helpiþ for þe evill in þe þiesse. || Crasse and gose gres y-mengid woll sle þe mytis and the tikys in þe hede.

---

290 þe] barm *deleted after this word.*   **292** garefill] garesill *MS.*
295 flewmatik] fewmatik *MS.*   **309** crasse] Crasse *written on the upper margin.*

---

300 crasse] Nasturcium *written by Hand C over the line, then* 23 *written by Hand E immediately after.*   **308** baryes] w *written by Hand B over* ry.

Þe levis i-stampid and sodyn wiþ gotis mylke and vsid rennith þe brest and sowbliþ and abatiþ the cough.

Costmaryn his leuys ben namely hote [and drye]. Who-so etith ham hit makiþ him well to defye his mete and to make vryn, & helpiþ to þe eyne, and a-batiþ the cogh. Stampe hem with hony: hit clensiþ þe body fro þe spotis and þe frantykles. The rote sodyn and stampid will draw oute brokyn bonys yf hit be laide þere-to. The sede ther-of sodyn in wyne will hele venum bat. Hit and oxis gall mengid to-gedir helpiþe þe morfue and a-noynte the bakke þere-with: hit shall sesse evill strokys. Hit is gode in sause. Who-so etith hit ofte hit hansiþe lecherye.

Celedony: þis maisteris saiþe that þere ben two maneres of hem, þe more and þe lasse, and boþe ben gode to þe eyne. Plenius saiþe þat | the swalowis byrd may nought se till þe modir brynge of that erbe and tuche hir eyne þere-wiþe, and þen þei takiþ þere sight, and þere-for þe swalowe is callid [yn] grewe "celedonie" þere-of þat erbe he hase his name. Þe juis of þe flour and hony y-sode to-gedir in a clene brasse pane well skemmyd till hit be þick no oynement so gode for þe eyne, yf þei be oftyn a-noynted þere-wiþ. Þe rote of hit temperid with wyne oiþer wiþ aisell i-vsed helpiþ for þe jandis and toþe-ache, & þat will sle þe worme in þe toþe if þe rote be done in þe mouþe be-twene þe toþe. Þe levis þere-of stampe ham in wyne, in maner of a plastre: hit doþe a-way þe blacke spottis of the body.

---

313 and drye] *om. MS.*   **316** rote] sta*m deleted after this word.*   **324** þat] þere ben two maneres of hem *deleted after this word.*   **326** yn] þr *MS.*

---

313 costmaryn] 24 *written by Hand E in the gap between entries.*   **322** celedony] 25 *written by Hand E in the gap between entries.*   **332** toþe] no*ta written by Hand B on the outer margin.*

Lelamour Herbal

Centory is ij man*er*, the more and þe lasse and, for þe more is 335
not well knowen, we takyn þe lasse, whiche is drye. Yf hit be
stampid hit makeþ wondis to go to-gedir that haþe ben evill
helid, yf þu lay hi*m* ther-to. The ‖ watir that hit is sodyn inne 18va
sessiþe akyng of þe senowys. Þe juis þ*ere*-of drinkyn in wyne
oþ*er* ale spurgiþ the floures and castiþ oute abortyve, and þe juis 340
in wyne castid all [dotovs] medicynes þrowe þe wombe. In
hervyste gadryt and make of pouder i-drowid ayene þe sonne,
and that vsid stryeth all venyme.

Colombyne ys hote and drye on þe þerde degre. Þ*er* ben two
man*er*, white and blewe, *in* flowres and o man*er* in levis; boþe 345
ar gode. Þe juis y-dronkyn w*ith* wat*er* castiþ oute abortyue an[d]
a-batith þe cogh, and helpiþ all evill brusi*n*g. Vse hit wiþ aysell,
hit dryeth þe splene. Drinke hit wiþ wyne, hit clansiþ þe flour*is*,
and hit helpiþ at þe begynyng for þe dropsye. He is gode to hele
wou*n*dis. Take þe juis and a litell hony, and that is gode to 350
a-noynte sore eyne. Stampe hit wiþ oyle and anoynte þe body
þ*ere*-wiþ and hit shall put a-way coldnes and sett the in gode
hete and gode temper. |

Coriandrum 18vb
Coryandyr is of colde nature. Galien seiþ: "take coryandyr and 355
drynk hit & he sleythe þe wormys in þe wombe." Take hi*m* and

341 dotovs] to do vs *MS*.   346 and] an *MS*.   354 coriandrum] *written on the upper margin.*

---

335 centory] 26 *written by Hand E in the gap between entries* ‖ The mor [by som boke *over the line*] is cleped erthegall & is leke to the lesse [but *written over the line, then deleted*] it haþe a yelow flo*ur* and it dronk w*ith* white wyn helpeth moch in eu*er*y desease *written by Hand C on the outer margin.*
344 colombyne] 27 *written by Hand E in the gap between entries.*
345 maner¹] This herbe is good for the qvincie. *written by Hand C on the outer margin.*   354 coriandrum] 28 *written by Hand E after this word.*

rosyne, aysell and hony to-ged*er*: hit swagiþ all swellynge and namely of þe balokk*is*. Drynke þe sede in water: hit stanchiþ the wombe that rennyth oute. Take þe cro*m*mes of white brede and þe juis þ*ere*-of hit a-batith all man*er* of akynge yf hit be laide þ*ere*-to. Take the sede of hym to drynke that haþe þe feu*er* cotidian*e*, and yf he drinke hit or þe feu*er* come hit helppith hi*m*. Autours saiþe that so many daies shall woman flouris stonde as she etiþ cornys of coryandry.

Camamilla

Camamyll is of iij man*er*s, an[d] all haþe v*er*tue. Þe levis ben dry and wete in þe firste degre. Drinke hit in wyne: hit makiþ vryn and brekiþe the stone in þe bladder, and spurgiþ þe floure of a woman*e* in hir mater yf she be weshyn || ther-wiþe. Seþe hit and drinke hit w*ith* wyne: hit a-batith hurlyng in the stomake and þe swellyng. Þe juis and hony to-gedir doþe a-way þe schalis of þe adeleth. Þe decoccio*un* þ*ere*-of helpiþ for þe jandis. And þe veccys in ma*n*nys sid*is* þ*at* is calliþ ypocandria hit goþe a-way wiþ þe oyneme*nt* and hit be dronke wiþ wyne. Plenius saiþe of xl daies take eu*er*y day v peny-wight of camamyll and xl peny-wixte of white wyne and drinke hit, and hit clensiþ þe splene of all man*er* evilles. Yf þ*u* ete hi*m* he helpiþ all evill bleynes in þe white of the eye that is callid egill pace in grewe. Make a plaster of hi*m* and hit clensiþ wondis. And that plaster is gode also for þe hede-ake yf þe hede be washe þ*ere*-wiþ þ*at* watir that camamyll was soden inne.

---

366 and] an *MS*.

365 camamilla] 29 *written by Hand E after this word.* **367** wete] hote *emended by Hand C.* **368** bladder] brekyth þe yelow jandes *written by Hand C over the line.* **379** wondis] & it is good for bityng of an adder or oþer venemos þyng *written by Hand C over the line.*

Calament

Calamynte ys an herbe þat | is of stronge sauoure, and þere bethe iij speces of þis erbe: þat one is stony, þat oþer is hery, and þe þride watrye, and al þay as Ypocras seiþe þat þay distroy a manys talent, and all beþ hote and dry in þe þirde degre. Þe vertu of him is: drinke þe juis wiþ hote mylke and þat will make all þe body to swete. Also seþe him in oyle and þere-wiþ anoynte a man that haþe þe feuerys. Also brayd grene: that brennyth þe skyn and dryuyth a-wey all leþer humourys and þe sore, and þe menstrue hit helith y-ete oþere y-dronke and clensiþ ham. Also þe lepir þat mon calliþ elefancia, þat is þe worste lepir, at þe begynyng drinke þe juis wiþ wyne: hit shall hele and distroy the humourys. Also stampe hit and lay hit to an nadder stynggynge and hit will hele hit. And yf one drinke þe juis wiþ wyne, þat heliþ all venym and scleith wormes in the wombe and || heliþ the evill of þe geser & an olde evill of þe sides. Also stampe hit and lay hit to black wondys: hit doþe a-way all þe blacknesse and bryngiþ hit to his gode colour, but myche bettir yf þe erbe be sodde in wyne and layde þer-to as a plaster. Also y-dronke wiþ wyne that confortiþ þe stomake and lettiþ yoxing and stopith þe appetide of lecherye. Also stampe him and þe sauor of him shall make naddris and venym wormes fle fro that house. Also drinke þe juis of þis erbe and of mogwort iij dayes, and that heliþe þe wondis wiþe-oute doute.

Caruium

Carwey is a gentill erbe, for comyn lesiþ his streynthe while þat carwey is þere-by, for þis erbe is hote and drye. Þe vertu of him

---

383 is of] Calamentum *written on the upper margin.* **402** yoxing] yoying *before emendation.*

---

382 calament] 30 *written by Hand E after this word.* **392** calliþ] lepire wenem wormes in þe wombe & woundes *written by Hand B on the outer margin.* **406** caruium] 31 *written by Hand E after this word.*

is þis: stampe him and drinke him with stale ale and þat distroieþ wekyd wyndis of one-is bowellys. Also that drynke put|tiþ a-way the cough and heliþ men þat ben take wiþ frenesy oþer i-bitt with venym wormes oþer bestis. Also þis erbe i-medlid with vynegre heliþ scabbis and makeþ here to growe that goþe a-way yf hit be a-noynted ther-with. Also yf he be dronke he heliþe þe menstrue and swelling of þe flaunke and he causiþ digestioun y-ete oþer i-dronke he sleyth wormes in þe bowelis. Also hit will hele castinge that comyþ oute from flewme. Also hit will hele þe wynde of þe wombe and sore kyrnyng that comith þere-of. Also he makiþ moiste þe stomake and he makiþ one to pisse. Also yf he be ete he stroyeth scabbis and clawynge.

Caulus domesticus

Caule is a comyn erbe. Þe vertu of þe erbe is that he will hele all freshe wondys and olde wondis. Also washe him in water and stampe him rawe wiþ wyne and hit doþ a-way þe cankyr, but washe || þe sore fyrste with hote wyne. Also take barly mele and þe juis of caule, rewe and coryandyr; mell þis well to-geder i-stampid, and hit helpith for the potagir. Also hit helpiþ for sore tone þat ben sore þrow clawynge. Also y-leide to [in] a plaster-wyse hit swagith swellynge. Also þe vryn of him þat vsiþ caule ys a nobill þinge to ham that havyth synowis y-dryd to washe ham hote þere-wyth, and childryn ben washen in suche vryn hit shall kepe ham in gode hele. Also who that vsiþe grene caule hit shall kepe his sight fro derknes. Also hit norshith mylke to norysys. Also þe mete ther-of clensiþe menstrue and castiþ oute dede childe of þe wombe, and hit is a grete comford to þe stomake. And yf hit be myche soden, þat stopiþ þe wombe, and

---

425 þe sore] Caulus domesticus *written on the upper margin.* **428** in] *om. MS.* **431** þere-wyth] þere water *before emendation.*

421 caulus domesticus] 32 *written by Hand E after this word.*

yf hit be litell soden & grene, that neschith þe wombe and makiþ laxatife. Also alym, vynegir and caule y-brought in-to one, medlid and stampe þat to-geder, and þat helpiþe | gretly a-yayne þe lepir. And wiþ þe same medicyne þu myght helpe ham þat har hare falleþ a-waye. Also hit helpiþ a-yayne swellynge and namely of man or of woman-is priuete, and myche þe bettir and she seþe hit wiþ benys. Also in plaster-wise of caule, fenecrek and vynegir that helpyn to al sorys of synewys and to þe potagir. Also bren stalkys of caule and þe askys medlid with olde grese þat heliþ all olde sekenesse of þe rynis and of the sidis. Also medill þe sede with vynegre, drink þat and hit will caste wormys oute of his wombe. Also bren þe rotis of drye caule in-to pouder and vndir-pitt hitt heliþe þe evill of þe strechillis. Also caste þe juis of caule in a manys nosse-þrellis: that castiþ oute flewme of þe hede. Also who-so will chewe and swellow hit a-downe that helpiþ for þe voce & narthe of þe brest. Also ete of þe pithe of þe stalkys and hit kepiþ one ‖ from dronknesse. Also take vp þe rote and let hit tuche no grownde, honge sum of him a-boute his nek that haþe þe strechillis, and hit saviþ him.

Ci[clami]num

[E]arthnote, that is an erbe that haþe levis like to fenell and wiþ flouris and smale stalkys. He growiþ in wodis, also in medis. The vertu of this erbe is þis: that and he be stampid & laid to a sore he will feche a-wey all dede fleshe and helpiþe renewe the quyck fleshe. Also stampe this erbe and put him to þat place þat lackiþ here: he shall restore hit a-gayne with-in schorte tyme of plaster layeng.

---

457 ciclaminum] cidanum *MS*. **458** earthnote] carthnote *MS*.

457 ciclaminum] 33 *written by Hand E after this word.*

Cardiaca

465 Cardiake is an erbe þat sum men calliþ cilsper. Þis erbe haþe levis somdell like to blynde-nettill and he will prikk sumdele vpon þe tonge, and he berythe litell sedis in smale coddis. The vertu of þis erbe is þis: that he is gode to grene sause. Also for to ete him or drinke | him for þe fallyng evill.

Herba cruciaca

Croswort is an erbe that beryth litell levis, somdell like to cokkyll, and a smale stalke, and he beryth a white floure y-like to a crosse and o branche haviþ many white flouris. And he is gode to hele woundis boþe olde and newe.

Cummin

Comyn ys an erbe of stronge sauor. Þe lyvis of him ben like to coryandyr and he haþe many branches comyn oute of a stok. Þe vertu of him is: take in metis oþer to drinke þe sede and þat will defye a-way all liþer wyndis oute of þe stomake and of þe bowellis. Also he makeþ gode digestioun. Also hit makiþ one to pisse and makiþ one well colourde. Also yf one ete hit or drinke hit, that stopiþe the flux and hit lettiþe lecherye, but hit is gode to hele venyme bytyng. Þis erbe is hote || and dry. Also take an handfull of þe sede and stampe hit to pouder, seþe þat in gode wyne fro a potell till a quarte let on, drinke ther-of als hote as he maye boþe, at morowe first and laste at evyn, and that is souerayne for him þat haþe stynking brethe.

---

467 prikk] þrikk *before emendation.* **483** that] sr *deleted after this word.*
484 and dry] Cumine *written on the upper margin.*

---

465 cardiaca] 34 *written by Hand E after this word.* **471** herba cruciaca] 35 *written by Hand E after this word.* **476** cummin] 36 *written by Hand E after this word.*

Consolida maior

Confery ys an erbe þat beriþ grete levis brode and longe. Þe vertu of him is þis: yf a man be brusid oþer broke with-inforþe take þe rote of þis erbe and ro[s]te him well amonge hote askys, and take that to þe seke wiþ hony and let him ete hit all fastyng, and he shall be hole. Also drinke þe juis of him and that heliþ brokyn bonys. Also yf a vayne be broke in a bodyes nose, stampe comfery and yf him þe juis to drinke in stale ale, and þe blode schall stanche. Þis erbe is hote and moiste.

Herba Petri

Cowslope is an erbe that his blossum is well like to prymrose, but þer growiþ on one stalke | many to-gedris, and this herbe is hote and drye in the þirde de-gre. The moste strenþe of him is in þe se[d]e and in þe rote. The vertu of him is þis: that he is gode for þe stomake þat swelliþ and makiþ gode digestioun. Also he helpiþ all sekenes that is wiþ-in the body, þe juis y-dronke. Also that drinke makiþ one to pisse and clensithe menstrue, that is womanys flouris. Also drinke him with wyne and that heliþ all maner of venym bitynge, oþer y-braied and laide þer-to. Also þe sede is gode for all maner lectuaryis to make digestioun, but he is not vertuus to a shelowe body in sauour ne in drinke.

Pes columbe

Coluyr-fote is an herbe, his levis beþ like to maworte, but þe levi[s] beþ more white and his flour is like to maworte, but þe stalke is not so rede ne so tendir. The vertu of him is þis: stampe

---

502 sede] seþe *MS*.   **512** levis] levill *MS*.

---

489 consolida maior] 37 *written by Hand E after this word.*   **498** herba Petri] 38 *written by Hand E after this word.*   **510** pes columbe] 39 *written by Hand E after this word.*   **512** levis] *The letters* ll *of the original MS reading were deleted and* s *written by Hand C over the line.*

him and a-noynte watery eyne w*ith* þe juis ofte-tymes and he
sesith hit. This is drye and hote. ||

21va

Persicaria

Cvlrage is an herbe that su*m* men calliþ arsmeche. Þis erbe
haviþ levis y-like to wythe levis, and þe*r*e be two spic*is* þe*r*e-of.
The ve*r*tu of þis erbe is þis: þ*at* þe watir of þis erbe istillid is
gode for the goute.

Consolida mi*nor*

Daysye is an herbe that su*m* men calleþ hi*m* brisewort oþ*er*
bon-worte. Þe ve*r*tu of þis erbe is þis: stampe hi*m* and lay hi*m*
to a boche and he will breke hi*m*. Also who that haviþ any
bonys broke, stampe þis erbe and drinke þe juis and vse hit,
and hit shall knyt ham faire, & þ*at* drinke is gode for to sese
aky*n*g and swellynge. Also yf one be brusid wiþ-in-forþe w*ith*
horting, late make potage of þis erbe & of conferye wiþ porke,
and late hi*m* vse that potage, and he shall fare well. This erbe
is a spece of confery.

Daucus asinin*us*

21vb Dauke is an erbe þ*at* su*m* men calliþ birdis-neste. This | erbe
haviþ levis y-like to he*m*loke, and he berrith a white flour. Þis
erbe is hote and drye. The ve*r*tu of this erbe is þis: he is gode to
hele þe dropesye and all venym bitinge of wormes and bestis,

516 persicaria] *written on the upper margin.*

---

514 eyne] or wassh the forehed *written by Hand C over the line.*
516 persicaria] 40 *written by Hand E after this word.*   **519** vertu] goute *written by Hand B on the outer margin.*   **521** consolida minor] 41 *written by Hand E after this word.*   **524** breke him] breke a boche for to seche akynge *written by Hand B on the outer margin.*   **531** daucus asininus] 42 *written by Hand E after this word.*   **533** flour] leke a birde nest *written by Hand C over the line.*

and hit be stampid and y-dronke. Also þe same drinke vnbyndiþ
the stopping of þe lyuer and þe mylte and also þe wombe.

Dragancia femina

Dragancia femall is an erbe þat beryth levis like to all-moste
ivy, but þes levys haviþ white blottis apon ham, and he berith a   540
yelowe flour and a stalke of two cubitis in leynthe in þe maner
of a crokid stafe i-like to a snake, and he beriþ his sede a-boue
like to a cluster of grapis, and when þe seide is ripe hit is
yelowe. The vertue of him is þis: powne the sede and medill hit
wiþ oille and put þat in one-is heryn & that helpiþ for evill   545
herynge. Also þe juis of þis erbe with a litell wolle y-put in-to
one‖-is nostrillis clensith the nosse of all filthe. Also stampe þe   22ra
rote of þis erbe and þe rote of þe white wyne and hony to-gader
and that is gode to hele cancre and woundis. Also who-so
a-noynte his honde with þe juis of þe rote of this erbe, he may   550
take naddres with-oute perell. Also take þe juis of þis erbe and
a-noyn[t]e a manys eyne, and þat puttiþ a-way derknes of ham.
Also who-so drinkiþ þe juis wiþ wyne that stireth a man to
lechery. Þis erbe growiþ in moiste placis and in drye.

Dens leonis   555

Dent de lyon is an erbe þat the levis beþe like to a lyonnis tothe,
and he brokyn þe stalke will drope mylke. The vertu of hym is
þis: stampe and drynke þe juis in clere ale and he is gode to hele
þe cotidiane feuer. Þis erbe growiþ in many placis.

---

552 a-noynte] a-noyne *MS.*

537 wombe] maky[n]g lax. hit is hote & drie. *written by Hand C after this word.*   **538** dragancia femina] 43 *written by Hand E after this word.*
547 one-is] Drogance [or dragans *over the line*] with adder-wort in juse dronke driveth a-way venym & akyng of þe erys distroyeth þe goute and [it *over the line*] sleeth a canker and hit is hote & drie. *written by Hand C on the lower margin.*   **555** dens leonis] 44 *written by Hand E after this word.*

Lappa

560 Dokkys ben in iij kyndis and all hauyth vertue | in medicyne, and þei ben hote for to vse hamme. Þey confortiþ þe stomake and castiþ oute evill wyndis. Etyn ham colde hit stroiþe the wombe. Soden water and washe the in: hit helpiþ þe rewme and
565 þe scabbe that brekiþ on þe body. Sethe hit in wyne and stampe hit: that brekiþ bilis and swagiþ brenyngis, and þat wyne is gode for þe hede and þe tothe-ake iff hit be ofte dronkyng. Hit helpiþ for þe menysoun and for the flankys. Hit doþe a-way akynge of þe erys yf þe juise be done ther-in. Dokk rote soden
570 in wyn oþer in aysell and stampe, hit helpiþe for þe swellinge splene. Seþe hit in wyne oþer in water and vse: hit castiþ oute þe flours of a woman and castiþ oute þe stone with-oute faile.

Diptanum

Ditander is dry of nature. Stampe him wiþ oyle and rosyn and
575 a-noynte þe seke mannys hede þer-with, and hit will a-bate the hede akynge. Þe oþer of þe levis makiþ ‖ venym humers to fle and doþe a-way glete a-boute the herte.

---

562 confortiþ] for þe skabbe & brekiþ bilis & toþe ake and þe swelling splene and þe stone with-oute faill *written on outer margin.*   567 gode for] for glat a-bote þe hert and þe hede-ake *written on outer margin and then deleted.*   574 stampe] for glate aboute aboute þe herte and þe hede-ake *written on outer margin.*

---

560 lappa] *id est.* the Clote *written by Hand C after this word, then* 55 *written by Hand E immediately after.*   561 dokkys] *id est.* þe Clotes *written by Hand C over the line.*   568 helpiþ] Lappa *id est.* the clote haþe brode leves & þyk & a hygh toppe roghe grete sede & clevyng to clothes & scharp with a gret eyre and þe juse þer-of dronke with stale ale is good for axes. *written by Hand C on the outer margin.*   573 diptanum] 46 *written by Hand E after this word.*   574 ditander] vel ditanie *written by Hand C over the line.*   nature] & hote *written by Hand C over the line.*   576 venym] ditanie stamped & leyd plaster-wyse draweth out iron or thorn in eny part of mannes bodie and þe juis dronke deliuereth a woman of hir dede child in her. *written by Hand C on the outer margin.*

S[o]latrum

Doworte ys an erbe that su*m* men calleþ dowechs oþ*er* lesior oþ*er* more morell. Þis erbe haviþ leuys y-like to hou*n*d-bery but þai beþ more, and þes haþe a more bustous flour and a longe stalke full of branchis, and hit berith grete bayes, gret*er* þen hou*n*d-bery. The ve*r*tu of this erbe is þis: yf a man ete þ*ere*-of hit will make hi*m* well to speke. Þ*is* growiþ in garthines and in wodis.

580

585

Ele*n*acampana

Elenaca*m*pana ys an erbe þ*at* som men calleþ horshele. He beryth grene levis and longe stalkys, and berith yelowe flou*r*es. The ve*r*tu of hi*m* is þis: yf a man haþe a wawing toþe þ*at* is not faste in þe go*m*mes, ete of þis rote and hit will faste h*a*m. Also yf one drinke þe juis of hi*m*, that is holsome for þe ston | and helpiþ one to pisse. Also that drinke will delyu*er* a woma*n* of dede childe. Also yf one be laxatife þis erbe will make one harde þe wombe. Also he is gode for þe cogh. Also hit a-batiþ þe tysain, þ*at* is þe evill of þe hede. Also seþ in wyne þe rote and vse: þ*at* doþe gode to all newe-ffratikys, þ*at* is þe evill of þe reynes. Also make pouder of þe rote and medill þ*at* w*ith* hony: þ*at* helpiþ the cough & hit heliþ longis. Also þe juis of hi*m* and of rwe helpiþ h*a*m that beþ broke-vylmyd. Also take of þe levis of hi*m* and levis of þe rede dokk, bugill and waybrede, of eu*ery* i-liche myche, stampe and frye ham w*ith* May buttyr and a litell alym þ*ere*-wiþ, strawe hit and put hit i*n* a box: þis is sou*er*ayne

590

22vb

595

600

---

578 solatrum] Salatrum *MS*.   **589** the vertu] for wauing teþe þe stone and wome*n* of dede childe *written on outer margin*.

---

578 solatrum] 47 *written by Hand E after this word*.   **584** þ*ere*-of] To make men to speke well *written by Hand F on the outer margin*.   **587** ys] 48 *written by Hand E after this word*.   ys] hote & drie moyst *written by Hand C over the line*.   **590** þis rote] and it is good for þe govte *written by Hand C on the outer margin*.

for scabbis. Also wat*er* y-stillid of þes tendir leuys rowmyth þe brest and doþe a-waye þe narthe.

Endiuia

605
23ra Endyue ys an erbe that ‖ som men calliþ horse-þistill. Þ*is* erbe haþe prykkys with-oute. Þe lefe ar longe, and when he is brokyn he dropiþ mylke, and he haþe a litell yelow flo*ur*, and his sede blawiþ a-waye w*ith* þe wynde as doþe dent de lyon. The ve*r*tu of
610 hi*m* is þis: take þe juis þ*er*e-of and medill hit w*ith* hote wat*er* and drynke hit, and þ*at* heliþ þe stoppinge of þe mylte and þe lyu*er*. Also þis erbe is gode y-dronke for þe jau*n*dys and for þe feu*er* tercian and for þe hote postem. Also þis erbe a-swagith þe grete hete of þe lyu*er* and of þe stom*a*ke, for he is colde & moiste.

Eufrasia

615
Eufrase is an erbe that growiþ in medis and be faire grene wayes, and he berith a litell white flour and smale endi[n]td leuys. The ve*r*tu of þis erbe is þis: who that eu*er* drinke þe juis of hi*m* wiþ clere ale, þ*at* is gode and p*ro*fitable for all sore
23rb eyne, | and þe water stillid for þ*e* same is gode.

Herba C*hris*toferi

Erbe C*hris*tofyr male ys an erbe that hauyþe leuys to crowesope þe lasse, but þei beþ more white and nought fullich so longe. He growiþ in dry grou*n*dis and in watri placis. Þe ve*r*tu of þis erbe

---

606 som men] Endiuia *written on the upper margin.* þis erbe] þ*is* erbe þis erbe *MS.* **615** eufrasia] eufracia *before emendation.* **617** endintd] enditd *MS,* endite *before emendation.* **618** vertu of] for sor*e* eyne *written on inner margin.* **623** fullich] for evill eire *written on outer margin.*

---

605 endiuia] 49 *written by Hand E after this word.* **615** eufrasia] 50 *written by Hand E after this word.* **621** herba Christoferi] 51 *written by Hand E after this word.*

is þis: that he is gode i-dronke for evill eire of the pestilence and   625
for frenesy. Also take þe rote of him and pigill and stampe hem
to-gedir and drinke þe juis wiþ clere ale, & that heliþ þe stiche
by a gode fire.

Herba Waltery

Erbe Waltir is an erbe þat hauyþ leuys like to persily [b]ote þei   630
beþ litell leuys, and þey beþ faire grene a-bove and vndir þe
leuys þay seme as bryght as siluer, and in Februare he is vp and
in June he goþe his waye. The vertu of him is þis: þat he is a
gode clenser and helere of wondis. ||

Herba Roberti   23va

Erbe Robert hauyth leuys like herbe benet, þe stalke rede,
comunly with a litell rede flour hauyng a stronge sauour as aftir
þe chafynge of a fox. The vertu: he is a gode heler of wondis.
His pouder sleys þe cancre and growiþ in dichis.

Herba benedicta   640

Erbe benet is like hemloke. Þe vertu of him is that he kepis
mayden pappis for grete wexing. The juis of þis erbe with
spume of siluer, with swynys grece a-swagiþe the hote potager
and all maner of hote evillis. And hit is colde and drye.

---

625 gode] for þe stiche *written on outer margin.*   **630** bote] hote *MS.*
631 and þey] To clere and to hele wondis *written on outer margin.*   **635** herba
Roberti] *written on the upper margin.*   **637** hauyng] A gode herbe for
woundis and sleis þe cancre *written on the outer margin.*   **641** þe vertu] To
kepe mayden pappis smale *written on the outer margin.*

---

626 also] for þe pestelens *written by Hand F on the outer margin.*   **627** &
that] for þe stychy *written by Hand F on the outer margin.*   **629** herba
Waltery] 52 *written by Hand E after this word.*   **635** herba Roberti] 53 *written
by Hand E after this word.*   **640** herba benedicta] 54 *written by Hand E after
this word.*   **644** drye] and þe juse þer-of dronke destroyeth lecherie *written by
Hand C after this word.*

645

Fuga demonum

Erbe Joha*n*n ha*þ*e leuys like to lasse centorye, and su*m* call hit þe more centuary. And he ha*þ*e yelowe flouris and a longe stalke oute of þe whiche com many stalkys. The ve*r*tu of hi*m* is that þe breth and the odyr of hi*m* stampe hit dryvi*þ* wickyd | venym fro that place. Also gad*er* this erbe in-to [þe] house in þe vigill of Saynt Joha*n*n Bapt*ista* or þe son aryse, and stik *þat* erbe in þe corners of þe house sayng þis word*is*: "in no*min*e p*at*ris *etc*.", makynge a crosse w*ith* þe erbe, and in so*þ*e hit will soffyr none evill spiret ne wekid goste to a-bide in that house.

23vb
650

655

H*erba* Plenius

Erbe moyntayne is an erbe riseth vp apon a stalke oute of þe rote and berith his lefe vpon þe toppe of þ*e* stalke and *þat* is passyng þick lefe and large and brode and slyt in v partes, but comenly þe levis lodde*þ* to-ged*er* and in Jule he is gon*n*e. Þe ve*r*tu of hi*m* is þis: iff a beste haue a sekenes callyd þe montayne euyll stampe this erbe and yf the juis to hi*m* for to drinke.

660

Filex campestris

Ferne is an erbe that is comovn to knowe, for he ‖ growis in all placis. But ye shall vndirstond that þ*ere* beþ iij spec*is* of this erbe. One that is callid polypody, and he growi*þ* bi oke treise. That is the firste spice for *þat* erbe is gode to make a man

24va

665

---

649 and the] and the and the *MS*. hit] and drinke hit *deleted after this word*. wickyd] wormes *deleted after this word*. **650** þe¹] & *MS*.

---

645 fuga demonum] vel H*er*ba Joha*nn*s *written by Hand C after this word, then* 55 *written by Hand E in the gap between the Latin heading and the ME text*. **647** he haþe] none evyll spiret ne wekid gost *written by Hand B on the outer margin*. **655** herba Plenius] 56 *written by Hand E after this word*. **662** filex campestris] 57 *written by Hand E after this word*. **663** for he] polypodi one off the sayd fernes good to make a man laxatyve *written by Hand F on the lower margin*.

laxatife. And that oþer ferne is calliþ osmou*n*de, and he growiþ
in dichis and in grippis. Þ*at* is þe seconde spece, for he is gode
to hele wondys and brokyn bonys. The þerde is callid
euere-verre[n]e, and he growiþ apon wallis. His v*er*tu is to hele 670
þe potager and strenth the synowys.

Filipendula

Filipendula, oþ*er*-weys callid dropwort, is like to mylfoly but
his leuys beþ more large. And he growiþ by þe grownde as doþe
mylfoly and he haþe a smale stalke and a flo*ur* somdell white. 675
The v*er*tu is: stampe þe juis and drinke h*it* w*ith* wlake wyne
oþ*er* al[e], and that will distroye wekid wyndis a-bote a manys
lyu*er* & his mylte. Also hit is a nobill | drynke for the stone. Þis 24rb
erbe is hote and drye.

Fum*us* terr*e* 680

Fvmyter ys an erbe that som men calleþ wilde rewe, for his
leuys be ney goynge to rewe. His flo*ur* is purpur*e* colour. Þe
v*er*tu of hi*m* is this: drinke hi*m* in wyne oþ*er* in ale eu*er*y day,
fro þe first thorsday in maye in-to þe ende of þe same moneth,
and that makiþ one haue a gode stom*a*ke and comfortith þe 685
herte. Also hit opynyth stoppinge of þe lyu*er* and puttiþ a-way
all evill humouris of a body w*ith*-in and w*ith*-oute. Also hit
distroieth þe swellynge of þe hede and hit norshith þe brayne.
Also hit is a nobill medsyne to put a-way the lepir and clense þe
blode and hit doþe a-way iching and skabbis. Also hit makyth 690

---

670 euere-verrene] Euere-verrewe *MS*. **677** ale] ald *MS*.

---

672 filipendula¹] 58 *written by Hand E after this word.* **678** þis erbe] for wyckyd wynd*is* & for þe stone *written by Hand F on the outer margin.* **680** fumus terre] 59 *written by Hand E after this word.* **688** distroieth] lepir*e written by Hand B on the outer margin.* **689** put] blode *written by Hand B on the outer margin.* **690** iching] iching *written by Hand B on the outer margin.*

one to pisse and brekiþe the stone in þe bladder, and yevith a mane gode appetide to his mete.

Feniculum ||

Finell is hote and drye in oþer de-gre. Drinke hit and hit sleith venym and inhansith lechery. The juis with hony clensith þe eyne. Þe juis do on the ere or in the ere sleyth þe wormes. Þe rote soden in tysain laid to þe eryn helpith. Drinke hit wiþ hony: hit castiþ a-way swellynge of þe dropsye, and helpiþ for the attributis and for þe longone & the gisser. Þe juis dronkyn makyth þe noryse haue mylke [yn] hir pappis. Drinke the juise wiþ wyne: hit helpith the bladder that is callid newffratik, and clensith þe vryne and lowsithe flouris in a woman. Stampe him and bynde hit to þe stomake in maner of a plaster: that a-batiþ castynge. Drynke hit with water: hit relowsith brennyng of þe stomake. Seþe hit in wyn: hit releuyth akynge of þe pyntill. Hit and oyle and aysell to-geder swagith all maner of swellinge for drinke, and who-so vsiþe hit myche hit makith | hym seme yongliche.

Sacrefolium

Full in englishe tonge, yn romayne jubarbe. Yf þe flewme smyȝth þe ere or the eyne with gounde, take þe juis and a-noynte þe eyne and hit makiþ relesse.

694 finell] Feniculum *written on the upper margin.* sleith] veym *deleted after this word.* **697** in] on *before emendation.* **700** yn] þn *MS.*

---

694 finell] 60 *written by Hand E after the word* Feniculum *that Hand A had repeated on the upper margin.* **696** juis do] venym *written by Hand B on the outer margin.* soden in] wormes *written by Hand B on the outer margin.* **698** þe dropsye] dropsye *written by Hand B on the outer margin.* **699** the gisser] mylke *written by Hand B on the outer margin.* **701** the bladder] bladder *written by Hand B on the outer margin.* **703** castynge] castynge *written by Hand B on the outer margin.* **704** of...stomake] stomake *written by Hand B on the outer margin.* **708** sacrefolium] 61 *written by Hand E after this word.*

Febrefuga

Fethirfoy is an erbe that som men calliþ hersgall. Hit haviþ many branchis comyn oute of on rote and white flouris, and þis erbe is bittir. Þe vertu of him is þat he conford a manys stomake. Also yf he be dronke he will a-swage the feuer cotidian and þe crampe and a colde stomake. Also bray him and ley him to þe sore bityng of eny venym worme and hit heliþ him. Also this erbe y-tempryd wiþ vynegir doþe a-waye þe mvrfue. Also stampe him and lay that to wondys in þe whiche yf þere be bonys i-brokyn: that shall brynge || oute the bonys and faire hele the woundis. This erbe is hote and drye.

Iris

Flour delice ys an erbe that is lyke leuyr, but this erbe beryth a blewe purpure colour and the levir beryth a yelowe flour. The vertu of this erbe is this that he is gode to hele akynge of the synowys and also he distroieth þe cogh. Also drinke þe juis wiþe wyne and that will put a-way þe wekyd humourys of onys breste. Also that helith bityng of venym wormes and bestis. Also that drinke distroyeth the crampe. And yf a woman haue a dede childe wiþ-in hir let hir drinke of the juis of this leuys in wlake wyne and she shall be delyuerde. All þis for-saide vertues haþe this erbe. Saue ma[y] done as well as hit, but floure delise is a souerayne worcher fo[r] the dropsy as þis: kyt the rote dounwarde and he shall de||lyuer be-nethe, and yf one

---

714 branchis] þe sto⟨make⟩ þe feuer cotidian þe crampe þe colde stomake þe morfue *written on the inner margin.*   721 brynge] oute þe bonys *written on the lower margin.*   oute] Febrefuga *written on the upper margin.*   724 is] is is *MS.*   733 may] many *MS.*   734 for] fo *MS.*

712 febrefuga] 62 *written by Hand E after this word.*   723 iris] 63 *written by Hand E after this word.*   734 for] r *written, probably by Hand F, over the line.*   735 delyuer] akynge *written by Hand B on the upper margin.*

kytt hym vpwarde he shall caste vpwarde, and that is a sore labo*ur*, ther-for when he is kytt downwarde stampe the rote and fill an egge-schill full of the juis and yf that to hi*m* that is in the dropesy, and hit will make hi*m* to rene oute all clene.

Linu*m*

740 Flax or lyne is an erbe of this ve*r*tu: that þe sede þ*er*-of medlyd wiþ schepis talowe is a souerayne medicyne to make of a laxatife, yf hit be sodyn in water to-ged*er* and dronke. Also oyle made of the sede called paynter oyll is gode to a-noynte for fire
745 brenynge. The ve*r*tu of dodyr, þ*a*t growiþ a-monge flax, is to spourge a man of the color*e*. Also a gode quantyte of hit medlid w*ith* myr*e* and oyle olyue in a plaster is gode for the reynes and the brest and dyu*er*[se] akyn*g* of þe ly*m*mes that hit is laide.

Fenigre[c]u*m*

750 Fenygreke is drye in the firste degree and hote in the seconde. ‖
25va The ve*r*tu: put to hym þre spicis of maloue and lynsede, this will dissolue all harde thingis & gad*er* to-gedir. Also he is gode to hele the potagre. Also take the rote of fenell and of centory þe lasse, fenigrek and hony, of eu*ery* like myche, sethe that in water
755 and w*ith* þe water washe onys eyne, and that is p*re*cious for ⸤þe⸥ sight. Also take this erbe and barly mele and lynsede, and seþe hame in wyne to-gadir, and that helith þe menstrue.

---

748 dyuerse] dyu*eres MS.*   **749** fenigrecum] Fenigretum *MS* ‖ A p*re*cious for þ*e* sight *written on the outer margin.*   **755** onys eyne] p*re*cious for the sight *written on the outer margin.*   þe²] *written over the line.*

---

736 kytt] breste crampe dede childe dropese kytte the rote *written by Hand B on the outer margin.*   **740** linum] 64 *written by Hand E after this word.*
745 brenynge] for fyer*e* brenyng *written by Hand F on the outer margin.*
747 reynes] for þ*e* raynes *written by Hand F on the outer margin.*
749 fenigrecum] 65 *written by Hand E after this word.*

Alium domesticum

Garlek ys hote and drye [in] þe fourthe degre. The vertu of him is to hele the bitynge or styngyng of all addrys. Also anoynte a body wiþ the juis, and all venym wormes fleith ther-fro. Also bray garloke with hony and that is a worþi plaster for houndis bytinge. Also the same oynement is gode for him that is hurte oþer brusyd, oþer his bladyr be boyled oþer swell: hit will relesse and sese akyng. Also hit will brynge oute þe seconde borþen of a woman, iff garlek be brent in a pan | of hote colis and set hit vndir a womans preuy membris. Also yf he be sodde or dronke wiþ mylke oþer y-ete all rawe hit helpiþ all the sekenys of þe longis. Also wiþ centory i-sode that helith for þe dropsy and dryeth wekyd humours of the body, and frentekill men and for þe fallynge evill. Also with coryandyr and wyn hit helpiþ for þe jaundys, and yf hit be sod wiþ benys and þer-wiþ rubbe þe hede in the templis for the hede-ache. Also wiþ swynes grece y-made hote for to put in-to a bodyes ere, þat helpiþ the hede of evill. Also y-sod that helpiþ the cogh and lettith all sykynge. Also boþ sodyn and rawe hit clerith ones voise—but better soden þen rawe. Also seþe hit well with fat porke in grewell, and that is holsum for þe wombe. Also braye hit wiþ swynes grece: þat is gode for swellynge. Also seþe him wiþ swete mylke and vynegir, and slethe wormes in þe wombe. Also who-so etiþ hit in þe morowe tyde ‖ first mete, hit helpiþ a man from evill eyre of pestlens and malady.

Granum solis

Gromyll ys like to mount syon, with a litell white flour and sede like to a perle. The vertu is that þe sede braide and dronke

---

759 in] *om. MS.* fourthe] A howndis bytinge *written on the outer margin.*
784 gromyll] Gromylsede *MS,* sede *then deleted.*

---

758 alium domesticum] 66 *written by Hand E after this word.* **783** granum solis] 67 *written by Hand E after this word.* **784** gromyll] hote & drie *written by Hand C over the line.*

helpiþ for the stone and for þe evill of þe bladder. Also stampe
þe herbe and drinke þe juis, & that wyll make one to pisse.

Galanga

Galynga, hote and drye, beriþ longe levis as wilde grasse. The
vertu of him is to caste oute flewme of þe stomake and lyþer
wyndis; makeþ to defye mete, and makiþ gode sauour in oneis
mouthe and in his brethe, and helyth þe reynes, and encresith
appete to lechery.

Gryniswelly is hote. Þe rote ther-of is done in [non] medicyne.
The floures and þe levis, stampid in wyne and rykkylles mengid
[in maner of a plaster] and laide to lwke-warme, hit swagiþ the
swellynge of the | ballokis, and makiþ the synewis harde and
heliþ woundis. Some maistres de[f]endith for to drinke him.
Stampe hit with salt and lay hit to a womanys shappe: hit helpiþ
and drawith the evill þat is in a woman-is matrice. Plenius seiþ
that yf ye take him vp with-oute eny [yryn] touche þe toþe that
akyth, hit will sesse akynge.

Genciana

Gencyan ys of hote nature, and his rote is bittyr. Hit helpiþ þe
evill of the stomake and till þe lyuer and till þe splene. He that
vsiþ hit he shall not be ciaticus ne he shall not haue no evill
cogh. Hit helpith for the hosnesse and for þe dropsy. Hit helpith

794 non] *om. MS.* **796** in…plaster] *of a plaster in a maner MS.*
797 synewis] *Swollyn ballokys to hele moundis toþe-ake written on the outer margin.* **798** defendith] *desendith MS.* **801** yryn] *om. MS.* **804** hit] *For þe brest for þe splene for the cyaticus written on the outer margin.*

---

786 helpiþ] *for þe stone written by Hand F on the inner margin.*
788 galanga] *68 written by Hand E after this word.* **791** wyndis] *& written, apparently by Hand C, over the line.* **794** gryniswelly] *69 written by Hand E in the gap between entries.* **798** woundis] *it with talewe olde written by Hand C over the line.* **801** that²] *for þe toth-ache written by Hand F on the outer margin.* **803** genciana] *70 written by Hand E after this word.*

for all evill of þe brest and of þe sidis, and to hem that han stynkyn brethe, and castith oute all evill humours of þe body þrow vryn, and spurgiþ þe rede gall, and castiþ oute venym, and helpiþ þe nerues.

Germandir haviþ sede like to a peny and makiþ grete ‖ noyse when he is ripe. Pouder made ther-of and yf one drinke þer-of with hote water, hit helith þe potager with-oute doute. Þe juis with olde wyne i-dronke helipe a man for þe stynge [of] a naddyr. He growiþ in medis. Also he delyuereth woman of dede childe. Drinke with watir for the cogh. Þe juis dronke with vineger soudith brokyn bonys, and þe dropsye at the begynynge. Stampe & lay to all venym bitte hit helith. Stampe with hony hit heliþ olde woundis. Medill þe juis with hony and that is gode for to a-noynte eyne. Also þe juis and oyle, anoyntyd a body with that, casteth oute colde and settiþ one in gode hete, for he is hote and drye in þe þirde [degre].

Growndswelow is hote and drye, oþer-weysse callid swython. Þe levis er like to tesyll & a litell yelowe flour. The vertu of him is, as Pleni[u]s saith, "yf non yrne to[l]e haþe twchide him, towche þe toþe þat akiþ þere-wiþ þrise and hit shall be hole." Þe rote þere-of is done in no medicine, but stampe | the leuys oþer the flourys with franke-encence and wyne and make as a plaster and lay that [to] swellyng ballokys leuke-warme: þat swagiþ ham and that will make synewes harde and helith wondis. Also stampe hit with salte and lay to a woman prevy membris, and hir helpiþ and helith for the matrice. Some maisters forbede to drinke hym.

814 potager] for þe potagre delyuer dede childe for woundys for eyne *written on the outer margin.* **815** wyne] with *before emendation.* of] *om. MS.* **821** Also] oyle *deleted after this word.* **823** degre] drege *MS.* **825** a litell] for þe toþeake for swellyng ballokys *written on the outer margin.* **826** Plenius] plenis *MS.* tole] toke *MS.* **830** to] *om. MS.*

812 germandir] 71 *written by Hand E in the gap between entries.*
824 growndswelow] 72 *written by Hand E in the gap between entries.*

Gladiolus

835 Gladoyne ys hote and drye in þe secounde degre, and þe moste vertu of him is in þe more. The rote y-dronke wiþ wyne helipe the cogh and yeueth gode sauour, and with swete mylke hit delyuereth leþer colour. And wiþ vynegre hit delyuereþ the wombe of akynge. Also hit is gode for all venym. Also þe water 840 y-dronke is gode for þe narthe. Also þe juis y-dronke heliþ lymmys that beþe shronke wiþ colde. Also þe rote put in a wounde stanche blode.

Gariofilum

27ra Garofull is hote and drye in the secounde degre. Þe iuse ‖ is
845 gode for the stomake and make gode digestion, and helpiþ to all thingis wiþ-in a man. Also a dram stampid and dronke with freshe mylke confortith and multiplieth a manys kynde.

Altea

Holyhok, or wilde malowe, haþ leuys as hit were like hockis
850 and so he berith his sede. Iff he be schrede with tallowe he helipe þe potager with-in þre daies. Also all doctorys afferme that yf þis erbe be sode wiþ vyneger and lynsede and laide to a manys side, þat will departe and hele all wekyd wyndis and all evill gaderinges that beþ engendrid in a manys body.

---

835 drye] þe cogh for þe lemmys stanche blode *written on the inner margin*.
836 y-dronke] y-dronke y-dronke *MS*. **846** thingis] colour kynde *written on the outer margin*. **851** þe potager] for þe potagere for all evill in a manns body *written on the inner margin*.

---

834 gladiolus] 73 *written by Hand E after this word*. **843** gariofilum] 74 *written by Hand E after this word*. **848** altea] 75 *written by Hand E after this word*. **849** hockis] *id est.* malowes tame *written by Hand C over the line*. **854** body] & it groweth in moyste places & is hote & moyste in ii *gradus written by Hand C after this word*.

Amarusca

Houndfynell, or maythen, or dogfynell, is like to camamyll in all degre. The juis y-dronke is gode to quell þe cancre and the pipis of the emrodys. Also wiþ the juis of this erbe anoynte þe quynacy a-yene a gode fire ij or þre tymes and hit shall be hole. Also for him that sodeynly lese speche take this erbe | stalke and al pone & with water yf drinke.

Balsa[m]ita

Horsmynte, oþer medemynt, oþer water-mynte, hit is wonder stronge of sauour. The juis of him confortith a bodies stomake and maketh well for to defye mete, and purgith with-in the body and makiþ well to speke. Also þe juis and a litell hony and wyne y-dronke dothe a-way colde oute of the stomake and oþer leþer woundis. The juis soden in wyne and yeue to a woman in travaill of childe makeþ hastely the childe to be borne. Hit is hote and drye.

[Cicuta]

Hemloke is colde, and þe rote of hit etyn in stede of pasnepis makiþ one oute of harr witt, but yett þere-for a souerayn medicyne is to drinke stronge wyne. The vertue of him: stampe

---

858 also] for þe cankyr emrodis quynacy loste speche *written on the inner margin.* **862** balsamita] balsanita *MS.* **866** hony and] for þe stomake for to speke colde in þe stomake to delyuer þe childe *written on the outer margin.* **871** cicuta] Crenta *MS.* **873** of harr] for a sore hede for blerid eyne for a woman-is tittis lechery polucyon þe potagire *written on the outer margin.* harr] half *before emendation.*

---

855 amarusca] 76 *written by Hand E after this word.* **862** balsamita] 77 *written by Hand E after this word.* **866** speke] & spete *written by Hand C over the line.* **870** drye] & þer be ij spices of hem *written by Hand C after this word.* **871** cicuta] vel cicuta *id est.* Herba benedicta *written by Hand C after this word, then* 78 *written by Hand E.*

875 the grene levisse and lay that to a sore hede and he helith hi*m*.
27va Also a-noynte the eye-liddys w*ith* that juis ‖ and that heliþ the blether of ham, and helpiþ a sekenys callid þe holy fire and in latyn herpe[t]a. Also put þe juis till a womanys tittis that swagith swellynge of ham and dryeth a-way þe mylke. Also
880 make a plaster of þe sede grette w*ith* silu*er* fome and grece y-medlid þ*er*-with: þ*at* is a medicyne for to pute oute þe hete of lechery and for polucyon of kynde. Also a plaster made of hi*m* and laide to al hote, that helpiþ þe potag*er* and all wekyd hetis.

Horeworte, or chauuede, oþ*er* wey-hor, growith in hard land and
885 berith no floure, but at þe top he berith his sede. Þe juis of hi*m* w*ith* hote mylke of a cowe of a colour ix daies, first at morowe and laste at evyn, schall stanche þe flux of blode. Also þe juis y-dronke w*ith* white wyne, first and laiste, heliþ cankris and
27vb fistula, yf the wou*n*des be washe w*ith* juis of planteyn*e*, | and
890 lay vpon the sides woundes þe levis of rede cawle oþ*er* of molayn*e* leuys.

Edera t*er*restris

Heyhofe has levis like to calamynte but þey be not so myche, and in the crope he beryth blewe flourys. Yf he be shred in
895 potage a-monge olde fleshe he will m*a*ke hit neshe. Of hit boyled in þe sekys vryn make a plaster, and lay to as hote as he may suffyr, for the stiche. Also þe juis secis toþe-ache yf hit be put in-to þe ere of þe same side that þe tothe is.

---

878 herpeta] herpera *MS.* **887** schall stanche] for þe flux of blode Cankris and fistula for wound*is written on the outer margin.* **895** potage] to m*a*ke olde fleshe tend*ir* for þe stiche þe toþe-ake *written on the inner margin.*

---

884 horeworte] 79 *written by Hand E in the gap between entries.* **892** edera terrestris] 80 *written by Hand E after this word.*

Horshele ys hote and wete. Hit nesheith þe wombe. Hit a-batith þe tysayne, that is þe evill of þe hede. The rote sodde in wyn and vsith doþe gode to all newe-frantikes, þat is þe evill of þe reynes. Make of the rote pouder and medill hony ther-with: þat a-batith þe cogh and helpith þe longis. Þe juis of him and rewe helpith hem that er bresten in yongthe.

Henbane ys in iij manerys: one beryth white sede, þe secunde rede sede, the þirde berithe black sede. The white is beste of all, but for defaute of the white men dothe the rede in medicynes, and the black not. Stampe the levis of þe white in maner of a plaster and hit stanchiþ swelyng and he helith potager. The juis done in the erys sleith þe wormys in ham and abatiþ þe hede-ake. Also stampe þe white sede and take þe juis ther-of and washe the eyne: hit castith oute byndynge and hote re[w]me. Seþ him in wyne and stampe hit, and hit swagithe swellynge of þe b[al]lokkys and of women pappis. Washe woundis with juis and hit helith. Take him and ache and juis of morell þat haue black berys and smale (hit growis in clostris) and rounde in levys, and barow-ys gresse y-medlid þere-with: is gode for þe hote goute.

---

901 newe-frantikes] for þe reynes þe coȝ and brestyn in youthe *written on the inner margin.* **912** hote] reaw *deleted after this word.* rewme] reame *MS.* **914** ballokkys] blokkys *MS.*

---

899 horshele] 81 *written by Hand E in the gap between entries.* **905** henbane] Jusquiamus *written by Hand C in the gap between entries, then* 82 *written by Hand E immediately after.* manerys] hote & drie *written by Hand C over the line.* secunde] The seid seed of henbane vsyd on a ho[t]e [hole *MS*] tyle & the smoke þer-of restryned into a mannes movthe destroyeth all the wormes in the tethe and oyle made þer [j *deleted after this word*] of will destroye all maner goutes *written by Hand C on the lower margin.*

Fraxinus

Hertwort, oþer [wodebroune], oþer silfehale, Stampyd and laide
to a sore heliþ hit anone. Hit haþe levis sharpe as a hert, a flour
blewe as bugill, and a shorte stalke. |

Lingua cerui

Hertis-tonge, oþer cerelonge, haviþ levis like to þe tonge of an
hert. Þis erbe, sode with oyle of rosse, will ripe and breke a
postom. Also þe juis dronke with olde wyne hardiþ þe wombe
that ys renyng oute and heliþ a man of þe [c]ow. Also take þis
erbe, sauge and percily in þe monthe of Maye, and make pouder
þere-of, and vse hit in metis and drinkys for þe colik.

Lingua canis

Houndystonge hathe a flour of purpill colour, almoste like to
confery flour, and he is gode for þe cough and postem for to
drynk him. Also stampe him oþer lay the levis to bochis oþer
bilis and that helith hame.

Marubium

Horehounde, oþer morall, oþer howndbene, ys like blynde-
nettill but þe levis ben whitter and hit haþe a godely sauour.
This erbe or þe sede sodyn helpiþ gretly for the tisike and þe

---

919 hertwort] to hele a sore a-lone *written on the inner margin.* wodebroune] edebreune *MS.* **922** lingua cerui] *written on the upper margin.* **925** postom] ripe and breke an postem hardiþ þe wombe þe colrik *written on the outer margin.* **926** cow] sow *MS.* **930** almoste] The co3 postem bochis bilis *written on the outer margin.*

---

918 fraxinus] 83 *written by Hand E after this word.* **922** lingua cerui] 84 *written by Hand E after this word.* **923** haviþ] This erbe haþe neþer sede ne stalke *written by Hand C on the outer margin.* **926** cow] *emended to* cogh *by Hand C.* **929** lingua canis] 85 *written by Hand E after this word.* **934** marubium] 86 *written by Hand E after this word.* **937** sodyn] with licoryse *written by Hand C over the line.* tisike] the coghe *written by Hand C over the line.*

narthe, but myche bettir yf þu drinke þe juis of gladoun oþer centory þer-with, and helpiþ a woman hastely to ber hir childe in travaill || and þe seconde borþen. Also stampe hit with hony: hit helith freting bocchis and clensithe wondis. Also hit helithe sore sides and al aboue-saide, yf the juis be dronke. Also þe juis of him with wyne and hony is a precious oynement for eyne that dyrkyn for febilnes. Also with oyle of rose hit helpith eris. Also water of horehound is gode for the cold spasum, but he is not gode to ham that havith sore in the reynes and in the bladrys of ston. Also, yf a man haue a wekyd colde, let this erbe rest a while in a tobbe of water, than late þe beste drinke of that water and she shall be hole. Also yf one haue a seke stomake drinke the juis of this erbe and he schall be holee. Also drinke of þe water that þe erbe is sodyn in for the feueres. Also the juis of this erbe wiþ wyne drinke for all venym. Also yf a man haue scabbis oþer tetterys seþe this erbe well in water and washe þe body in that water. Also yf one haue any hardnes in his body | stampe this erbe and swynes grece and lay to the sore in maner of a plaster and hit will a-mend. This erbe is hote and drye. Also the water of horehound y-stillid is gode for þe colde spasom and for synowys stoyned. Also sethe juis of this erbe with wyne and gotis mylke in like quantite till halfe be wastid: drinke þere-of onys in a monthe and þu shalte neuer haue sekenes but yf hit be of superfluyte.

Pes pulli agrestis

Horsho[ue], fole-fote, coltisfote, oþer diuee, this erbe is grene in that one side and white in that oþer. This erbe y-ete will stanche the flux and hele one of þe feuerys. Also þe grete hete of þe

---

947 yf a] Tysike and narthe to bere a childe and bocchis & woundys eyne and a wekid coȝ stommak þe feueres tetteris *written on the outer margin*. **963** horshoue] horshon *MS*.

---

962 pes pulli agrestis] 87 *written by Hand E after this word*.

son*n*e shall do no harme to hi*m* þ*a*t etith hi*m* and hit will hele one of þe s[to]ne. Also yf onys eyne be swell with evill blode ete þ*is* erbe and he shall be hole. This erbe is hote and drye.

Rubia minor ||

29ra Hayreff, clyu*er*, oþ*er* aron, is like to wodruff and þe sed tuchid will honge in one-is cloþis. Wiþ the wat*er* of þe e*r*be a-noynte a wounde and hit shall close w*ith*-in shorte tyme. He will make geese and hennys fatte yf hit be broke small. Hit grow*ith* ovir-all in dichis.

Portulaca

975 Helow is dry and colde. The v*er*tu of hi*m* is this: lay the levis y-stampid as a plaster to þe stom*a*ke oþ*er* ete ham or drinke ham, and that stopith þe flux of blode and hit stopith the wombe. Also stampe hit and do hit to eyne that ben y-swell and hit swagith
980 ham. Also ete hi*m* in som*er* and þe hete of the sonne shall do one none harme, and wiþ white saltt hit makiþ þe wombe al neshe that is harde. Plenius saithe who-so will ete hit ofte shall done a-way akynge of þe bladd*er* and in all vertues that is like to þe soure-docke, and su*m* men calliþ hym portulake, oþ*er* horshoo. |

Isopus

29rb Isope is hote and drye in þe ij. degre. Þe juis þere-of delyu*er*yth women of dede childe w*ith*-oute p*er*ill. Also drinke hi*m* ofte

966 etith] for þe flux hele þe feu*er*es stone for eyne *written on the outer margin.* **967** stone] sitne *MS.* **970** hayreff] Rubia minor *written on the upper margin.* tuchid] to close a wou*n*de *written on the inner margin.* **977** þe stomake] for þe flux of blode for swollyn eyne *written on the inner margin.* **985** isopus] *written on the upper margin.*

---

969 rubia minor] 88 *written by Hand E after this word.* **975** portulaca] 89 *written by Hand E after this word.* **985** isopus] 90 *written by Hand E after this word.*

fastynge and that makiþ one well colourde and of gode sight, and sleyth wormes in þe wombe, and is gode for the lyuer and the longis. Also ofte y-dronke hit doþe a-way þe dropsye. Also seþ him in wyne fro a potell till a quarte: vse þere-of at evyn hote and at morowe colde for a streite breste. Also medill þe juis with aysell and put that to a sore mouthe, and that will hele all sores þere-in. Also seþe him wiþ hony and dry figis: that helpith for hosnes and þe mylt, and clensith wormes, and helpith the cogh and tysik. Poudyr y-made of him and medlid with hony y-vsid will do this aboue-saide. Also do him grynde wiþ hony and seede of toune-carse, and that neshith þe wombe and dryvith oute flewme and leper wyndes. Also dronke with wyne hit makiþ rome the breste and helpith all swellyng of þe ‖ stomake. Also seþe him in vineger and fret well a tothe that akiþ with that aysell, and hit heliþ him. Also þe juis þere-of puttiþ a-way hosyng of one-is [eris], and yf hit be sod and y-laide þer-to hit doþe away all swellyng of ham.

Edera nigra

Ivy ys an erbe that berryth black beryes, and he hathe to him an herbe that is callid bryony, and that erbe beryth frute as hit were bayes. The vertu of this erbe is, yf he be sode in wyne and laide apon a boche, hit will hele him. Also who þat haviþ þe hede-ake take þe juis of þis erbe and oyle of rosis and sethe that to-gadir in wyn and a-noynte þe hede þere-with & he shall be hole. Also yf þu wilt kepe þi hede fro akynge of þe son, take þe levis of this erbe and stampe ham smale, þan temper ham with aysell and oyle of rosis, and þere-wiþ a-noynte well þe forhede and hit

---

990 hit] To delyuer dede childe wiþ-oute perill well colord and gode of sight for þe dropesye *written on the outer margin.* **1003** eris] *om. MS.* **1007** as hit] to hele a boche hede-ache for þe stone *written on the outer margin.*

994 all] sore in þe mowthe *written by Hand C on the outer margin.*
1005 edera nigra] 91 *written by Hand E after this word.*

1015 shall be hole. Also þe beryes of ivy that grow*ith* on a roche,
29vb y-made to poud*er* and vse | hit, brekith the stone.

Ostragium

Ive, oþ*ere* herbe yue, oþ*er* hertishorne, hauythe leuys lyke to the tyndes of a hert, and growiþ be þe grownde a-brode and þe rote
1020 goþe evyn downe. This erbe, sodyn in wyne w*ith* oyle w*ith* comyn and þ*ere*-of a plaster made of þis rotis and vse hit in met*is*, makiþ a man laxatyfe. The knobbys of þe rotis of þis erbe, layde in rose water in þe son till þe wat*er* be consumyd, will make þi face or any oþ*er* parte of þi body white and faire,
1025 yf þ*u* rubbe ham ther-with ij or þre tymes. Also poudyr of this erbe vsid puttith a-way sup*er*fluyte of fleshe. Also, for þe blody menysou*n*, seþe this erbe i*n* wat*er*, þan let þe seke holde boþe his fete in þe watir till þe ancles—but no deppir—as hote as he may suffyr. Þis erbe is hote and dry.

1030 ## Barba Jouis

30ra Jubarbe, oþ*er* houseleke, with || a þikk lefe, growith comynly vppon house. The v*er*tu of this erbe is, yf a man haue a postem w*ith*-in hi*m* gadryd w*ith* hote mat*er*, take þis erbe at þe begynynge of þe postem & talowe and [s]ede coryandyr, stampe
1035 þes to-ged*er* in man*er* of a plast*er* and lay hit to þe posto*m*, and hit shall distroye hi*m*. Also yf one be scallyd w*ith* hote water oþ*er* brent with fire take þe juis of þis erbe and oyle of rosys and wax, and make an oyntment and a-noynte þe sore but þre of þe fyrst daies aftir that he ys scallyd or bre*n*t. Also this erbe is
1040 gode to hele wikkyd hetis. Also þ*is* herbe ys gode for bolnynge

1022 the knobbys] for erys laxatife white faire þe blody menisou*n* to m*a*ke faire white *written on the inner margin.* 1031 a þikk] Barba iouis *written on the upper margin.* 1034 sede] rede *MS.*

1017 ostragium] 92 *written by Hand E after this word.* 1030 barba Jouis] 93 *written by Hand E after this word.*

Lelamour Herbal

& hardnes. Also þe juis ther-of tempird wiþ þe cromys of white brede and swynys grese and coryandyr y-stampid to-gadyr woll hele a-yene all swellyng sekenes. Drinke þe juis of þe rote of [jubarbe] for brokyn bonys, and | he shall knyt ham one.

H*erba* Plenius

Þis erbe is like to verne, but þe leuys be like to kayre. Þis erbe grow*ith* moche in more & medoys.

Spica celtica

Kalketrap ys cold in the first degre and moiste *in* þe secounde de-gre. He y-ete neshith þe wombe. Also a enplaster made þ*ere*-of and laide to þe sore nayles helpiþ ham. Also hit doþe a-way the blott*is* a-boue þe nayles in þe quyk.

[Resta] bouis

Kammok haþe levis like to þre-levid-grasse, and he haþe a rede stalke full of levis, and he growiþ crokyng by the grownde, and a flour of purpur colour, and when he is of grete age he havith p*ri*kkis as hit were forse, and þen comenly he will lett þe plowe. Þe v*er*tu of hi*m* ys þ*at* he, sode in wyne and dronke, hit [sleeþ a man]. ||

Apiu*m* risus

Kerwell is hote and drye, oþ*er*-wais called cheruell. He stampid w*ith* hony helith þe cankyr. Also y-soden with wyne hit helpith

---

1044 jubarbe] *om. MS.*   **1045** herba Plenius] þe postom þe blad*er* or brent or scaldid w*ith* fire or wat*er written on the outer margin.*   **1053** Resta bouis] Beta bouis *MS.*   **1059** sleeþ a man] *om. MS.*   **1060** apium risus] *written on the upper margin.*   **1061** he stampid] þe canker for akyng of þe hede for þe side and þe colik woundis for casting wilde fire *written on the outer margin.*   **1062** helpith] man *deleted after this word.*

1048 spica celtica] 94 *written by Hand E after this word.*   **1053** Resta bouis] 95 *written by Hand E after this word.*   **1060** apium risus] 96 *written by Hand E after this word.*

and a-batith [mal de flaunke]. Also y-dronke in mouste [helith] gl[e]ttis bowndyn in the mouthe. Also kerwell, barowes grece and virgyn wax y-stampid to-gedir heliþ all maner of swellynge. Hit etyn with vynegir makiþ the wombe lax and stroyeth vomyt. Also washe þe hede with þe juis luke-warme and that sesith akyng of þe hede. Also who that drynkyth the juis with wyne hit makyth him to pisse and deliueryth ache of þe reynesse and the bladder. Also drinke him with wyne: he lattiþe oute and vnbyndith leþer wyndys fro þe side, and þe stoppinge from the colik, and of þe lyuer, and of all maner of wondis. Also hit with-holdith castinge. Also a plaster, y-made of the erbe | and temper hit with aisell, distroith wilde fire and helithe þe cankyr and oþer wondis, and puttiþ a-way colde of all wondis. And hit is hote and drye.

Lollium

Kokkyll ys of ij maners: þe one is gode that oþer is not. That one havith foure hornys tawarde þe walkyne and lokkyd to-gader in the topys. Greynes amendith brede. Þe vertu of this erbe is, yf he be grounde with a litell radich and salt, that is gode to hele cankyr and oþer woundis. Also hit confortith þe stomake and þe lyuer, and vnbyndyth leþer wyndis that beþ in a mans wombe, and helpiþ a man to pisse, and is gode for sore eyne. Also þe subiugacioun of hit shall helpe a woman to ber hir childe liȝtly with-oute perill oþer harme. Also hit swagith þe paynes of the akynge of lepir. Also þe || woman that vsith hit shall haue plente of mylke and will make þik humouris thyn. Also þere is cokkill cumy[n] to wete and helpinge to medicyne, for he clansith þe cankyr i-write hit is a-boue whate maner. Also

1063 mal de flaunke] maudeslamylke *MS*.   helith] *om. MS.*   **1064** glettis] glottis *MS*.   **1078** oþer is] for cankir and woundis sore eyne to ber a childe with-oute perell þe squynacy & postomms cietica pascio *written on the inner margin.*   **1089** cumyn] cumy *MS*.

1077 lollium] 97 *written by Hand E after this word.*

Lelamour Herbal

medill hit w*ith* brymstone and colueris donge and wyne as a plaster, and that will hele the squynacy and postomys and bolwyngis. Also þe sede, y-grounde and boyled in wyne and franke-encense and safron, helpis sekenys vndir þe sidis þ*at* men calliþ scietica passio, that is be-twene þe rige and þe navill. This is hote and drye. 1095

M[ir]tus

Knotwort, oþ*er* gasar, ys like in colour to whityngtre and beryth rede beryis, but þei beþ not so grete. And he growith in woddis a-longe comynly by a-noþ*er* tre. The v*er*tu ys that yf a body haue an arme or eny bone brokyn in his body take the first day | and bray iij of þes beries and drinke ham with stale ale, and þe secunde day stampe vj beryis and drynke ham, and hit shall knyt ham wiþ-oute more helpe. 1100

31rb

Kerwell is hote and drye, & stampe hit w*ith* hony: hit helith þe cankyr. Sodyn in wyn hit helpith and a-batith [mal de flaunke]. Dronkyn in moust helyt the gl[e]tt*is* boundyn in þe mouthe. Keruell and barois grece and virgyn wax done to-gedir hit helpith of all man*er* of swellynge. Hete hi*m* w*ith* aisell: hit swagith and makyth solubill and stroyth vomyt. Þe iuse ther-of luke-warme weshe the hede ther-with and hit swagith akynge. 1105

1110

1097 mirtus] Mutus *MS*. **1098** whityngtre] to knyt brokyn bonys *written on the inner margin*. **1102** and bray] and bray and bray *MS*. **1105** kerwell] Lerwell *MS, even though* k *was written as a guide-letter below the Lombardic letter*. **1106** mal de flaunke] maudeslamyke *MS* || Cankyr hede-ache *written on the outer margin*. **1107** glettis] glottis *MS*. **1110** stroyth] *apparently*, stroytt *before emendation*.

1097 mirtus] 98 *written by Hand E after this word*. **1105** kerwell] 99 *written by Hand E in the gap between entries*.

Lekys. Ypocras byddith to take juis of þe leke and þe appill of þe oke and þe floure of rikylle, myrre and wyne and make þere-of a drinke, and yf þat to þe body that castith blode for brusynge and þu shalte wariche, and with that medicyne men may stanche blode at þe nose. ‖ If þu kytt eny place of þi body a-non take the levis and stampe ham with a lytell salt to-gedir to þe sore and hit sesith akynge, and stanchith to a woman-ys shape that is sore with brenynge with-in. A-noynte hit wiþ þe fyrst medicyne and hit helith. Maiden þat etith ham hit makyth ham haue her flour. Stampe pore and boyle hit in hony in maner of a plaster and ley hit to a febill hede, and yf þe humouris of flux commyth of þe hede hit spurgith women that etith þere-off and makiþ ham to contayne and helith hame. The juis ther-of with tysaine made of bere helpiþ þe longis and the breste and þe voice well to singe, and a-batiþ the cogh. The juis of pore sodyn in wyne helpith for cost[if]nys and hit helpith for naddrys styngyng. Women mylke and the juis of leke helpith for þe cogh and for þe lonngis. The juis of lekys & þe gall of a catte with wyne other mouste mengid to-gedyr and don lawe in his eris delyuereth the hede-ake and þe stoppinge of the eris. | The juis þere-of and wyne, sodyn to-gedyr and vse hit, doþ gode for akynge of þe lendys and knetith veynes and harde þinge hit makiþ neshe. Grynde hit with salt and ete hit: hit kepith a man from dronknes & hansith lechery. And who-so vsith hit ofte rawe hit makiþ hym solibyll.

Lylly the leuys þere-of stampid and plastride to harde synowis hit makiþ neshe, and helpiþ brenyng of membris, and helyth þe

1112 þe appill] for casting of blode for kyttyng and stanche blode þe brest and þe voice hede-ake knyt veynys *written on the outer margin.* 1117 lytell] *written on the outer margin.* 1127 costifnys] costnys *MS.*

1112 lekys] Porrum *written by Hand C in the gap between entries, then* 100 *written by Hand E in the outer margin.* 1116 þe nose] Also þe ius of hit dronk with wyne swageth dronkenes *written by Hand C on the outer margin.* 1136 lylly] 101 *written by Hand E in the gap between entries.*

stang of an nadder oþer other wormes. Sethe þe rote in wyne
and lay hit to biles in maner of a plaster þre dayes & hit helith.
The rote sodyn in wyne with schepis talowe y-mengid makyth
here to growe in brennyd place. The rote dronkyn in wyne
spurgith evill blode þrowe the wombe, and helpith þe splene,
and helpithe womenys schappe, and spurgiþ hir flouris. Stampe
hit with hony: he helpith veynes and synowys kytt in two. The
juis of the lefe, aysell and || hony drieth wondis and helpiþ
sursanouris. The juis puttiþ a-way black spottis of the face,
flewme and frantiklys in the face. The juis done in womanys
schappe neshes þe flouris.

Lawreoll and sporge ys of one vertue: þei ben don for to make
men delyuer a-boue othir by-nethe, or þei perys the bowelis.
Ther-for, take þe levis and drye ham in an ovyn, than make
þere-of pouder, and yf ther-of to stronge men v peny-wight, to
febler [iij peny-wight,] and to harde boundyn men more, and to
la[s]e bund men less, in coule, oþer in grewell, oþer in ne[sch]
eggis, oþer in ale, other in wyne. The sede ther-of ys nought so
myghty as the lefe. But yf þu wilt clense eny man take iij
peny-wight of þe sede and done a-way þe hoyles and stampe
hit with wyne and meng hit with wyne, and yf hit to drinke:
that ys a purgacion for delicious men; oþer put hit in an appill

1138 oþer] to make here growe in brent placis splene veyne senowys knytt *written on the inner margin.* **1151** and drye] for porgacions vpward or downe *written on the outer margin.* **1153** iij peny-wight] *om. MS.* **1154** lase] late *MS.* nesch] nechs *MS.*

1149 lawreoll] Lauriola *written by Hand C in the gap between entries, then* 102 *written by Hand E immediately after.* **1154** lase] *emended to* lasse *by Hand C.* **1155** wyne] & also it purcheth of flewme & colre *written by Hand C over the line.*

32rb and yff hym to ete with mylke. | The levys juis a-noynte þe with hit, [hit] makeþ the seme mesell.

Lovache ys hote and drye. The moste strey[n]the ys in the rote and in the sede, for bothe hathe maistrey in wirchinge medicynes. Dronkyn in wyne hit helpith þe stomake of swellynge, and that
1165 drinke makeþ a man to defye his mete, and hit doþe gode to all evill*is* of þe entrellys. Also hit makith vryn and spurgith flourys. Stampe h*im* and lay hit to þe woundys: hit helith. The rote oþ*er* the sede soden in water and dronkyn*e* helpith the foundeme*n*t that is callid coly[k]. Plenius saithe that men shall done the sede
1170 i*n* all medycynes that men makiþ solibyll.

Lauandula

Lauandyr y-sodde in wat*er* and y-dronke ofte is gode to hele the palesy. Also þe flou‿e‿ris of h*im* yf a nobyll sauo*ur* a-monge cloþis. He is hote and drye.

32va Lavandyr coton grow*ith* in gardynes, || and his colour is white-horyd. He berith yelow flourys and is of swete sauor for to smell to. The smell of this erbe putteþ a-way the pestelens, and þe juis will distroy lyse w*ith* a-noyntynge.

1161 hit[2]] *om. MS.*   **1162** streynthe] streythe *MS.*   **1169** colyk] coly *MS.*
1173 floueris] flouris *before emendation,* e *written over the line.*

1160 mylke] And if the leves of laureol to be yeve for p*ur*gation be gad*er*ed or plukked dou*n*ward þe p*ur*gation schall be dou*n*ward and if they be plukked vpward the p*ur*gation schall be vpward p*r*oved certeinlie. *written by Hand C on the lower margin.*   **1162** lovache] 103 *written by Hand E in the outer margin.*   **1171** lauandula] 104 *written by Hand E after this word.*
1175 lavandyr coton] 105 *written by Hand E in the gap between entries.*

F[l]amula min*or*

Las[se] sper-wort hauith leuis shapid like a sper*e*. He sta*m*p hit and laide to a wownd heliþ hit anone.   1180

Lingua bouis

Longe de [be]ffe, oþ*er* oxetonge: þe juis y-dronke w*ith* hote water makyth a man to haue gode mynde and witt. Also he will put a-way þe rede colo*ur*. Also he y-dronke wiþ wyne helpith to distroy the cardiacle and wekyd humourys of a ma*n*is lon*n*gis. This erbe ys hote and moiste. Also wondirly he heliþ a-yene the evill y-callid scietica passio, and also þe narthe of þe brest. Also mell þe juis of hi*m* wiþ wyne and drinke hit and caste of þe same in the hall: h*i*t makiþ all that be þ*er*e-in mery | and gladde.   1185

32vb

Lupinus fabe

Lvpyne ys like to þe v-levys but, for the more p*ar*ty, þ*er*e be vj levis and a white floure and white brode sede, as hit were pese in coddys. The sede y-stampid and medlid w*ith* hony & etyn avoyden wormes oute of the wombe. A plaster made of þe mele of lupyne & wermote laide to the stom*a*ke dothe þe same. Or els make paste (a kake) of this sede and wermote for the same, and ete hit for þe wormes, and also hit will distroy the dropsye. Also take the mele of lupyne and þe juis of smert and medill ham to-gadir and put in-to the erys, and that wil clense ham of all stynke and sle wormes þ*er*-in. Oþ*er* els make paste of that and ete hit. Also mell of lupyn and juis of leke tempird to-ged*er* and y-put in þe erys clensith ham of al stynche and hore. Also mell   1195

1200

1179 flamula minor] famula min*or* MS.   **1180** lasse sper-wort] lassper wort MS.   shapid] woundys *written on the outer margin.*   **1183** longe de beffe] Longedeffe *MS.*

1179 flamula minor] 106 *written by Hand E after this word.*   **1182** lingua bouis] 107 *written by Hand E after this word.*   **1183** beffe] be *written by Hand C over the line.*   **1191** lupinus fabe] 108 *written by Hand E after this word.*

33ra of lupyne with hony will rippe and breke || all man*er* postemes,
1205 for þ*is* erbe is hote and drye.

Lacctuca

Letuse is colde and moiste in [the] þerde deg*re*. Stampe hi*m* and drinke the juis w*ith* wyne, and h*i*t stanchith the flux and colyth vnkynde hetis. Also who-so etiþ hi*m* rawe oþ*er* sod, hit gendrit
1210 gode blode and yevith mylke to the norys largely. Also hit is gode for the feu*er*ys. Also sethe hi*m* in aisell and do safron þ*er*-to and drinke that, and hit vnbyndith stoppinge of the lyu*er* and þ*e* mylt. Also a plaster made of the poud*er* þ*er*e-of with womans mylke and white of an egge and y-laide to þe templis
1215 of his hede makeþ a man well to slepe. Or else drinke þe poud*er* w*ith* cowe mylke all hote, and that is gode for slepe. Also take þe sede and oyle of rosys and m*a*ke a plaster and do þ*at* vppon the stomake, and that shall put a-way the hote posteme. Also
33rb who that etith þe sede h*i*t doþe a-way ydell dremys. | Also
1220 stampe the sede with watir and drinke hit, and h*i*t puttith a-way polluc*i*onys. But who that vse hit myche in mete or in drinke hit a-peireth þe sight.

Eleborus

Longwort, oþ*er* elebyr, oþ*er* piletir of Spayne: þ*er* beþe ij
1225 spic*es* of this erbe: one ys white (that purgiþ vpwarde), and a-noþ*er* is black (that purgith dounward), and þay beþ hote &

1207 the] *written on the inner margin.* **1216** cowe] colde *before emendation.*

1206 lacctuca] 109 *written by Hand E after this word.* **1223** eleborus] Albus *written by Hand C after this word, then* 110 *written by Hand E immediately after.* **1224** longwort] vel michellworte *written by Hand C over the line.* elebyr oþer] Elebor*us* niger is called pedelione & he hath a yelow flour [bredder þen a penye *over the line*] of whom is mentiou*n* made after in P. it is leke to longewort but þe leves of longewort be not slitte *written by Hand C on the outer margin.*

dry in the þirde degre. And the white is more violent þen the black. The white put in a womanys priuete delyuereth woman of dede childe. Also þe juis of him put in-to a mans nose oþer the pouder makyth him to fnese and clensith þe hede. Also medill þe poudyr of him with rattys and myse floure and that quellith rattis & myse. Also he is gode with all þinge that helpith for the sight. Also þe poudyr medlid with mylke sleith flyes. Elebure black is gode for the herynge whan the juis ‖ is put in the ere. Also he is gode for to hele scabbys and tetirrys and for the morfue. Also sethe him in vynegre, hold som of þe aisell in one-is mouthe, and that helithe tothe-ake. Also he helithe a man of þe emorodys yf þei be brusid and laide to, and he purgith colour [and] flewme.

Epatica

Levirwort ys an erbe that [g]rowith apon moiste wallis, and he cleuyth faste to þe stone. This erbe hathe no stalke ne flour, and he will distroye and clense the hardnes of onys lyuer. Also medill þis erbe and barowis grece to-gadyr, and that is gode to hele a wounde and þe feuer quarteyn. Also seþ him in wyne and that helithe brokyn rybbis. And he is hote and drie in iij degre.

Liquericia

Lycorys will make moiste kyndely the grete hete of man, and ther-for he is | gode for þe cogh, and makyþ þe þrote, þe breste and the longis moist. Also sethe hit in freshe water, till hit be all-moyste y-consumyd: that water y-dronke puttith a-way þerst.

1234 elebure black] *underlined in red as a lemma.* **1239** and] of *MS.*
1241 erbe] apon moiste wallis *deleted after this word.* growith] rowith *MS.*

1240 epatica] III *written by Hand E after this word.* **1247** liquericia] 112 *written by Hand E after this word.*

[Astericon]

Lvnary growith a-monge stonys. This erbe shyneth be nyght and hathe yelowe flourys and rounde, as hit were cokkyll oþer flouris of fox-gloue, and the levis of him ben ynde blewe. In the medill of þe lefe ys the merke of the mone, as hit were in iij-levid-grasse, but his levis ben more and rounde. Þe stalke is rede, þe juis yelewe. He incresith withe levis and wanyth as þe mone dothe, and þer he growith in grete quantite. Who-so etith of his bayi[s], oþer else of the erbe, in the wanyng of the mone whan he is in the synge virginis, that shall saue a body for þe fallyng evill. Also who that hauyth this evill, ber this erbe a-bute his nek ‖ and he shall be hole.

Magirona

Magiron is an erbe of swete sauour. Make pouder ther-of and caste sum in-to ones nose-þrillys, and that will clense the brayne. Þe same pouder caste in-to grewell ys gode for þe stomake. This erbe in podyngs of shepe blode yevith gode apetyde, for this erbe ys hote and dry.

Rubia maior

Madyr, oþer warance, haþe a rede rote and ys gode to clense and oppyn the stoppynge of the lyuere and þe mylte. Also he is

---

1252 astericon] astericion *MS*. **1260** bayis] bayith *MS*. **1267** þe¹…pouder] þe same pouder þe same poudir *MS*.

1252 astericon] vel Asterion *written by Hand C after this word, then* 113 *written by Hand E immediately after.* **1253** growith] in hygh places *written by Hand C over the line.* **1254** flourys] hole *written by Hand C over the line.* cokkyll] vel as a cokkysbyll *written by Hand C over the line.* **1255** blewe] and *written by Hand C over the line.* **1257** rounde] as a peny *written by Hand C over the line.* **1258** levis] sume every day of xv. i lefe *written by Hand C over the line.* wanyth] after *written by Hand C over the line.* **1259** growith] he groweth *written by Hand C over the line.* **1263** nek] Lunarie is most founde by scheperdes *written by Hand C on the outer margin.* **1264** magirona] 114 *written by Hand E after this word.* **1270** rubia maior] 115 *written by Hand E after this word.*

a wo[r]þy drynke for woundys and will clense and kepe a mannes lymes fro rottynge. Also boyle madyr and mastik to-geder in wyne, and drinke that for þe stomak and þe lyuere. Also he is leder | and knytter of bonys, yf he be dronke. Also seþe him in watir and washe the hede þer-with, and that makeþ rede here. Also make a plaster of him and lay to þe navyll, and will sle wormes in þe wombe y-callyd lymbrykys. Also take þe grete rote & shaue hit clene with-oute and a-noynte that wiþ hony, strowe þere-vppon powdir scamony, bynde a þrede a-boute an ende of hit, put þat in a womanys priue membris, sone after drawe hit oute be the þrede, and hit delyuereth hir of childe. This erbe ys hote and drye.

Spicarius

Maworte haviþ levis like to coluyrfote, and hit havith a rede stalke and rede flour, and he is gode to vpyn þe stoppinge of the leure and the myl[t]. ||

Malua minor

Maloys, oþer hokkys, ofte y-vside in wortis, but Plenius for-bedith that in þe monthe of February for venym. The levis y-stampid and laide vpon þe stomake will breke an hote posteme in þe begynynge. Oþer stampe þis erbe with freshe swyness grece and hete hit vpon a tyle, and so hote do vpon a stomake, and þat shall rippe a postem. Also this plastir is gode for to distroye hardnes of one-ys lyuer and hys mylt. Also this erbe sodde in potache is gode to make a body lax, for he is

---

1273 worþy] woþy *MS.* **1285** spicarius] maworte oþer warance haþe a rede rote *written in the following line, then deleted.* **1288** mylt] mylk *MS.* **1289** malua minor] *written on the upper margin.* **1296** this] thir *before emendation.*

1285 spicarius] 116 *written by Hand E after this word.* **1289** malua minor] 117 *written by Hand E after this word.*

colde and wete. Also make poudir of hi*m* and drinke that wiþ wyne, and that will caste blode oute of a wound.

Capilli Ven*e*ris

1300

Maydenhere, in watry valeys, and hit hathe levis lyke verne, and in þe medill of þe leve þe*r*e is as were a smale black here. The ve*r*tu of þ*is* | erbe is that hit is a sou*e*rayn þinge for the stone, yf he be dronke and hit will distroy venym, for hit is hote and dry.

34vb

Morsus diaboli

1305

Mor*r*e y-bitt is like to dent de lyonne, and hit hauyþ yelowe flowris. The p*ri*ncipale rote of hi*m* is bitt a-waye. The ve*r*tu: stampe hi*m* and drinke the juis wiþ stale ale, and that helithe þe feu*e*rys þ*a*t com*ith* eu*e*ry day oþ*er* eu*e*ry þirde day. Also þe juis and þe poudyr of hi*m* y-made is gode to hele wondys.

1310

Mercurialis

Mercury, papwort, or smere-worte, beryth his sede like bete. Þe juis of this erbe y-dronke clense the stomak of all filthe. Poud*er* of the sede y-dronke clense the stomake of wekkyd humouris. Þe juis of þe erbe w*ith* olde white wyne tempird and stillyd fai*r*e is gode for the ‖ eyne. For a worme cropyn in-to a ma*n*nys ere, hete þ*is* juis and all warme put in-to þe ere.

1315
35ra

Mynte is dry and hote. In drynke hit helpith for to defye, and confortith the stomake, and castiþ oute wormys of þe wo*m*be. Seþe hit in watir and that will helpe all sore ballokys, and hit

1320

1300 capilli Veneris] 118 *written by Hand E after this word.* **1305** morsus diaboli] 119 *written by Hand E after this word.* **1311** mercurialis] 120 *written by Hand E after this word.* **1318** mynte] Menta *written by Hand C in the gap between entries, then* 121 *written by Hand E immediately after.* **1320** seþe hit] þe juis put in þe nose distroyeth þe wormes The poud*er* of it in potage schall make good digestio*n written by Hand C on the outer margin.*

brekyth þe mylke in a womanys pappis. Þe juis and hony done
in þe ere be-nymeth the akynge. Fro[te] the tonge þere-with: Hit
takyth a-way bittirnes. With salt and aysell hit helpith houndes
bitte. Yf a womanys shappe be smerid þere-with ar she dele
with a man she shall not consayue. Washe woundys with þe
iuse: hit sauyth hym from [festerynge].

Mostarde ys dry and hote, & drawiþ oute gle[t]ous humourys.
Set hit to þe hede and he brennyth him wiþ his hete. His moste
streynth is in þe sede. He sharpith þe witt. He mevith þe wombe.
He brekyþe the wombe & makyth vryn. He clansith þe florys.
He castiþ oute evill flewme of | the hede. He confortith þe
stomak. He helith wormes stynge. Temper hit with aysell: hit
helpith the eyne, and þe humerys of the hede, and þe longis, and
stomake, and þe host wher-of the tysik comyth, and olde akynge
of the reynes. Hit drawith oute þe bladder all evill, that is callid
tyasyne yn grewe, and relesith hert swellynge of þe splene and
of the geser, and for all olde evillys of þe body hit helpith. And
for he ys so gode to so many encheysones, lechis deuerse make
plastris þere-with. The maistrys comaundiþ to take mostarde
sede and bete hit to pouder in a morter and þird parte as myche
of crommys of white brede, and dry figis, hony, and aysell as
myche as hit will aske, and make þere-of a plaster and lay to all
evillis that we haue to-for saide. Plenius biddith to take þe sede
and þe rote, and stampe ham with new muste, for when hit is
come to wyne hit is not so gode ne so holsom, and drynke for
the eyne, for þe || splene, for þe stomake, for þe hede. Oyle
made of þe sede is gode to a-noynte the lendys and the synewis
that akith. Þe sede stamped with ale and borys grece doþ to þe
veynes of the nek moche gode, yf hit be a-noynted þer-with.

1322 frote] fro *MS*. **1326** festerynge] fretrynge *MS*. **1327** gletous] glecous
MS.

1327 mostarde] 122 *written by Hand E in the gap between entries.*

1350 The levys and þe stalke y-brent is gode for the fallynge evill. The sede and figis stampid to-gedir beþ gode for that man that havith þe litarge, þat is hevy and sclepy. The sede and barowis gresse growndyn to-geder helpiþ þe lepir yf þei be a-noyntid þere-wiþ, and puttiþ a-way all evill scroffe and scabbe.

1355 Medewort ys of iij manerys and hauyth one vertue, for all ben hote and dry in boþe degreis. The levis dronkyn helith wysillis bytt and venym bytte, and brekiþ in woman that childire is in longe stekyd [if it be drounkyn] wiþ pepir and myr to-geder. Yf þu a-noynte the gomys ther-wiþ hit doþe a-way the stenche of 1360 þe tethe, and þe hardnes of the splene, and akynge of þe sidis. Drinke hit wiþ water: hit helpiþ for þe feuer, and for þe 35vb potagir, | and þe fallynge evill, and for akynge of þe wombe, and helpiþ þe paralityke. The rote y-stampid and laid ther-to clensyth þe fester. Anoynte þe bene-hyve wiþ þe juis and þe 1365 swarme shall neuer fle. Stampe hit and a-noynte þe ther-wiþ and hit helpiþ for waspis bityng, for ben, for attercoppis. The juis þere-of clensith woundys & lousith þe evill of þe joyntes. Stampe hit wiþ stale ale & layde to, hit helyth houndys bitte. Hold hit in þy mouthe: hit helith þe toþe-ake. Plenius saiþe that 1370 iuse helyth þe sight.

Morell. Þe juis þere-of done in erys abatith þe hede-ake. Weshe þe scabbe wiþ þe juis and hit helis. The juis þere-of stanchis þe flux of women yf hit be done in her schappe. Morell, and [blankett], and þe [scome] of siluer, oyle, and rosyn stampid 1375 to-gedyr in a plastyr and laide to helpiþ for the fu de inferne.

1358 if it be drounkyn] drynke hit *MS*.   **1374** blankett] blay *MS*.   scome] setine *MS*.

1355 medewort] 123 *written by Hand E in the gap between entries.*
1371 morell] 124 *written by Hand E in the gap between entries.*

Myllefoly haþe smale raggid levis and many, and for hit ys mylfoly. Some men calliþ h*i*t yarowe. Þe vertu is suche: take || the juis of hi*m*, and of waybred, and þe flour of whete, and makiþ forthe to ete: hit stanchiþ all man*er* of menysou*n*. Put hit in the nose: hit makiþ to blede and delyu*er*þe the hede stopynge. The sede of mylfoly, avance, and centory, in wyne y-vsid delyu*er*eth þe childe of javndys, and makys the gall, & swagith the swelli*ng* of þe dropesy.

Arthemesia

Mogwort ys hote and drye in þe þirde de-gre. Þe ve*r*tu of hi*m* is, stampe hi*m* and late a woman drinke that juis w*ith* wlake wyne in tyme of flo*ur*ys, and that shall make hir conceyue. Also seþe hit and hit helpiþ for þe menstrue, a plast[*er*] y-laide oþ*er* y-dronke in wyne. Also y-dronke hit delyu*er*eth women with childe. Or else put in hir pr*i*uete and that helpiþ þe modir of swellynge & hardnes. And who-so drinkeþ hit with wyne hit is gode for | þe javndis, and that same drynke will make a man well y-collourid. Also make poudyr of hym and of horehound, and strow þ*er*-of apon þe tittis of emerodys, and that shall hele ham. But first late the seke garse hi*m* in þe boþe helys, and after strawe þe poud*er*. And for to delyu*er* a dede childe fro*m* a woman take and make a plaster of mogwort and lay that to þe navill all cold. Also y-dronke he helpith one to pisse and helith

---

1382 gall &] fwagith *deleted after this word.* **1388** plaster] plast *MS.* **1396** to delyuer] To conceyue to ber childe þe mother jandes well colou*r*d tittys of emerodis delyu*er* dede childe stone not be wery clawyng ycchinge hond*is* that quakith *written on the outer margin.*

1376 myllefoly] Millefoliu*m written by Hand C between entries, then* 125 *written by Hand E immediately after.* **1377** take] The jus of milfolie w*ith* wyne or ale stoppeth the flyx *written by Hand C on the lower margin.* **1379** hit¹] bake *written by Hand C over the line.* **1384** arthemesia] 126 *written by Hand E after this word.* **1385** mogwort] or moderwort *written by Hand C over the line.*

grevance of þe stone *in* þe raynes. Also and þ*u* wilt go in any jornaye ber su*m* of this erbe wiþ the, & þ*u* shalt not be wery. Also yf þ*i*s erbe be in an house þ*er* may no wikkyd spirite to bide inne that house. Also stampe [the] gres and that is gode for clowyng & ychchyng of hondis, and yf hit be y-braide w*ith* talowe that helpiþ sore akynge of onys fete. Also poudir of hi*m* y-dronke wiþ luke wat*er* heliþ þe akynge of onys guttis. Also who that drinkeþ hi*m* hit saviþ hym fro all venym ‖ and bytinge of lether bestis. Also stampe hi*m* grene and put þe juis ther-of a-monge muste: that is gode for many evilles, for hit helpith þ*e* stomake and conforte þe harte and inner membris of þ*e* body. Also anoynte the body w*ith* the juis of oyle olyfe iij dayes, and that doþe a-way the feu*er*ys. Also make an oynement of hi*m* and oyle olyfe, and þ*er*-w*ith* a-noynte hondis that quakiþe. Also put hi*m* vndir a seke-manys hede and yf he may slepe he shall lyve, but lat hi*m* not be war*e* of the erbe and but he sclepe e *con*trario.

Mandragora

Mandrake ys an erbe of male and fe*m*malle. Þe male haþe leuys like to bete, þe female haþe levis y-like to letuse. The v*er*tu of this erbe: y-sodyn tellyth yf the rynde of this erbe be y-sodde in wyne and yf to a body for to drynke, hit will make one to slepe so | faste that þey may come to kytt hym and vnneth he may fele ham. Also the juis of this erbe i-temp*er*id w*ith* womanys mylke and y-dronke makeþ one to slepe wondyrly stronge. But hit is for-bode that men shall not take to myche in medicynes, for hit may be cause of onys dethe. This erbe hathe grete streynthe of koldnes and distroyenge of manys kynde. And for this erbe ys so gretly colde the juis of hit sleyth and quenchith wylde fyre. Also hit qwynchithe þe grete brenyng hete of the colre. Also

---

1402 the] and *MS*.

1402 stampe] it *written by Hand C over the line.*   **1415** mandragora] 127 *written by Hand E after this word.*

that same drynke will hele a man of the flux. Placeus saiþ that
this erbe haviþ no man*er* shappe of man ne woman, but hit
takyn in dew tyme and du maner*e* will kele a woman that ys
hote and dispose hir well to consayve a childe; but a woman
that is well disposid hit will distroy yf she vse hit. Also hit will
distroy || all maner swellyng in onys body. Also all venym
bitynge of wormes and bestis this erbe helith. Also for þe hede-
ake bynde the levys to þe templis of the hede, oþ*er* els take oyle
of mandrag and menge hit with oyle olyue, and boyle hame
to-gedyr a litell. Strayne hit þan þrow a cloþe and this callid oyle
of mandragge, that is gode to a-noynte a seke hede and a manys
po[uc]ys that haviþ the feu*er*ys. Also hit is gode to a-noynte at
the begy*n*neng þ*at* hauyth an hote postem. Also poud*er* y-made
of þ*is* erbe ys gode to all medicynes yf hit be medlid w*ith* þe juis
of eny colde erbe, for þis erbe is colde and drye.

Moleyne, oþ*er* tap*er*wort: take þe levys, and bray ham smale,
and fry ham [with] shepis talowe, and þen do hit opon a lyn-
cloþe and, as hote as þe seke may suffyr, lett hi*m* sit | vpon hit
that hauyth the emorodis. And when hit is colde hete hit ayene.
Also þe levis ben gode to saluys.

Melilote, oþ*er* hony-sokyll, oþ*er* þre-levid-grasse, ys i*n* iij
spicis: one yelowe, an-oþ*er* white, and a-noþ*er* black. The juis
of hym ys gode to hele sore eyne, and so beþe all þe spicys of
ham. Also yf the sede ther-of be put a-monge mete, hit shall
make all þe mete sauery and swete. Þ*is* erbe is hote and drye.

1433 distroy] *written on the lower margin.* **1439** poucys] pomys *MS.*
1444 with] *om. MS.* **1446** when hit] Emerodis *written on the outer margin.*
1450 to hele] Sore eyne sau*er*y mete *written on the outer margin.*

1443 moleyne] 128 *written by Hand E in the gap between entries.*
1448 melilote] 129 *written by Hand E in the gap between entries.*

Menta romana

Mynte ther ys of a-noþer kynde: som men calliþ him white mynte. That erbe ys stronge of sauoure, and sum calliþ him horse-mynte for he growiþ in bankys of watrys. The vertu is to sle wormis in the wombe yf the juis be dronke. And þe juis dropid in-to þe nestryllis will sle wormes in the nesse. The pouder ‖ in mete makyth one well to defye. Also the juis of this erbe with warme wyne will sle wormes crop in-to the ere.

Osmunda

Mistilte oþer arbuste growith vpon okys tre and oþere treys. He beryth many branches and bayis. He is gode to distroy the fallynge evill. Also for þe hede-ake take þis juis with oyle of rosis, this erbe stampe hit and bynde hit to þe for-hede. Drynke him iij tymes fastinge for the feuer. He is hote and dry.

Auricula muris

Mowsere growith lowe by the grownde and berith a yellowe floure. Drinke þe juis with wyne oþer ale and a-noynte þe reynes and the bak wiþ the blode of a fox for the stone. Also stampe him and mylfoly to-gadyr and drinke that juis with white wyne, and that will make one to pisse. | Also drinke the juis with stale ale a seke man that is woundid and, yf he holdiþe that

---

1456 of watrys] sle wormys in þe wombe wormes in þe nase *written on the outer margin.* **1459** defye] Sle wermis in þe eris & in þe nese-þrellis *written on the outer margin.* **1463** the fallynge] fallyng evill feuer *written on the outer margin.* **1469** a-noynte] þe stone to pisse to lyfe or dye *written on the outer margin.*

1453 menta romana] 130 *written by Hand E after this word.* **1461** osmunda] 131 *written by Hand E after this word.* **1467** auricula muris] 132 *written by Hand E after this word.* **1471** that juis] The pouder þer-of made in month of may is good for hem þat may not holde theire water. & soo doeth þe pouder of myntes. *written by Hand C on the outer margin.*

drinke, he shall lyfe. And yf he caste hit, he shall dye. Also drinke the juis of this erbe for the squynacy.

Vrtica

Nettyll is hote in þe third de-gre. Þe juis y-dronkyn helpyn a-yene the colde cogh. Also make poudir of him and mell hit with hony, and that helpiþ þe colde of the matryce and þe swellinge of the wombe. Also make a plaster of the levis with salt, and that clansith wondis olde and newe, and that is gode for a wode houndys bytinge. And the levis soden er gode for þe cancre, and hit will helpe to bringe a-yene the fleshe that sleith fro the bone. Also hit drieth al evill humouris. Also bray the rote of hit with vynegir and that helith swellynge of the splene and helpith potager. || Also sethe this erbe in oyle for sore tone yf hit be laide ther-to. Also put the erbe to one-is nosthrill and that will draw blode. And yf þu wilte stanche blode of the nose, stampe this erbe and frett the forhede wel wiþ the juis, and hit shall staunche. Also with wyne i-dronke and hony hit helpith all sore sidis and makyth to pisse. Also þe sede ther-of y-dronke is gode for the fallynge evill. Also this erbe y-sode in wortis that nesheith the wombe. Also þe juis þere-of y-holde in the mouthe will heve vp the strichell. Also seth [in] oile, anoynte a body þer-with, and that will make one swete. Also a-noynte þe hede with this juis and lettiþ the here to fall a-waye. Also for him that lose his speche stampe an vnce of the rede nettill and drinke hit with water. Also for marice of a woman drinke þe juis wiþ wyne. Also stampe þe sede with pouder of pepir, & that wiþ wyne oþer hony: drinke oþer ete of that, and hit will take a-way

---

1486 for sore] for cold cogh to clense woundis wode hounde bytyng cancre stanche blode fallyng evill laxatife strichillis in þe mouþe for speche to let lechery *written on the inner margin.* **1494** in] *om. MS.*

1476 vrtica] 133 *written by Hand E after this word.* **1494** in] the *deleted and* in *written over the line perhaps by Hand C.*

þe will and | the luste of a body, that he haue no luste to lechery. If þu wilt preue hit, yf hit to a beste that is in saute.

Nepta

Nepte ryall, oþer catt-mynte, for cattis will ete hit and stroy hit. Drinke the juis in wyne and hit will make a body to swete strongly. Also sethe hit in oyle and þer-with fret well a man that hauyth þe feuerys, and hit shall put a-way all the colde, and oftymes hit doþe a-way al þe feuerys. And yf a wounde akith sore stampe this erbe and yf him to drinke wiþ wyne, and hit sesith akynge. Also þe same medicyne may caste oute blode of a wounde with-oute lettynge. Also this erbe y-dronke wiþ wyne will distroye al maner of venym. Also hit will a-swage þe grete paynes of þe lepir and hit sleith wormis in one-is wombe. Also he helith þe jaundys and all evillis that is a-boute a body-is throte. And so the sauour of this erbe || dryvith a-way naddrys and oþer venym wormes fro the place. Also y-dronke in wyne he distroyeth the yox. This erbe is hote and drie.

Morella medica

Nyght-shade, oþer pety morell, oþer houndbery, haþe leuys like to d[wa]le, with a litell white flour and a yelow with-inne, and at Our Lady day in harviste hc berith black bayis in clustris and stynkis. The vertu: he is gode to encha[f]e the levir and the mylt

---

1506 sethe hit] To swete for þe feueres for akyng jawndis for wormys for þe yox *written on the outer margin.* **1520** dwale] dawle *MS.* white flour] iche and emerodis *written on the outer margin.* **1522** enchafe] enchase *MS.*

1503 nepta] 134 *written by Hand E after this word.* **1504** catt-mynte] Thys erbe hath leves leke dede netles but þe sauour is moche after mynte *written by Hand C on the outer margin.* **1509** drinke wiþ] Et dicitur nepta facit dentem cadere tactum ipsa *written by Hand C on the outer margin.* **1518** morella medica] 135 *written by Hand E after this word.*

& distroieth akyn[g] of the eryn. Also þe bayes of this erbe ben gode to lay to þe emerodis, for he is colde and dry.

Rapa domestica

Nepis ys hote and drye. Drinke hit in hote muste, hit makiþ men to swete. Anoy[n]te the body wiþ the watir that hit is soden in, Hit a-batith þe accese of flourys, and also akyng of þe reynesse, and drieth vmeris | of þe splene, that is callid delle elefanciasys. As the olifant is more þan any oþer beste, so is the lepir more þan ony other evill. Hit helpith for addir stinge and a-batith venym & sleith all þe wormes in the membris. If þe juis be mengid with salt, hony, and woman with childe drinke hit or do hit in hir shappe, he sleith þe childe in hir wombe. Drinke hit with wyne, hit clensith the wombe. Drinke þe same, hit clensith þe stomake of all filþe. Made in maner of a plaster with wyne he helith black spottis, & all venym wormes þe smyl þere-of sleyth.

Nux muscata

Notemyge is a froite. Hit growith apon a tre in Inde. And he that will well chese this froyte take þat whiche is playne and sumdele hevy, and loke that he be noȝte brokyn with-in and sumdele kene in taste, whiche ben þe beste for medicynes. Take in || the mornyng a notte and, yf hit be a litell not, hit is þe better. Also yf a man holde a notemyge in his nostrill, that confortiþ myche the brayne and all þe spiritis of the body. Also hit will make a manys moþ savery, and dryve oute wekyd wyndis that ben stopid in his body, and distroy the swelling a-boue a bodyes lyuer. This frute is hote and drye.

1523 akyng] akyn *MS.* 1526 hit in] to swete for þe accesse þe splene wormes in þe wombe *written on the outer margin.* 1527 anoynte] Anoyte *MS.* 1540 this] iter. *MS.* 1543 hit be] brayn *written on the outer margin.*

1525 rapa domestica] 136 *written by Hand E after this word.* 1538 nux muscata] 137 *written by Hand E after this word.*

Crassula maior

1550 Orpyn growith in garthynes. Yf he be stampid and laide to a wonde, he will hele that wounde wiþ-‿oute‿ eny helpe.

Origanu*m*

Origanu*m*, oþ*er* broþ*er*-worte, ys in the þerd degre hote and drye. This erbe i-sodde in wyne and ofte y-dronke helpith 1555 venym bityn*g* boþ of wormes and of bestis. Also ete this erbe oþ*er* drynke his juis, and that heliþ all brusynge. Also the poud*er* | made of hi*m* and dronke helpith þe cogh and all man*er* of icching and clawynge. Also the wat*er* that he is soden in y-dronke helith þe jau*n*dyce. Also þe grene juis of this erbe 1560 helpiþ the stricchilys and þe bolwing wombe. Also þe juis of this erbe and cowe mylk put in-to the eris helith all sore of ham. Holde the juis in thi mouthe and that helith sorys of þe mouthe. Also vse hit with white wyne and that makyth gode digestion. Also drinke hit and hit sleith wormes in the wombe and makiþ 1565 gode digestiou*n* and to pisse. Also bray hi*m*, and lay hi*m* to the toþe that akiþ, and that swagith þe sore. Also the juise y-dro*n*ke helpiþ all þe in-warde sekenys. Also stampe hit and drinke hit, that makyth one to swete. Also þe juis w*ith* floure laide to sore sidys heliþ ham. ||

Ostriciu*m*

Ostriciu*m* is hote and drye. The v*er*tu of hi*m* is this: drinke the rote w*ith* wyne and þ*at* helith þe geser and þe swellynge of the

---

1551 wiþ-oute] oute *written over the line.*   **1558** the water] venym bityng ecching clawing jau*n*dis sore of eris *written on the outer margin.*   **1563** digestion] and to pisse *deleted after this word.*   **1570** ostricium¹] *written on the upper margin.*   **1571** drinke the] þe swelling of þe splene breke þe stone þe jau*n*dis dede childe whelk*is* scabbis *written on the outer margin.*

1549 crassula maior] 138 *written by Hand E after this word.*   **1552** origanum¹] 139 *written by Hand E after this word.*   **1570** ostricium¹] 140 *written by Hand E after this word.*

splene. Also hit brekyth þe stone of the bladder, and brekyth oute the flourys of a woman, and helpith to pisse, and a-batiþ the cough, and helith þe jaundis. Also vndirlaide to a womanys privete delyverþe hir of dede childe. Also hit, mengid with vyneger, heliþ the scabbe. Also þe juis and flour of barly, y-laide as a plaster, this helith all postomes of whelkys oþer scabbis. Also put þe juis to þe nose-þrelle, and that helith all þe leþir sorys of the hede, and makeþ a man to fnese.

Oynown[e]is ys an erbe that lechis acorde not all in his vertuis, for som say that he grevith the eyne and the hede. And Galyan saythe | that he is nought gode to þe body that havith sekenys in þe gall, but to flematik men he profitith. Hote in the iij degre and moyste in the fourthe degre. The vertu of this erbe is this: Plenius saith þat hit is gode for the blode wiþ-in a man and makeþ gode colour and nesheth þe wombe. Also stampe hit with hony or vynegre, oþer sethe hit in wyne and with-in þre daies hit will hele the bolwyng of an howndis bytinge and all postomys. Also stampe oynonys, salt, and rewe [to-gedder], and that helith addris bytinge. Also juis of oynonys and womanys mylke y-put in-to a sore ere helithe dyuerse sekenes in þe erys. Also þe juis y-dronke with water helpiþe ham to speke that shortly haþ loste her speche. Also þe juis y-put in the nese-þrellys dryvith a-way evill humouris || of þe hede. Also y-ete oþer y-dronke hit purgith women flouris. Also for hirte fete with frotinge take þe juis of oynon and mell hit with caponys grece and hit helith. Also anoynte one-is tethe erly with þe juis & hit savith ham from akynge. Also al soris with-in the mouthe

1576 with] watir *deleted after this word.*   **1581** oynowneis] Oynowndis *MS.*   lechis acorde] houndis biting sore eris for þe speche for þe fete for þe moiþe emerodis *written on the outer margin.*   **1590** to-gedder] to-gredder *MS.*

1581 oynowneis] 141 *written by Hand E in the gap between entries;* Cepe *added by Hand D on the outer margin.*

1600 Oynon sode in oyle & ete hit w*ith* brede hit helith. Also þe same medicyne helith þe flux wiþ blode. Also þe juis þ*er*-of is gode to a-noynte that place that lackith here. And þei ben gode for stynkyng movthe and leþer appetite. Also stampe hit oþ*er* broyse hit, þei beþ gode to ley to þe emerodis. Also þe juis is gode for
1605 to a-noynte eyne for dyrknes of the sight. Also þe juis w*ith* vynegyr dothe a-way blott*is* yf hit be ofte a-noynte þ*er*-with.

Oy[n]one gresse haþe a rounde more and growiþ myche i*n* bankys of the see. He y-dronke will make a body to caste.
40rb Þis | erbe sodyn in aisell and y-dronk helith þe dropsye. Also
1610 hit helith bityng of naddirs and oþ*er* venym bestis. Hit is hote and drye.

Osmunda

Osmu*n*de, oþ*er* diche verne, will hele brokyn bonys and is gode to salvis h*it*.

1615 ## Oculus *Christ*i

Oculus *Christ*i, oþ*er* wilde worte, oþ*er* scabwort, havith a blew floure and rownde sede. The v*er*tu: yf a man haue a webbe in his eyne or eny oþ*er* sore, take the sede of this erbe and pute o corne in his eye and late h*im* ly downe to slepe. Also in potage
1620 hit makyth a gode stomake and will defye grete metis. Also this erbe will distroye the cardiacle þ*at* genderith of black colour

---

1607 oynone gresse] oytone gresse *MS.*   **1616** a blew] for a webb *written on the outer margin.*

1607 oynone gresse] 142 *written by Hand E in the gap between entries.* **1612** osmunda] 143 *written by Hand E after this word.*   **1615** oculus Christi] 144 *written by Hand E after this word.*   **1617** webbe] or here *written by Hand C on the outer margin.*   **1618** eyne] or oþer mote *written by Hand C over the line.*

oþer flewme, and will opyne þe stoppynge of one-is lyuer, and of the brayne, and of the nase-þrellis. This erbe ys hote and drye.

Paratorum

Paratory, oþer lithwort, other hem[er]worte, is hote and dry || and growith apon wallis. The vertu: for an yl stomake oþer akynge with-in, this erbe y-sodyn in potage helith. Also he is gode to distroye all swellynge that beþ engendrid in ones reynes oþer in a manys pintill. Also he is gode for the stone, for to make a bathe of him. Also boyle him and lay him to þe emrodis.

Pulyoll monten, oþer hilwort, oþer wilde tyme, ys gode to distroye all wekid humouris in the body. And ys a nobill erbe for wondys.

Pygele is hote and drye in that þirde de-gre. Seþe hit in wyne and vse, hit helpith evill bitt. Drinke hit in muste, hit dothe gode for all maner venyme. Drynke hit oþere ete hit, hit is gode for brenynge. Hit castith þe ydrop, and a-batith swellynge and black colour. Hit spurgith flours yf hit be stampid and dronkyn, or hit be washen in watir that hit is soden in. The pouder þere-of and hony | abatithe the cogh and dothe a-way spottis fro the body. The water that hit is sodyn in helpith for the jaundis yf the

---

1625 hemerworte] hemworte MS.   **1626** akynge with-in] stomake reynes pintill stone emrodis *written on the outer margin.*   **1631** oþer wilde] for woundis *written on the outer margin.*   **1632** distroye] nota *written on the outer margin.*   nobill] ere *deleted after this word.*

1624 paratorum] 145 *written by Hand E after this word.*   **1631** pulyoll monten] 146 *written by Hand E in the gap between entries.*   **1634** pygele] 147 *written by Hand E in the gap between entries.*

seke be washen ther-in. The juis helith swellinge chek*is* and, yf þ*u* holde hit longe in thi mouthe, hit helith all wondis with-in þe mouthe. The juis þ*er*-of, hony, and rose, put to-ged*er* like myche yn a basyn and sett in þe hote sonne xl dayes till hit be pouder, and þ*er*-of caste in þe place þ*er* þ*u* haste doute of venym bestis, and all shall flee. Drinke hit [&] wyne to-ged*er* and hit makith gode degestion. The juis, and oyle of rose, and aysell to-gedir y-vsid abatith þe akynge of þe sidis. The juis and hony vsyd abatith þe dryeth of the long*is* that bethe watry. The juis dronkyn in wyne castithe oute venym and helpith all entraulis. The juis is gode for the eyne that ben dym.

Pulyoll is hote and drye in the þirde de-gre. Woman ‖ with childe that etith hit oþ*er* drynkeþ hit delyu*er*eth hir of childe. Dry[n]ke hit w*ith* wyne, hit m*a*keþ hir to haue flouris and brekith þe h[a]yme that þe childe liþe in. Stampe hi*m* w*ith* hony and salt, hit helpith for all evill of the crampe. The poudyr ther-of and hony to-ged*er* y-vsid doþe gode for the breste and maketh caste oute glettis humoris. That sam helith the brenynge of þe stom*a*ke and holdith fomyte. Dronkyn in wyne abatith malencoly & venym. If the seke man fille þrow forse of feu*er*, oþ*er* ovir-myche bledynge, oþ*er* eny sodeyn enchison that lechis calleth maufete, stampe pulioll and vyneg*er* to-gad*er*, and hold hit to his nose that he may haue the sauour, and he shall warishe. Vse hit in poudyr and hit fastith þe gomys. Stampe hit grene and hit helpyþ þe potag*er*, and swagith swellin*g*, and doþe a-way franticles of þ*e* body. Ete hit w*ith* salt, hit helpiþ þe

---

1642 seke] jaund*is* *written on the inner margin.*   **1647** &] ¶ *MS.*
1650 abatith þe] akynge *deleted and expunctuated after this word.*   **1652** that ben] eyne *written on the inner margin.*   **1655** drynke] Dryke *MS.*
1656 hayme] hyme *MS.*   **1666** helpyþ] heliþ *before emendation.*

1647 hit] & *written by Hand C over the line.*   **1653** pulyoll] 148 *written by Hand E in the gap between entries.*

splene. Seþe hit in water and washe þe ther-with, hit sleiþ | the wormys of the body and swagith swellinge of the matrice. Dronkyn in luke-warme wyn abatiþ the cogh and makiþ to make vryn.

Pyany is hote and drye in that oþere de-gre. Drynke hit in muste, hit helpith þe splene. Stampe hit and almondys and vse hit, hit spurgith the flouris and stoppith þe flux of the wombe. Sethe hit in wyne and ofte dronkyn abatith þe akynge of the blader and helpith for the jaundis. The sede dronkyn ofte delyuereth þe childe from þe stone. Galean seiþ that hit helpith children of þe fallyng evill and he telliþ that he sawe a childe of viij wynter olde that was in that evill and was wonyd to ber the branche with the levis, & that savid him & sone aftir he lett that be and a-none he fell wiþ that evill. Men toke of that same erbe and did a-boute his neck and sone he rose vp hole. Diascardias saith that hit is gode boþe to yonge and to olde || to ber vpon ham, oþer drinke hit. Take xv cornys of the sede that is rede and drinke ham when ye gothe to bed. Ther is ij. maner of this erbe, male and female. The rote of the female is many smale branches and that clensith þe womane after she is delyuerd yf she drinke hit in wyne. The rote of the male ys longe, grete, and rownde, and that helpiþ to all oþer þinges aforsaide. Ete euery day v cornes of þe sede fastynge, hit helpith a man fro the palsy. Stampe hit and menge hit with watir & put hit in the mouthe of the man that has loste his speche sodeynly, and shall speke sone.

1674 flux of] Splene jaundis stone Falling evill palsy loste his speche *written on the outer margin.* **1681** that¹] the *before emendation.* **1682** vp] a *deleted after this word.* hole] Diaca *deleted after this word.*

1672 pyany] 149 *written by Hand E in the gap between entries.* **1673** þe splene] þe mawe & þe reynes of all diseases *written by Hand C on the outer margin.* **1680** &²] *written by Hand B on the outer margin.*

Papauer

Papy is hote and drye and ben of iij manerys. The first ys white, þe seconde ys black, þe þerde is rede. Some men calliþ hit chessboll. Þe white flouris ys best of all. Take þe tendryn[s] of the hede and shere hit lightly of the vtmost hyde and ther comith | oute mylke. Kepe that mylke for hit is gode for many medicynes. That oþer the floure is rede and men makiþ oyle of the sede, that is gode for to ete and makeþ men to slepe. The þirde is blak and yevith gode odure yff hit be dronkyn. The man that drinkiþ one of þis þre that is seke, oþer weshid his hede ther with one of ham, he shall slepe but yf that deth be him ney. The sede of the black, dronkyn in wyne, stanchith þe wombe and þe flux of þe woman, and hit makiþ him slepe and abatith evil coȝ. And a penny-wight shall men take at onys of the sede, and who-so takiþ more hit norshith þe evill that men calliþ þe litergy. The levis of hit made in a plaster sleyth the fire of helle. The white papy is better þan þay oþer two. When that tendryn hathe flourys with mylk, þen take þu ham and seþ ham in water, and þe þirde parte hony and that reseyvid ys gode || for many thingis, and makiþ men to slepe, and batiþ the coȝ, and stroiethe the [w]omme, and dryeth the reynes. Take my[l]ke þer-of and oyle of rose & a-noynte thi hede þer-with, and hit takith a-way the akynge and makiþ a man to slepe. Put sauery ther-to and hit makiþ a man to slepe the bettir. Take that mylke and womannys

---

1696 tendryns] tendrynge *MS*.   **1704** the sede] slepe *written on the inner margin*.   wombe and] flux *written on the inner margin*.   **1705** and hit] for akyng *written on the inner margin*.   **1708** of hit] Slepe *written on the inner margin*.   **1713** womme] romme *MS*.   mylke] myke *MS*.

1693 papauer] 150 *written by Hand E after this word*.   **1694** white] slepe [slepee, *then emended*] flux for womanys pappes slepe *written by Hand B on the outer margin*.   **1702** is seke] or stampe hit with oyle & anoynt þe temples. *written by Hand C on the outer margin*.   **1711** gode] resset ys good *written by Hand B on the lower margin*.

mylke to-gedir w*ith* savoray, puttiþ a-way the hote potogary.
And a-noynte women papis þ*ere*-with, hit makiþ ham slepe.

Pasti[nac]a domestica

Pastyrnepe is an erbe þat som men callith pasnepe. The v*er*tu of
hi*m* is only in his rote and in his sede. Take þe rote of hi*m* &
braid, & sod, and y-dronk the brothe, that helpiþ the splene, the
mawe, and the lendys. Also the rote i-sodd in mylk ys gode for
hi*m* that castiþ myche. Also the | rote y-bore with a body savith
hi*m* of stynge of s*er*pentis. And yf a man bere hit, hit kepiþ for
swellyng of ballokys. Also rubbe tethe with the rote and that
sesythe akynge of ham. Also sethe the rote in wyne and drynke
that for styngyng of venym worm*is*. And that drynke woll
aswage þe grett wombe of a woma*n* that semyth w*ith* childe.
Also stampe the rote and mell h*it* w*ith* hony, and that helith the
cankyre. Also drynke hi*m* & that helith akyng in onys mylt, and
of his sidis. And yf a man haue the flux, take the rote of this
erbe and seþ hi*m* in mylke and drinke that. Also y-fried in oyle
hit is holsome and stirryth a body to lechery.

Arnoglossa

Playnteyn, oþ*er* waybrede, is colde and dry in the þirde de-gre.
Stampe hym w*ith* ‖ hony and he clensith wete woundis and hory
and heliþ. Also y-sod w*ith* salt, as wort*is* in vyneg*er*, that
restreyneth the flux of þe wombe. And stampe hit and y-laid to
that stopith renynge blode. Also hit helith black blott*is*. Also the

1719 pastinaca domestica] pastita MS.   **1725** serpentis and] splene for casti*ng*
for swelling of þe ballok*is* toþe ake grete wo*m*be of wome*n* þat semi*th* w*ith*
childe canker*e* flux *written on the outer margin.*   **1737** woundis and] wond*is*
flux breny*ng* soris hou*n*dis byting*e* tetteris dropsy þe mouþe eris toþe-ake ters
þe feue*r*ys bochis whelkys kerving*is* of þe wombe *written on the outer margin.*

1718 slepe] And w*ith* þe jus anoynt þe py*m*ples aboue the ighen *written by Hand C after this word.*   **1719** pastinaca domestica] 151 *written by Hand E between the Latin heading and the ME text.*   **1735** arnoglossa] 152 *written by Hand E after this word.*

juis of him and oyle of eryn helpith to all brennyd sorys. Also he will hele al houndis bytinge y-dronke, and all maner venym bytynge & swellynge, & with salt he distroyeth teterys. Also y-sode as wortis and ete that heliþ the dropsye. And y-dronke hitt helpith for þe fallyng evill and for ham that ben lunatike. Also þe juis of him heliþ the foule sore of the mouthe. Also he helith the pipe if the juis be holde longe in the mouthe. Also y-stampid and laide to he helith all w[e]r[k]ys of the eris and þe vretyng evyll. Also y-dronke that heliþ | ham that spitt blode. Also with aysell and hony hit heliþ the tisik. Also hit helith the swelling and the hete of the eyne. Also chew this erbe and that makiþ the fleshe a-boute þe gomes clene and puttiþ a-way toþe-ake. Also i-sodde and y-dronke in wyne with tansy stanchith þe menstrue. And yf þe modir purge to fele, stampe the juis and put in hir priue membris. Also þe sede of him to all þingis aforsaid, and to the sorys of the bladder, and to þe reynes þe same medicynes helpith. Also the rote y-bore aboute one-is nek will kepe him fro tetterys. Also take iij rotis of this erbe and put þer-to iij soppis of wyn and iij soppis of water, and yf that to drynk to him þat [haþe] þe feuerys or þe quakynge com, and hit shall not greue hym the tercian. Also iiij rotis of this erbe and iiij sopis of wyne || and iijj sponys of watir for to drink hit helith þe feuer quarteyn. And þe lesse playnteyn i-callid rubwort may do all þes vertues aforsaide. Also juis of playnteyn with neshe woll will hele all the bochis and whelkys that wexith in þe face and all a-boute þe eyne and in ix dayes shall be newid. Also rub the wombe with þe juis and that sleith wormis in onys body. Also a plaster þer-of and of olde swynys grece helith swellynge of woundys. Also drinke þe juis ij ana for the quakyng of the feuer and that shall hele þe quarten. Also yf the juis till a woman in trauayll to drynke wyth wyne, and that shall delyuer

1748 werkys] wrys *MS.* **1750** hit heliþ] ham that spit blode *expunctuated.* **1760** haþe] *om. MS.* **1767** the] the the *MS.* **1768** olde] grece *deleted after this word.* **1770** þe] quaking *deleted after this word.*

hir of the seco[n]d borþen. Also stampe him and vyneger and lay that to all sore fete for trauayll. Also þe juis of him y-dronke ys gode for the passyon in the bladder. Also | the rote of plantoyne ys as gode dry as grene. And yf a body haue the hede-ake, honge þis erbe a-boute his neke and he shall be hole. Also the sede of this erbe made in pouder let springe þer-of in-to a wounde and that helith with-oute payne. Also yf a body be neshe in þe wombe, take x peny-wight of þe juis and temper hit with aysell oþer wyne and drinke hit, and he shall be harde y-nowe. Also ete this erbe & he distroieth all maner venym and styng of naddrys. Also yf a man haue eny potager oþer swellynge in his synews, ponde þe levis of this erbe with a litell salt and to that place. Also yf ther beþe eny woundys oþer eny swellynge sore be by one-is eyne oþer by his nose, take the juis of this erbe and softe woll and washe þe sore ix dayes ther-with medicina vt supra. Also he stanchith þe menisoun boþ in drynke and wiþ plaster y-made with || pouder of Armany, and sa[nk]e dragon, and of barly mele, with white of eggis y-leide to the wombe as a plaster. Also seþe him in watir and washe all þe mouthe ther-with þat is sore and hit helith him. Also drinke þe juis of him for bledyng at þe nose. Also stampe him & with þe juis a-noynte all sore akynge and hit sesith. The juis and venegir, hony, and pouder alym helith þe cankyr in the mouthe. The juis of hym and juis of letuse y-temperid with aysell, a plaster y-made and laide to þe right side, þis helith þe jaundys with-outyn doute and hit be oftyme y-vsid.

Petrocillium

Persely ys hote in the þirde degre. The vertu of him ys that þe sede of him vnbyndyth dyuerse wyndes in þe medicyne. Also hit clensith the menstrue. Also make | a plaster ther-of and hit helith þe scabbe and teterrys. Also he is gode for þe dropsy.

1772 second] secomd MS. **1789** sanke] saule MS.

1798 petrocillium] 153 *written by Hand E after this word.*

And he clensith þe lyuer, and helpiþ the reynes, and þe sore of
þe bladder. Also all bilis an[d] welkys on a bodyes leggis þis
erbe helith. Also stampe and put hit to a womanys priuete, that
bringith oute hir flouris and dede childe of þe secounde borþen
of a woman. And yf a woman drinke þe juis, that shall clense
the childe with-in and the stomake wlatynge. Sethe percell,
hokkys and marche with wortis and that makiþ gode digestioun.
Also wortis off percill and of coule is gode for sidys, and to þe
reynes, and to all in-warde euyllys. Also yf one be bytt with an
naddyr, take a dram, that is a peny-wight of the pouder of this
erbe, and yf to drinke, and hit heliþe hym, but stampe ‖ the erbe
and ley ther-to. All hit is gode to distroy the cardiakyll. Also for
the stone drinke þe sede or ete hit and hit esiþ myche. Also this
erbe distroyeth the coȝ and hit multiplyeþ blode. He stroyethe
the tysike and þe feuer tercian. He comfortiþ þe stomak and the
harte ofte vsyd.

Piretum domesticum

Pelletir ys a gode erbe for grene sause. The vertu of him ys this:
iff a body haue þe toþe-ake, chewe this erbe and hit sese akynge.
Also yf one haue þe pallesy in his tonge, chew well þis erbe and
he shall fare well. Also yf one haue þe feuerys, ley this to his
breste er that þe axcesse come. Also sethe him in vyneger and
after medill hym with oyle of rose and anoynte the hede þere-
with, and hit doþe a-way the hede-ake. Also he that etith þere-
of dar not dred venym wormys. Also all venym bytinge hit
stroiþe | yf hit be dronke and þe erbe y-stampid and laide to.
Also hit makiþ one to pisse and, mellid with vinegre and laide
to, hit helith þe splene. And drinke hit with wyne, hit make
norysis to haue plente of mylke. Pyretum is hote & drye in þe

---

1804 and] an *MS.* **1816** multiplyeþ] multiplyeþe *before emendation.*

1819 piretum domesticum] *id est.* pinedoke *written by Hand C over the line, then* 154 *written by Hand E between the Latin heading and the ME text.*
1820 pelletir] *id est* peleter comen *written by Hand C over the line.*
1831 hote &] Peleter of Spayn *written by Hand C on the outer margin.*

Lelamour Herbal 191

iiij degre. He ys gode for the body hauyng cold in his teþe to holde and chewe in his mouþe. Also w*ith* aysell i-holde hote in the mouthe doþ a-way flewme and bolowyng of þe tonge and helpith oþ*er* sorys of þe mouthe. Also w*ith* hony y-dronke hit helpith for þe fallyng evill, oþ*er* hong piretu*m* a-boute a childes nek and hit sauyth hi*m* from the same evill. Also þe oyle that hit is sod in ys gode to a-noynte one w*ith* er*e* the acces com, and that oynement ys gode for þe renys and the palsy. 1835

Ligustru*m*
Prymerose is gode i*n* potage. Also yf a manys pyntyll || be swell and akiþ, stampe þ*i*s erbe and ley ther-to and hit helith. Also þe juis of þis erbe and of cowesloppe y-like myche put in a pen, and þ*a*t y-blawe in-to the nose-þrill for the mygrane, and hit puttiþ a-way þe pose, and þe rewme, and evill stoppyng of þe hede. Also yf one haue loste his speche sodenly, put þe juis of p*r*imerose in his mouthe & he shall speke. Also þ*e* flours of hi*m* makith yolowe toþe white. Also þe juis of hi*m* i-dronke is gode for sore of þe bowell*is*. Also he esithe þe toþe-ake. 1840 44va 1845

Eleborus
Pedelyon, oþ*er* clofe-tonge, ys hote and drye and berith a yelew flour. And yf one ˬchewe˯ hym, he will bite angrely. The v*er*tu of hi*m*: is gode for a skallyd hede, for he will fret well dede 1850

1852 chewe] bite *deleted, then* chewe *written over the line.*

1840 ligustrum] 155 *written by Hand E after this word.*   **1841** potage] a pyntyll *written by Hand B on the outer margin.*   be swell] The rotes of hit sode in water & þe wat*er* þ*er*-of dronke colde on eve & warm*e* on mornyng*es* clereth þe voyce *written by Hand C on the outer margin.*   **1850** eleborus] 156 *written by Hand E before this word,* niger *written by Hand C after this word.*   **1851** pedelyon] Thys elebor*us* niger is leke to elebor*us* alb*us id est.* longeworth but þe leves þ*er*-of is nat slytte as ben þe leves here-of. & þ*i*s herbe hath a v*er*ie blacke rote. *written by Hand C on the outer margin.*   **1852** flour] breder then a peny *written by Hand C over the line.*   **1853** for a] For a skallyd hede for dede flesch *written by Hand B on the outer margin.*

fleshis. Also a beste that pissith blode yff hym this erbe a-monge oþere | gresse and he shall be hole. Also make pouder of hym and mell that weth grewyll oþer with mele of whete, and þat will sle rattys.

Ippia maior

Pympirnell, oþer [wa]yworte, oþer wolshele, oþer kennyngworte, goþe a-longe by the grond and he beryth a rede sangwyne colour. The vertu of him ys, yf a worme hafe bitte on, drinke þe juis of þis erbe and hit will distroye all þe venym. And þe same erbe will hele a man of þe postem. Also he ys gode to hele woundys. Also drynke hym, and brekiþ the webb in a bodyes eye. Also drynke hym with rewe and rede wyne ofte, and that kepiþ one fro sekenys.

Pes pulli

Portulake is an erbe that is moiste in the thirde degre and [colde] in þe secounde. || He helith þe hote feuerys yf he be braide and y-do opon þe stomak. Also drinke the juis oþer ete the erbe in wortis, hit doþ þe vertu a-boue saide. Also y-ete or i-dronke hit stanchithe þe blody flux and swagith þe hete of the wombe. Also teþe that ben an eghe chew þis erbe and hit shall a-wey a-none. Also y-stampid and laide to hit helpith for swellynge of eyne. Also y-hette hit letteþ the hete of þe sone to noy a body. Also with salt and wyn hit makiþ the wombe neshe. Also hit is gode to men that spetiþ blode. Also ete hit and that doþe a-way

---

1859 wayworte] yworte *MS.*   **1866** and...kepiþ] and þat kepiþ and þat kepiþ *MS.*   **1868** colde] *om. MS.*

1854 yff hym] sle rattys *written by Hand B on the outer margin.*   **1858** ippia maior] 157 *written by Hand E after this word.*   **1861** colour] and leves leke to chekwede *written by Hand C over the line.*   **1864** gode] nota *written by Hand C on the inner margin.*   **1866** sekenys] Et dicitur quod facit vera responsa haberi portanti ad interrogationes sue *written by Hand C after this word.*   **1867** pes pulli] 158 *written by Hand E after this word.*

sorys of the bladd*er*. And in so þe h*i*t havith þe same v*er*tuys that hathe þe souredok that comeþ after.

Policaria

Polycary ys an erbe that ys like to ferne, and hit havith a smale floure and | su*m*dell rede and a stalke full of brau*n*ches, and he beryth coddis w*ith* sede. The stalke and þe levis bethe somdell rede and he growith in watry plac*is*. The v*er*tu of this erbe ys that he will comford a bodyes stomak yf he be y-dronke. Also who-so vsithe hi*m* myche in poud*er* he stirry a body to lechery. Also yf he be dronke hit is gode for the black colo*ur*.

P[s]iliu*m*, þe erbe som men saithe policarya. Þe sede [of] this erbe is colde in the first de-gre and moiste in þird degre. The v*er*tu of hi*m* ys that he ys a gode plaster for bren*n*y*n*g synowys. Also he quenchith grete thurste and hetis. Also take þis erbe and oyle of rosys w*ith* aysell, stampe hit to-ged*er* and make a plaster, and that will hele postomes opon the tonge and apon þe fete. Also take þis erbe and ronde astrologi, betony, and savyne, || boyle this in wyne and drink the wyne, and that helith a sekenys that lechis callith fustula, that is in the pipis of a manys breste.

Polipodiu*m*

Polipody, oþ*er* oke-verne, for he ys like vnto verne þ*at* grow*ith* vpon okys. This erbe ys gode to clense black colour and þe

1888 psilium] philiu*m* MS. of] om. MS. 1891 grete] hete *expunctuated*.
1894 astrologi] *underlined in red as a lemma.*

1880 policaria] 159 *written by Hand E after this word.* 1888 psilium] 160 *written by Hand E in the gap between entries.* 1895 the wyne] helith a seke-nes þ*at* lechis callith fustula *written by Hand B on the outer margin.* 1896 of a] .no*t*a. *written by Hand B on the outer margin.* 1898 polipodium] 161 *written by Hand E after this word.*

grete flewme. Also yf a man be laxatife, take a fatte hen and stofe hir w*ith* þ*i*s erbe small y-c[h]oppid and lett that boille well. But bett*er* ys to grynde the erbe smale, þan stufe hir with þis erbe and freshe grece a gode quantyte, boyle till þe birde be tend*ir* and let one drinke of that brothe as hote as he may.

Pes arietis

Ram-ys-fote ys an erbe þ*at* is like to crowe-fote and su*m* men calliþ hi*m* lode-worte, and beryth a yelowe floure as dothe crowe-fote, so a man shall haue | vnneth knawleche whiche is crowe-fote oþ*er* ra*m*mys-fote. But this ra*m*mys-fote hathe a knobe in þe rote and he grow*ith* myche in harde grownde. The v*er*tu of hym ys for to drawe a goute to whate place of the body that ye will haue hym. And þ*er*-for yf hit be the toþe-ake and come of þe gowte, take this erbe w*ith* þe rote and sta*m*pe hi*m* w*ith* spettill of a manys mouthe, take that in your hond and begyn at the cheppe that is sor*e*, and drawe so a-down for þe vndir the chyne opon þe nakyd fleshe, and so do alonge the arme of þe same side till þu com to þe ureste of the honde, and þ*er*e bynde hit all that nyght. On the morow þ*u* shalt fynde ther a bladder. Late oute þe wynde or þe wat*er* of hym and hele hit vppe w*ith* salue and so w*ith* this erbe vt sup*r*a.

Rappan[us]

Radich is an erbe that haþe a grete rote wonder strong ‖ in etynge. He beryth a white flour. The v*er*tu of this erbe is that he ys gode to hele bochis i[n] a manys mouthe. Also he will putt a-way akynge in þe wombe and in the stomak. Also yf a body haue an hard mylt and a sore, boyle this erbe in wyne and oyle

---

1902 y-choppid] y cloppid *MS.*   **1922** rappanus] rappaner *MS.*   **1925** in] i *MS.*   will] pull *deleted after this word.*

1906 pes arietis] 162 *written by Hand E after this word.*   **1922** rappanus] 163 *written by Hand E after this word.*

and make þer-of a plaster and lay that to his side, and he shall be hole. This erbe is hote and drye.

Ragworte, oþer fly-fo, berithe yelowe flouris like tansy and stynkith foule. The vertu of hym is, stampe hym & marche like myche to-gedir. Take flour of whete, hony, mylke, shepis trodlys, and shepis tallowe. Fry þes to-geder, þan strayne hit in-to a box. Let this be done in þe ende of maye and this is souerayne for to sle any felon or whate rysynge be by onys nose or any oþer place of his body.

Lanceolata

Rybwort, oþer launcell, woll hele þe cankyr and woundis. Also all þe vertues that playnton | may do þe same, vt supra de vertutibus planteyn.

Solsequium

Rodewort, oþer marygoldye, yf a man be bit with any venym beste oþer worme, hit heliþ him yf he ete hit. Also yf a body be stopid a-boute the lyuer, drink þe juis of this erbe and he shall a-mend. Also this erbe haviþ mo vertues as endyue haþe, vbi supra.

Rewe ys hote and drye & dothe gode to the stomake. Hit doþe a-way conseyvyng. Hit castiþ oute lechery. Hit spurgiþ the

---

1940 vertutibus planteyn] *written beyond the margin-line.* **1942** venym] venyn *before emendation.* **1946** vbi supra] *written beyond the margin-line.*

1930 ragworte] .nota. *written by Hand B in the gap between the lines, then* 164 *written by Hand E immediately after.* **1937** lanceolata] 165 *written by Hand E after this word.* **1938** rybwort] .nota. *written by Hand B on the inner margin.* **1941** solsequium] 166 *written by Hand E after this word.* **1947** rewe] 167 *written by Hand E in the outer margin.*

flourys. Hit a-batith þe cogh. Yf hit be soden in water and in aysell hit helpith for gryndi*n*g of þe wombe. Hit helpe the long, and þe breste, and the sidys. Take rwe and oyle of rosys and a-noynte the seke or þe accesse comythe, and hit shall passe & that oynement helpith þe archangeles that is curnelid fyngris. That same doþe gode to a woman yf hit be put in hir shappe w*ith* a dosell that is callid enclyse. Rew & cromyn sodyn in || wyne, this [is] gode for þe dropsy. The juis of rewe and of rose and eysell helpith þe hede for akynge. The juis of rewe in the nose-þryllys stanchith blode, and put law in the erys, a-batiþ þe hede-ake. The juis of rew, of rose and of aysell done to-gedir as an oyneme*n*t doþ a-way the hote scabbe and bilys rennand of quyter, and for the hede and for the nose stynkande. Rewe oue*r*comyth venym. The kynge Perys taȝte one to take xx levis of rewe and ij vnc*es* of figis, and þ*er*e-of ete eue*ry* day fastynge, and that shall distroy all venym in mete and in drinke and that day shall don none harme. Hit helpith for the wesyll bitt. Rew sodyn in but*ter* and done in womanys shappe amendith the evill that is w*ith*-in the body. That oynement w*ith* levis of lorrey swagith the ballok*is* that ben*e* swellyd.

Rosse ys floure of all flourys. Hit is colde and dry in the fyrste degre. Hit helpith to the | fu de inferne and to brenyng of the stomak and of entraly[s]. Drynkyn in wyne hit revith þe flux of þe womanys shapp*e* and þe wombe. The po[u]dir ther-of helpith the mouthe. Rede roses sesyth all brenynge jyf hit be stampid wiþ hony. Oyle made of rose leues ys gode to many medycynes. If þ*u* drinke hit, þ*at* helpiþ þe wombe and a-batiþ*e* myche hete

1956 is] *om. MS.* **1971** entralys] entraly *MS.* **1972** poudir] podir *MS.*

1957 the nose-þryllys] stanchith blod*e* þe hed*e*-ake *written by Hand B on the outer margin.* **1960** the hote] the hote scabbe *written by Hand B on the outer margin.* **1967** oynement] oynement *written by Hand B on the outer margin.* **1968** swagith] For*e* ballok*is* *written by Hand B on the outer margin.* **1969** rosse] 168 *written by Hand E in the gap between entries.*

of þe stomake, and wiþ aysell he helid myche akyng and brenyng of the hede. Hit is gode for the brynnyng of the fyr. Holde hit longe in the mouþe, hit a-batith þe toþe-ache. Hit helpiþ þe eye-breri*s* that ben harde yf they be a-noynted þer-with. Palydius techith one to make oyle off rede rose on this man*er*: thou shalt take su*m*-whate of roysyng, and an vnc*e* of oyle olyfe, and a pounde of rose, and stoppe to-ged*er* in a fessell of glasse, and honge hit vij dayes in the hote sonne. And that ys callid oyle of rosys.

Rose-mary. Take the flouris of || the rose-marye, and bynde hym in lynclothe, and seþ hi*m* in clene water vnto halfyndell, and drynke þe water, and hit shall hele a man of all man*er* sekenys. Take þe levis of that erbe, and seþe ham in wyne, and washe þi face, þi berde, þy brewys, and þine hede, and þi here shall not fall a-way & hit shall make þy face white and clere. Take the flour of þe erbe, and dry hi*m*, and make poud*er* of hi*m*, and put hit vnd*ir* þi right arme-hole in lynyn cloþe, and þ*u* shalt be light and mery as longe as þei ben þer*e*. Take þe stalkys of þ*e* erbe, and bren ham, and make þ*er*-of colis and bynde hym [in] clene lyncloþe, and rubbe þi teþe, and þei shall be white, and sle the wormes in the teþe. The ryndys of the erbe take and lay ham vpon colys so that hit smoke, and holde [o]u*er* thi nose, & that is gode medicyne for the colnes þ*at* is y-take on the hevede. Take þe rotis of the erbe, | and put ham in vynag*er*, and washe þi fete þere-in, and þ*u* shalt haue streynth in thi leggis & hele. Take the lefe of this erbe and do hi*m* vnd*ir* þi bedd, and þ*u* shalt haue no meting. Take þ*is* erbe and ete hym fastinge wiþ brede and hony, and þ*u* shalt haue no swelli*ng* nothir bo[cc]his. Make a baþe of hym and styve þe þ*er*-in, and hit shall make the seme

1985 the rose-marye] for all man*er* sekenes *written on the upper margin.* **1994** in] *om. MS.* **1997** ouer] eu*er MS.* **2003** bocchis] botthis *MS.*

1985 rose-mary] 169 *written by Hand E in the gap between entries.*

2005 yonge, and make the haue vertu and streynth þat þu hadest bifor, and hit confortith all thi lymes. Take þe levis of this erbe, and stampe hem, and lay ham apon a cancre, and hit shall sle him. Take þe erbe and stik him ovir a dor, and þer ne shall non adder done none harme ne oþer wekyd worme to none of the
2010 house. Take þe levis and put hem in a ton of wyne, and hit shall not torne to no vyneger ne oþer evill savour till hit be opende.
47va Take þe stalkis of þe erbe, and make þere-of a vessell, || and put þere-in wyne, and late stonde longe ther-in, and vse that wyne, and þu ne shalt drede of none postem and hit distroieþ all maner
2015 evillis in man and woman-is body. Yf þu be febill be way of sweting, take the levis of this erbe and seþ ham in water, and with þe water washe þine hede and þu shalt be delyuerd of sweting and for þe cogh. And yf þu puttiste this erbe in thi gardyne and kepist hit euer fresh, hit shall make all þi gardyne
2020 ber well his frute. Also yf a man may note ete, take þe levis of that erbe wiþ wyne and water, and make þere-in soppis of brede, and ete þe soppis, and þu shalt haue gode appetide to þi mete. If þu haue þe flix, take þe levis of this erbe and seþe hym in stronge vinegre, and when thei ben y-sod well bynde ham to
2025 þine wombe, and a-none þe flux shall stanche. Also yf a body
47vb be oute of his witt, take þe levis of | this erbe, and seþe hame in water, and washe ther-with his hede, and he shall be hole. The erbe wiþ his levis & þe flouris make ham smoke in an naddyr-is hole and þe adder shall dye in the hole. Iff a manys lemys beþe
2030 y-swell be the way of goutis, take þe levis of this erbe, and seþe ham in water, and take þe levis all hote, and lay to þe sore, and he shall be hole. For stomake that is hote by eny cause oþer that þu soferist þorst, take þe levis of this erbe and seþ ham in water, and whan he is hote medell hym with a pomigarnet and vse hit
2035 ofte, and þu shalt fare well. Take this erbe and do amonge cloþes and he savith hem from mothis. Take þe floure of this erbe, and seþe him in water, and yf him to drink that haþe the tysik, eiþer ete þe levis and he shall be hole. Take þe erbe while
48ra he hathe the flour and his levis || full of dewe, and still hym, and

take the water, and a-noynte thi face and thi body, and ye shall seme yonge & lenthe þi lyfe. Take the flo*ur* of this erbe, and sethe hym in gotis mylke, and let hym stond all nyght, and yf hi*m* to drinke that hathe the tisike, and he shall fare well. Take the stoke of this erbe and make þere-of a spone, and the mete that þu etiste ther-w*ith* shall do the gode. Amen.

Savory is hote and drye. The juis with wyne he makyth vryn and clensiþ the flouris and castiþ oute abortive of a womanys entrayles. The poud*er* of h*i*t, and hony, and wyne sodyn to-ged*er* makiþ caste oute glett y-holde yn the brest þrow spvyng. Drynke hit in lowe wyne, hit swage the grynd*ing* in the wombe. Sethe sau*ery* in water and washe the hede | ther-w*ith*, hit doþe a-way the hede akynge and that ys gode for literge, þ*at* is evill that makeþ men to slepe till þay dye. Woman that etiþ hit with childe, hit distroieþ that childe and sleyth hit. Drynke hit wiþ hote wyne, hit a-batith castinge; and yf þ*u* drinke myche there-of and vse hit, soþly hit movis lechery. Vse sauery, hony, and pepyr to-gadir & that makith brennand in lechery.

Sawyn ys hote & drye. H*i*t an[d] hony mengid to-gedris drieth woundys and clensith ham of filth. Savayn dronkyn in wyne drawith oute flouris and spillith conseyvynge yf the skape be washen w*ith* the juis. Sethe saveyn in hony oþ*er* in water and washe þe hede, hit slakiþ the hede-ake & sleithe the nytys þer-on. An autor of medicyne co*m*mau*n*deþ to take saveyn, and canell, || and hony, and do hit a medicyne for the hede-ake: for

---

2046 the juis] to cast out glat *in* þe brest for þe hede-ache to sle a childe *in* a woman *written on the inner margin*.   **2058** and] an MS.   to-gedris] to drye and clense wou*n*dis þe hede-ake *written on the outer margin*.

2046 savory] 170 *written by Hand E in the gap between entries.*
2058 sawyn] 171 *written by Hand E in the gap between entries.*

2065 to seþe hit in watir and washe the ovy[r]-hede w*ith* þe wat*er*, and of the erbe make a plast*er* and lay hit to the tempill*is* and the forhede.

Savygill ys hote and dry in nature. The rote y-sta*m*pid and [dronkyn] in wyne helpith for the geser, and for the jaundis, and
2070 for the hard swellyng of the splene. And on that ilke man*er* hit brekith þe stone. Hit stirreth þe flour*is*, and helpith for the cogh, and delyu*er*eth women of dede child and, yf she do hit in hir shapp*e*, hit lousith flour*is* that longe ben hardyd in hir body. Þe juis, and vinegre, and flour of ber*e*, made in a plaster, clensiþ
2075 the lepir and a-batith well akynge wher*e*-to he is layde. The juis and hony to-gad*er* y-vsid spurgith all evill humouris of the
48vb hede. Caste of | the same in thi nose and hit will make a man to nese. The juis and womanys mylke helith children*e* fro the jaundys of eyne.

2080 Sagge ys of ij man*er*, tame and wilde. The wilde ys callid ambros, oþ*er* eupatorye, and boþe ben v*er*tus yn medicyne. Take þe juis of þe tame sauge and drink w*ith* wyn, hit helpith þe mawe. Hit castiþ owte abortyue and purgith the flourys. Stampe hit in man*er* of plaster w*ith* shepis talowe, hit helith venyme.
2085 But þe levis stampid and layde to þe bledyng wou*n*dis hit

---

2065 ovyr-hede] ovyn hede *MS.* **2068** savygill] savygill *MS.* in nature] for jau*n*dis for the splene for þe co3 þe lepyr*e* fo[r] þe jaund*is* of eyne *written on the outer margin.* **2069** dronkyn] dronking *MS.* **2077** of] of of *MS.* **2080** wilde ys] to sta*n*che bledyng wou*n*dis þe cou3 and tesik ache in onys sidis to make þe here black þe axes hele wou*n*dis *written on the inner margin.* **2084** venyme] venyne *before emendation.*

2068 savygill] 172 *written by Hand E in the gap between entries.* **2080** sagge] w *written over the line by Hand B with a caret before* gg, *then* 173 *written by Hand E in the gap between entries.* **2083** flourys] and is good for the dropese *written by Hand C over the line.* **2085** but] the poud*er* or *written by Hand C over the line.*

stanchith ham. Drinke the juis w*ith* hote wyne, and hit dothe a-way the cogh, & openyth þe voise, and brekithe the tisyke and þe akyng yn onys sydis. The juis dronke in wyne oþ*er* anoynte þe woma*n*ys shapp*e*, that doþe a-way the sore þ*er*-of and of manys pyntill. a-noynte thi hede wiþ the juis || and hit makiþ thi here black. Ete eu*er*y day sauge fasti*n*g and vse hit in thi drinke. Sage stampe hit and þe juis dronkyn ys gode for the lyu*er* and swagith the hardnes ther-of. The erbe stampid w*ith* olde wyne and layde to wondys hit helpith ham. Ete that erbe oþ*er* drinke þe juis þ*er*e-of or þe accesse com, and hit shall noughte greue the.

49ra

2095

Irios

Safe ys like to flour delys. He grow*ith* in wat*er* and beryth a white flour. He will hele the akynge of synewes and distroy the cogh. The juis y-dronke wiþ wyne hit distroieth the humouris that ben wekyd of one-ys breste, and hit helpiþ the bitynge of venym wormes and bestis, and heliþe the crampe. Also the juis of this erbe y-dronke delyu*er*eth a woman of dede | childe.

2100

49rb

Crocus

Safur ys holsom for þe stomake, and for þe body, and for the evillis of þe body with-in-forth, and for the jaund*is*, and distroieth abho*min*acion of a body-ys stomake, & hit will make a man to slepe well. Also who that hathe a sore eye put o þrede of safur þ*er*-in and hit shall hele hym, be hit webb or kenynge w*ith*-in iij nyghtis & eu*er*y nyght put on þrede þ*er*-in.

2105

_{2090 juis] A-yene the son*n*e *written on the lower margin.* 2097 delys] the cra*m*pe and wo*m*men of dede childe *written on the inner margin.* 2105 þe body] to hele a webb or a kenyng *written on the outer margin.* 2108 safur] safu*r*e *before emendation.*}

_{2086 ham] & helith *written by Hand C over the line.* 2090 and hit] bledyng. wondes. a-yene þe son*n*e *written by Hand C on the upper margin.* 2096 irios] 174 *written by Hand E after this word.* 2103 crocus] 175 *written by Hand E after this word.*}

Abrotanum

Sowtheryne-wode ys hote and drye in the þirde de-gre. The vertu of this erbe ys that yf the sede of hym be brayed and dronke with water, hit helith ham that havith þe stone oþer the palsy. And dronke the sede with wyne, hit helith bytinge of venym wormes. Also poudir of this erbe y-medlyd with || barly mell vnbyndeth and brekiþ the harde postem. Also bren this erbe, and þe pouder medill hit with woll oylle, and ther-wiþ anoynte the place þer that lakkyth here, and hit shall growe a-yene. Also sethe him and vse hit, and that helpiþ the synewis and þe brest. Also hit distroieth ichinge and clawynge. Also y-dronke with wyne hit helpiþ to the reynes and helith the sore of a woman-is preuete. Also he makiþ a body to pisse and clensse the brest & closith flouris. Also þe savor dryvith a-wey serpentis and venym wormys, and hit sesith the colde feuerys yf hit be dronke with water, oþer sode in oyle. And with that oyle a-noynte the body or þe accesse come. Also drinke the juis and that sleiþ wormes in the body. Also y-sodde in water wiþ myys of brede and a frute that is callid malacidonia, hit doþe a-way | þe sekenys of the empatyk. Also stampe him with talowe & that shall drawe oute spikynterys and þornes. Also drynke him in wyne and he stirreþ a man to lechery. And yf þe erbe be laide vndir a manys hede, hit doþe the same yf he be not ware ther-of. Also yf a man speke myche in his slepe, drinke þe juis of this erbe wiþ wyne whan he goþ to his bed, and that shall saue hym.

2111 þirde de-gre] for þe ston þe hard postem to make here to growe jching and clawing & þe boches *written on the outer margin.*   **2123** a-wey] a-wel *before emendation.*

2110 abrotanum] 176 *written by Hand E after this word.*   **2114** palsy] & wormes in a manes wombe *written by Hand C over the line.*

Apium siluaticum

Serfoyle is an erbe that is hote and dry in the þirde degre. He is a maner of wodebynde and beryth a white flour like to the lyly, but þey beryth hongynge. The vertu of hym is, stampe him and [t]emper him wiþ hony, and that is gode for cankyr in the mouthe. Also drinke him with wyne and he sesith akyng in the wombe. Also seþe hym in water and washe the hede ther-in, and that helith the evill that || ys callid vertyne. Also drinke the juis with wyne and hit sesith akynge in the sides [&] in the wombe. Also sethe hit in watir and washe the hede þere-in, and that helith the evill callid vertyne. Also fry hit with oyle olyfe and freshe shepis talow, and that plaster is gode for synewes and all the lymmes that ben take with colde. Som men say that cheuer[fo]ill may be the same.

Crassula minor

Stonecrop ys an erbe þat growith lowe and som-tyme vppon moiste wallys and moiste housyn. The vertu of hym ys this: that yf a body drynke him with whate lycour him liste, hit shall kepe him fro lechery.

Centinodium

Sparowe-tonge ys an erbe that is hote and drye, oþer-wyse callys swynes-carsse, oþer stryle. This erbe ys noþinge to garthines, for his branchis goþe lowe & wide and þey beþ full of knottys. He distroyeth þe stone. |

2140 temper] emper *MS.* **2143** the juis] for þe cankyr in þe mouthe for synewis take with colde *written on the inner margin.* **2144** &] om. *MS.* **2149** cheuerfoill] cheuerill *MS.* **2151** stonecrop] for lechery *written on the inner margin.* **2156** that is] for þe stone *written on the inner margin.*

2136 apium siluaticum] 177 *written by Hand E after this word.* **2143** ys callid] .nota. *written by Hand B on the upper margin.* **2150** crassula minor] 178 *written by Hand E after this word.* **2154** lechery] & it will make a sike mane to vomette *written by Hand C after this word.* **2155** centinodium] 179 *written by Hand E after this word.*

Eruca

50rb

Sky[r]white ys hote but noȝte drye. The juis holde in the mouthe helith all sorys ther-of. Also this erbe y-vsid ys holsom for the stone. The juis y-dronke distroieth þe black colour and helpith to pisse, & with stale ale hit delyu*ere*the men of the cogh. Also this erbe y-ete make gode digestion and is *p*rofitable for childryn. Also medill hit w*ith* hony, hit doþe a-way spottis vpon a man-ys skynne and makeþ the face clene of all frekylnes. Also the rote y-sodd and laide to brokyn bonys, that shall draw ham oute. Also þe sede y-stampid and y-dronke in wyne helith all venym bitynge. Also with oxys gall anoynted hit helith black wennys. Also y-dronke largely he sharpith and hardith wonderly the wytt. Also in all man*er* potage hit makiþ gode sauour, and y-fryeþ he grevith a man to lechery.

2165

2170

F[l]amula maior

50va

Spereworte ys hote and drye, oþ*er* launcell, oþ*er* ‖ sper-hede. Oute of the toppe come many smale stalkys havinge a white flour and growyng in watris. Yf a manys pownce be a-noynted ther-with, he shal be hole. Also the lefe of hym ys gode to breke bilys & bochis and for to drawe oute the quyter*e*.

Fragra

2180

Strawbery will hele blered eyne, and þe juis will distroy the webbe and the kenynge in the eyen. And this erbe helith

---

2160 eruca] *written on the upper margin.*   **2161** skyrwhite] skywhite MS.   juis holde] for þe stone þe coȝ to drawe oute brokyn bonis for frekilles *written on the outer margin.*   **2174** flamula maior] famula maior *MS.*   **2176** white flour] for bochis and bilis *written on the outer margin.*   **2178** to] bylis *deleted after this word.*   **2182** kenynge in] wond*is* blerid eyne þe web þe kenyn*n*gis of a bodis eyne *written on the outer margin.*

2160 eruca] 180 *written by Hand E after this word.*   **2174** flamula maior] 181 *written by Hand E after this word.*   **2180** fragra] 182 *written by Hand E after this word.*

greuous woundys. The juis with hony dronke helith akynge of a manys mylte w*ith*-oute fayll.

Feniculus porci[n]us

Swynes-fenyll ys hote & drye, o*þer* wormesede. The sede y-ete distroieth wormes in the wombe.

Lab[r]u*m* Ven*e*ris

Sowe-þistill y-broke droppiþ mylke. He hathe a yelowe flour, and his sede ys callid Seynte Mary sede. The juis wiþ hote wat*er* y-dronke heliþ the feu*e*rys. Also this erbe, dried | to poud*er* and mellid w*ith* wyne y-dronke, castiþ all venym oute of the body.

Saturion maior

S[t]andilgose, oþ*er* ȝekesterris, oþ*er* s[t]andylwelkys, ys hote and drye, and havith knobbis in the rotis lyke ballok-stonys. He will distroy wikkid wyndis with-in a man. Also yf a man haue a greuance wounde, stampe the rote of þ*is* erbe and lay hit to his wou*n*d*is*. Wiþ the juis and hony a-noynte bleryd eyne.

Saxifragia

Saxfrage ys an erbe that ys colde and dry. His levis bethe lyke to dauke but þey beth more black and a lytell white flour, and his

2185 feniculus porcinus] feniculus porcius *MS*. **2188** labrum Veneris] labiu*m* veneris *MS*. **2189** flour and] for þe feu*e*rys *written on the outer margin*. **2195** standilgose] scandilgose *MS*. standylwelkys] skandylwelkys *MS*. **2196** he will] he will he will *MS*. **2197** wikkid] blerid eyne *written on the inner margin*. **2201** levis] þe ston i*n* þe bladd*er* and reynes *written on the inner margin*.

2185 feniculus porcinus] 183 *written by Hand E after this word*. **2186** drye] wormesed*e written by Hand C on the outer margin*. **2188** labrum Veneris] 184 *written by Hand E after this word*. **2194** saturion maior] 185 *written by Hand E after this word*. **2200** saxifragia] 186 *written by Hand E after this word*.

sede ys like to carwy. The juis y-dronke brekith the stone in the bladd*er* and reynes.

Scabiosa

Scabyeus. y-broke, the lefe will hyng to-gad*er* by a þrede, and ys colde and moyst. || The juis of hym, aisell, and oyle, y-boyled to-gadir and ther-of made an oynement, shall distroye the skabbe. The juis will restore here a-yene. Also þe juis, y-dronke with wyne, all maner of posteme w*ith*-in oþer with-oute esyle. Hit brekith and clensith his brest, and all old*e* sorys þ*er*-of he helith, and also venym. Also stampe hi*m* and lay hi*m* to a fellon, and he shall hele hi*m* wiþ-in iij dayes. Stampe scabyous and sethe that in wyne and drynke, þ*at* is gode for the leu*er* and that distroyth evill humourys of the stomake.

Elactuericu*m*

Spurge will make a man laxe, for to delyu*er* a-boue oþ*er* by-nethe, oþ*er* he will pers the bowellis. And þ*er*-for dry his levis in an ovyn, þen bete h*a*m to poud*er* and yf þere-of to strong men v. peny-wight, and to febill men lasse, and to men that beþe harde y-bounde þu moste | take more, & to lite bounde men lasse, in caule, oþ*er* in growell, oþ*er* in neshe egis, oþ*er* in ale, oþ*er* in wyne. The sede of this erbe is nought so myghty as the þ*at* is callid catapusia. Laureoll and sporge ben of a vertu.

2211 olde] *written on the inner margin.* **2217** oþer by-nethe] to m*a*ke a man laxatif *written on the inner margin.*

2203 juis] w*ith* white wyne *written by Hand C on the outer margin.* **2205** scabiosa] 187 *written by Hand E after this word.* **2216** elactuericum] u *deleted and expunctuated, probably by Hand C;* 188 *written by Hand E after this word;* .nota. *written by Hand B on the inner margin.* **2221** bounde men] *id est.* anabulla mylke of spurge wylle destroy fistula in ano. *written by Hand C on the outer margin.*

[Stafisagria]

[Stafisagre] is hote and dry, and berith levis like to wilde vyne. The ve*r*tu of þ*is* erbe ys þ*at* yf one haue wekid humeris in his body, take xv cor[n]ys of this erbe, and grynde ham in vlake watir, and drynke that, and he shall caste, but aftir he hauyth y-dronke latte hi*m* warke a while er*e* he caste, and all was as he castith lat hi*m* soupe of þe wat*er*, oþ*er* þe strey[n]th of þe erbe will bren his chekys. Also yf a man haue eny scabbis oþ*er* ycching*is*, stampe the sede of this erbe w*ith* portulake and w*ith* oyle, and a-noynte the body ther-with and he shall be hole. ||

Quinq*ue* foliu*m*

Synkefoly, oþ*er* quynfoyly, is colde and drye in þe secounde degre. He crepith lawe bi þe grownde. The ve*r*tu of hi*m* is, sethe this erbe in white wyne and late drinke ther-of, first at morowe and laste at eve, and that heliþ ache in onys lendys, and for the hede-ake, and for sore mouthe, and sore tonge, oþ*er* þrote. Galean sayth, "stampe hi*m* and te*m*p[*er*] h*it* wiþ clere ale, drinke that and hi[t] heliþ all sor*e* akyng." Also yf one spit blode, seþ hy*m* with wyne and drinke that. Also he is gode y-dronke to hele the stone, oþ*er* stampe this erbe and olde talowe and lay to þe sore place. Also yf one haue akynge in his wombe oþ*er* swelling, drynke þe juis of this erbe w*ith* clere ale, [oþer] seþ hit in wyne. Also make poudyr of this erbe & þ*er*-with frete well the mouthe and the tonge, and that doþe a-way all sore ther-of. Also yf one haue bledyng at his | nose, drinke well the juis of þis erbe and washe well þe forhede ther-with, & hit shall stanche and holde þe mouthe þer-ovir. Also yf one be bitt with an naddyr, drynke the juis with wyne and hit shall distroye the venym. Also yf a body be brennyd in eny lym of hym, stampe þis erbe and drinke þe juis, and he shall be all hole. Also washe him well in fayre water, sprynge oute þe water clene, þan stampe him & boyle him in water. Than take som þer-of and do hit to the toþe that akyth as hote as one may suffyr, and holde hit so the space of ij Credis, Þen spitt oute all. And take so myche a-yane viij tymes oþer ix, and that shall distroy the toþe-ake with-oute doute.

Acedula

Souredok is an erbe that ys colde and drye in the þirde degre. The vertu of him ‖ is, in somertyme i-ete hit makith a gode stomake. Also sta[m]pe him and lay him to the freting evyll, hit helpith. And in maner of a plaster hit helpiþ the swellyng of þe eyne, and crepynge goutys, and brennyng of þe potager that is hote. Also the grene levis sod in oyle olyfe helith the olde hede-ache yf hit be laid to þe hede. Also drinke hit [with] wyne oþer ete hit, and he restreyneth all maner flix of the wombe and sleyth wormes of þe wombe. Also he ys gode a-yene all venym. Also a-noynte þe eyne wiþe the juis, hit clerith ham. Also he that berith him dar not drad bytinge of scropionys. Also the juis ther-of done in oneis eryn. Also þe juis stampid anoynte the eyne-lyddis with þe juis that ben y-lok to-geder be-cause of flewme, that helith.

2249 at his] at his at his *MS*. **2263** is in] swelling of eyne and brenyng guttis þe flux to clere þe sight *written on the inner margin*. **2264** stampe] stape *MS*. **2268** with] *om. MS*.

2261 acedula] 191 *written by Hand E after this word*.

Lelamour Herbal

Sigilum Sancte Marie |
Seynt Mary seall, oþer godhishond, ys hote and drye. The juis y-dronke stopith the hete of lechery, as dothe tisayne. He ys a gode erbe for to helpe make pyment. Also yf an ox be seke with-in him, a-none yf him the water to drynke that þis erbe lay in, and anone he shall be hole.

Tanacetum
Tansy. Drynke the juis for wormys in the wombe. Also þe juis of tansy and of fedyrfewe y-dro[n]ke ys gode for the axes. Also fry tansy and talow of a shepe, and lay that to swellinge fete. Also stampe tansy with mogwort and drinke the juis to-geder with wyne oþer clere ale, and that is gode for the stone in the raynes. Also juis of tansy with wyne y-dronke ys remedy for all maner venym bytinge. Also þe juis is holsum in metis. ||

Agnus castus
Tutesayne is hote and dry, and som men callith him pa[r]k-levis. He berryth black bayes; when thei ben ripe the smyll of hym makes men & women caste. Also hit will opyn the po[rr]ys and lat oute wekyd wyndis and humoris of manys body. Also this erbe distroieth manys kynde, as Places saith, but he seiþ: "sethe this erbe and fenell sede with a lytell aysell, and that is gode to distroye the colde dropsy." Also seþe this erbe and smalache

---

2277 oþer] for a nox *written on the outer margin.* **2283** the juis] for þe accesse þe stone *written on the outer margin.* **2284** y-dronke] y-droke *MS.* **2289** in metis] *written beyond the margin line.* **2290** agnus castus] *written on the upper margin.* **2291** tutesayne] þe colde dropsye *written on the outer margin.* park-levis] pak-levis *MS.* **2293** porrys] pomys *MS.*

2277 Seynt Mary seall] 192 *written by Hand E over the line.* **2282** tanacetum] 193 *written by Hand E after this word.* **2290** agnus castus] 194 *written by Hand E after this word.* **2291** park-levis] he hath leves leke to arage & hath a yelow flour as moche as a peny. *written by Hand C on the outer margin.*

and sage in wat*er*, and washe the hinder part of onys hede strongly þ*er*-with, and that vnbyndith þe evyll of litarge. Also þe bayes y-gaddryd by-twyx our Lady daies, and stampe v oþ*er* vj of ham, & drynke hit w*ith* rede wyne, and þ*at* helith þe bledyng of the fondement. Also he is gode to distroy the hardnes and þe stoppyng of the lyu*er* and þe mylte. Also a plaster y-made of hy*m*m is gode | to do away the ache of onys hede that is gadrid of lethir humouris.

Bursa pastoris

Totheworte, oþ*er* herdys purse, oþ*er* stanche, oþ*er* sanguynary, ys hote and dry. The ve*r*tu of hi*m* is, yf one be in the flux of blode, yonge oþ*er* olde, sta*m*pe this erbe and drinke hit with wlake wyne, and hit will sese bledynge. Also yf ther be eny veynes kyt a-two, drynke þe juis of this erbe. Also þ*is* erbe ys helynge all festrynge sorys & he helith wou*n*dys.

Epetimu*m*

Tyme ys hote in [þe þyrde] degre. Drynke the juis þere-of w*ith* wlake white wyne for the stone, yf hit be ofte y-vsid. Also þe juis y-dronke wiþ wyne makiþ one to pisse, and clensith þe flouris of a woman, and castith oute the secund wher-in the childe lieth. Also the juis and hony y-||sode in wyne kestiþ oute glett y-holde in the breste þrow spewynge. Also drinke hit with wyne, hit helpith kernyng in the wombe. Also seþe hit in wat*er*

2299 vnbyndith] vndbyndith *MS*.   **2300** by-twyx] b *deleted after this word*.   **2307** sanguynary] for þe flux of cold old oþ*er* yong for bledi*n*g for vey[n]*i*s kytt and al fest*er* sores and wond*is* *written on the inner margin*.   **2314** þe þyrde] *om*. *MS*.   **2315** wlake] wyne *deleted after this word*.   wyne] for þe stone for glett in þe brest þrowe spewyng *written on the inner margin*.

2305 humouris] & þ*er* be ij spices of hit *written by Hand C after this word*.   **2306** bursa pastoris] 195 *written by Hand E after this word*.   **2313** epetimum] 196 *written by Hand E after this word*.   **2318** hony] þrow. spewyng. no*ta*. *written by Hand B on the lower margin*.

and washe the hede in þat water, and that voideth hede-ake and
þe lytarge. All oþer vertus havith savery.

Tana[s]etum

Turmentile ys an erbe þat creppith a-brode in many smale
braunchis, and beryth yelowe flourys and smale levis, and
havith a grete knob in þe rote. Þe juis y-dronke with eny maner
of lecour distroyeth al poyson of wormys and venym. And yf a
childe haue kennyng in his eye, temper þe juis with gotis mylke
and yf the norysse to drynke. Also drynke iij vnces of powder
tarmentill with swete mylke for the flux.

Anabulla

Tvtymallys, oþer wilde spurge, ys hote and growyth vpon | a
playne stalke, and berith no leve but at the croppe, and þer he
growith brode and rounde compas, and he y-broke dropith
mylke. Take him while he is yonge and olde barowis grece, and
boyle hame in white wyne till þe wyne be ny sodyn all yn, let
hit kele a while, put þere-to quyk-sy[l]uer, þat flayne wiþ thi
spotill and askys, medyll thes well to-gedris and a-noynte þer
any dry scabbe-ys.

Hastula regia

Woderofe ys hote of kynde and swete of savour. He heliþ wiþ
oile of almondis scabbid leggis and fete. Also þe juis of þe rotis

2323 tanasetum] tanafetum *MS.*   **2324** creppith] for kenynngis in a child-is eye for þe flux *written on the outer margin.*   **2333** and þer] for a drye scabb *written on the outer margin.*   **2337** quyk-syluer] quyk-syuer *MS.*
2341 savour] for scabbid leggis and fete to stanche blode þe potagyr þe flex and sore þrote *written on the outer margin.*

2323 tanasetum] 197 *written by Hand E after this word.*   **2331** anabulla] 198 *written by Hand E after this word.*   **2340** hastula regia] 199 *written by Hand E after this word.*

w*ith* wyne y-dronke ys gode for the stom*a*ke. Also þe juis y-dronke stanchith blode. Also y-sodd in met*is*, that doþe a-way the rewme of one-ys body. W*ith* quyk brymstone and hony hit is gode for the potagyr. Yf þe rotis be poundid w*ith* wyne, he helithe sore in the mouthe. Also ‖ this erbe stampe þe sede and y-dronke with soure vyneg*er*, staunche the flix. Also þe juis y-dronke wiþ stale ale heliþ a sore throte.

Wermode stroyeth þe stom*a*ke on whate man*er* hit be resceyved, but þe bett*er* hit ys yf hit be sodyn*e* in rayne wat*er*, and þ*er*-to lat stond all a nyght w*ith*-oute and let þe mouthe of þe vessell be vppyn for to take the humerys of þe ayre, and þ*at* he be in faire stede þ*er* noþing com ther-to. And on the morowe take ther-of all fasting a quantite, and faste þ*er*-vpon*e* in till mydday, and þen ete freshe mete and done þis iij dayes, and hit will sle wormes in the wombe, and will swage the wombe of swellyng, and takiþ a-waye sore of the stomake, and coloure, and flewme, and glat, and yfith oute vryn, and spurgiþ flouris longe holdynge in woman-ys body. Oþ*er* make a tentur*e* of woll and | wete hit in that lecour*e*, and put hit in womanys shappe, and hit castith oute abortife. Cerementayne, spyknard, and aloyne, and boyll hit well with aysell, and þe juis of wermode drinke þ*er*e-of, and hit doþ a-way all gnawynge evill a-boute the herte that is callid cardiaca, of þe lyu*er* that ys callid epatica. The juis dro[n]kyn ys gode for the jaundys. The levis tempirde with aysell ys gode for the mydryd. The gris þ*er*-of helpith all

---

2346 potagyr] *apparently,* potag*er* *before emendation.* **2366** dronkyn] drokyn *MS.*

2350 wermode] Absinthium *written by Hand C in the gap between entries, then* 200 *written by Hand E immediately after.* **2358** and takiþ] and clenseth the here & doeth a-way dronkenes. & it te*m*pered w*ith* hony heleth the sore of þe mouth & it stomped & te*m*pered w*ith* þe galle of a veale put in a ma*n*nes yere putteth a-way þe sondyng of the hede. *written by Hand C on the outer margin.*

Lelamour Herbal

venym bytynge. Meng þe gus w*ith* hony and a-noynte the eyen, hit makeþ hem bright and h*it* helpith all brusynge that co*m*yth of betynge. Wormod soden and laid to þe er*is* stoppid [þrow] the evill of the hede hit helpiþ, and yf they ren with quyter, put hony ther-with, and make a plaster, and sett þ*ere*-to. And þe gresse plaster ys gode for the sqyna[c]e and sleithe nit*is* yn the hede yf hit be washe wiþ || the juis. The odour of the gres will make sekmen slepe yf they wote note that hit ys vndyr her hede. The erbe y-brent and askyn made ther-of take that askyn and virgyn wex, and anoynte the hede, and that m*a*kiþ the hede black yf hit be oftyn anoynted.

Wolde ys hote and drye, and makiþ a man*e* to make vryne, and spurgith þe flouris. The wat*er* that hit is soden in helpith for eny evillis of the skap yf hit be washe ther-w*ith*. The gresse dronkynge helpith for þe jaundis, and that clensith þe entr*a*ill þrow vomyte as hit were walworte, but hit is not so violent ne so douto*us*.

Walworte ys in two man*eris*: that one white, that oþ*er* blak. Þey beþ boþe of hem hote and dry in þe þirde degre. The white is more violent then þ*e* black. And whate woman doþ | hit in hir shape hit castith oute abortife. The poud*er* of the gress done in the nose puttiþ a-way evillis of the hede. And menge of the poudyr w*ith* juis of celydonu*m* and rew, hit clerith the sight. The powd*er* done in the grewell of fleshe sodyn therin myse do note ete, and do of that poud*er* in mylke, and hit sleys fleys that light ther-on. And that reseyte castith oute wekyd humer*is*

2370 þrow] helpiþ *MS*. **2373** sqynace] sqynare *MS*. **2375** yf] yf yf *MS*.

2378 anoynted] & this herbe is hoot & drie *written by Hand C after this word.*
2379 wolde] 201 *written by Hand E in the gap between entries.*
2385 walworte] 202 *written by Hand E in the gap between entries.*

þrowe vomyte and olde evillis. Sethe hit in watir and drinke
ther-of, and hit helpith for ham that beþe wode. At þe
begynyng of þe dropsy hit will helpe ther-for, and malencoly,
and to þe falling evill, and clensyth the lepir, & helpith þe
gryndynge in the stomake. Ypocras and Plenyus comaundith
that þu yf noȝte but x *peny*-wight to the man that þu wilt clense,
and that þu yf hit nought to olde men, ne to childryn, ne to
women but to ham that ys off stronge nature. The levis sodyn in
watir ‖ wyth wilewe levys, and ache, and lovache, betony, and
vervyn, i-put in a bathe, and let a body baþe him ther-in: hit
helpith for olde brusynge, and akynge of þe longis, and for all
sorys of the body.

The blak is also mekyll to doute as the white. The maistres
comandeþ to do sede in coule and vse hit, and hit helpith wode
men, and the potagir, and the dropsy, and also the feuer. Stampe
hit in wyne and drinke hit, hit is gode for the palsy and to all
evillis that drawith to-geder þe humeris. Hit castith oute the
blacke colour and the flewme, and amendith þe sight. Stampe
the rotis and do hem to-gedir in maner of a plaster, hit swagith
and drieth swellinge of þe dropsye. Put þe same plaster to a
woman-is shappe, hit makiþ hir haue hir flouris, and delyuereth
abortive, and helpiþe defe eris yf hit be laide to ham ij dayes,
and clensyth þe lepire, & doþe a-way skabbe. Sodyn in aysell
and longe holde in his mouþe | puttith a-way toþe-ake. Plenius
biddith that men shall noȝt haue at onys but v peny-wight of
the rote.

Wylwe. The rote sodyn in wyne clensith wondis. And wiþ wyn
y-stampid and laide to womanys pappe, hit reviþ the akynge
and helpith the brenynge. The rote sodyn & stampid and mengid
with wyne anoynte ham, hit helpiþ all swellinge of the mawe,
and makiþ syneous harde, and brekiþ bilis. And þe water ther-

---

2420 wylwe] 203 *written by Hand E in the gap between entries.*

Lelamour Herbal 215

of helpiþ for many evillis of the body. The rote i-sode in wyne 2425
doþe gode for the menysoun and for the flix that is longe
holdyn. Hit helpith all þe evill*is* of the bladyr. The sede
y-sta*m*pid with oyle of olyfe and wyne doþe a-way all man*er* of
foule spott*is*. Hit is gode for venym. Þe levys sodyn in oyle
helpiþ brenynge. 2430

Verveyn is in ij man*er*ys, and || bothe ben of one vertu. Drynke 55ra
hit in wyne, hit helpith for the jaundys. Sta*m*pe hit and lay hit in
all venym bitte. Þe juis and wyne stampid to-ged*er* in þe mouthe
helpith the woundys yn the mouthe. Sta*m*pe hit and ley to, h*i*t
helith wou*n*d*is* to-ged*er*. Stampe hit and drinke hit w*ith* wyne, 2435
hit doþe gode for all [m]an*er* venym. The wat*er* that hit is sodyn
yn, yff he be caste a-monge pepill that fastith, hit makiþ hame
be blythe and gladde. Take þe levys on thi right honde & take a
seke manys right honde in thi right honde and aske howe he
faryth, and yf he say that he shall lyfe trowe hit trewly. And yf 2440
he say that he shall dye, so he shall w*ith*-oute doute. Make a
garland of þe levys and hit a-batith hede-ake. Plenius
comau*n*diþ to drinke hit in wyne, and that doþe gode to þe
entrayles, and till þe sidys, and till the | gisser, and to the longis, 55rb
and to the brest, and hit dothe gode for all evill*is*. Drynke the 2445
juis and a-noynte the þere-w*ith* and all folke shall loue the the
while hit laste vpon the. Take vervyne, betayne, mylfoly and
wyne, drinke the juis, hit brekyth þe stone noþinge soner*e* and
dothe gode for the feu*er*. And yf a veyne be smyte þrowe oþ*er*
in two, [take] vervyne, and barow-is grese, and cro*m*mys of 2450
white brede, and stampe to-gedir and lay ther-to, and hit helith.

2436 maner] naner *MS*.   **2446** folke] *apparently,* fooke *before emendation*.
2450 take] *om. MS*.

2431 verveyn] 204 *written by Hand E in the gap between entries*.

Nasturcium aquaticum

Watyr-cars stampe and stife in a pot all drye, and make a plaster ther-of, and lay to the emerodis. Also shrede þis cars smale, then do hem in-to a newe erþen pott, put þere-to wyne drestis, and whete branne, and wedders talo, of euery y-like myche by wiȝt, boyle this well to-gadyr till ‖ þay be right þik. Lay that to the sore als ho[t]e as he may suffyr hit, y-bownde with lyncloþe o nyght and a daye vnremevid. Than take that a-way and ley to a-noþer a-yen all hote, and this shall aswage swellynge of leggis oþer of fete, and do away sore akynge. Also sethe cars & horehound in wyne and drynke that, at evyn hote and at morowe colde, for straitnes of the brest. Also stampe þis erbe and wrynge oute the juis and so myche of the juis of elisaunder, late boyle ham to-gedyr with a quantite of hony. Scome þis clene, strayne that lecour in-to a clene vessell. Drynke euery morow fastyng iij sponefull for the stone.

Alleluya

Wodesoure ys an erbe þat is hote and drye. Som men calliþ hit stokwort, oþer sorell de boys, oþer cokkowe-|brede. He growyth in moiste placys and hathe but iij levs foldyng donwarde and a litell white floure. The vertu of him is, yf that he [be rostid] apon the colis i-wrappid in þe levis of þe rede dokk, lay that to dede fleshe and hit will frett the dede fleshe a-way, and wertis. Also he will drawe oute a corne that growith vppon the to. Also gadyr a gode quantite of this erbe with-oute rote, stampe ham and wringe oute the juis in-to a clene saucere. Take softely and poure oute the clere white water fro the grene, take a faire keuerchiff oþer brode cloþe that haþ ire-molys a-pon a bord in

---

2458 hote] hole *MS.* **2472** be rostid] berostid *MS.*

2452 nasturcium aquaticum] 205 *written by Hand E after this word.* **2453** stampe and] And thys herbe is good for the dropesie to destroye. *written by Hand C on the outer margin.* **2468** alleluya] 206 *written by Hand E after this word.*

þe hote sonne, and w*ith* a feþ*er* a-noynte that lecou*r*e apon þe moyle, and eu*er* as he drynkiþ in, do mor to till þe moyle wax white as the cloþe.

Caprifoliu*m*

W[o]debynd, oþ*er* cheuyrfoyle, ‖ oþ*er* withwynde, ys hote and drye. This erbe will hele wondys that cankerith, and bladdrys, and akynge of tethe, & sore in a bodyes tonge. Also he is gode to hele the stynge of beeys oþ*er* waspis. Also stampe hi*m* and lay to wondis, he drawith oute blode.

Camelion

Wolfe-ys þistill berith a rede floure, and the levis ben sharpe. The vertu of this erbe ys, take hym while the sone is in Cap*ri*cornis with þe newe mone, and bere hi*m* vpon the, and þ*er*e shall no myschefe fall to þe.

Canabaria

Wylde hempe ys an erbe þ*at* som men callyth holy rope, oþ*er* donnetyl. His levys ben like hempe levis. The ve*r*tu of this erbe ys, yf the pounce of a man that havith þe feue*r*ys be frettid well w*ith* þe levis of this erbe, he shall be [hole]. Þ*is* | growith moche by wate*r*s.

Iacea alba

Wylde tansy, oþ*er* gose gresse, and som men callith ham whityn mor*e*. His levis ben like tansy, but thei ben white. The levis of

---

2484 wodebynd] wedebynd *MS*. **2493** þe] c *deleted after this word*.
2498 hole] holde *MS*.

2483 caprifolium] 207 *written by Hand E after this word*. **2486** tethe &] bladd*er* or *written by Hand C on the inner margin*. **2488** blode] & it hath white floures *written by Hand C after this word*. **2489** camelion] 208 *written by Hand E after this word*. **2494** canabaria] 209 *written by Hand E after this word*. **2500** iacea alba] 210 *written by Hand E after this word*.

this erbe will kepe the that þu shalt not chafe, and ys gode to clene manys lymmys.

Rapistrum domesticum

White pepir ys hote and dry, and his levis ben like mostarde but þay ben slyttid. The sede here-of is white. He is gode for sauce, & to clense woundys, and hele ham, and makyth olde wondys fayr.

Salix

Wythi is dry in kynde. Take the tend[ryns] of him and stampe hit, and hit stanche blody woundys. Also drinke the erbe in water, and hit stopyth the flourys of a woman. ‖ The askys tempird wiþ aisell doþe a-way the sore of the solis of þe fete. Also hit dothe a-way wartis. His flour sodyn in water y-dronke distroyeth lechery.

Viola alba

Vyolett ys moiste & colde in the firste de-gre, and iij specis þere-offe, almoste a-corde in vertue. For brenynge stampe this erbe & lay to. The sauour of the flouris is gode for þe hede. Also drinke þe juis with water for the fallyng evill. Also the rotis and myre with safyr y-mellyd and layde to the eyne be nyght takyth a-way the bler of the eyne. Also þe levys y-stampid with hony ys gode to hele þe skall and þe skabbe. Also þe juis y-dronke with clene water doþ a-way the cogh fro childryn. Oyle made of the erbe ys gode to quynche all hote evillys. Also the rote of | the white vyolett y-holde in a bodyes

---

2511 tendryns] tendyrst *MS.* **2512** stanche] bro *deleted after this word.*
2523 takyth] takyth takiþ *MS.* **2526** hote] evllis *expunctuated.*

2505 rapistrum domesticum] 211 *written by Hand E after this word.*
2510 salix] 212 *written by Hand E after this word.* **2517** viola alba] 213 *written by Hand E after this word.*

mouthe, þe juis y-swolowyd downe, stanchith blody woundys. The juis of p*ur*pur violet will brynge oute brokyn bonys. The sede of violet, the sede of marche, and annys-is sede, boyle to-gad*er* with white wyne till hit wex þick, ete here-of, first & laste, for the cogh. Also yf þe skolle bon be dryfe a-downe w*ith* a stroke so that a man lesith his speche, anone stampe violet and yf hi*m* to drinke þe juis w*ith* wyne. And yf he be hirt apon the right side of the hede, take þe same erbe y-stampyd and bynde to þe sole of þe lyfte fote *et* eq*ua* si eo*rum* alia p*ar*te.

Lolliu*m*

Wylde sanagrene, oþ*er* cokkyll, stampid and laide in a cloþ bryngith oute the secound of a woman. Also the woman that vsith hit shall haue plente || of mylke. Also hit will make þikk humouris thine. Also stampe hit and hastely hit [h]elyth wekyd wynd*is* with-in a man and his juis be y-dronke þ*ere* y-stampid y-leyde þ*ere*-to. Also he amendith breth.

Explicit Mac*er*

God g*ra*cious of g*ra*untis havyth y-yeue and y-grauntid v*er*tuys in wordys, stonys, and herbis, of the whiche erbis Mac*er* the philizofur made a boke in Latyn. The whiche boke Joh*ann*es Lelamour, scolemaister of Herforde Est, þey he vnworthy was, in the yer of our Lord a*nno* Mccclxxiij tournyd in-to Ynglis. And yff ther be eny þinge myssaide in the tornynge of the langage, the wise reder and godely vndirstond*er* he prayeth wi[th] all his hart the fautys to amende.

2536 et...parte] *apparently written in a second stint, after the text was completed.* **2541** helyth] lelyth *MS.* **2552** with] will *MS.*

2537 lollium] 214 *written by Hand E after this word.*

Explanatory Notes

1 ache. The entry derives from the entry *apium* in *DVH* 332–365 as translated in *DVH(NME)*. Identification of the species treated here with wild celery (*Apium graveolens* L.) is traditional and seems sure on account of the pharmacological virtues of the species, cf. its perceived powers as an ophthalmic and analgesic (**3** = *DVH* 341–344), antacid and alexipharmic (**4** = *DVH* 345, 351), antitussive (**5** = *DVH* 353), antidiarrheic (**6** = *DVH* 354), febrifuge (**8** = *DVH* 358–359), cosmetic (**8** = *DVH* 356) and splanchnic (**10** = *DVH* 360–361). Some other virtues of celery provided in *DVH* are missing in the ME text: anti-inflammatory (*DVH* 345), carminative (*DVH* 346–347) and diuretic (*DVH* 348–350), although the latter virtue is recorded in the other MSS of the tradition. Oppositely, the galactogenous virtue of the species (**6**) is missing from the original Latin text: in fact, according to *LS*, celery is aphrodisiac and hence should not be eaten by nurses "quia incitat eis libidinem & abscindit lac earum". This is probably due to confusion of *Apium* with parsley (see the appropriate remarks in Tu).

> **Literature**: WILD CELERY (*Apium graveolens* L.): *HP* i.2.2 (σέλινον); *MM* iii.64 (σέλινον κηπαῖον); *NH* xx.112–115 (*apium*); *SM* xii.118 (σέλινον); *RM* ii.257; *Grad.* 379; *OEH* 120 (*herba apium. merce*); *Dur.Glos.* 299 (*apium. mearce*); *DVH* 332–365 (*apium*); *LS* 280 (*karphs* [كرفس *karafs*], *apium*); *EPN* iii (*apio. merce*), v (*apium. ache*); *Cl* A.8 (*apium. merche*); *TH* 8 (*appium*); *Pand.* 47 (LA*apium*, GR*selinum*, AR*kaspar, karfi*); *DVH(NME)* 246v.7 (*ache*); *DVH(SME)* 7b.5 (*ache, smalache*); *Alph.* 11–12, 202 (*apium domesticum sive ortolanum*. GA*mennache*, AN*smalache*), 194, 235 (*xilenum*), 211 (*charasis*), 212 (*elimon*), 216 (*gaxit*); *Sin.Bart.* 11 (*apium simpliciter*, AN*smale ache*); *AC* 158.18 (*apium*) ⚜ *GH* 8 (APIUM, *smalache, stammarche*); Fu 283 (ΣΕΛΙΝΟΝ ΚΗΠΑΙΟΝ, *apium hortense, apium satiuum*); Tu I.308 (SMALLAGE, *elioselinon, paludapium, marche*); DL 437 (WILDE PARSELY, σέλινον ἄγριον, ὑδροσέλινον ἄγριον, *apium syluestre*); Ge 860 (PARSLEY, σέλινον κηπαῖον, *apium hortense, petroselinum*).
>
> C (*SM, RM*) | C²S³ (Fu, Ge) | C³S³ (*Grad., DVH, LS, Cl, TH, GH, DL*)

1 brede y-made of whete. A *lectio facilior* in AS_1, cf. *B*.246v/8 ⟨whytt bred⟩ (and similarly *W*.31r/1), rendering *DVH* 341 *candida mica*. *P*.270/15 simply reads ⟨bred⟩.

2 swellinge. This translates *DVH* 342 *sedare tumores* correctly. Still, this cannot be an authorial reading, since the other MSS of the tradition make no references to tumours: they mention pain in the eye. On the other hand, S_1 omits the word *BOLNYD that must have followed *PAPPIS in Ω (cf. *B*.246v/9

⟨þe pappis þat ere bolnyd⟩, and similarly *W* and *P*). It seems that the scribe realized, immediately after writing ⟨swagiþ swellinge⟩, that these words actually belonged to the antimastitic, rather than to the ophthalmic, virtue that he almost missed, and tried to make the best of the whole passage without having to delete the wrong fragment.

4 brenynge of þe stomake. The reference to swollen stomach is missing in this text (cf. *DVH* 345 *fervorem stomachi* […] *tumorem*); *W*.31r/2–3 ⟨bolny*ng* of þe stomak*is*⟩ does keep that part yet misses the reference to heartburn. The Bodley and Pepys versions provide the complete passage.

6 hache… 13 sursanouris. Explanations as to why the latter half of the entry was copied immediately after the entry *Anisum* are difficult to provide and range from a faulty exemplar, where the two entries were mingled, to a mere copying mistake by the scribe of S_1, who may have inadvertently skipped part of the entry. Be as it may, the scribe realized his mistake and indicated the correct way to read the entry by writing a letter ⟨a⟩ at the end of the first line of the revisitation of *ache*, and a letter ⟨b⟩ before the Lombardic letter of *Annys*.

The spelling *ache* with initial **h** seems to be privative to this MS, according to MED: *s.v.* ache *n.*², but can hardly be a mistake, as the allograph appears three times in the entry. Note moreover the odd spelling ⟨sache⟩ **11**, which is probably due to contamination from *sage*.

10 dropsy. Aphetic form of *ydrop(e)sy(e)* (whence the synonym ⟨ydrop⟩ **1637**), this is "a morbid condition characterized by the accumulation of watery fluid in the serous cavities or the connective tissue of the body" (OED: *s.v.*). The medieval doctrine pointed to an aposteme of water or air in the bowels because of a liver fault in the second digestion as the cause of this disorder, cf. *Chir.(ME)* 163:

> Ydropisis, after Brune, is saide of ydrops, þat is water, and of pisis, þat is a passioun, as it were a watry passioun, namely in þe wombe. Wherof ydropisis, forsoþe, als mykel as longeþ to a cirurgien, is an aposteme and bolnynge of þe wombe gendred of a watry and wyndy mater wiþyn þe wydenesse of þe wombe by errour of þe vertu digestyf of þe lyuer. Wherof, in 5° De Interioribus, soche a sekenesse forsoþe is neuer made wiþoute disese of þe lyuer. The lyuer forsoþe is sometyme disesed for neyghenesse and sometyme for fastnynge togedre […]. Soche a sekenesse forsoþe is errour in þe lyuer and colynge or lessynge of kyndely hete þerof, made by itself euenly of colde and of hete forsoþe by accident and vneuenly, in resoluynge þe kynde hete of þe lyuer.

Different types of dropsy were distinguished in medieval medicine (→ **2295**).

11 fernticlys. The emendation rests on the reading in *DVH(NME)* (cf. *B*.246v/16 ⟨ferntikyll*is*⟩, *W*.31r/10 ⟨francicles⟩, *P*.270/25 ⟨frentikles⟩) and is ultimately based on *DVH* 360–362, where it translates *lentigo*.

12 doust of myll. *Ω* probably read *DUST OF MILN(E) (cf. *B*.246v/16–17 ⟨þe dust off the mylne⟩ and similarly *W*.31r/10–11), which by then was probably a Northern form (cf. its dialectal distribution in EDD: *s.v.* miln *n.*). The original spelling must have been rendered as *DOUST OF MILLE in the Southern dialect of *Λ* and miscopied in S_1 due to the similarity of **l** and **k** in Anglicana scripts. *P*.270/26 ⟨flour of whete⟩ looks like an innovation due to the scribe's failure to recognize Northern *MILNE. *Dust of mill* is explained by the MED as "fine floury dust thrown out by a grain mill, mill dust" (*s.v.* dŭst *n.*, § 1.*d*). The fragment translates *DVH* 363: *farris cum polline*, i.e. finely ground flour of emmer (*Triticum dicoccum* Schrank).

12 eggis by even porcion. "even portion" may arguably be a translation of *DVH* 365 *more frequenter* and hence belong to a different phrase from *eggis* altogether, particularly if the sentence was corrupt in the exemplar. But comparison with other witnesses from *DVH(NME)* and the position of the phrase within the sentence suggest that this in fact stands for *DVH* 364 *ovi lacrymo* (→ **174I** for another rendering of the same expression). *Lac(h)rymus* (not included in du Fresne 1938) is medieval Latin for Classical *lacrima* when referring to the exudations of certain plants such as poppy or pinetrees (see OLD: *s.v.* lacrima *n.*, § 3), but here it seems to be a transparent metaphor to describe the more watery part of the egg, i.e. the albumen, cf. *B*.246v/17 ⟨whytt of eggi*s*⟩, *W*.31r/11 ⟨egge whit⟩. The MHG translation similarly offers "wissem des eies" (Schnell/Crossgrove 2003: 334).

15 annys. The entry does not record the medical virtues of anise (*Pimpinella anisum* L.), a plant not treated in *DVH*, but those of dill (*Anethum graveolens* L.) as translated in the *DVH(NME)* tradition (*DVH* 395–428). Comparison of the entry in S_1 with the other members of the family suggests a faulty reading in some subarchetype, cf. *P*.271/1 ⟨Loueache⟩ here. Perhaps the original reading should be reconstructed as *ANECE instead of the more correct *a n e t e (cf. *B*.248r/24 ⟨Anece⟩), which would explain the transmission to *ANIS in Branch γ more easily (cf. *W*.31r/10 ⟨Anis⟩; see Moreno Olalla 2013b: 955). The reading in Pepys could be explained directly from *ANECE through the frequent confusion between **n** and **u** and a not impossible confusion between **A** and **lu**, particularly if the Lombardic letter in its exemplar had a squarish shape, which is more than likely, cf. *FINEL rendered as *P*.267/16 ⟨Auel⟩. The species will be treated again, this time under its expected ME name (→ **105**, with discussion).

Most of the usual virtues allotted to the species are mirrored in the translation: galactogenous (**16** = *DVH* 397–398), diuretic (**19** = *DVH* 403), against gripes (**17** = *DVH* 398), flatulence (**18** = *DVH* 400–401), vomit (**19** = *DVH* 402) and sicknesses of the uterus (**20** = *DVH* 404). The dangers of dill against the sight and sperm (**22** = *DVH* 409–410) are also mentioned in medical literature.

 Literature: Dill (*Anethum graveolens* L.): → annete [**105**]. ¶ Anise (*Pimpinella anisum* L.): *HP* i.11.2 (ἄνησσον); *MM* iii.56; *NH* xx.185 (*anesum*); *SM* xi.833 (ἄνισον); *RM* ii.194; *Grad.* 376 (*anisum*); *LS* 242 (*aneisum* [آنیسون *ānaīsūn*], *anisum*); *EPN* xi (*hoc anisum. a cvlrayge*); *CI* c.18 (*anisum, ciminum dulce*); *TH* 21 (*anisum*); *Pand.* 44 ($_{AR}$*aneisim, aneisum,* $_{GR,LA}$*anisum*); *DVH(SME)* 14a18 (*anyse*); *Alph.* 10 (*anisum*), 40 (*ciminum dulce, anisum,* $_{AN}$*anyse*); *Sin.Bart.* 16 (*ciminum dulce, anisum*); *AC* 165,15 (*anisoum. anyse*) ⚘ *GH* 21 (Anisum, *aneisum, anys, swete commyn*); *Fu* 19 (ἌΝΙΣΟΝ, *anisum*); *Tu* I.235 (anyse, *anison, anysum*); *DL* 194 (anise, ἄνισον, ἄνησον, *anisum*); *Ge* 879 (anise, *anisum,* ἄνησον).

 C²S (Tu) | C²S¹ (Ge) | C³S³ (*SM, RM, Grad., TH, LS, GH, Fu, DL*) | C⁴S⁴ (*CI*)

19 and vomyte. This fragment, which translates *DVH* 402 *nausea*, and must therefore be authorial, is only found in the southern MSS (S_1 and *P*).

19 helpiþ þat is in womanys schappe. The sense of the passage is distorted in S_1, cf. *DVH* 404 *matricem iuvat*. The other MSS from the tradition provide correct versions: *B*.248v/3–4 ⟨helys þe matras þat is þe womans schape⟩, and similarly in *W*; *P*.271/5–6 offers ⟨heleþ þe moder þat is to seye þe matrice⟩.

20 washen… 21 ballokis. This fragment renders *DVH* 405–406 but the original sense of the passage is altered, partly due to the Latin version which served as exemplar to the Middle English translator (*Q*). There is no reference to ale in the Latin text, which only gives *tepida*—probably referring to water. The reference is not an alteration by Lelamour or the copyist of S_1, since the reference is recorded in all known witnesses. In some Renaissance editions of the Latin text (sigla δδ, εε, ηη and θθ in Choulant's edition), though, the word *aceto* "vinegar" appears instead of *anethum*, but ζζ (which is closest to *Q*, see Moreno Olalla 2018), is canonical here. It is possible that *aceto* answers to an editorial emmendation (which means a further correction to *tepido*) to make a clearer sense.

 Similarly, there is no reference to testicles in the Latin text, which offers *intestinorum* (406). Choulant's apparatus remains again silent about a possible variant here. The fragment is missing in MS *B*, so only *RH* provides parallel readings (*W*.31r/20 ⟨sore ballok*is*⟩, *P*.271/7 ⟨þe ballock*is*⟩).

 The fragment also shows traces of deterioration during the transmission of the ME text. While a reconstructed form *w e t t e could perhaps have been acceptable for S_1 ⟨wethe⟩, the parallel readings from the other witnesses suggest the convenience of assuming an exemplary *WASCHEN, cf. B.248v/4 ⟨weschyne⟩, W.31r/19, P.271/6 ⟨waschen⟩.

22 stoppyth þe yate of the engendir. This translates *DVH* 409–410 *genitale / claudit iter*. Therefore ⟨yate⟩ here is not etymologically related to OE *geat* "gate", as assumed in MED: *s.v.* gāte *n*.¹, but is a Southern formation deriving from ON *gata* "path" translating La. *iter*, cf. (Northern) B.248v/5 ⟨gatte of þe engenderure⟩, W.31r/21 ⟨gate of engendurare⟩, (SE Midlands) P.271/9 ⟨ʒate of engendrynge⟩.

24 grynde him. This is missing in all MSS of the tradition: the fragment is not in *B* or *P*, while *W* misses the whole virtue. The relative position within the entry suggests that it could be a translation of *DVH* 418 *cinis infusus*.

26 the¹...eyne. Two different virtues have been conflated here. The first one (*DVH* 419–420) deals with the properties of roasted dill seed against hiccups if they are inhaled, while the second (*DVH* 421–422) states the value of ground dill root against burning eyes. The error can be traced back to the scribe of *RH* as it is found in all three MSS belonging of that branch, while the Bodley version renders the text correctly: B.239v/8–9 ⟨þe odure þer-of reuys þe mannys ʒyskynge. Þe rott brynt in powder helys þe brynnyng of þe eyne⟩.

27 knottys...stomake. This fragment should deal with hemorrhoids and condylomata, in accordance with *DVH* 423–424. Perhaps *Q* had some lines rearranged and offered here *DVH* 401, where *os stomachi* is mentioned, but it is perhaps more likely to assume that the scribe of *Ω* mistranslated *condylomata solvit* (424). Note very particularly the choice of the Latin verb *solvo*, which may have suggested the translator the idea of knots.

30 avance. The Latin heading, the ME name and the physical description provided for this plant strongly suggest that the entry is devoted to wood avens (*Geum urbanum* L.). The same species will be treated again under *garofull* (→ **844**). The synonym *hare-fote* is recorded in a substantial number of medieval sources (see the Literature apparatus, and also PNME: *s.vv.* avancia, gariofilata, osmius, pes leporis, sanamunda) even though this name actually refers to several clovers (in particular *Trifolium arvense* L. and *T. sylvaticum* Gérard *ex* Loisel.). Confusion between both species probably originated from the burred fruits of *Geum*, which must have been assimilated to the inflorescences of the *Trifolium*, and the hairy stalks of both species.

The entry derives from *AC*, hence identification is sure on textual grounds, but pharmacographically the medical qualities of the *Trifolium* as provided in the entry λαγώπους (literally "hare's foot") in *MM* iv.17 (febrifuge, **34** and stomachal, **35**) have been blended with that of the *Geum* (a vulnerary, **36**), cf. "[t]he decoction of auens made with water [...] cureth all inward wounds and hurts. And the same decoction cureth outward wounds if they be washed therewithall" (DL). The digestive virtue, which is common to the *Trifolium* and the *Geum*, is recorded in none of the MSS used by Brodin.

> **Literature**: WOOD AVENS (*Geum urbanum* L.): *NH* xxvi.37 (*geum*); *Grad.* 357 (*gariophyllatum*); *DVH* 1–2146 (*garofilus*); *EPN* vi (*avencia. avence, hare-fot*); *Cl* G.6 (*gariofilata. auaunce*); *TH* 205 (*gariofilata*); *Pand.* 276 ($_{LA}$*gariofilata, erba benedicta,* $_{GR}$*lapagum*); *Alph.* 17, 70, 141, 162 (*avencia, pes leporis, gariofilata, sanamunda, zimis.* $_{GA,AN}$*auense*); *Sin.Bart.* 22 (*gariofilata, avancia*), 24 (*harefote*), 33 (*pes leporis*), 37 (*sanamunda*); *AC* 164.19 (*auencia. auence*) ⚜ *GH* 90 (GARIOFILATA, *auens*); *Fu* 143 (CARYOPHYLLATA, *herba benedicta, sanamunda*); *Tu* 2.389 (AVENES, *geum, gariophillata, sana munda, benedicta*); *DL* 94 (AVENS, *sanamunda, hearbe bennet, garyophyllata, benedicta, nardus rustica*); *Ge* 841 (AUENS, *herbe bennet, caryophyllata, sanamunda, herba benedicta, nardus rustica*).
>
> CS (Ge) | C^{2}S^2 (*TH, Grad., DVH, Cl,* Fu, DL)

36 cankyr. During the Middle Ages, the word *cancer/cancre* designated two different, if related, ailments according to its outward aspect, cf. "[t]he cancre is euen-voycely parted to two, þat is to saye, þe cancre þat is aposteme [...], and to þe cancre þat is a bocche" (*Chir.(ME)* 127). That is, cancer could mean a swelling (of a malignant type) or an ulcer. The first type was more precisely called *cancre nouȝt vlcerate*, while the second was *cancre vlcerate*, and was actually an ulcus, the consequence of a badly cured non-ulcerated cancer ("[t]he festred cancre is caused of an vnfestred cancre and of vlcers ygreuede and vnwisely curede" *Chir.(ME)* 299) that could degenerate into a severe gangrene (hence the early by-form *cancrene*, created by popular etymology) or even necrosis (Norri 1992: 197). This is the sense in *cankyr in the mouthe* (**1794**), where it must refer to a canker, that is a gangrenous stomatitis, an infection in the mouth and gums characterized by small fetid sloughing ulcers.

The word is normally used without any precision in the text and might mean either of the two ailings, although the context helps in the correct identification sometimes.

38 addyrworte. While PDE *adderwort* as a rule refers to the *Persicaria bistorta* (L.) Samp., the Latin name, the ME evidence and the brief physical description point towards quite a different plant, the one usually called δρακόντιον in Greek and *dracunculus* in Classical Latin, and which is traditionally identified with the dragons, *Dracunculus vulgaris* Schott, an Eastern Mediterranean plant (→ **539**, which offers an extremely detailed physical description of the plant). Comparison of the ME entry with the usual Latin sources makes it clear that, other than the antiarthritic virtue (about which, → 47), the entry derives from a translation of *DVH* other than *DVH(NME)* and *DVH(SME)*.

Identification with that species is sure on textual and pharmacological grounds, cf. its value as an alexipharmic (**42** = *DVH* 1733–1735), antiotalgic (**44** = *DVH* 1736–1737), ophthalmic (**46** = *DVH* 1741–1746), anticancerous (**46** = *DVH* 1740), antiabortive (**48** = *DVH* 1747–1749), antitussive and expectorant (**50** = *DVH* 1750–1755), and antipernius (**53** = *DVH* 1761–1765). The entry misses the virtues of the plant against polypus (*DVH* 1738–1739) and an as anthemoptyic (*DVH* 1752). A missing fragment in the original Latin text (*DVH* 1756–1760) could explain that the virtues of the plant as an aphrodisiac, diuretic, vulnerary and cosmetic are not recorded in the ME text, while a rearrangement in the lines of the poem is probably behind the fact that the benefits for the eye (*DVH* 1741–1744) are presented before, rather than after that one against *cancer magnus* (*DVH* 1740).

Literature: DRAGONS (*Dracunculus vulgaris* Schott): HP vii.12.2 (δρακόντιον); MM ii.166 (δρακόντιον); NH xxiv.149–150 (*dracunculus*); SM xi.864; RM ii.267; OEH 6 (*herba viperina. nædderwyrt*), 15 (*herba dracontea. dracentse*), 131 (*herba basilisca. nædderwyrt*); Dur.Glos. 300 (*basilisca. nedre-vyrt*), 302 (*dracantea. dracentia*); DVH 1728–1765 (*dragontea, colubrina*); LS 43 (*luf* [لُوف *lūf*], *dragontea*); EPN ix (*hec dragansia. a dragauns*); Cl s.33 (*serpentaria, dragontea, colubrina. dragance*); TH 451 (*serpentaria, colubraria, dracuntea*); Pand. 510 (_{AR}*luf, dragontea, belda, saredarecon, asclepias,* _{GR}*dragontium,* _{LA}*serpentaria, viperina, collum draconis*); DVH(SME) 25b.9 (*dragaunce. nedretunge*); Alph. 48, 167, 205 (*draguncea, asclepias, uiperina, pentaria, serpentilla, colubrina, basilica, cocodrilla.* _{GA,AN}*dragaunce*) 82 (*herpentaria*); Sin. Bart. 18, 23 (*dragantea, serpentaria, herba colubrina*), 39 (*cocodrilla*); AC 180.23 (*dragansia. dragauns, oderwourt, serpentyn*), 182,6 (*dragancia femina. dragans femel*) ✥ GH 410 (SERPENTINA, *dragons, snake grasse*); Fu 86 (ΔΡΑΚΟΝΤΙΑ ΜΕΓΑΛΗ, δρακόντιον μέγα, *dracunculus maior, serpentaria maior, colubrina*); Tu 1.305 (DRAGON, *dragontion*); DL 230 (DRAGONS, *dragons woort*, δρακόντια μεγάλη, *dracunculus maior, serpentaria, colabrina, serpentaria maior*); Ge 681 (DRAGONS, *dragon woort*, δρακόντιον, *dracunculus, serpentaria maior, bisaria, colubrina*).

CS (*Cl, TH, GH,* Fu) | C¹S¹ (*RM, LS,* Ge) | C³S³ (DL)

40 hote and drye. The Latin poem does not provide with the temperament of this species, while *AC* states that the plant is "hot *and* weet" (181.4–5).

47 the goute and þe festeryng of a wonde. This is not in the Latin poem, but seems to have been taken verbatim from *AC* (which, other than here, offers a wholly different text for this entry), cf. "Also þis he*r*be is good to dystroye þe gowte *and* þe cancre *and* festrynge of wou*n*dys" (181.2–4). According to Brodin's apparatus criticus, *gowte* is variant of *cowȝhe*, recorded in MSS

HRBL of the tradition and which may be authorial (cf. the antitussive quality of the species mentioned in **50**).

56 agrymony. The entry records the virtues of the agrimony (*Agrimonia eupatoria* L.) as given in *AC*. Pharmacological evidence does not support such claim, since the entry in *MM* provides with wholly different medical virtues (vulnerary, antidysenteric, hepatic, and alexipharmic), while *SM* commends it as a deoppilant. A few of the virtues found in the ME text are recorded in the corresponding entry of the *Spuria Macri*: as an anticolic (**59** = *SpMa* 23), splenetic (**64** = *SpMa* 30), and, most obviously, vulnerary whenever the patient was hurt with an iron tool (**61** = *SpMa* 28). This, together with the reference to the burred seed that will stick to animals or people touching the plant, which is rutinely repeated at least since Dioscorides, and the fuller physical description provided in *AC*, including the colour of the flowers and the (passing) resemblance of its serrated leaves to those of tansy, makes identification sure. The virtue of the species as an antiphtheiriac (**65**), which is not in *AC* nor *SpMa*, seems an addition.

The same species seems to be treated later in the herbal (→ **133**, with discussion).

Literature: AGRIMONY (*Agrimonia eupatoria* L.): *MM* iv.41 (εὐπατόριος); *NH* xxv.65 (*eupatoria*); *SM* xi.879 (εὐπατόριος); *RM* ii.212; *Grad.* 346 (*eupatorium*); *OEH* 32 (*herba argimonia. garclife*); *Dur.Glos.* 299 (*agrimonia. garcliue oththe clif vyrt*); *LS* 77 (*cafat* [غافث *ġāfiš*], *eupatorium*); *EPN* ii (*agrimonia. styc-wyrt*), v (*agrimonia, car-clife*); *Cl* E.13 (*eupatorium*); *TH* 162 (*eupatorium*); *Pand.* 54 (*argemonia, volucrum minus,* GR*arascelen,* LA*agrimonia, ferraria minor*), 247 (GR,LA*eupatorium, eupatorion, volucrum maius,* AR*ġafir*); *Alph.* 6, 201 (*agrimonia, ferraria, lappa inuersa, adiascordion, filantropos*), 3 (*agimonia.* GA,AN*egremoigne*), 204 (*ascella, sacrogrion, stephilon, pinaca agrestis*), 232 (*sarcocolla | sinon elauer*); *Sin.Bart.* 9 (*agrimonia. egremoyn*), 22 (*gasith. eupatorium*), 26 (*lappa incisa*); *AC* 164.6 (*agrimonia. egrimonye*) ⚭ *GH* 38 (AGRIMONIA, *egrymony*); *Fu* 90 (ΕΥΠΑΤΩΡΙΟΝ, ἡπατώριον, *eupatorium, hepatorium, agrimonia*); *Tu* I.314 (AGRIMONIE, *eupatorium*); *DL* 41 (AGRIMONIE, εὐπατώριον, ἡπατώριον, *hepatorium, agrimonia, ferraria minor, concordia, marmorella*); *Ge* 575 (EGRIMONIE, εὐπατώριον, *eupatorium, hepatorium, lappa inuersa, philanthropos*).

CS (Ge) | C¹S¹ (*LS*) | C¹S² (*Grad., Cl, TH*)

67 astrologie. An evident *lectio facilior* instead of *a r i s t o l o g i e, the text describes the medical properties of the several species called *aristolochia* in Latin as provided in *DVH*. The writer follows the teachings of *MM* when stating that there are three different species, rather than *NH*, where a fourfold division was made, or *Grad.*, where only two subspecies are distinguished. These are not described in the text but are traditionally taken to be the sarrasine

(*Aristolochia longa* L.), the smearwort (*A. rotunda* L.) and the European birthwort (*A. clematitis* L.). *A. longa* was also referred to as the male species on account of the form of its double root, which resembles two testicles, so that *A. rotunda* was, by opposition, its female counterpart. Only these two species were described and used in the ME medical corpus (see for instance Chauliac, Trevisa, and also secondary literature such as synonyma) and in the Renaissance: *GH* wrote that there were only two species, while Fu states that "Germanie officine solam longa*m* aristolochia*m* agnoscunt".

Identification with the several birthworts is sure on textual and pharmacological grounds, cf. its value as an alexipharmic (**70** = *DVH* 1402–1403), mazolytic and antiasthmatic (**71** = *DVH* 1404; see also note to **72**), vulnerary and anticaries (**73** = *DVH* 1410–1412), splenetic (**75** = *DVH* 1413), antipleurodynic, febrifuge, carminative, antipodagric, antiepileptic (**75** = *DVH* 1413–1418), for pain in womb and antiparalytic (**77** = *DVH* 1419–1420), demonifuge and exhilarant (**78** = *DVH* 1421–1422). The deoppilant, carminative and antidysenteric virtues of the species provided in **80–83** are not in the Latin text, while some medical qualities from *DVH* are missing: emmenagogue (*DVH* 1405–1406), calefacient (*DVH* 1407), antipleuritic (*DVH* 1408) or as vulnerary for fistulas (*DVH* 1423).

A par of the virtues of these species (up to ‹lettiþ› **77**) was included as well in an entry devoted to a different species (*Melissa officinalis* L.), but drawing the information from a different translation (→ **1355** for details). Some birthwort, probably *A. clematitis* L., seems to have been faultily described also elsewhere in the herbal (→ **919**).

Literature: BIRTHWORTS (*Aristolochia* L. spp.): *HP* ix.13.13 (ἀριστολοχία); *MM* iii.4; *NH* xxv.95–96, xxvi.154 (*aristolochia*); *SM* xi.835; *RM* ii.195; *Grad.* 356; *OEH* 20 (*herba aristolochia. smerowyrt*); *Dur.Glos.* 300 (*aristolochia. smerevyrt*); *DVH* 1395–1436 (*aristolochia*); *LS* 171 (*zaraund* [زراوند *zarāwand*], *aristologia*); *EPN* iv (*aristolochia. smert-wyrt*); *Cl* A.22 (*aristologia*); *TH* 27 (*aristolongia*); *Pand.* 7 ($_{AR}$acanug, carabuth, $_{GR}$ariston, fetalogos, apiston, panodracia, $_{LA}$aristologia); *DVH(SME)* 6b.19 (*smerewort*); *Alph.* 14 (*aristologie longa/rotunda*), 107 (*malum storacis*), 179 (*strongilis*), 202 (*aricalomi*), 227 (*ponadatria*); *Sin.Bart.* 11, 33 (*aristologia, paciens*); *AC* 162.13 (*astralogia longa. redemadur*), 162.26 (*astralogia rotunda. astrologie þe rounde, ganyngale*) ❧ *GH* 26 (ARISTOLOGIA ROTUNDA, *accange, carabuth, fetalagos, apiston, pauodricia, smerwort, meke galyngale*), 27 (ARISTOLOGIA LONGA, *reed mader, erratica, ephesta, petricomis*); Fu 31 (ἈΡΙΣΤΟΛΟΧΙΑ, *aristolochia, aristologia*); *Tu* 1.241 (ARISTOLOCHIA); *DL* 225 (ARISTOLOCHIA, ἀριστολοχία, *birthwurt, hartwurt*); *Ge* 696 (BIRTHWOORTS, *hartwoort*, ἀριστολοχία).

C (*RM*) | C²S¹ (*DVH*) | C²S² (*Grad., LS, Cl, TH, GH,* Fu, Tu, DL) | C³S³ (Ge)

67 rede mader. Given as a synonym for *Aristolochia longa*, this name usually refers to a different plant, *Rubia tinctorum* L. (→ **1271**). The same synonym is provided in a number of works, including *AC* and several synonyma (C26, C32, C41 in PNME: *s.v.* aristolochia).

72 nature of þe brest. This corresponds to *DVH* 1407 *asthmaticis prodest*, ⟨nature⟩ surely being a *lectio facilior* for *NARTHE "constriction" (< OE *nearu* "narrow" + *-th*). The word is usually spelt right in the ME treatise (cf. **453, 604, 938,** etc.), although the original sense may have been kept in just one passage (→ **840**).

83 Ipocras. Hippocrates of Kos, a contemporary of Socrates (469–399 B.C.) and frequently referred to as the Father of Modern Medicine. The most famous of all Greek physicians, he was the founder of the eponymous Hippocratic School and traditionally identified as the author of the *Hippocratic Corpus*, a collection of ca. 60 medical works which are in fact fully or partially anonymous.

The reference in *LH* is a very distorted version from *AC* 163.1–4, where the plant is said to be good for people suffering from oppilation in the breast if drunk with hot water. This is perhaps a very simplified reference to a passage in the treatise Περὶ νούσων (*De morbis*) iii.16.12 which deals with pleuresy (Potter 1980: 90–91):

> ἢν δὲ πρὸς τῇ ἐν τῇσι πλευρῇσιν ὀδύνῃ καὶ τὰ ὑποχόνδρια ἀλγέῃ, ὑποκλύσαι τε καὶ πιεῖν νήστι δοῦναι ἀριστολοχίαν καὶ ὕσσωπον καὶ κύμινον καὶ σίλφιον καὶ μήκωνα λευκὴν καὶ ἄνθος χαλκοῦ καὶ μέλι καὶ ὄξος καὶ ὕδωρ.

> In case that, apart from the pain in the side, the hypochondria are hurting too, you must use an enema and make the sick person drink birthwort, hyssop, cumin, laserwort, white poppy, a solution of blue vitriol [*or else* "copper ore"?], honey, vinegar and water with an empty stomach.

85 alixsandir. The Latin heading and the ME synonyms indicate that the entry must deal with horse parsley, *Smyrnium olusatrum* L., as described in *AC*. This tradition offers the same synonym and a similar, yet fuller, physical description than *LH* (where only the reference to the species's large black seed capsules is kept, cf. ⟨seme*n* nigru*m* magnu*m*⟩ *Sl*.3r/19). Identification seems therefore sustained on textual grounds, but the edited version of *AC* does not provide any virtue, and those provided in the Latin text (lithontriptic and antiverrucous) do not tally with the ones in the ME text, nor those in the descriptions by Dioscorides (emmenagogue and antihematuric) or Pliny (alexipharmic, anticolic, diuretic, lithontriptic, antilumbalgic and calefacient; the emmenagogue value of other *Apiaceae* such as *heleoselinum* and *oreoselinum* is also mentioned). Only the supposed spasmolytic qualities of the species are common to the Greek and the ME texts, but even here the Dioscoridean passage connects the shaking to fever, while there is no reference to that in the corresponding ME fragment. It is possible that the exemplary text was corrupt: it is not easy to see how taking horse parsley in a broth will cure apostemes, which were normally healed by external application of unguents. The fragment may therefore answer to a scribal conjecture.

> **Literature**: HORSE PARSLEY (*Smyrnium olusatrum* L.): *HP* ii.2.1 (ἱπποσέλινον); *MM* iii.67; *NH* xx 117 (*olusatrum*); *SM* xii.118 (σέλινον); *RM* ii.217; *Grad*. 379 (*petroselinum*); *OEH* 108 (*herba olisatra. oliastrum*); *LS* 280 (*karphs* [كرفس *karafs*], *apium*); *EPN* ii (*petrosilion. stan-merce*), iv (*sigsonte. stan-merce*), vi (*closera. alisaundre*); *Cl* p.6 (*petrosilinum*); *TH* 359 (*petrosellinum*); *Pand*. 573 (*petroselinum, apium petre, apium macedonicum, sinonum*); *Alph*. 5, 128, 139, 202, 222, 225 (*alexander, olixatrum, petrosillinum macedonicum.* ᴳᴬ*alisandre,* ᴬᴺ*stanmersh*), 11 (*apium siluestrum/montanum*), 108 (*macedonia*), 169, 230 (*silonum, sinonum, simonum*); *Sin.Bart*. 29 (*macedonicum, alexandrinum*), 33 (*petrocelinum macedonicum. stanmarche*); *AC* 168.15 (*alexandrum. alysaundre, stanmarch*) ⁊ *GH* 331 (PETROCILIUM, *synomum*); *Fu* 122 (ʹΙΠΠΟΣΕΛΙΝΟΝ, *olus atrum, petroselinum macedonicum, hipposelinon*); *Tu* 2.471 (ALEXANDER, *hipposelinon, olus atrum*); *DL* 439 (SMYRNIUM, σμύρνιον, *petroselinon, hipposelinon agreste, wilde alexander*); *Ge* 865 (ALEXANDERS, *wilde parsley,* ἱπποσέλινον, σμύρνιον, *olus atrum, syluestre apium, petroselinum macedonicum*).
>
> C (*SM*) | C²S² (*Cl, GH*) | C²S³ (*Fu*) | C³S³ (*Grad., LS,* Tu, DL, Ge)

88 postome. An abscess. According to Trevisa's translation of *De Proprietatibus Rerum*, "a posteme is gaderinge of superfluyte of humours in som membre, and makeþ rotynge and swellinge" (Seymour *et al.* 1975–1988: i.415). Norri (1992: 120) expands on this by quoting from Andrew Boorde's *The Breuiary of Helthe* (1547; f. 20r) "a postume is no other thynge but a collection or a ronnynge togyther of euyll humours. And some be internal, and some be exteryall.' Apostemes were considered the usual container of superfluous humours, so that it is then a cause of little wonder that they are so frequently mentioned in *LH*: they were the cause of both psychical and physical ailments, according to the place where they appeared and the humour contained in them. The following excerpt (*Chir.(ME)* 75) exposes concisely the several general types of apostemes distinguished by a Medical scholar of the time:

> And þe differences of þe qualite and quantite folwen suche differences taken of þe mater, nameliche i-ioyned togidre, when þay beeþ of þe bosome of þe mater, as it is saide in þat faculte. And þerfore moste and principally þai ben saide in þe book, þe Differences of Feueres. The whiche was wont to be saide by oþer wordes in oure comune scole of Mountpilers: þat of apostemes, some ben made of a mater nouȝt aduste (i. brente) neyþer corrupte (i. roten) and some of corrupte and aduste. And of eyþer, some ben sanguine, some colrik, some flewmatik, some melancolique, some watry and wyndy, symply and compownedly. The firste

were saide by oure felowe Maistre Iohan Iames oneliche euel. Þe secoundes ben euel wiþ an addicioun of deceyte and of euel manere.

91 affodill. While the species described in the text, displaying yellow flowers and long, narrow leaves is probably a daffodil (*Narcissus pseudo-narcissus* L.), and the ME synonym refers as a rule to the ramsons (*Allium ursinum* L.), comparison with the Classical pharmacopea indicates that the medical virtues provided here correspond to those of the summer asphodel (*Asphodelus aestivus* Brot.), as suggested by the Latin heading. See a fuller explanation in Moreno Olalla 2015: 61–67. The text follows *AC* closely, including the exact temperament of the species, which is missing in Brodin's edited text.

> **Literature**: SUMMER ASPHODEL (*Asphodelus aestivus* Brot.): *HP* i.10.7 (ἀσφόδελος); *MM* ii.169; *NH* xxi.109 (*albucus*); *SM* xi.842; *RM* ii.198; *Grad.* 366 (*asphodelus*); *OEH* 33 (*herba astularegia. wudurofe*); *LS* 211 (*cheunce* [خنـﺶ *hanšā*], *aphodillus*); *CI* A.14 (*affodilus, centum capita, albutium. affodill*); *TH* 17 (*anfodillum*); *Pand.* 17 (*affodillus, albutium, lappa, astula regia*); *Alph.* 3 (*affodillus, centum capita, albucium, albutron.* ₐₙ*ramesen*), 37 (*hermodactilis*), 209 (*cruco leucodio*); *Sin.Bart.* 9 (*affodillus, centum capita*); *AC* 161.26 (*affadilla. affadille, belle brome*) ❧ *GH* 17 (AFFODILLUS, *centum capita, albutium, porcus cerinus, aspilidos, poliortis, asucus, ampularia, affodylly*); Fu 40 (ἈΣΦΟΔΕΛΟΣ, *asphodelus, affodillus*); Tu 1.223 (RIGHT AFFODYLL, *albucum, hastula regia, asphedelos*); DL 464 (AFFODILL, *daffodill*, ἀσφόδελος, *albucus, hastula regia, affodilus*); Ge 85 (WHITE ASPHODILL, *asphodelus, albucum, hastula regia*, ἀσφόδελος).
>
> CS (Fu) | C²S² (*Grad., LS, CI, TH, GH, Ge, DL*)

96 þe juis of his leuys. *AC* adds myrrh to the list of ingredients: ‹modico murra [*sic*] & modico croco› *Sl.*IV/24. The words were dropped in *LH* probably due to a homoioteleuton *LITEL...LITEL, cf. "wi*th* a lytyl myrre *and* a lytyl safrou*n*" (*AC* 162.4).

102 the morfue. Morphew, an obscure skin disease, which the Latin text assimilates with impetigo: ‹morphea vel petigo› (*Sl.*IV/26). On the basis of the ME texts studied by Norri (1992: 120), the term probably referred to a leprous or scruffy eruption appearing in patches without pustules. The colour of these patches varied according to the humour that caused it. Cf. the following (*Chir. (ME)* 390):

> The morphewe þerfore is a spotty defoulynge of þe playne skynne. Of þe whiche, þogh þat ther be als many spices as of þe lepre, neuerþelatter þere ben two moste famouse (i. kowþe), þat is to say, þe blakke and þe white. Þe cause of þe whiche ben flewme of þe whyte and an humour of melancoly of þe blakke, as it was saide in 6ᵗᵒ De Egritudine et Sinthomate.

Norri has suggested that the white type might be vitiligo, "in which areas of skin lose their pigment and become white" (1992: 193; see moreover Wilson 1868: 585–591, where it is connected to elephantiasis) while the black variety probably indicates some type of skin cancers or ulcerations: "a blacke morphewe [...] is with vlceration" (Johannes de Vigo, *The Most Excellent Workes of Chirurgerye* 1543, f. 139va; quoted in Norri 1992: *ibidem*). Wilson 1868: 591 on the other hand suggests that rather than ulceration there is in fact a process of hyperpigmentation (in opposition to the hypopigmentation typical of vitiligo), which would explain the usage of the word to translate *nigras maculas* in → **319**.

105 annete. An account of the virtues of dill (*Anethum graveolens* L.) according to *AC* with additions from another source, akin to *DVH*, from **115** to the end of the entry. The medical virtues of the species had already been reviewed under a different plant name (→ **15**, with discussion). Identification is sure on textual and pharmacological grounds, cf. its value as a diuretic (**107**), carminative (→ **108**), antisingultus (**109**), vulnerary, particularly in the genitals (**111**), and antihemorrhoidal (**115**). A second source, very close to *DVH* but where the virtues seem to have been abridged and probably rearranged, must have provided the references to this species as a good galactogenous (**116** = *DVH* 397–389), stomachal and eupeptic (**116** = *DVH* 407–408), calefacient, anticephalalgic, and relaxant (**119** = *DVH* 425–428). The reference to the dangers to the sight and sperm is also taken from Macer Floridus's poem (*DVH* 409–410), while the properties of the species as an emmenagogue and nephretic (**117**) must derive from *DVH* 403–404, where the womb and urine are mentioned.

> Literature: DILL (*Anethum graveolens* L.): *HP* i.11.2 (ἄνηθον); *MM* iii.58; *NH* xx.196 (*anetum*); *SM* xi.832; *RM* ii.194; *Grad.* 363; *OEH* 123 (*herba anetum. dile*); *Dur.Glos.* 299 (*anecum. dile*); *DVH* 395–428 (*anetum*); *LS* 316 (*xebeth* [شِبِش *šibiš*], *anethum*); *EPN* iv (*anethum. dile*); *Cl* A.13 (*anetum. dille*); *TH* 16 (*anetum*); *Pand.* 673 ($_{A}$R*uebet,* $_{LA}$*anetum*); *DVH(NME)* 248r.24 (*anece*); *DVH(SME)* 14a.18 (*anyse*); *Alph.* 11 (*anetum agreste*), 174, 230 (*sister, meu*), 210 (*cinco*), 229 (*raticus*); *Sin.Bart.* 10 (*anetum.* $_{AN}$*dile, dille*), 30 (*men, anetum agreste*); *AC* 159.6 (*anetum. anete, dille*) ⚭ *GH* 16 (ANETUM, *dyll*); *Fu* 9 ('ANHΘON, *anethum*); *Tu* 1.235 (DYLL, *anethon, anethum*); *DL* 193 (DILL, ἄνηθον, *anethum*); *Ge* 878 (DILL, *anet,* ἄνηθον, *anethum*).
>
> C¹S² (Tu) | C²S¹ (SM, Fu, Ge) | C²S² (RM, Grad., DVH, Cl, TH, GH) | C³S² (DL) | C³S³ (LS)

108 kyrnyng. Norri (1992: 344), probably following *MED*: *s.v.* kirnel *n.*, § 4, suggested that *kernyng* must derive from OE *cyrnel* and therefore should be interpreted as a "morbid formation of rounded form, especially swollen gland", but the context here and in **418, 2320** makes it clear that this is in fact some digestive ailment connected to flatulence. Comparison with the ultimate source of the passage (*MM* iii.58 στρόφους τε καὶ ἐμπνευματώσεις παύει, "stops colic and inflations") proves that this assumption is correct, and that the actual sense must be "the unpleasant sensation in the bowels due to gastric winds". The direct source (AC 159.11–12, "Also þis erbe makyth a man to swage of rowelynge and wycked wynd in mannys body") supports this interpretation as well, since *rowelynge* must then be a spelling variant of "rolling" (cf. OF *rouler* < Vulgar L **rotulō*), rather than "revelling", as Brodin thought (1950: 289). Further support for this interpretation will be found on **1950**, where ‹gryndi*ng*› translates *DVH* 273 *tormina*, a Latin word that *P*.266/13 rendered as ‹kernyng›. The word *kirning* is not in MED but must be a velarized variant of *chirninge*, an obvious metaphor of the movements of the gas in the bowels and the borborygmi and those felt and heard while turning milk into butter.

124 ameos. The entry describes the medical properties of bishopsweed (*Ammi majus* L.) according to the *AC* tradition. Identification is sure on textual and pharmacological grounds: cf. its powers as an anthelminthic (**126**), carminative (**127**), lithontriptic (**128**), calefacient, hepatic and nephretic (**128**), and antiseptic and alexipharmic (**129**). Comparison in the text of this species with the danewort (*Sambucus ebulus* L.) is quite apposite as both display a big clusters of white flowers at the top, and have slightly serrated leaves.

> **Literature:** BISHOPSWEED (*Ammi majus* L.): *MM* iii.62 (ἄμι); *NH* xx.163 (*ami*), xx.264 (*ammi*); *SM* xi.824; *RM* ii.192; *Grad.* 369 (*ameos*); *OEH* 164 (*herba ami. miluium*); *LS* 287 (*nanochach* [نانخواه *nānḥawa*], *ameos*); *Cl* A.33 (*ameos*); *TH* 52 (*ameos*); *Pand.* 547 (_{AR}*nachana*, _{GR,LA}*ameos*); *Alph.* 8, 9 (*ameos agreste*, _{AN}*wodewhisgle*), 30, 206 (*carui agreste, cumnella, cordumeon, cordumeni*), 62 (*fraxinaria*), 202 (*ammi, cyminella, pe perdium* | *vmurcula, redi domum*), 223 (*muriula*); *AC* 163.19 (*amieos. amiyis*) 🕉 *GH* 48 (AMEOS, *pypercula, caruy agrestis, curcumela, woodnep, peny wort*); Fu 21 (*'AMMI, ammi, ameos*); Tu 1.231 (AMI, *ameos*); DL 195 (AMEOS, *ammi*); Ge 880 (BISHOPS WEEDE, *herbe William, ameos, comin royall, bulwoort*, ἄμμι, *cuminum Æthiopicum, cuminum regium, ammios*).
>
> C³s³ (*SM, RM, Grad., LS, Cl, TH*, Fu, Ge, DL)

129 clansiþ. Cf. "clensy3t" *AC* 163.28, and ‹mundificat› *Sl*.2v/13.

132 euperatorium. This seems a probable *lectio facilior* for *EUPATORIUM (cf. Gk εὐπατόριον), as if the word was related to "emperor" (the script makes no difference between **n** and **u**, and hence an alternative reading *e n p e r a t o r i u m is possible). This plant name referred as a rule to the agrimony (*Agrimonia eupatoria* L.) and rarely to the white horehound (*Marrubium vulgare* L.) in (post-)Classical Latin (see André 1985: *s.v.* eupatorium). In many Medieval and early Modern works, on the other hand, the name seems to have meant different species, including hemp agrimony

(*Eupatorium cannabinum* L.) or wild basil (*Clinopodium vulgare* L. = *Satureja vulgaris* (L.) Fritsch; see details in Stirling 1995–1998: *s.v.* eupatoria).

133 ambrose. An uncertain entry made worse by the lack of a physical description. While the Latin heading was used to refer to a number of separate species, agrimony in particular (see preceding note), three of the four ME plant names (⟨ambrose⟩, ⟨wilde sauge⟩ and ⟨hyndale⟩) are normally taken to refer to the wood sage (*Teucrium scorodonia* L.; → **2081**, where several of the synonyms are repeated). The connection between *eupatorium* and wood sage is found in many works of the period, including synonyma such as *Alph.* and *Sin.Bart.*, even though already Simon Januensis wondered why "medici nostri ipsis non advertentes verba Dyascoridis et Auicenne creduli herbulariis salviam agrestem eupatorium dicentes que nec in sapore nec in odore cum eo conuenit" (27r). As for the last synonym, ⟨wode-merche⟩, as a rule this refers to either the sanicle (*Sanicula europaea* L.) or wild celery (*Apium graveolens* L.). While this might be just a copy error for *w o d e - s a u g e—yet another known synonym for *T. scorodonia*—its Latin equivalent, *apium silvaticum*, is given as a Latin synonym for *ambrosia* by Isidore of Seville (*Etym.* xvii.9.80) and Pseudo-Dioscorides (iii.114). Identifications of *ambrosia* (see Stirling 1995–1998: *s.v.* for details) include, *inter alia*, species as diverse as yarrow (*Achillea millefolium* L.), chicory (*Cichorium intybus* L.), houseleek (*Sempervivum tectorum* L.), several *Artemisia* L., and both garden and wild sage, which explains its presence in *LH*.

Unfortunately, identification with any of the species quoted in the preceding paragraph or those mentioned by Stirling in the entries *eupatoria* and *ambrosia* is not supported by the usual pharmacological literature. According to the entry, the species is a purgative (**135**), vulnerary (**137, 144**), consolidative (**142**), deoppilant of the liver (**143**), spasmolytic (**145**) and antihematuric (**148**). Of all these, only the vulnerary and hepatic qualities are also found in the chapter devoted to the agrimony in *MM* (the relation between agrimony and liver diseases surely explains why some Medieval sources rendered εὐπατόριον as *Hepatorium*), the virtues of the other candidates being even more dissimilar from the ME text. The sentence ⟨yf ye bray hit with egrymony⟩ (**136–137**), yet, makes this equation impossible, unless this is a scribal emendation for *YF YE BRAY EGRYMONY.

   Literature: *WOOD SAGE (*Teucrium scorodonia* L.): *HP* i.10.4 (πόλιον); *MM* iii.110; *NH* xxv.63 (*scordotis/scordion*); *SM* xii.106; *RM* ii.253; *Grad.* 357 (*polium*); *OEH* 58 (*polion*), 151 (*omnimorbia. polios*);] *Dur.Glos.* 299 (*ambrosia. hind helethe*); *CI* p.22 (*polium*); *TH* 377 (*polius*); *Pand.* 37 (_LA_*ambrosia, athanasia*, _GR_*aysdo*); *Alph.* 8, 54, 98, 161, 212,

219 (*Ambrosia, lilifagus, eupatorium, saluia agrestis.* $_{GA}$*ambreise,* $_{AN}$*wildesauge*), 60 ($_{A}$*eufrasie*); *Sin.Bart.* 20, 28 (*esbrium, saltica, lilifagus, eupatorium, agresti salvia*), 10 (*Ambrosia. wilde sauge*) ❧ *GH* 152 (EUPATORIUM, *saluia agrestis, wylde sawge*); Fu 320 (ΤΕΥΚΡΙΟΝ, χαμαίδρυς, *teucrion, chamædrys*); DL 180 (WILDE-SAGE, *wood sage, ambros, saluia agrestis, ambrosiana*); Ge 535 (*wood sage, garlicke sage*). ¶ AGRIMONY (*Agrimonia eupatoria* L.): → agrymony [56].

CS (DL) | C¹S² (*GH*) | C²S² (*Grad., Cl,* Ge) | C²S³ (Fu)

149 betania. A *lectio facilior* instead of expected *b e t o n i c a*, as if ML *Bethania*, i.e. Bethany, the site of several well-known incidents in the New Testament including the raising of Lazarus (Jn 11:1, 18) and the Ascension of Jesus (Lk 24:50). In opposition to other, more exotic phytonyms, the Latin name for this species seems to have been extremely current at the time, and therefore unlikely to have passed unrecognized to any scribe competent in the copying of medical *Fachprosa*. The error is therefore intriguing and may be suggestive of a scribe who may have been more at ease copying religious texts (→ **188**, **784**, **1953**, and perhaps **282**, **708** for other instances of emendations with religious nuances). Note yet that the scribe did spell the word right over the top margin of 15va («Betayne») and 16ra («Betany»).

150 betayne. The entry describes the virtues of betony, *Stachys officinalis* (L.) Trevis., a plant extremely popular during the Middle Ages as a medicinal component, as given in *DVH(NME)*. No physical description of the actual species is provided but identification seems sure on account of the entry contents, cf. the supposed medical qualities of the betony as a diuretic and lithontriptic (*DVH* 430), anthydropic and anthemoptyic (**151**, **170** = *DVH* 431–432, 467–468), ophthalmic (**153**, **159** = *DVH* 433–434, 445–452), antiotalgic (**153** = *DVH* 435–436), antitussive and against hiccups (**155**, **166** = *DVH* 438, 462), stomachal (→ **155** = *DVH* 439–441), vulnerary (**157** = *DVH* 442–444), anti-inflammatory (→ **161**), splanchnic (→ **162**), laxative (**167** = *DVH* 462), febrifuge (**168** = *DVH* 463–466), phlegmagogue (**173** = *DVH* 470–473), alexipharmic (**174** = *DVH* 476), anticteric and emmenagogue (**175** = *DVH* 479), eupeptic (**178** = *DVH* 480–481), herpetofuge (→ **178**), and tonic (**184** = *DVH* 490–491).

The ME translation missed the value of betony against hysteroptosis (→ **173** = *DVH* 474–475) and the first reference to its laxative powers (corresponding to *DVH* 441), while on the other hand adds analgesic and soporific qualities (→ **184**) that are not in the canonical Latin text.

Literature: BETONY (*Stachys officinalis* (L.) Trevis.): *MM* iv.1 (κέστρον); *NH* xxv.84 (*vettonica*); *SM* xii.23; *RM* ii.200 (βεττονίκη); *OEH* 1 (*herbe betonica, biscopwyrt*); *Dur. Glos.* 300 (*betonica. se lease bisceop vyrt*); *DVH* 429–491 (*betonica*); *LS* 312 (*kastara* [كَسْطَرَ

kastara], *betonica*); *EPN* ii, v (*seo læssa biscop‹wyrt›*), iv (*byscop-wyrt*), vi (*bethonica. beteine*), ix (*hec betana. betany*); *Cl* B.7 (*betonica. beteyn*); *TH* 65 (*bectonica*); *Pand.* 81 (_AR_*bastarem, castaron,* _GR_*vectonicon,* _LA_*betonica*); *DVH(NME)* 252v.20 (*vetone*); *DVH(SME)* 14b.24 (*betoyne. castreon*); *Alph.* 21, 189, 207 (*betonica, betonia, vetonica, cestos, cestrum.* _GA_*betoine,* _AN_*betonyke*), 36 (*cestronidum*), 206 (*bibone*), 208 (*confinice*), 210 (*chestu*), 223 (*nici flos*), 234 (*troicutes*); *Sin.Bart.* 13 (*betonia major. selfhele*), 40 (*smirtus*), 43 (*vetonica. betyne*); *AC* 168.19 (*betonia, betonye, boyschopyswort*) ℞ *GH* 61 (BETHONICA, *bethony*); Fu 131 (ΚΕΣΤΡΟΝ, *betonica, vetonica*); Tu 1.251 (BETONIE, *betonica, kestron, psychotropon*); DL 208 (BETONIE, κέστρον, ψυχρότροφον, *betonica, vetonica*); Ge 578 (BETONIE, κέστρον, *betonica, vetonica*).

C^1S^1 (Fu) | C^2S^2 (DL, Ge) | C^3S^3 (*LS, Cl, TH, GH*)

150 colde. The original Latin poem never mentioned the temperament of this plant, but only stated that *Betonicam soliti sunt Cestron* [i.e. κέστρον] *dicere Graeci* (*DVH* 429). Moreover, betony was universally taken to have a warm, rather than a cold, temperament (see previous note, and the marginal scribbling by Hand B). The appearance of ‹colde› here is actually due to a mistaken scribal reading of the verb *CALD* "called" in the exemplar (answering to *soliti sunt* [...] *dicere*, cf. *W.*38r/25 ‹is cald costron i*n* gru›; this passage is missing in the Bodley version) as if the Northern ME adjective *cāld* "cold" by the Southern scribe of either *A* or S_1. See Moreno Olalla 2017: 677–678 for details.

151 þe empetik. This misinterprets *DVH* 431 *haemoptoicis* "suffering from hemoptysis, i.e. spitting of blood". The whole sentence is a shambles in Branch α of *DVH(NME)*, and unfortunately MS *P* does not keep this entry, but the mistake must have been already present in Branch γ of the tradition, as it is also found in the Wellcome version of the herbal, cf. *W.*38r/27 ‹þe empetik*is*›. The word is apparently misused again in → **2129**, that time to refer to some eye disease.

153 erys. Reading emended after *B.*252v/22 ‹errs› and *W.*38v/1 ‹heris›, and ultimately *DVH* 436 *auribus*.

155 þe ʒiskynge. Cf. *B.*252v/24 ‹ʒyskynge› and *W.*38v/2 ‹ʒisky*n*g›, translating *DVH* 438 *suspiria*.

156 hit helpiþ for feuer. A mistaken translation of the Latin original (*DVH* 440–441), which actually states that the species should be taken for the stomach-ache mentioned in the previous sentence if the pain is accompanied also by fever, and with wine if there is none.

161 hit addys voymett. The meaning of the original fragment in *DVH* 453 *Purgatur vomica dira* "it removes the dire abscess", seems to have posed problems to the ME translator, or else it was faultily written in Ω: in any case, each of the two main branches of *DVH(NME)* provide different readings here:, cf. *B*.253r/6 ⟨helys weme*n*⟩ vs. *W*.38v/10 ⟨addes vomit⟩.

162 take... 165 wombe. This sentence translates *DVH* 456–461 very faultily. The original Latin text, for example, indicates that one must use four ounces of betony (*uncia betonicae* [...] *quaterna*) for each three cyathi of old wine (*vetusti / cum vini cyathis tribus*), and makes reference neither to the spleen nor the liver, but only to the kidneys (*renes*). Moreover, while the same dosis is also provided for stomach ache, *DVH* 460 actually recommended a different posology, viz. one ounce of betony for each two cyathi of old wine.

All witnesses of *DVH(NME)* agree in this, but S_1 moreover adds a phrase ⟨of þe eyen⟩ (**165**) that is missing both in the original Latin text and in the other ME versions. It is possible that the scribe spotted a diplography *AKYNGE OF ÞE REYNES OF ÞE REYNES in his exemplar, emended what he assumed to be a copy mistake for **of* þe eyne*, and turned it into ⟨eyen⟩, which may have been closer to his own dialect.

167 with... 168 þere-to. Comparison with the Latin original indicates that this fragment, which corresponds to *DVH* 464 *Uncia iungatur plantaginis una duabus*, is syntactically misplaced and should appear immediately after ⟨juis of betayn⟩ in the section describing the febrifuge virtues of betony. Since both Branch α and Wellcome provide correct versions of this passage (*B*.253r/9–10 ⟨an vnce of plantane done to ij vnce off veto*n*⟩, *W*.38v/16–17 ⟨a nounce of plantayn don*e* to two vnceys of betoyn*e*⟩), it is likely that the copyist of either *A* or S_1 misunderstood his exemplar, hence the scribal need to add a coda ⟨put þ*e*re-to⟩, which refers back to the ⟨wombe⟩ that had just been mentioned.

169 helpiþ. The ME text misses *DVH* 466 *Antea quam febris praenuncia frigora fiant* that should appear immediately after this word. The fragment is recorded in both the Bodley and Wellcome versions, although the syntax and wording are widely divergent (*B*.253r/11 ⟨& he sall a-schape þe axeys⟩, *W*.38v/18 ⟨be-for þe access of schakyng⟩).

170 most & þe rote estampit. The reading in S_1 has been emended after *B*.253r/12–13 ⟨rot stampd & dronkyne with must⟩ (similarly *W*.38v/20–21), and ultimately *DVH* 469 *Radicum pulvis cum mulsa tritus et haustus*. Note that the scribe of *A* mistook the noun *MUST as a verb in the imperative and had to rearrange the ingredients.

171 Plenius commaundith. Gaius Plinius Secundus, known as Pliny the Elder (23/24–79), uncle of Pliny the Younger and commander of the Roman fleet at Misenum, but best remembered today as a polymath, particularly as the author of the monumental *Naturalis Historia* in 37 volumes, designed as an encyclopedia of all contemporary knowledge of the natural world.

The fragment quoted here, which corresponds to *DVH* 471–473, is obviously a loose rendition of *NH* xxv.127: "vettonicae semen in mulso aut passo, vel farina drachma in vini veteris cyathis quattuor; vomere cogendi atque iterum bibere". Macer Floridus's alterations of Pliny's original text include *DVH radicum* vs. *NH* "semen" or *bis binas dragmas* vs. "cyathis quattuor", and the omission of wheat flour and old wine from the list of ingredients.

173 vomyte. A translation of *DVH* 474–475, containing the assumed medicinal powers of ground betony leaves drunk with must against hysteroptosis (i.e. prolapse of the uterus), should have appeared after this word. While of course a mere scribal oversight cannot be ruled out, Macer Floridus's usage of medieval La. *steras* "uteri" probably played a part in this omission, since this was a learned word (cf. Gk ὑστέρα, with addition of the Latin plural accusative ending -*as*) that the ME translator must have not recognized.

178 Plenius saiþe. The passage translates *DVH* 482–485, which is parallel to a section of the *Regimen sanitatis Salernitanum* (de Renzi 1852–1859: I.462). The text of the *Regimen* is in turn based on *NH* xxv.101: "vettonica […], cui vis tanta perhibetur, ut inclusae circulo eius serpentes ipsae sese interimant flagellando". Note moreover that ‹grete venym with betony› is a scribal mistake for *DVH* 482 *de betonica viridi.* cf. *B*.253r/20 ‹grene veton›, and similarly *W*.39r/1.

180 the maister of medecynes. This stands for *DVH* 486 *Menemachus*. Menemachus (Μενέμαχος) was a physician from Aphrodisias whom Galen mentioned several times. No works by this physician are now extant, so Macer Floridus must be dropping names here, probably because the foot structure of the name, mistakenly assumed to present a sequence ⌣ ⌣ – ⌣, suits him (→ **1682** for another probable instance of the same policy).

It is not clear why the translator of *DVH(NME)* came to this reading instead of simply copying the name on the Latin text (cf. *B*.253r/21–22 ‹Maystres of medcyns›, *W*.39r/3 ‹þe maister of medycyns›), but it may be worth mentioning here that Tradition δ in Choulant's edition reads ‹Medeacus› here, which lends itself well to what would then be but a *lectio facilior*. Perhaps *Q* read together with δ here. See **1339** for another example of the same.

182 Plenius saiþe. This mistranslates *DVH* 488–489, by turning the drug (*nocuo medicamine*) of the original text into an evil beast. The passage ultimately rests on *NH* xxv.128: "qui cotidie gustent eam [i.e. pulvis vettonicae], nulla nocitura mala medicamenta tradunt". Explanation of the change is doubtful since none of the several versions in Choulant's edition records anything of the sort, but it is worth noting that whereas Branch α mentions adders (*B*.253r/24 ‹edders›), *RH* refers more generally to beasts (*W*.39r/6 ‹best›). Perhaps it should be put down as a faulty reading in Ω, which led the scribes of α and *RH* to conjecture.

184 take... 187 sclepe. This fragment is missing in the canonical text of *DVH*, and is mentioned neither by Choulant in his apparatus nor in *DVH(SME)*. The Bodley and Wellcome versions moreover add at the very end of the entry an extra virtue, this time as an anticephalalgic: *B*.253v/1 ‹& dos a-way the hedwerke›.

188 beata. A *lectio facilior* instead of *b e t a , as if the feminine form of La *beatus* "happy, blessed", a word frequent in religious contexts (→ **149**, **784**, **1953**, and perhaps **282**, **708** for other possible examples). The scribe wrote the name right as ‹Beta› over the top margin of f. 16rb.

189 beatis. Checking the medical qualities included in this article against *DVH* reveals that this translates lines 1087–1126 of the Latin treatise, which are devoted to the virtues of the onion (*Allium cepa* L.), a species that will be treated again in the herbal (→ **1581**, with discussion). Besides the reference to the onion's different effects on choleric and phlegmatic people, cf. the value of the species as a stomachal and cosmetic (**192** = *DVH* 1093–1094), against hound-bite (**195** = *DVH* 1099) and muteness (**196** = *DVH* 1107–1108), sternutatory and anticallus (**197** = *DVH* 1109–1114), ophthalmic (**199** = *DVH* 1124–1125) and antiephelic (**200** = *DVH* 1125–1126). In opposition to the other version of the text included in *LH*, here the soporific qualities are recorded, albeit faultily (→ **193**). On the other hand a substantial number of verses, where the medical properties of the species as antiodontalgic, antiaphthic, antidysenteric, antialopecic, antihalitosic, orectic, and antihemorrhoidal, is missing (*DVH* 1115–1123). The text moreover includes a few virtues at the end that look like an interpolation (**200–203**: refrigerant, soporific, galactogenous, antidysenteric and ophthalmic). The soporific and ophthalmic powers of onion had already been treated in the entry, hence the interpolated section might have shared a common origin with Macer Floridus's poem.

Identification with the onion also allows to explain the different plant names used in the several MSS of *DVH(NME)* (*B*.245r/10 ‹letus›, *W*.33r/13 ‹Betys›, *P*.277/12 ‹Letuse›) as due to misspelling from a reconstructed form *LEK*IS*, which could still mean several alliaceous species in late ME, and particularly the onion (just like in the North Germanic languages, see Moreno Olalla 2017:

685–686). The reading ⟨betys⟩, common to MSS of the same branch (W and S₁), suggests moreover that Subarchetype γ must have been written in a minuscule script, thus making **l** and **b** confusable because both letterforms have an upper loop. (Of course the confusion between **t** and **c** in *BP* is too widespread to allow the drawing of any conclusions).

Literature: ONION (*Allium cepa* L.): → oynowneis [**1581**]

189 some... hede. This passage is a faulty translation of *DVH* 1088–1089 *Namque Dioscorides inflare caputque gravare / Atque sitim Cepas dicit succendere mansas*, and the flatulent and dipsetic qualities of onions are indeed listed in *MM* ii.151, § 1; [κρόμυα] ἔστι δὲ ἅπαντα [...] πνευματωτικά, [...] διψώδη "all [onions] are [...] apt to cause flatulence, [and] thirst-making." As for the Dioscoridean claim that onions are bad for the head, cf. ἔστι δὲ καὶ κεφαλαλγές (*MM* ii 151 § 2, "[b]ut it also causes headaches").

189 Galyen saythe. Claudius Galen of Pergamon (129–200/216) was personal physician to the Roman emperors Commodus and Septimius Severus, a skilled surgeon, and also a philosopher praised by Marcus Aurelius. A very prolific writer, his extant medical works were avidly studied in the Middle Ages both in Europe and the Muslim world and served as the basis to Galenic medicine, which rests on the assumption, already sketched by the Hippocratic Medical School, that illnesses originate when the four body humours (blood, phlegm, bile and black bile) were unbalanced or else became corrupt. His anatomical ideas too went virtually unchallenged until well into the 16th century.

The passage renders *DVH* 1090–1091 (another translation in → **1582**). The idea that alliaceous species such as onion, garlic or leek are damaging to choleric temperaments but beneficial to phlegmatic ones can also be found in the *Regimen sanitatis Salernitanum*, 453–461 (de Renzi 1852–1859: V.801–802), and ultimately stems from Galen's Περὶ τροφῶν δυνάμεως (*De alimentorum facultatibus*) ii.71 (Kühn 1821–1833: vi.659):

> φείδεσθαι δὲ χρὴ τῆς συνεχοῦς ἐδωδῆς ἁπάντων τῶν δριμέων, καὶ μάλισθ᾽ ὅταν ὁ προσφερόμενος αὐτὰ χολωδέστερος ᾖ φύσει. μόνοις γὰρ τοῖς ἤτοι τὸν φλεγματώδη χυμὸν ἢ τὸν ὠμὸν καὶ παχὺν καὶ γλίσχρον ἠθροικόσιν ἐπιτήδεια τὰ τοιαῦτα τῶν ἐδεσμάτων ἐστίν.
>
> It is necessary to refrain from the continuous eating of any of these pungent foods, and above all if the receiver is of a very bilious nature. Such meals are in fact convenient only to those that gather the fierce, thick and sticky phlegmatic humour.

191 gode and holsome. This expands on the original *DVH* 1091 *salubres*. Only the two Southern MSS read together here (cf. *P*.277/14 ⟨good and holsom⟩), in opposition to *B*.245r/12 ⟨haylsum⟩ and *W*.33r/15 ⟨god⟩. Since the exact ME translation of La. *salubris* is "wholesome" (as suggested by the Bodley version), it is possible that the addition of *good* is not authorial but due to the scribe of *RH*.

191 he affirmeth. The claimed benefits of onions to the stomach and skin colour are not found in any Galenic treatise. The Latin text (*DVH* 1092–1093) states that these virtues come from the teachings of none other than the god Asclepius—which of course makes but very little sense. The original quotation, which derives from Pliny, and a full explanation will be found later in the treatise (→ **1586**). Subarchetype γ must have turned the exemplary *ASCLEPIUS into *AFFIRMES, for Wellcome reads together with S_1 here. Only Pepys reads correctly here, cf. *P*.277/16 ‹asclepyng seyþ› (the confusion between **us** and **ng** is of course usual). As for Bodley, the whole passage is simplified: *B*.245r/13 ‹& it is hailsym to þe stomake›.

DVH 1095–1096, which describe the analgesic virtues of onions if eaten each day and should immediately follow this passage, seem to be missing in the ME translation.

193 he… 194 wombe. All witnesses read together with S_1 and therefore the sentence can be safely taken to have appeared already in Ω, yet there is nothing in the canonical version of the Latin passage about vinegar or good taste: rather, the text (*DVH* 1097–1098) reads *affirmant omnes mansas inferre soporem, / et dicunt illas mollire salubriter alvum*. (Note moreover that S_1 innovated, since Wellcome and Pepys did translate *affirmant omnes* correctly: *W*.33r/16–17, *P*.277/17–18 ‹all þai con*ferme*›.) Other than as due to a muddled MS, the reference to vinegar is difficult to account for until *Q* or an akin version be found, but the change of original *soporem* to *SAPOREM, which is obviously behind ME *sauor*, is supported by at least one tradition in Choulant's apparatus (MS η) and may therefore have also appeared in the Latin exemplar.

194 hony and eysell. The variant *melle* […] *et aceto* for *DVH* 1100 that underlays the ME version is found in Tradition θ.

195 heliþ. Emended after *W*.33r/19 ‹helis›, even though *BP* offer ‹helpis› here, because S_1 normally reads together with Wellcome (Moreno Olalla 2013b: 948–950) and is moreover in accordance with *DVH* 1099 *curare*.

198 ete… bilys. The ME sentence is obviously nonsensical, and seems to blend two different virtues (praising the onion as an emmenagogue and anticallus), cf. *DVH* 1111–1114:

> Mausae vel potae tardantia menstrua purgant.
> Triturasque pedum, soleae quas vel caligarum
> Duriciae faciunt, succo sanabis eodem,
> Cum gallinarum pingui si saepe perungas.

The Wellcome and Pepys versions offer the full fragment (*W.*33r/22–23 ‹Etyn or drunken it sp*ur*ges þe floures of woman*e* stamp it & lay to þe biles›, *P.*277/24–26 ‹etyn or drunkyn it purgeþ þe flo*ur*es of wymmen. stampe it and ley it to þe beuyles›), suggesting that there was a homoioteleuton in S_1 (*or drinke... it and lay it).

199 take... 200 frenteklys. This fragment should appear at the very end of the entry since it translates the last two virtues alloted to this plant (*DVH* 1124–1126), but is placed in the same position in all versions of *DVH(NME)*. These lines must have been transposed in *Q*, probably after *DVH* 1113.

200 who-so... 202 mylke. Comparison with other versions of *DVH(NME)* indicate that the text in S_1 is faulty here, cf. *W.*33r/25–29:

> who-so et*is* it it abat*is* bry*m*ny*n*g of ou*ir*-mich hete. Soden i*n* jus & etyn is god for þe stomak þe sede dru*n*kyn*e* i*n* wyne gers men*e* slepe & þe norris to haue mylk in h*ir* pappis.

The fragment is similar in *B* and *P*, but Bodley reads ‹myntt› instead of ‹jus› and Pepys gives a nonsensical ‹frennyng*is* ouer-mechel etyng› instead of the burning sensation of heat. The lines seem an interpolation in *Q*, as these virtues are missing in the canonical version of *DVH*.

202 and³... 203 sighte. This virtue seems misplaced. The other versions of *DVH(NME)* offer this before the antidysenteric powers of onion that immediately precedes it (and which renders to *DVH* 1119). The scribe of S_1 must have realized his previous mistake and emended it by copying it at the end of the entry.

205 bvgill. Notwithstanding the Latin headword and ME name, the medical qualities of this entry do not correspond to that of the bugle (some *Ajuga* L. spp., probably *A. reptans* L.; → **223** for that species) but to those included in *DVH* 1127–1138, which deals with the plant *buglossa*—borage (*Borago officinalis* L.) rather than alkanet (*Anchusa officinalis* L. or *A. arvensis* (L.) M.Bieb.)—as translated in the *DVH(NME)* tradition. The confusion between *bugula* and *buglossa* was not infrequent in medieval times (see OED: *s.v.* bugle *n.*²) and must have been already present in Ω. The same Latin entry will be translated again under different names (→ **214** and **1183**, with discussion).

Identification is sure on pharmacographic grounds too, cf. its properties as an anticholeric and cardiac (**206** = *DVH* 1128–1131), pulmonic (**208** = *DVH* 1132–

1132), anamnestic (→ **209**) and exhilarant (**212** = *DVH* 1137–1138). Missing from this account is the supposed antisciatic value of the species (*DVH* 1133–1134).

    Literature: BORAGE (*Borago officinalis* L.): → borage [**214**].

205 hote and drye in that oþer de-gre. The temperament of the species is never consigned in *DVH*, and is broadly given in *B* (it misses the exact gradation), so this could be an addition of *RH* since all three MSS read together here. Medical *auctoritates* considered this species to be hot and moist, rather than dry (→ **1183**).

209 helpeþ... 210 vsed. The missing fragment, due to a homoioteleuton *v s e d ... v s e d in the *AS*₁ branch, is kept in the other versions of the *DVH(NME)* tradition and stands for *DVH* 1135–1136. The reading is taken from *P*.271/28–272/1.

214 borage. The Latin headword and ME name point naturally to the borage (*Borago officinalis* L.), while the medical virtues provided in the entry demonstrate that this is an abridged version of the entry *Buglossa* (a plant name generally identified with the alkanet, *Anchusa officinalis* L.) as rendered in *DVH* (note the reference to "þe wordis of Macer"). Whether the *Borago* or the *Anchusa*, the species was treated several times in the herbal with mostly the same medical powers (→ **205**, and **1183**, with discussion): exhilarant (**217** = *DVH* 1137–1138), cardiac and anticholeric (**219** = *DVH* 1128–1131). Missing from this account are the properties of the species as a pulmonic, antisciatic and anamnestic. On the other hand, the value of the species as an alexipharmic (**217**) and anticteric (**221**) must be an interpolation from another source: the former virtue is recorded in the chapter devoted to the different buglosses in DL, while the latter appears in *Cl*, *GH*, and in Renaissance treatises in connection with bugloss.

    Literature: *BORAGE (*Borago officinalis* L.): *Grad*. 348 (*borrago*); *Cl* B.4 (*borago*); *TH* 62 (*borrago*); *Pand*. 101 (*borrago*); *Alph*. 23 (*borago*. $_{GA,AN}$*borage, bourache*); AC 171.10 (*boragia. borage*) ⚜ *GH* 58 (BORAGO, *borage*); Fu 51 (ΒΟΥΓΛΩΣΣΟΝ, *buglossum, bubula lingua, bouis lingua, borrago*); Tu 1.256 (BORAGE, *borageo, buglossum*); DL 10 (BORAGE, *oxe tongue*, βούγλωσσον, *lingua bubula, libanium, lingua bouis*); Ge 652 (BORAGE, *borago*, βούγλωσσον, *lingua bubula, euphrosinum*). ¶ ALKANET (*Anchusa officinalis* L./*A. arvensis* (L.) M.Bieb): → longe de beffe [**1183**].

223 browne bugill. Brown bugle is traditionally taken to be the bugle (*Ajuga reptans* L.). Identification is supported textually, since the entry follows AC closely (even in the misspelling "bigula" instead of expected *b u g u l a) yet misses the physical description offered in the exemplar, where the plant is said to have rough blue flowers and ovate brown leaves (these physical features do appear in a revisitation of the same species, → **919**). Pharmacographically as well, identification with *A. reptans* is very likely: the species is praised as beneficial to the head, being an excellent vulnerary (**224**), anticatarrhal (**225**), deoppilant and analgesic (**226**) to that area. The vulnerary qualities of the bugle were rutinely extolled in Medieval and Renaissance texts (cf. the synonym ‹silfe-hele›, which was applied to a number of species, and such Latin synonyms for the species as *solidago, consolida media*).

Besides the heading, the entry offers two synonyms, both of which are missing in *AC*. ‹Silfe-hele› was applied to a number of vulnerary species, in particular to refer to *Prunella vulgaris* L. (which similarly displays purple flowers but has lanceolated leaves, and hence cannot be the species intended here; see DL, where both are treated under the same heading), but the apparition of ‹hart-worte› is unexpected since "heart-wort" as a rule refers to the birthwort (*Aristolochia clematitis* L., → **67**, and particularly **919**). Note incidentally that, while *hart-worte* could also stand for a number of Apiaceae (hart-worts, *Tordylium* L. spp.), this name is a post-Medieval calque of German *hartzwurt* (see OED: *s.v.*) and hence can be safely ruled out as be the species described here.

Literature: BUGLE (*Ajuga reptans* L.): *Dur.Glos.* 300 (*buglosse. foxes gloue*); *EPN* vi (*buglosa. bugle, wude brune*); *Alph.* 25 (*bugla.* $_{GA,AN}$*bugle*), 190 (*venti media*); *Sin.Bart.* 13 (*bugla. bugle, uodebroun*); *AC* 171.16 (*bigula. brounbugle*) ⚘ Fu 146 (CONSOLIDA MEDIA, *solidago*); DL 92 (BUGLE, *prunel, cerpenters hearbe, self heale, hookeheale, consolida media, prunella, brunella*); Ge 506 (BUGLE, *middle comfrey, sickle woort, herbe carpenter, consolida media, bugula, buglum, browne bugle*).

CS (Fu, DL, Ge)

230 bornete-is. The Latin heading, the ME synonym and the distinction made in the text between two different species make it quite possible that the entry was intended to describe the medical qualities of two *Sanguisorba* L. species: the one that grows in grasslands would be *S. officinalis* L., while the one found in dry ground would then be *S. minor* Scop. (= *Poterium sanguisorba* L.). Textually, the entry follows *AC* very closely, omitting just a few details such as the size of the leaves of each species.

Still, the physical description of the plant cannot grant such identification, since the flowers of the *Sanguisorba* are either pink or red, rather than blue as stated in the text, and phytomorphologically are not reminiscent of that of ‹heyhofe›, i.e. ground ivy (*Glechoma hederacea* L.), to which they are compared. Similarly, the leaves of the *Sanguisorba*, as most Rosoideae, are broad, pinnate and display serrated edges, while those of the tansy (*Tanacetum vulgare* L.) are markedly lobed—as usual among Asteraceae—and resemble those of a fern (cf. "sideritis... folio filicis" in *NH*).

Pharmacographically as well, the virtues given in the entry are unexpected. The two *Sanguisorba*, as suggested by their binomen, were generally commended as vulnerary and hemostatic plants, particularly if the effusion of blood was due to a weapon wound (cf. the Greek name, derived from σίδηρος "iron"), but the species here are assumed to be good to dissolve humours in the body—hence its value as a laxative (**232**, deoppilant (**233**), and diuretic and anticteric (**235**)—and as an analgesic in the thorax (**236**). *RM*, where the vulnerary effects of σιδηρῖτις are suprisingly not mentioned either, is yet in complete opposition with the ME text, since the plant is said to be good to staunch fluxes (τοῖς ῥοώδεσιν ἁρμόττει πάθεσιν).

Literature: *BURNETS (*Sanguisorba* L. spp.): MM iv.34 (σιδηρῖτις ἄλλη); NH xxv.44 (*sideritis... folio filicis*); SM xii.121 (σιδηρῖτις); RM ii.258; EPN vi (*borneta, sprungwurt*); Alph. 25 (*burneta.* GA,AN*burnete, burnette*); Sin.Bart. 13 (*burneta, camepiteos*); AC 171.22 (*burneta. burnet*) ⚘ Fu 303 (SANGUISORBA); Tu 2.731 (BURNET, *pimpinella (italica), bipennula, sanguisorba*); DL 97 (BURNET, *pimpinell, pimpinula, bipennella, pampinula, sanguisorba, solbastrella*); Ge 888 (BURNET, *pimpinella sanguisorba, sanguinaria, bipennula, solbastrella*).

S (Fu) | FH (*SM*) | FS (Ge, Tu) | F²S³ (DL)

231 and. A missing verb, probably *HAUYÞ, is expected after this word, cf. AC 171.23 "haȝt".

240 bellyre. The Latin heading, the physical description of the plant, which compares it to a skirret (probably, *Sium sisarum* L., → **2161**, even though that entry actually describes the medical qualities of *Eruca vesicaria* (L.) Cav.), and its habitat make it quite likely that the entry describes the medical virtues of the narrow-leaved water-parsnip, *Berula erecta* (Huds.) Coville (= *Sium angustifolium* L.), as provided in the *AC* tradition. Note that some Medieval and Renaissance works (cf. the use of the common synonym *fabaria* in the Literature apparatus for this and the next entry, or the plate-title *Sium* in Fu) seem to have confused this species with *Veronica beccabunga* L.

While there are good textual and botanical reasons to assume that the entry describes de healing properties of *Berula erecta*, identification is not really sustained from a pharmacographic point of view. According to the Classical evidence, the species—just like any other *Apiaceae*—is an excellent diuretic, lithontriptic, emmenagogue and oxytocic, but none of these virtues are mentioned here. Rather, the species is taken to be good against furuncles (→ **242**).

Literature: NARROW-LEAVED WATER-PARSNIP (*Berula erecta* (Huds.) Coville): *MM* ii.127 (σίον); *NH* xxii.84 (*sium*), xxvi 50 (*lauer*), 80 (*silaus*); *SM* xii.123; *RM* ii.259; *OEH* 136 (*herba sion. laber*); *Alph.* 21 (*berula. bilus*); *Sin.Bart.* 13 (*berula, fabaria, levick*); *AC* 172.12 (*bursula. billere*) ❦ Fu 276 (*ΣΙΟΝ*, ἀναγαλλίς, ἔνυδρος, *sion, lauer, anagalis aquatica*); Tu 2.573 (SION, *sium, laver, water cresses, belragges, water/salat persely*); DL 448 (WATER CRESSES, *lesser water cress*, σισύμβριον ἕτερον, καρδαμίνη, *sisymbrium alterum, cardamine, sium, flos cuculi, nasturtium aquaticum*); Ge 199 (WATER CRESSES, *brown cresses, sium, sisymbrium aquaticum, lauer*).

CS (Fu, Ge) | C²S² (DL)

245 brokleuys. The Latin heading, the ME name, and the description of the leaves, which are compared to those of mint, point to brooklime (*Veronica beccabunga* L.). *Fabaria* seems to have been used in some sources to refer to *Berula erecta* (Huds.) Coville (→ **240**), but the leaf shape makes that equation very dubious. The entry follows *AC*. The species seems not to have been treated by Classical pharmacopeia but identification is supported pharmacographically by at least one Renaissance writer: according to Ge, the species is a good anti-inflammatory if mixed with grease and applied as a poultice, just like in the ME text (**248**).

Literature: BROOKLIME (*Veronica beccabunga* L.): *EPN* vi (*fabaria. faverole*); *Alph.* 21 (*berula.* ɢᴀ*berles,* ᴀɴ*bilus*), 61 (*faba, faberia inversa, fabaria aquatica,* ᴀɴ*brolemoderwort, lempke*); *Sin.Bart.* 13 (*berula. fabaria. levick*); *AC* 186.22 (*fabria minor. waterlingke, faurole*) ❦ DL 415 (BROOKELIME, *anagallis aquatica, becabunga,* κηπαία, *cepaea*); Ge 495 (BROOKELYME, *water pimpernell, anagallis aquatica, becabunga, berula, cepaea,* κηπαία).

C² (DL) | CS (Ge)

251 brome. The Latin heading indicates that the plant must be one of the several species called *Genista* or *Genistella* in Latin. The text provides no physical description, so strictly speaking we can go no further that to assume that the species must belong to the tribe Genisteae, composed by a number of genera—including *Genista*, *Cytisus*, and *Spartium*—all of which are usually called "brooms" in English (see Stirling 1995–1998: *s.vv.* genista, genistella for details). Traditionally, though, the species is taken to be the common broom (*C. scoparius* (L.) Link).

According to the entry, the species is anthydropic (**256**), antiarthritic (**257**), lithontriptic (**261**), consolidative (**262**) and dentifrice (**265**). The quality of the plant as stone-breaker is also recorded in *GH*, together with an antiepileptic virtue; and similarly in Fu, where the plant is also praised as particularly good against illnesses of the bladder (such as dysury and strangury), podagra and scrofula. The ME text is closest to DL and Ge, where the anthydropic, lithontriptic, and antiarthtitic qualities of broom are mentioned.

I have not been able to trace a source for this particular entry. The consolidative quality of the species, which is missing in all Renaissance accounts of *genesta*, appears in *AC* but is in fact the sole point of contact between both texts. In any case, the style of the section, where the recipes are described minutely and quantities are given is distinctly different from the more casual style of the usual sources. This can be seen also in the syntax of the fragment, which is reminiscent of that of a receptarium, rather than the one of a text on materia medica. Another striking feature of this entry that opposes it to most sections of the herbal is the use of both *Dreckapotheke* (→ **258**) and inorganic compounds (‹alyme i-brent› **264**, i.e., burnt alum): for most entries of *LH*, the stress is on juices and parts of plants.

> **Literature**: COMMON BROOM (*Cytisus scoparius* (L.) Link): *HP* ix.7.3 (ἀσπάλαθος); *MM* 1.20; *NH* xxiv.11 (*aspalathus*); *SM* xi.840; *RM* ii.197; *Dur.Glos.* 303 (*genesta. brom*); *EPN* ii, iii, iv (*genista. brom*), v (*genesta. brom*), vi (*genesta. genest. brom*); *Cl* G.11 (*genestula*); *TH* 214 (*genestra*); *Pand.* 278 ($_{LA}$*genestra, bul, filex,* $_{GR}$*spartus, spargamum,* $_{AR}$*mabrahinch*); *Alph.* 73, 74, 117, 221 (*genesteola, mirica, genesta.* $_{GA}$*geneste,* $_{AN}$*brom*), 203 (*alocis*), 215 (*filibon*); *Sin.Bart.* 22 (*genesta, genestula, mirica, reubis agrestis*) 36 (*reubarbarum agreste*); *AC* 189.22 (*Genescula. genestres, broum*) ⚜ *GH* 196 (GENESTA, *brome*); Fu 79 (GENISTA, *genestra*); DL 477 (BROOME, *genesta, genestra*); Ge 1130 (BROOME, *genista*).
>
> C^2 (DL) | C^2S^2 (*TH, GH,* Fu, Ge) | FS (*Cl*)

256 mylke. The meaning conveyed here seems to be 'extract (sap, latex...) from a plant'; it seems therefore be the oldest example in the English language of this particular sense, antedating the earliest instance quoted by OED: *s.v.* milk *v.,* § 7 (dated 1746) by about 280 years. The meaning seems moreover to be isolated in the ME corpus, since it is not included in the MED: *s.v.* milken *v.*

258 ynnyrer pithe of pichon-is geserys. The MS reading ‹ynnyter› has been emended following MED: *s.v.* innerere *a.,* with the sense "inner" in the comparative. The passage makes reference, therefore, to the tough lining (called *cutica gastrica*, composed of a keratin-like material called koilin) that protects the ventriculus from the gastroliths (grit and small stones that birds ingest and keep inside this muscular stomach to help grind the foodstuffs; Dyce/Sack/Wensing 2010: 796).

267 balme. "Balm" is used to refer both to some Lamiaceae, mainly *Melissa officinalis* L. (common or lemon balm, balm-mint), and to the aromatic resin of the *Commiphora gileadensis* (L.) C.Chr. (balsam-tree, balm of Gilead), a

Burseraceae species native to the Arabia Felix. The Latin heading suggests that it is the second species that is dealt with here, since *melissa* was the usual Latin way to refer to the Lamiaceae. There is some pharmacographic support for that identification, since several of the characteristics and properties of βάλσαμον according to Classical and Medieval evidence are mirrored in *LH*: cf. its value as a eupeptic (**269**), anticephalalgic (**272**), antisingultus and mazolytic (**274**), antiepileptic (**279**). In any case, many of the qualities of *Commiphora* routinely commended by medical writers of the period (alexipharmic, antiasthmatic, ophthalmic, antiotalgic, or emollient, among many others) are missing from the ME account.

Moreover, the compiler of *LH* might have blended the virtues of this plant with those of *Melissa officinalis* (→ **1355**, with additional literature): *DVH(SME)*, for example, offers a parallel (if extended) version of a couple of properties mentioned in the text, viz. that balm is beneficial to an ailing bladder (**270**), and as a febrifuge (**268**, **277**). The remaining virtues provided in the text (antiemetic, **273**, antipodagric, **276**, and relaxant, **281**) are apparently not recorded in any account of the species. The source of this entry remains untraced.

Literature: BALSAM-TREE (*Commiphora gileadensis* (L.) C.Chr.): *HP* ix.6.1 (βάλσαμον); *MM* i.19; *NH* xxiii.92 (*balsamum*); *SM* xi.846; *RM* ii.199; *Grad.* 356; *LS* 160 (*belesem* [بلسان *balasān*], *balsamus*); *Cl* B.1 (*balsamus. bame*); *TH* 59 (*balsamus*); *Pand.* 367 (ARi*elessem, yesse*, GR,LA*balsamum*); *Alph.* 19 (*balsamum*); *Sin.Bart.* 12 (*balsamum*) ⚜ *GH* 55 (BALSAMUM, *bawme tree*).

C²S² (*SM, RM, Grad., LS, GH*)

274 þe laste burþen. This is one of the two ways used in *LH* to refer to the placenta, the other being *seco(u)nd(e) borþen* (→ **765**, **940**, **1772**, **1806**). Both of them, and particularly the last one, are slavish renderings of Latin *secundinae* (ultimately from Gk δεύτερα) and seem privative to this herbal. In ME the expressions *afterburden*, akin to PDE *afterbirth*, and *second birthe* were also used (for example in *DVH(SME)* 29b.24) but neither is apparently recorded in MED.

282 basilica. An obvious mistake for *b a s i l i c o n (Gk. βασιλικόν). While inferences from religious language are frequent in the text (→ **149**, **188**, **784**, **1953**, and perhaps **708**) and may explain this spelling, influences from medical vocabulary cannot be ruled out (cf. La. *vena basilica* in the forearm). Note moreover the existence of *basilica* in several ME works instead of *b a s i l i s c a to refer either to *Persicaria bistorta* (L.) Samp. or *Dracunculus vulgaris* Schott (PNME: *s.v.*; → **38**).

283 basilicon. Identification of the species described in the entry with basils (*Ocimum* L. spp.) seems granted on textual, botanical and pharmacographic grounds.

The tripartite distinction made in the entry appears to have been unknown to Classical writers but is frequently encountered in Medieval and Renaissance texts. As seen from several 16th-century works, the division seems to have been based (totally or partially) on the size of the leaves (so Fu and DL) or the comparative height of each subspecies (so Ge). Other authors of the period, such as Constantinus Africanus or the author of *Cl*, followed a division between *o. garyophyllatum* and *o. citreum/citrinum* (*citratum* in Ge), depending on whether the scent of the species reminded that of cloves (or frankincense, as mentioned in the text) or lemon. DL blends garden and wild basils in the same entry, although the wild species was traditionally taken to correspond not to the Dioscoridean ὤκιμον but to ἄκινος (*MM* iii.43), a plant of dubious identification, perhaps *Clinopodium acinos* (L.) Kuntze or *C. graveolens* subsp. *rotundifolium* (Pers.) Govaerts.

Since the text provides no real physical description of each type other than the different colours, the two first types of basils of the entry may be mere varieties or cultivars of *Ocimum basilicum* L., one displaying purple petals, the other—one can safely assume—white. The ‹garifilatum› subspecies, which *auctoritates* took to be smaller in size than the other two, is probably *Ocimum minimum* L., the species sometimes called Greek basil. *LS* called it *scexabram* or *ozimum carmenum*, corresponding to *bush basill* and *ocimum minimum gariophyllatum* in Ge. The temperament (faultily) given in the entry should lead us to believe that the section deals with this particular subspecies.

Phytomorphologically, while the leaves of basil are sometimes compared with those of *mercurialis*, i.e. the Euphorbiaceae *Mercurialis annua* L. (so Fu, DL, Ge), the reference to rue is unexpected, since basils display nothing like the spatulate leaves of *Ruta graveolens*.

Identification with basil is also reassured on pharmacographic basis. According to the text, basils—and particularly the *garyophyllatum* subspecies—are exhilarant (→ **288**), comfortative to the stomach and the brain (**290**), soporific (**291**), anti-inflammatory and ophthalmic (**292**, **299**), eupeptic, cardiac and anticholeric (→ **290**, **295**), antiphlegmatic and deoppilant of the brain if used as an sternutatory (**295**), and analgesic (**298**). Of these, only the assumed exhilarant and soporific virtues are not present in *MM*, but the former is mentioned in several medieval sources, including *Grad.* and Συν (→ **288**), and the latter might similarly stem as well from Συν, or else be due a distorted rendering of a passage in *NH* (→ **291**). Other virtues usually attached to the species are on the other hand missing from the ME account (for example, its alexipharmic, emmenagogue, diuretic, or anticteric qualities). Although the ultimate origins of most virtues can be traced to Classical and medieval pharmacographic texts, the direct source of the entry remains unknown.

> **Literature**: BASILS (*Ocimum* L. spp.): *HP* i.6.6 (ὤκιμον); *MM* ii.141; *NH* xx.119 (*ocimum*); *SM* xii.158; *RM* ii.274; *Grad.* 349; *OEH* 119 (*herba ocimus. mistel*); Dur.Glos. 304 (*ocimus. mistel*); *LS* 73 (*scexabram* [شاهسفرم *šāhsifrim*], *ozimum carmenum, basilicon garyophylatum*), 156 (*berengemisch* [نجمشك *baranġamašik*], *ozimum gariophilatum*), 157 (*berendarog* [بادروج *bādarūġ*], *ozimum non gariophilatus*), 175 (*hamehim, amachim* [حمأحم *himāḥim*], *selichi, ozimum domesticum*); *EPN* iv (*ocimum. mistel*); *Cl* o.1 (*ozimum. basilicon*); *TH* 339 (*ocimum*); *Pand.* 94 (ₐᵣ*berengemisch,* ɢᵣ*oçimum,* ʟₐ*basilicon gariofilatum*), 565 (*ocimum, basilicon*); *Alph.* 18 (*basilicon. semen est maiorane, ozimus idem*), 133 (*ozimum. i. basilicon*); Sin.Bart. 12 (*basilicon. ozimum idem*) ⚭ Fu 207 ('ΟΚΙΜΟΝ, βασιλικόν, *ocimum gariophyllatum*); Tu 2.469 (BASIL, *ocimon, basilicon*); DL 172 (BASILL, *basil-royall, basil-gentle, garden basil,* ὄκιμον, ὄξιμον, *ocimum gariophyllatum, basilicum | bush basill*); Ge 548 (BASILL, *garden basill, basill royall,* ὄκιμον, ὤκιμον, βασιλικόν, *ocimum, basilicum | basill gentle, bush basill, cloue basill, basilicum gariophyllatum*).
>
> CH (DL [garden]) |C²H (*SM, RM, LS*₁₅₇, Fu, Tu, Ge) | C¹S¹ (*Grad.* [citreum], *Cl* [citreum], *TH* [citreum]) | C¹S² (*Grad.* [garioph.], *Cl* [garioph.], *TH* [garioph.], *LS*₇₃) | C²S² (*LS*₁₅₆, ₁₇₅, DL [wild])

283 and. A missing adjective (likely to be *d r y e) is expected after the conjunction. The text has not been emended since, as seen from the preceding note, some *auctoritates*, including Galen, considered that basil had some humidity.

288 make...290 colour. This fragment follows closely—if faultily—a passage in *Grad.* dealing with the citric-smelling subspecies of basil: "Galenus tristia cordia lætificans uocauit [...], cordis defectionem amputat. Vigilias & timorem & suspitionem & cordis tremorem, quæ sunt propter nigram choleram & adustam, expellit." Note that Constantinus's text has been rearranged: ⟨defautis⟩ must logically correspond to *defectionem*, rather than *tremorem*, and so it is unlikely that the ME text is a direct translation from the Latin source.

291 to slepe esily. A soporific virtue is not recorded for basil in the Classical pharmacographic literature, but Pliny did make some references to the actual action of basil on lethargy (→ **1352**). According to his account, the Greek physician Chrysippus (i.e. Chrysippus of Cnidos, 4th century BC) thought that basil caused madness, lethargy, and liver diseases (*NH* xx.119: "insania facere et lethargos et iocineris vitia"), but a second generation of doctors thought that basil actually could be of value against such illness (*NH* xx.121: "salutare esse [...] lethargicis"). But perhaps a more direct source is Συν 29, which states that basil invites sleep (ὕπνον ἐπάγει).

300 crasse. The entry derives from the entry *Nasturtium* in *DVH* 988–1015, as rendered in the *DVH(NME)* tradition. The species treated here is traditionally taken to be the garden cress (*Lepidium sativum* L.). Identification is also positive on account of the medical qualities mentioned by the text, most of which are also recorded in the appropriate entry in *MM*: cf. § 1 with the value of cress as a splenetic (**308** = *DVH* 1002), abortifacient (**305–306** = *DVH* 998–999), vermifuge (→ **306** = *DVH* 999) and aphrodisiac (**300**, = *DVH* 989), and § 2 with cress as expectorant (**311–312** = *DVH* 1010–1012), alexipharmic (**306** = *DVH* 1000), herpetofuge (**306–307** = *DVH* 1001), antialopecic (**304** = *DVH* 995–996), antianthracic (**301** = *DVH* 991–994) and antisciatic (**309** = *DVH* 1004–1005). The analgesic and antiodontalgic (**303** = *DVH* 996–997), antiphtheiriac (**310** = *DVH* 1006) and antitussive (**312** = *DVH* 1015) qualities of the species, on the other hand, are not to be found in the Dioscoridean account.

> **Literature**: GARDEN CRESS (*Lepidium sativum* L.): *HP* i.12.1 (κάρδαμον); *MM* ii.155; *NH* xx.127 (*nasturtium*); *SM* xii.11; *RM* ii.220; *Grad*. 384; *OEH* 21 (*herba narstucium. cærse*); *Dur.Glos*. 304 (*nasturcium. vilde cerse*); *DVH* 988–1015 (*nasturtium*); *LS* 349 (*norph* [حرف *ḥurf*], *nasturcium*); *EPN* ii (*tun-kerse*), iii (*leac-cersan*), vi (*kersuns, cressen*); *Cl* N.1 (*nasturcium. carces*);*TH* 327 (*nasturcium*); *Pand*. 136 (_{GR}*cardamus*, _{AR}*iorbalsathefe, madiera*, _{LA}*nasturtium*); *DVH(NME)* 246r.1 (*cressis*); *Alph*. 122 (*nasturcium ortolanum. cresse idem*. _{GA}*cresso‹uns›*); *Sin.Bart*. 11 (*araseth. nasturtiun*), 31 (*nasturcium ortolanum*) ※ *GH* 303 (NASTURCIUM, *gusium, anthonaes, tame cresses, gardyne cresses*); *Fu* 135 (ΚΑΡΔΑΜΟΝ, *nasturtium satiuum, cressio hortensis*); *Tu* 2.467 (GARDEN CRESSES, *kardomom*); *DL* 447 (CRESSES, *towne kars*, κάρδαμον, *nasturtium, cressio*); *Ge* 194 (GARDEN CRESSES, *town cresses, garde karsse*, κάρδαμον, *nasturtium*).
>
> CS (DVH) | C⁴S⁴ (*SM, RM, Grad., LS, Cl, TH, GH, Fu, DL, Ge*)

300 hansith lecherye. The Latin text means the exact opposite of its ME rendering, cf. *DVH* 989 *Venerem* [...] *coercent*. The different words used by each scribe (*B*.246r/2 ‹prok*is*›, *W*.29r/21 ‹proch*is*›, *P*.267/7 ‹helpeþ›) strongly suggest a faulty reading in Ω, which may have been *PROKIS in case that the wrong translation derives from the original. The translator has moreover omitted the comparison of the anaphrodisiac powers of cress with those of the rue, and its posology(*ceu ruta* [...] *si sumpta frequenter DVH* 989–990).

300 stampe...301 mele. *DVH* 990 *siccando semen*, which explains how cresses actually quell sexual desire (see above), was mistaken by the ME translator as if part of the antianthracic quality of the species. The whole fragment is built on a forced interpretation in *Ω* of *semen* as the object of *terendo* "rubbing" (but which can also mean "bruising, grinding", hence *STAMPID) that appears at the end on the following line. La. *fermento* "yeast" is moreover mistranslated as "barley flour". The other MSS of the tradition are surely closer to the original reading in *Ω* as they still keep the word *DRY that must once have been part of the fragment: *B*.246r/2–3 ⟨þe drye seyd stampid & mengid⟩, *W*.29r/22 ⟨þe drie sede stamp it & meng it⟩, *P*.267/7–8 ⟨þe dreye seed stamped and medled⟩.

301 antracas. Anthrax is a fatal infectious disease of farm animals, caused by the *Bacillus anthracis*, that can be transmitted to man and attack the lungs—that is, pulmonary anthrax, known popularly as woolsorter's disease—or the skin. In medieval times, however, the word referred to a skin condition (*Chir.(ME)* 94):

> Antrax, after William de Saliceto, is no þing elles but a wicked carbuncle. Þe mater forsoþe of antrax is grete blood, strongely boylynge in so moche þat for his grete boylynge it haþ geten venyme. It is cleped forsoþe *bona buba* (i. a good byle) by contrarie speche, for it [is] werste and most perilouse.

The mention of ⟨quitter⟩ (i.e. pus, translating *DVH* 993 *furunculus*) makes it likely that the ⟨vncomes in þe face⟩ (*DVH* 992 *bona* [...] *ulcera*, cf. La. *bona buba* in Chauliac's quotation) is actually a case of skin anthrax (in its modern sense), which produces a 'red, inflamed swelling with a blob of pus on top' (Norri 1992: 194).

Reference to anthrax is already in Macer Floridus's Latin text (*DVH* 992) but it is only kept in *RH*, cf. on the other hand *B*.246r/3 ⟨þat helys vncommys in þe face⟩. *ANTRACAS was rendered in Pepys as *P*.267/8 ⟨felouns⟩.

302 men riseth. A scribal conjecture from an original *RYNNYS "runs", cf. *B*.246r/4, *W*.29r/24 ⟨rynnys⟩. *P* misses the sentence altogether.

302 and a-batith all akynge. This is authorial as it translates *DVH* 994 *cum qua dolor ille recedit*, but the words are only kept in Branch γ.

304 þe²... 305 away. The virtue of cress against alopecia appears before, rather than after, those against toothache in the canonical version of *DVH*, which probably indicates that lines 995–997 may have been rearranged in *Q*.

306 from his modir wombe. A mistaken translation (kept in all MSS of the *DVH(NME)* tradition) of the Latin text, which refers rather to the anthelminthic properties of cress, cf. *DVH* 999 *ventrisque animalia pellit*. These were already mentioned in *MM*. Obviously the reference to La. *venter*, which may stand either for the intestines or the vagina, must have misguided the translator, who conjectured here.

308 baryes gres. *DVH* 1003 *polline*, i.e. fine flour. Branchs α and γ read together as "boar's grease" (*B*.246r/8 ⟨galtt greyse⟩, *W*.29v/3 ⟨galt smere⟩), while *P*.267/11 reads ⟨salt⟩, which can easily be traced back to an original *GALT just like the other MSS (→ **1108**; Moreno Olalla 2017: 683–684). The normal words in *DVH* for animal grease are *adeps* (cf. for instance ⟨gose gres⟩ **310** answering to *DVH* 1008) and *axungia* (⟨barowes grece⟩ **1064**, translating *DVH* 937), hence either *Q* was defective here or else the translator made a mistake.

309 þe evill in þe þiesse. *DVH* 1004 *sciasis* [...] *dolori*. ⟨Þiesse⟩ is probably a muddled scribal rendering of *THEYS, a Northern ME word for "thighs" (< ON *þjó*) which was unknown to the scribe of S_1, a speaker of some South Essex-North London dialect. Cf. on the other hand the correct Northern versions *B*.246r/9 ⟨euyll in þe theys⟩ and *W*.29v/4 ⟨euil in þe thees⟩ (→ **338**, **900**). Note as well that MED: *s.v.* thresse *n*., which appears to be a hapax based on this passage, is a ghost word based on a misreading in *WG*.

310 þe mytis and the tikys. An extremely free version of *DVH* 1007 *prurigo* [...] *aut ulcera turpia*. Some Latin traditions, including ζζ, read *porrigo* "scurf" here, but *prurigo* "itching" probably explains the ME translation better as an itching sensation in the scalp indicating the presence of the parasites. All MSS of the tradition read together with *B*.246r/9 ⟨neyttis⟩, i.e. "nits", instead of "mites", but the original reading in S_1 has been kept since it makes sense in the passage.

312 sowbliþ. Probably *DVH* 1014 *molliat*. The word seems therefore authorial, but it was kept only in Branch γ (cf. *W*.29v/6 ⟨solibles⟩, which suggests a reconstructed form *SOWBLIS) and then faultily, for it is not cough, but the stomach which is softened if cress seeds are drunk, cf. *duram* [...] *alvum*. MED: rublen *v*., § b, "to do away (with an ailment)", is based on a misreading of this word in *WG* and should better appear under the entry sŏuplen *v*.

313 costmaryn. The ME entry corresponds neither to costmary (*Tanacetum balsamitoides* Sch.Bip., → **1454**), nor to the aromatic *costus* of the Romans (*DVH* 2165–2181). The text in fact translates *DVH* 1016–1036, which deals with the properties of *eruca*, i.e. the rocket (*Eruca vesicaria* (L) Cav.; → **2161** for another rendering of the same plant), as translated in the *DVH(NME)* tradition.

Identification with the rocket is positive on account of its assumed medical properties, all of which are found in *MM* ii.140 and the Latin poem: eupeptic and diuretic (**314** = *DVH* 1017–1018), ophthalmic and antitussive (→ **315** = *DVH*

1019), cosmetic (**316** = DVH 1020–1021, and again in → **319**), consolidative (**317** = DVH 1022–1023), alexipharmic (→ **318**), indurant (→ **320**), aphrodisiac (**321** = DVH 1033), as well as its value as a condiment (**321** = DVH 1029–1032).

Literature: ROCKET (*Eruca vesicaria* (L.) Cav.): *HP* i.6.6 (εὔζωμον); *MM* ii.140; *NH* xx.125 (*eruca*); *RM* ii.212; *Dur.Glos.* 302 (*eruci. sinapis*); *DVH* 1016–1036 (*eruca*); LS 214 (*iergir* [جرجر *ǧarǧīr*], *eruca*); EPN ii (*eruca. calf-wyrt*), viii (*hec eruta. whytte pepyre*), ix (*hec eruca. a schynlok* | *hec eruca. a carlok*); *Cl* E.10 (*eruca. skiriwhitte*); TH 169 (*eruca*); Pand. 369 ($_{AR}$*iergit, iergir, ierir,* $_{GR}$*euzonium,* $_{LA}$*eruca*); DVH(NME) 245v.19 (*coste*); DVH(SME) 19a.3 (*white peper, white senuey. eruca*); Alph. 58 (*eruca*), 213 (*eucimus*); Sin.Bart. 20 (*eruca. skirwhit* | *sinapis albus, cherloc*); AC 183.17 (*eruca. skyrwyt*) ⚜ GH 160 (ERUCA, *skyrwort, wylde caules that bereth mustarde sede*); Fu 99 (ΕΥΖΩΜΟΝ, *eruca*); Tu 1.309 (ROCKET, *euzomos*); DL 445 (ROCKET, εὔζωμον, *eruca satiua, hortensis, syluestris*); Ge 191 (ROCKET, *racket*, εὔζωμον, *eruca, herba salax*).

C^2S^1 (*DVH*) | C^2S^2 (*LS*) | C^3S^3 (*Cl, TH, GH, DL, Ge*) | C^4S^4 (Fu)

313 his…drye. The reading ⟨his leuys⟩ in S_1 is opposed to *B*.245v/19 ⟨is a greyse⟩, *W*.33v/8 ⟨is gres⟩ and *P*.275/6 ⟨is an herbe⟩. Since the scribe of S_1 normally had not trouble with *GRES, this reading may be indicative of a faulty passage in Λ. This is corroborated by the omission of the dry quality of the species in this MS (as opposed to *B*.245v/20, *W*.33v/8 and *P*.275/7). While most MSS of the tradition stress the great heat of this species by using *nam(e)ly* here, *P* offers ⟨menely⟩, which translates *mediocriter DVH* 1016 correctly.

315 helpiþ to þe eyne. This does not translate *DVH* 1019a, as one would expect. In the original text Macer Floridus suggests eating rockets for children's health. The ophthalmic benefit does appear nevertheless in the ultimate source, *NH* xx.126: "subtrita eruca si foveantur oculi, claritatem restituit".

316 þe body. *DVH* 1020 *cutem*. Only the Wellcome version provides the correct reading here, cf. *W*.33v/11 ⟨þe hyd⟩ vs. *B*.245v/22 ⟨the heyd⟩ (unless this is taken as an indication of a late ME diphthongized *ī*, which is very dubious as it would be the sole example in the text; cf. also *B*.245v/25 ⟨hyde⟩). Pepys simplified the fragment into ⟨clenseþ þe spottes⟩. The reading in S_1, while probably not authorial, represents a scribal alteration, either stylistic or dialectal. Cf. also the appearance of ⟨body⟩ in **334** (also in *W*), rather than *B*.255v/1, *P*.278/23 ⟨hyde⟩.

316 rote sodyn and stampid. This passage was misread in *WG*, who apparently did not notice that the word written after ⟨rote⟩ (⟨stam⟩) was deleted by the scribe. This caused the inclusion of a ghost collocation *stamp rote*, that is explained as "the stalk growing out of the root of a plant" in MED: *s.v.* stampne *n*.

318 venum bat. *DVH* 1025 *quosvis pestiferos ictus*. The sense of the passage is not totally clear but probably refers to bites by noxious animals, cf. *NH* xx.125 "Erucae semen scorpionum venenis et muris aranei medetur". S_1 ⟨bat⟩ "stroke, blow" (OED: *s.v.* bat *n*.², § 14.a., MED: *s.v.* bat *n*., § 2.) is a scribal innovation from *DYNT*I*S*, cf. *B*.245v/23 ⟨dynttis⟩ (and similarly *W*.3v/14 and *P*.275/13). S_1 would predate the earliest known reference with this sense by more than a decade.

319 þe morfue. This translates *DVH* 1026 *nigras maculas*. S_1 innovates in opposition to ⟨blake spott*is* of þe hyde⟩, the slavish rendition of the original Latin given in *BWP*. It seems that the scribe of *Λ* possessed some medical knowledge and knew the foremost sign of the black morphew, originated by an excess of melancholy (*Chir.(ME)* 390 → **102** for the full quotation). It is unclear whether this represents an innovation by John Lelamour: if it were so, he was not consistent, for *DVH* 1708 *maculas* was translated as ⟨blacke spottis⟩ (**334**), and similarly in **1146** and **1537**.

320 hit shall sesse evill strokys. This is a clumsy rendering of *DVH* 1028 *Indurare ferunt hanc contra verbera sensum*. Each MS of the *DVH(NME)* tradition provides a different text here, suggesting that the fragment must have been unclear already in *Ω* (in fact, the poem states that the mixture must be drunk, rather than smeared, since *DVH* 1027 *illita* belongs to the previous sentence, which deals with black spots, see previous note). The one in Bodley is particularly nonsensical: *B*.245v/25 ⟨it shall be hard & for bolnynge⟩, while Wellcome fares slightly better, cf. *W*.33v/16–17 ⟨it sall hard again bityng⟩. Pepys, just as S_1, does manage to salvage somewhat the idea of the Latin text (⟨þat schal be hard aȝen þe betyng⟩) and is probably closest to the original ME text. Note that the other version of the entry also mistranslated this sentence (→ **2171**).

322 celedony. The entry derives from the entry *Chelidonia* in *DVH* (1690–1708), as rendered in the *DVH(NME)* tradition. The species treated here are the two celandines: to judge from the woodcuts in Fu, the *major* species must be *Chelidonium majus* L., while the *minor* seems to be *Ranunculus ficaria* L. Identification is traditional but also positive on account of the medical qualities mentioned by the text, most of which are also recorded in *MM* ii.180, § 2, not only their ophthalmic value for which the plant was renowned in Antiquity and the Middle Ages, but also its value as an anticteric and antiodontalgic (**331** = *DVH* 1704–1706) and antiherpetic (**334** = *DVH* 1707–1708).

Literature: GREATER & LESSER CELANDINE (*Chelidonium majus* L., *Ranunculus ficaria* L.): *HP* vii.15.1 ($χελιδόνιον$); *MM* ii.180 ($χελιδόνιον\ μέγα$), 181 ($χ.\ τὸ\ μικρόν$); *NH* xxv.89 (*chelidonia*); *SM* xii.156 ($χελιδόνιον$); *RM* ii.272; *Grad.* 381; *OEH* 75 (*herba cœlidonia*.

cylepenie); *Dur.Glos.* 301 (*celidonia. celitheme*); *DVH* 1690–1708 (*chelidonia*); *LS* 296 (*kauroch* [⚜ *kurkum*], *curcuma*); *EPN* vii (*hec celidonia. celydoun*); *Cl* c.32 (*chelidonia. celedoyne*); *TH* 121 (*celidonia*); *Pand.* 145 (_{LA}*celidonia*, _{GR}*chilidonion*, _{AR}*hauroch*); *DVH(NME)* 255r.14 (*seldone*); *DVH(SME)* 32b.17 (*celydoine*); *Alph.* 36 (*celidonia, herba petiginaria, glauca.* _{GA,AN}*celidoyne* | *celidonia maior* | *celidonia minor, taurion, piron agreste*); *Sin.Bart.* 15 (*celidonia agrestis. memithe idem*); *AC* 175.13 (*celidonie. celydonye, teterwort*) ❧ *GH* 115 (CELYDONYA, *celendyne, brighte*); *Fu* 331 (ΧΕΛΙΔΟΝΙΟΝ ΜΕΓΑ, *chelidonium maius, chelidonia, hirundinaria*), 332 (Χ. ΜΙΚΡΟΝ, *chelidonium minus, scrofularia minor*); *Tu* 2.395 (SELENDINE, *hirundinaria, chelidonion*); *DL* 23 (CELANDINE, χελιδόνιον, *chelidonium maius, hirundinaria maior, chelidonia, anemone*); *Ge* 911 (GREAT CELANDINE, *great celandine, common celandine, swallowe woort, tetterwort,* χελιδόνιον, *chelidonium maius, hirundinaria maior, chelidonia*).

C (*SM*) | C³ (*RM*) | C³S³ (*LS*, Fu, DL, Ge) | C⁴S⁴ (*Grad., Cl, TH, GH*, Fu)

323 Plenius saiþe. This is a translation of *DVH* 1693–1696, drawing from *NH* xxv.89.

331 wiþ aisell. The canonical reading is *DVH* 1704 *anetho*, but *aceto* appears in several traditions, including ζζ.

331 &... 333 toþe. This virtue, which appears in all MSS of the tradition, is not recorded in the canonical version of *DVH*, and seems an expansion in either *Q* or *Ω* on the antiodontalgic values of celandine that had just been copied.

335 centory. The entry is drawn from the *DVH(NME)* tradition, and renders the entry *Centaurea* as given in *DVH* 1709–1727. A *major* and a *minor* species of centaury have been customarily distinguished at least since Dioscorides (see Literature). According to the physical description provided in *MM*, the *major* species is probably an Asteraceae such as greater centaury (*Centaurea centaurium* L.) or black knapweed (*C. nigra* L.), while the *minor* counterpart is the common centaury (*Centaurium erythraea* Rafn), a Gentianaceae. Unfortunately, the text provides no physical description so identification remains traditional.

The medical qualities mentioned by Macer Floridus are indeed contained in the Dioscoridean account of the minor centaury (κενταύρειον τὸ λεπτόν), above all the vulnerary qualities for which this species was renowned since Antiquity (**337** = *DVH* 1715–1716), as an antisciatic (→ **338**), emmenagogue (**340** = *DVH* 1721), abortifacient (**340** = *DVH* 1722) and purgative (**341** = *DVH* 1722–1723).

Literature: CENTAURIES (*Centaurea centaurium/nigra* L., *Centaurium erythraea* Rafn.): *HP* iii.3.6 (κενταύρειον); *MM* iii.6 (κενταύρειον τὸ μέγα), 7 (κ. λεπτὸν); *NH* xxv.66 (*centaurium*), 68 (*centaurium cognomine lepton*); *SM* xii.19–20; *RM* ii.222 (κενταύρειον); *Grad.* 362 (*centaurea*); *OEH* 35–36 (*herba centauria maior/*

minor. curmelle seo mare/læsse); Dur.Glos. 301 (centauria. eorth gella, hyrd vyrt, curmelle); DVH 1709–1727 (centaurea); LS 304 (kanturion kibir [كبير قطريون] qanṭuryūn kabīr], centaurea maior), 305 (kanturion segir [صغير قطريون] q. ṣagīr], c. minor); EPN ii (certaurea major. curmelle | centurea minor. ban-wyrt), iv (centauria. eorð-gealle), v (felterre vel centauria. eorð-gealle); CI c.10 (centaurea); TH 96 (centaurea); Pand. 148 ($_{LA}$centaurea, centinen, $_{GR}$anuticen, $_{AR}$anturion); DVH(NME) 252r.13 (centory); DVH(SME) 24b.21 (centory þe more and þe lesse); Alph. 37 (centaurea maior | centaurea minor, ision); Sin.Bart. 15 (centaurea major, fell terræ | centaurea minor, febrifuga); AC 174.12 (centorie. centurie, erthegalle), 174.24 (centure minor. lesse centure, cristis leddere) ⚕ GH 91 (CENTAUREA, centory); Fu 144 (KENTAYPION MIKPON, λιμνήσιον, λιμναῖον, febrifuga, fel terræ, centauria minor, limnesion, limnæum); Tu 1.266 (CENTORY, centaurium magnum/minum, ruponticum, rupontike, centaury); DL 234 (CENTORIE, κενταύριον τὸ μέγα, ναρκή, μαρώνη, μαρώνιον, νέσσιον, λιμνήσιον, λιμνηστρις, πλεκτρονία, πλεκτρόνιον, χειρωνία, αἷμα Ἡρακλέους, centaurium magnum, centaurida, rha ponticum, Herculis sanguis, vnefera, fel terræ, polyhydion | κενταύρειον τὸ μικρόν, κενταυρίς, centaurium paruum, centaurium minus, febrifuga, fel terræ, multiradix, centauria minor); Ge 435 (GREAT CENTORIE, κενταύριον τὸ μέγα, centauris, rha ponticum, unefera, fel terræ, polyhydion, centauria), 436 (SMALL CENTORIE, lesser centorie, common centorie, libadion, fel terræ).

CS (Fu) | C²S² (Grad., CI, DL [small], Ge$_{436}$) | C³S³ (LS, TH, GH, DL [great], Ge$_{437}$) | C⁴S⁴ (CI)

338 ther-to. A portion of the ME translation, corresponding to DVH 1716–1719, is missing after this word. The passage, kept in the other MSS of the tradition that offer this entry, mentions antisciatic properties, cf. B.252r/16–17 ‹& þe decoccion þer-of done into þe fundment helpys for þe tyasyme, þat is þe euyll off þe theys›. The reading in Wellcome is slightly faulty, since ‹tiasin› is taken to be an ‹euil of þe teth› (W.36r/25). ‹Theys› "thigh" in B is surely the same word as ‹þiesse› used on **309**.

339 in wyne oþer ale. This is an addition of either Λ or S_1, for no beverage is mentioned in DVH 1721, and neither in B nor W.

341 dotovs. cf. DVH 1722 maligna, B.252r/20 ‹dowtus› and W.36r/28 ‹dotous›.

342 gadryt...sonne. The reading in the Bodley and Wellcome versions is slightly different, and syntactically preferable: B.252r/21 ‹men shall take þe gresse & dry it in þe son›.

343 and...venyme. A garbled passage. The Latin poem makes no reference to poison, but succinctly makes reference to rerum [...] quas diximus ante (DVH 1727). This is also stated in the remaining MSS of the DVH(NME) tradition, cf. B.252r/22 ‹& þat is gude to thyngis þat I haue sayd be-fore›, W.36r/31 ‹& it is gode to þing þat er be-for said›.

344 colombyne. This translates *DVH* 1903–1917, which deals with the properties of *Chamaedrys*, according to the *DVH(NME)* tradition. Another description of the pharmacological values of the same species, similarly derived from Macer Floridus's poem but mixed with information from *AC*, will be found later in the text (→ **812**). Identification of *chamaedrys* with the wall germander (*Teucrium chamaedrys* L.) is traditional, and comparison with *MM* iii.98 is moreover positive: cf. its qualities as an abortifacient (**346** = *DVH* 1905), antitussive (**347** = *DVH* 1906), splenetic (**348** = *DVH* 1907–1908), emmenagogue (**348** = *DVH* 1908), anthydropic (**349** = *DVH* 1909), vulnerary (**350, 351** = *DVH* 1910, 1912), ophthalmic (**351** = *DVH* 1914–1915) and calefacient (**352–353** = *DVH* 19016–1917). Still, there is important textual evidence suggesting that one of the scribes of Branch ΛS_1 must have thought that species intended here was actually the vervain (see next note).

> **Literature**: WALL GERMANDER (*Teucrium chamaedrys* L.): *HP* ix.9.5 (χαμαίδρυς); *MM* iii.98; *NH* xxiv.130 (*chamaedrys, trixago*); *SM* xii.153; *RM* ii.271; *Grad.* 374 (*chamedræos*); *OEH* xxv (*chamedris. heortclæfre*); *Dur.Glos.* 300 (*cameleon, camedris. vuluuescomb*); *DVH* 1903–1917 (*chamaedrys*); *LS* 180 (*damederios* [كامدريوس *kamādryūs*], *kamedreos*); *EPN* ii (*cynocephaleon. heort-clæfre*), iv (*camedus. heort-clæfre*); *Cl* c.17 (*camedreos, quercula maior*); *TH* 103 (*camedreos*); *Pand.* 123 (₍GR₎*camedreos, cameb, cameropa,* ₍AR₎*hamedreos,* ₍LA₎*quercula minor*); *DVH(SME)* 25a.18 (*gamodreos. gamadrea*); *Alph.* 28 (*camedreos, polion, serfulla minor, quartula minor, germa andrea minor, trisogus, erisosogus*), 74 (*germandrea minor, camedreos, quercula minor*), 147 (*polion, camedreos, quercula minor, germandria minor*), 187 (*trisogus, camedreos, polion, cerfulla minor, quercula minor, germandria minor*); *Sin.Bart.* 14 (*camedreos, quercula minor, germandria minor*), 22 (*germandrea minor, quercula minor, camedreos | germandrea simpliciter, camedreos*), 36 (*quercula minor, camedreos*) ※ *GH* 98 (CAMEDRIOS, *germaundrea, quercula minor, germaundre, the lesse quercle*); Fu 333 (*XAMAIΔPYΣ, trissago, quercula minor, serratula*); Tu 1.270 (GERMANDER, *Englishe triacle, chamedrys, trissago, chamedryos*); *DL* 19 (GERMANDER, *English treacle*, χαμαίδρυς, *chamædrys, trixago, quercula minor, serratula, chamædryos*); Ge 529 (GERMANDER, *English treacle,* χαμαίδρυς, *chamædrys, trissago, trixago, quercula minor*). ¶ VERVEIN (*Verbena officinalis* L.): → verveyn [**2431**].
>
> C^2S^2 (*LS*) | C^3S^3 (*SM, RM, DVH, GH,* Fu, DL, Ge) | C^4S^4 (*Cl*)

344 þer... 346 gode. This passage is an addition in Branch ΛS_1, found neither in *DVH* 1903–1917 (nor, for all it matters, in the appropriate chapters of *MM* or *NH* devoted to the wall germander) nor in any of the other versions of *DVH(NME)*. In fact there seems to have never been a botanical division among species called *chamaedrys* during Antiquity or the Middle Ages.

On the other hand, there *was* a division in the species diversely called *columbina, peristereon* (cf. Gk περιστερεών "dovecote") or *verbenaca* in

Latin. One of them was called περιστέριον in MM iv.59 and περιστερεών ὀρθός in the parallel entry of Ps.-Dios., while the other was called ἱερὰ βοτάνη, lit. "holy herb" or περιστερεών in MM iv.60 and περιστερεών ὕπτιος in Ps.-Dios. The names used in Ps.-Dios. were translated into Latin as *verbena(ca) (e)recta* and *verbena(ca) supina*, respectively (see for example Fu, where they are turned into German as *Eisenkraut mennle* and *E. weible*). The Latin names are of course behind the division between the *vpright* and *creeping veruaine* in Ge$_{580-581}$. What is relevant to the argument at hand is that, according to the *auctoritates*, the species designated *verbena(ca) (e)recta* displays whitish flowers (cf. MM ὑπόλευκα), while those of the *verbena(ca) supina* are mauve (cf. MM ὑπόγλαυκα). Identification of the *erecta* species is usually assumed to be *Lycopus europaeus* L., while the *supina* counterpart is *Verbena officinalis* L. The two species are mentioned again but not described elsewhere in the text (→ **2431**).

This has immediate consequences for the history of the transmission of S_1 as it proves that, while the virtues of the plant copied in this entry does certainly correspond to DVH *chamaedrys*, the scribe of $Λ$ thought that he was copying those of *verbenaca*.

346 þe...water. The original syntax was simplified in S_1, cf. DVH 1906 *Si mixta potetur aqua* and *B*.252r/23 ⟨it mengit with watter & dronkyn⟩.

355 coryandyr[1]. The entry derives from the entry *Coriandrum* in DVH (957–987), as translated in DVH(NME). Identification with *Coriandrum sativum* L. is traditional, although comparison of the medical qualities with those of MM shows that only a few of them are actually shared by both texts, viz. as an anthelminthic (**356** = DVH 959–960), anti-inflammatory (**357** = DVH 962–964, most particularly against orchitis), and as antiherpetic (**360** = DVH 974–975). On the other hand, the claimed powers of coriander as an antidiarrheic (**359** = DVH 965–966), febrifuge (**361–362** = DVH 979–981) and antiemmenagogue (**363** = DVH 984–987) are missing from the Dioscoridean account.

Literature: CORIANDER (*Coriandrum sativum* L.): HP vii.1.2 (κορίαννον); MM iii.63 (κόριον); NH xx.216 (*coriandrum*); SM xii.36 (κορίανον); RM ii.229 (κορίαννον); OEH 104 (*herba coliandra. celendre*); Dur.Glos. 301 (*coliandra. cellendre*); DVH 957–987 (*coriandrum*); LS 34 (*kusbor* [ڪُزْبَرَة *kuzbara*], *coriandrum*); EPN ii, iii (*coliandrum. celendre*), vi (*coliandrum. coriandre, chele priem*); Cl c.33 (*coriandrum. coliaundre*); TH 122 (*coliandrum*); Pand. 203 ($_{AR}$*baybora*, *cumbera*, $_{GR}$*corion*, *coriamium*, $_{LA}$*coriandrum*); DVH(NME) 248r.13 (*coriander*); DVH(SME) 20b.14 (*coriaundre. coriaundre*); Alph. 42 (*coriandrum agreste. coliaundre*); AC 176.10 (*coliandrum. colyandre*) ⚜ GH 116 (CORIANDRUM, *coryandre*); Fu 129 (*KOPION*, κορίαννον, *corion*, *coriandrum*); Tu 1.286 (CORYANDRE, *coriandrum, corianum, corion, corianon, colander*); DL 197 (CORIANDER, *coliander,* κόριον, κορίανον, *coriandrum*); Ge 859 (CORIANDERS, *coriandrum*).

CS (DL [seed], Ge [seed]) | C¹S¹ (*LS*) | C²S² (*Cl, TH, GH*) | FS (DL [leaves], Ge [leaves])

355 Galien seiþ. There seems to be no reference in the Galenic corpus to the anthelminthic qualities of coriander. In fact, this is a translation mistake: the reference to Galen in the Latin text belongs to the previous sentence, which deals with the temperament of the species. In the beginning of the entry κορίανον in *SM* xii.36 Galen discusses the actual quality of coriander as a cold species, as Dioscorides had stated (ψυκτικὴν ἔχει δύναμιν), to conclude that this is inaccurate, for this plant has an earthly, bitter quality (and as such had a cold and dry temperament) together with a hot moist juice that is somewhat astringent:

σύγκειται γὰρ ἐξ ἐναντίων δυνάμεων πολὺ μὲν ἔχουσα πικρᾶς οὐσίας, ἥτις ἐδείκνυτο λεπτομερὴς ὑπάρχειν καὶ γεώδης, οὐκ ὀλίγον δὲ καὶ ὑδατώδους ὑγρότητος χλιαρᾶς κατὰ δύναμιν, ἔχει δέ τι καὶ στύψεως ὀλίγης.

Auctoritates such as Paul of Aegina, Fuchs or Turner, all of whom appear to have drawn directly from that Galenic account, were equally unclear in their descriptions, while others (Dodoens, whence probably also Gerard) seem to have reached a compromise between the two opposing complexions suggested by the distinctly different taste of the pleasantly orangey seed and that of leaves, which was traditionally compared to that of bedbugs (popular etymology wanted the phytonym to come from κόρις, the Greek word for that insect, cf. for instance Fu: "Corio nomen fecisse cimices uerisimile est, quos folia & caules eius olent; κόρυς enim Græcis insecti, id genus est, quod Latinis cimex dicitur"; Chantraine 1999: *s.v.* κορίαννον).

357 rosyne aysell and hony. The original text only calls for *uva* [...] *passa* [...] *melque* (*DVH* 962). The addition of vinegar is probably due to a reading mistake, for this ingredient was to be used with the antihelminthic recipe immediately before.

359 that rennyth oute. A substantial number of lines from *DVH* (967–973), which provide the recipe of an ointment against *sacer ignis*, were probably missing already in Ω. S₁ reads together with *B*.248r/17 ⟨þat ry*n*nys⟩, while *P*.283/2 offers ⟨fro rennyng⟩. *W* misses the fragment altogether.

360 akynge. This corresponds to *DVH* 975 *calorem*. All MSS from *RH* coincide here, while *B*.248r/18 reads ⟨werke of þe heyd⟩: *Q* must obviously have read *DOLOREM, which is recorded solely in ζζ.

360 yf hit be laide þere-to. An addition of the $ΛS_1$ branch. Note moreover that three lines from DVH (976–978), describing the value of coriander as an antiscrofulous and which should appear immediately after this passage, were probably missing already in $Ω$.

361 feuer cotidiane. A copy mistake in $ΛS_1$: the other MSS of the tradition read ‹tercian› here, which is in accordance with DVH 981.

362 þe feuer. DVH 979 *tremorem*. The other MSS offer the correct translation "access" (*B*.248r/19, *W*.36v/16). Branch $ΛS_1$ moreover modified the passage that followed, cf. *W*.36v/16 ‹& he schal achap þe accesse›.

363 autours. The original Latin poem reads DVH 984 *Xenocrates*, although several Latin MSS read otherwise (*S(c)enocrates* $η$, $λ$, $αα$, $ββ$; *Ut Socrates* $θ$) or omit the name altogether (so $κ$), which may help explain the scribal conjecture. Xenocrates of Aphrodisias (*fl.* 1st century) was a physician quoted several times by Galen in works, frequently in connection with the use of disgusting ingredients in his remedies (*Dreckapotheke*; see for instance Kühn 1821–1833: xii.248–251).

366 camamyll. The entry describes the medical qualities of several composites generically called camomiles as rendered in DVH (549–591) and following the DVH(NME) tradition. A tripartite division on account of the colour of the flower, which was already present in MM, is also made in the ME text, although the entry is silent on the basis for the division. *Auctoritates* seem to agree in that a white, a yellow and a purple species must be distinguished. These are traditionally identified as the Roman camomile (*Chamaemelum nobile* (L.) All. = *Anthemis nobilis* L.; alternatively, this might be the field camomile, *Anthemis arvensis* L.), the golden marguerite (*Cota tinctoria* (L.) J. Gay = *Anthemis tinctoria* L.), and the purple marguerite (*Anthemis rosea* Sm.), respectively.

Identification is reassured on textual and pharmacographic grounds as well, since these species are taken to be diuretic (**368** = DVH 565), lithontriptic and emmenagogue (**368** = DVH 566–568), anticolic and carminative (**370** = DVH 569–570), detergent (→ **371**, **379** = DVH 570–571, 585), anticteric (**372** = DVH 572), splanchnic (→ **373**), splenetic (**377** = DVH 580–583), ophthalmic (→ **378**), and anticephalalgic (**380** = DVH 586–591). A missing fragment, corresponding to DVH 573–576, surely explains that the assumed hepatic, abortifacient and febrifuge qualities of the species were not recorded in any of the witnesses of the DVH(NME) tradition. DVH 578–579, which describes the alexipharmic value of the plant, appears to have left untranslated in this tradition as well.

Literature: CAMOMILES (*Anthemis* L. spp.): *HP* vii.8.3 (ἄνθεμον ἀφύλλανθες); *MM* iii.137 (ἀνθεμίς); *NH* xxii.53 (*anthemis*); *SM* xi.833 (ἀνθεμίς); *RM* ii.271 (χαμαίμηλον); *Grad*. 346; *OEH* 24 (*herba camemelon. magepe*); *Dur.Glos.* 301 (*camemelon. magethe*); *DVH* 549–591 (*anthemis, chamaemelum, chamomilla*); *LS* 22 (*debonigi* [بَابُونِج *bābūniğ*], *camomilla*); *EPN* iv (*beneolentem. mageðe | obtalmon, mageðe*), vī (*camomilla. camemille, maiwe*), viii (*hec camamella. camamelle*), ix (*hec camamilla. a camamy*); *TH* 131 (*camomilla*); *Pand*. 85 (_ARbebonig, bebonigi, bebonici, beborugi, bebunegiemara, GRarthemis, antimus, leucantimos, gamilla, heranthemiden, chamelon, melantemon, crisocomon, LAcamomilla*); *DVH(NME)* 253v.1 (*camamyle*); *DVH(SME)* 26a.11 (*camomille*); *Alph*. 28 (*camamilla. camamille*); *AC* 172.22 (*camomilla. camamylle*) ❦ *GH* 122 (CAMOMILLA, *camomyll, charmiere pertenicon, diacolefac, trystycos elyatos, aperytos, nypeos ieromatenus, alion patres, olerasa, superba, puxetos, vulenta, sapera, solifacium, oblandia, obulacia, amula, abiana, amulusta, alba bona*); *Fu* 8 (ἈΝΘΕΜΙΣ, χαμαίμηλον, *anthemis, chamæmelon, camomilla*); *Tu* 1.236 (CAMOMYLE, *anthemis, chamelum*); *DL* 131 (CAMOMILL, ἀνθεμίς, χαμαίμηλον, *chamæmelum, bene olens, camomilla*); *Ge* 614 (CAMMOIL, *chamamelum, anthemis, leucanthemis, leucanthemon*).

C¹S¹ (*SM, RM, DVH, LS, Fu, Tu, DL, Ge*)

367 dry and wete. *Auctoritates* agree in assuming that the plant is hot and dry in the first degree, but only Bodley kept the correct temperament: *B*.253v/2 ⟨dry & hotte⟩; just like *S*₁, Wellcome reads *W*.39v/2 ⟨drye & weth⟩. Unfortunately, this entry is not in *P*, so it is impossible to ascertain whether the copy mistake for exemplary *HOTE originated in γ or was already present in *RH*.

371 þe schalis of þe adeleth. This translates *DVH* 570 *squamas de vultibus*. Hence ⟨adeleth⟩ must mean "face, countenance" and derive from OE *andwlita*, rather than "excrement" as stated in MED: *s.v.* adeleth *n*. and treated as a hapax (Moreno Olalla 2007: 128, fn. 48 and 2011: 61, fn. 15). Note as well the mistaken transcription **sthalis* in the quotation, instead of MS ⟨schalis⟩. The reading in Ω was probably *ANDLETH, cf. *B*.253v/6–7 ⟨scalle of þe anleth⟩; Wellcome is of no use for the reconstruction as it offers *W*.39v/7 ⟨þe schales⟩ only. According to the evidence quoted in MED: *s.v.* anlĕt *n*., the word appears to have been kept only in Northern dialects during the ME period (*Ormulum*, the *Northern Verse Psalter*, and the lyrical poem "Wyth was hys…"), perhaps due to reinforcement for the ON cognate *andlit* (note the missing ⟨w⟩ also in all post-1200 quoted evidence, as opposed to its presence in the OE texts).

373 veccys in mannys sidis þat is calliþ ypocandria. This stands for *DVH* 577 *Unguine purgantur hypochondria turgida tali*. ⟨veccys⟩ must then stand for "swellings", and hence is probably a faulty spelling for *v e s c y s /v e c i e s (< OF *ves(s)ie*), with the sense "blisters" that enjoyed current use in Medieval French (see sense C, "ampoule, cloque", in DMF: *s.v.* vessie) but is unrecorded in MED: *s.v.* vesī(e *n*., where it is simply glossed "the urinary bladder"; note yet "blister" *s.v.* vēsĭc(e n., § b (< La. *vēsīca*). The word can be traced back to Ω (cf. *B*.253v/7 ⟨voce⟩, *W*.39v/8 ⟨baccis⟩), where it was perhaps spelt *VECCIS. The ME text is unclear as to whether these blisters are external or internal, but the original Latin text (which is in fact mistranslated, as it actually means that the ointment will cleanse the swollen viscera of the abdomen) probably favours the latter interpretation, so that ⟨veccys⟩ would be a container of corrupt humours—black bile, probably, see below—and hence a synonym for "aposteme". Be as it may, sense 2(d), "a pain, stitch", of MED: *s.v.* rak *n*.², where this passage is quoted, should be put down as a ghost word based on a misreading *reccys in *WG*.

As for ⟨ypocandria⟩, i.e. hypochondria, this is "the soft part or parts of the body below the [costal] cartilage and above the navel" (LSJ: *s.v.* ὑποχόνδριον *n*.), and, by extension, "the viscera situated in the hypochondria; the liver, gallbladder, spleen, etc." (OED: *s.v.* hypochondria *n*.). The abdomen was taken to be the seat of unnatural humours, especially black bile, whose fumes caused a general state of depression (whence *melancholia* < Gk μέλαινα χολή, lit. "black bile"). Metonymically, hypochondria came to mean a particular mental state of low spirits and morbid feelings which is now the usual PDE meaning.

374 Plenius... 375 saiþe. This translates *DVH* 580–584. There is no reference to that prescription in the section where Pliny dealt with camomile (*NH* xxii.53), but Choulant managed to trace back a passage where a similar recipe for diseases of the spleen was recorded: "splenicis prodest in vino potus radicis cortex duabus drachmis, dempto balinearum usu, feruntque XXXV diebus per urinam et alvum totum lienem emitti" (*NH* xx.166). Such identification is yet dubious because that fragment deals with *capparis*, i.e. capers, a plant very dissimilar to camomile, and moreover there are several substantial differences between both receipts: the number of days during which each prescription must be followed does not tally and the reference of the patient giving up the use of the bath is on the other hand not mentioned in the poem—although of course Macer Floridus might have been dropped this on purpose. There is a much better chance that the text in *DVH* is in fact a rendering of *NH* xxvi.76: "Cissanthemus drachma bis die sumpta in vini albi cyathis duobus per dies XL lienem dicitur paulatim emittere per urinam". In opposition to Choulant's suggestion, in this passage the references to white wine and the number of days when this treatment should be followed do run parallel with the ME text. Admittedly, the passage does not deal with camomile, but it is extremely easy to assume scribal confusion between *c i s s a n t h e m u s

(< Gk κισσάνθεμον), either the woodbine (*Lonicera periclymenum* L.) or else some *Cyclamen* L., and *c h r y s a n t h e m u s (< Gk χρυσάνθεμον), one of the several known plant names for the golden marguerite (André 1985: *s.vv.* chrȳsanthemum, cissanthemos).

378 egill pace. This stands for *DVH* 584–585 *aegilopas curat*, so ‹egill pace› is a misspelling of Ω *EGILOPAS, which must have been already split into two words in γ (cf. *W.*39v/14 ‹egole pas›); the words are missing in the parallel passage of the Bodley version (*B.*253v/13). According to *RM* i.175, aegilops (< Gk αἰγίλωψ) is an aposteme between the inner corner of the eye and the nose, which could become a fistulous ulcer and even corrode the lachrymal bone if neglected. This ailment appears to have been not well-known, even among the specialists: *Chir.(ME)* 307, for example, preferred the form "garab" (< Ar الغرب *al-ġarab*) that probably derives from the Greek name and which Chauliac must have borrowed from Avicenna (II.123.30; Vázquez de Benito/ Herrera 1989: 89), and the word is mentioned neither in Benvenutus Grassus's *De probatissima arte oculorum* (Miranda García/González Fernández-Corugedo 2011) nor Lanfrank's *Art of Cirurgie* (von Fleischhacker 1894), and it is not included in the list of sicknesses composed in Norri 1992 (*garab*, on the other hand, is). In fact, MED: *s.v.* egilopa *n.* only quoted the two translations of *DVH*, and in both cases the term was used without any precision: while *DVH(NME)* suggests that it was an aposteme in the sclerotic rather than in the lachrymal area, the author of *DVH(SME)* took it for a type of leprosy.

383 calamynte. This section describes the virtues of calamints (once *Calamintha* Mill. but now segregated into several families) as rendered in the *AC* tradition. The tribe Menthae, which the family *Calamintha* belongs to, is large and full of varieties, hybrids, and cultivars, so distinctions between species are frequently far from clear-cut unless a very accurate description is provided. This must have been already so in Antiquity, to judge from the different names used in Greek and Latin to refer to these plants (see Andrews 1958a, particularly 145–146 for an attempt to put some order in the mass of—frequently contradictory—evidence). A tripartite division, traditional at least since *MM*, was made on their overall physical similarity of these plants with basil (the mountain species, diversely identified with *Mentha pulegium* L., *Clinopodium alpinum* (L.) Kuntze and *Nepeta cataria* L.; → **283**), pennyroyal (→ **1504, 1526**; most scholars think this must be *Mentha arvensis* L.), or wild mint (→ **1454**; this is Berendes's *Clinopodium nepeta* subsp. *glandulosum* (Req.) Govaerts = *Satureja calamintha* (L.) Scheele, although the plate in Fu looks rather like the fleabane, *Pulicaria dysenterica* (L.) Bernh.).

The distinction between species in the ME entry, however, is based on the species's habitat and surely derives from *Grad.* 376–377:

> Est etiam quoddam semper nasce*n*s in ripa fluminu*m*, & aquosi locis. Est aliud quod inuenitur in siccis locis, & ab aqua remotis. Est & aliud nascens in mo*n*tanis locis. Quod cu*m* in diuersis partibus nascatur, diuersis nominibus nu*n*cupatur, petrosum, terrestre, aquosum.

It seems clear that ⟨stony⟩ (La. *petrosum*) is metonymic and hence must correspond to the Dioscoridean mountain species (→ **384** about the ⟨hery⟩ variety) but, since the entry provides no real physical description, positive identification of the actual three species is probably impossible.

Regardless of the actual species, identification with the species usually called *calamintha* in Latin is also reassured pharmacographically, as the plants are taken to be diaphoretic (**388**), febrifuge (**389**), corrosive (**390**), emmenagogue (**391**), leprostatic (**392**), alexipharmic (**395**), anthelminthic (**396**), splanchnic (**397**), detergent (**399**), stomachal, antisingultus and anaphrodisiac (**401**), vermifuge (**403**) and vulnerary (**405**).

> **Literature**: CALAMINTS (*Calamintha* Mill. spp.): *HP* ii.1.3 (σισύμβριον); *MM* iii.35 (καλαμίνθη); *NH* xx.144 (*mentastrum*); *SM* xii.4; *RM* ii.219; *Grad.* 376; Dur.Glos. 304 (*nereta. sea minte*); DVH 592–625 (*nepta, calamentum*); LS 301 (*calamentum*); EPN vi (*calamentum. calemente*); Cl c.9 (*calamentum*); TH 95 (*calamentum*); *Pand.* 120 (ₐᵣ*calamentum,* ɢʀ*calamitatis,* ʟₐ*nepita, menta non odorifera*); DVH(SME) 8b.24 (*nepis. calamentum*); Alph. 27 (*calamentum.* ₐɴ*semtositwurt*); Sin.Bart. 14 (*calamentum majus, quo communiter utimur | calamentum minus, nepita*); AC 173.3 (*calamentum. calamente*) ⚜ GH 90 (CALAMENTUM, *calamynt, nelpyte*); Fu 164 (ΚΑΛΑΜΙΝΘΗ, *calamentum*); Tu 1.259 (CALAMYNTE); DL 177 (CALAMINT, καλαμίνθη, *calamintha, mentastrum*); Ge 556 (MOUNTAINE MINT, *mountaine calamint,* καλαμίνθη, *calamintha, mentastrum, montana calamintha, calamentum montanum*).

C^3S^3 (*SM, RM, Grad., DVH, LS, Cl, TH, GH,* Fu, DL, Ge)

384 hery. Since all calamints are covered "with a verie thinne hairie down" or "woolley mossines" that resembles "hoarie or fine cotton" (Ge 556–557), it is unclear why one species only should stand out as the "hairy" one. This is in fact a mistake carried over from the exemplar of the *AC* tradition, cf. ⟨eorthy⟩ in MS *H*, ⟨erthi⟩ in *R*, answering to the original Latin *terrestre* (see preceding note). The interpretation of MED: *s.v.* airī *a.,* § c, which takes this as an allograph of *airy* "having the properties of the 'element' air"—probably induced by a correlation of the epithets ⟨stony⟩ and ⟨watrye⟩ with the elements earth and water—, is thus based on a wrong assumption.

385 Ypocras seiþe. This translates loosely a passage from *Grad.* 377 ("Vnde Hippoc*ra*tes Calamenthum, inquit, extinguit libidine*m*, quia ipsum sperma liquefacere in uoluntario fluxu necesse est"), but will not be found in any of Hippocrates's texts, nor seems to be part of the *Corpus Hippocraticum*. In fact no medical *auctoritas*, be it Classical, medieval or post-medieval, appears to have mentioned anaphrodisiac qualities in connection with calamints. The fragment is likely to be an interpolation, ultimately from the the Hippocratic treatise Περὶ διαίτης (II.54.4), where mint is said to cause seminal losses, hinder erection and weaken the body of those who eat it often:

μίνθη θερμαίνει καὶ οὐρέεται καὶ ἐμέτους ἵστησι, καὶ ἢν πολλάκις ἐσθίῃ τις, τὴν γονὴν τήκει ὥστε ῥέειν, καὶ ἐντείνειν κωλύει, καὶ τὸ σῶμα ἀσθενὲς ποιέει.

The idea seems to have been traditional: already Aristotle (*Prob* XX.2, 923a9–12) echoed a Greek saying that stated that mint should be neither eaten nor planted during wartime (μίνθην ἐν πολέμῳ μήτ' ἔσθιε μήτε φύτευε), for it cooled the bodies and caused corruption to semen, and so it opposed courage and warring spirit (καταψύχει τὰ σώματα; δηλοῖ δὲ ἡ τοῦ σπέρματος φθορά. τοῦτο δὲ ὑπεναντίον πρὸς ἀνδρείαν καὶ θυμὸν ταὐτὸν ὂν τῷ γένει).

A confusion between mint and calamint can be easily assumed, all the more so since both species are so similar. Moreover, the Hippocratic sentence immediately preceding the one quoted above deals with calamint and begins with the same verb θερμαίνει "warms" (καλαμίνθη θερμαίνει καὶ καθαίρει "calamint warms and purges"), so the possibility of a homoioteleuton already in the source text should perhaps not be ruled out.

392 lepir þat mon calliþ elefancia. Leprosy was an umbrella term in medieval medicine to refer to several skin diseases caused by burnt black bile that had become rotten. This black bile originated by the deterioration of any humour—including black bile itself—during the second digestion through a malfunction of the associative virtue in the liver, which became cold and dry. Galen, and similarly several Arabic scholars such as Haly Abbas or Serapion the Younger, thought that only bilious humours (yellow and black) were prone to it, but other medical schools in the Middle Ages assumed that in fact four separate types of leprosy could be distinguished, depending on the original humour from whence black bile was derived: *alopecia* (not to be confused with the falling of the hair) if from blood, *tiria* from phlegm, *leonina* if from yellow bile, and *elephantiasis* from black bile (Costantinus Africanus, *De morborum cognitione*, vii.17). Since black bile was in itself the final detritus of the several digestions and thus the least choice of all humours, leprosy derived from it was deemed particularly dangerous.

407 carwey. According to the Latin heading and the ME plant name, the entry must be a description of the medical qualities of caraway (*Carum carvi*

L.). Textually, yet, the entry does not tally with any of the usual medical traditions, but appears to be a blending from several sources, as suggested by the repetition of a couple of virtues. There is evidence that some of these sources were misapplied, as one would not expect a hot species such as caraway to moisten the stomach (**419**); its value against frenzy (→ **411**) is similarly unexpected.

Identification with the caraway is borne out pharmacographically, as *auctoritates* said that the species was, above all, an excellent carminative (**410, 418**), eupeptic and anthelminthic (**416**), and diuretic (**419**). The emmenagogue power of the species (**414**) does not appear in the usual sources but was recorded in *DVH(SME)*, while its antiscabious qualities (**413, 420**) are mentioned in *AC*. Some other virtues appear attached to cumin, an akin species not always well distinguished from caraway: for example *Cl* commends cumin as an antitussive (**411**). The following virtues on the other hand do not seem to have been recorded in the usual medical literature: alexipharmic (**412**), trichogenous (**413**), splanchnic (**414**), and antiemetic (**417**).

Literature: CARAWAY (*Carum carvi* L.): *MM* iii.57 (καρώ); *NH* xix.164 (*careum*); *SM* xii.13; *RM* ii.221; *Grad.* 372; *OEH* 155 (*herba quiminon. cymen*); *LS* 279 (*caruia* [كرويا] *karawyā*], *carui*); *Cl* c.19 (*carui. carewy*); *TH* 105 (*carvi*); *Pand.* 326 (_{AR}*haruncij, karu nacari*, _{GR,LA}*carui*); *DVH(SME)* 42a.6 (*carui*); *Alph.* 31 (*careos. carui*); *Sin.Bart.* 15 (*careos*); *AC* 175.6 (*carui. carawey*) ⚭ *GH* 100 (CARUI); *Fu* 149 (ΚΑΡΟΣ, *caron, careum, carui*); *Tu* 1.264 (CARUWAYES, *karos, karon, car(e)um, carui*); *DL* 196 (CARUWAYES, κάρος, *car(e)um, carui*); *Ge* 879 (CARUWAIES, κάρος, *car(e)um, carui, carnabadion*).

C³S³ (*SM, RM, Grad., LS, Cl, TH, GH, Fu, Tu, DL, Ge*)

411 frenesy. Frenzy was a type of mental derangement due to an aposteme in the brain (depending on the author, the aposteme would be located in the meninges or the front lobe), which originated by the accumulation of either burnt bile from the liver or else the fumes of boiling blood from the heart. The effects of the aposteme were slightly different according to its origins: blood fumes caused insanity and sleeplessness, while bile turned the patient into a very irritable person. The furious mania that is widely recognizable as the main feature of this illness was common to all types of frenzy. Since the disease was caused by the two hot humours, it was prevalent in summer, and among those of a hot and dry temperament or those who had to toil suddenly. This makes using a hot species such as caraway quite an unexpected remedy—if not downright counterproductive.

413 scabbis. Just like *lepra* (→ **392**), to which it is related, *scab* (La. *scabies*) is an umbrella term to refer to a number of separate skin conditions usually causing an itching sensation (→ **953, 1354, 2339**) and thought to be due to the rotting of the excess of blood in the body (so *LS* v.7) or, more generally, to an excess of any salty humours (Lanfrank's *Cirurgie* III.i.5; von Fleischhacker 1894: 191–193). Medieval physicians distinguished two types, depending on whether the cutaneous affection was accompanied by the apparition of pustules and vesicles (*scabies humida*) or of dry scales (*scabies sicca*):

> Scabbies sicca, & non saniosa cum prurigine, & punctura, & fissura, de cholericis chymis incensis esse significatur. Vulnerosa, & crassa in superficie corporis, neq*ue* prurigine forti, & cum scalpatur cutis excoriatur, sicut alba squama, signat salsum & incensum phlegma, & plurimum hęc innascuntur senioribus, propter collectionem salsi phlegmatis, & defectionem cutis. Scabies humida, & saniosa, & cum delectatione pruriginosa, sanguinem incensum cum cholera, rubea esse demonstrat. Si sanies sit crassa, maiorem abundantiam sanguis signat. Si subtilis aquosa & citrina, cholera abundantem offendit. (*Viat.* vii.20)

Modern interpretation of the medieval medical evidence suggests that La. *scabies* is simply the general designation for eczema. Wet scab, or simply *scab*, would correspond to Gk ψώρα and is generally interpreted as eczema vesiculosum, eczema ichirosum and eczema pustulosum, while the dry version (Gk ψωρίασις) is thought to mean eczema erythematosum, eczema papulosum and eczema squamosum (Wilson 1864: 569).

422 caule. Although a physical description of the plant is missing (maybe because the plant was so well-known), both the Latin heading and the Middle English plant name suggest this entry describes the properties of the several cole crops and particularly the cabbage (*Brassica oleracea* L.) and akin garden varieties/cultivars. The text is quite an accurate translation of *DVH* 1201–1263, but as per usual omits the synonymy of the opening lines and the references to the Latin sources quoted by Macer Floridus: Cato, Chrysippus (→ **291**), and "Melicius" (probably the Phrygian monk Meletius who wrote a theologically-laden Περὶ τῆς τοῦ ἀνθρώπου κατασκευῆς (*De natura hominis*); see Cramer 1835–1837: III.1–157, Choulant 1956: 145).

Identification is supported pharmacographically, as the plant is said to be vulnerary (**423** = *DVH* 1208–1210), anticancerous (**424** = *DVH* 1210–1212), antipodragric (**427** = *DVH* 1213–1216), anti-inflammatory (**429, 442** = *DVH* 1219, 1243–1245), ophthalmic (**433** = *DVH* 1226–1227), galactogenous (**433** = *DVH* 1228), emmenagogue and abortifacient (**434** = *DVH* 1228), stomachal (**436** = *DVH* 1229), antidiarrheic and—slightly paradoxically—laxative (**436–438** = *DVH* 1230–1231), leprostatic (**440** = *DVH* 1238–1241), trichogenous (**441** = *DVH* 1242), antiarthritic and antipodagric (**445** = *DVH* 1246–1249), nephretic and splachnic (**447** = *DVH* 1250–1252), anthelminthic (**448** = *DVH* 1253–1254), antiuvulitic (**450, 456** = *DVH* 1255–1256, 1261–1263), antiraucedo and antiasmathic (**452** = *DVH* 1257–1258), and acrepalous (**454** = *DVH* 1260). The value of cabbage to produce medicinal urine that can then be profitably used for sinews and children is also recorded (**429–432** = *DVH* 1220–1223), while on the other hand two virtues from *DVH* 1232–1237 (splenetic and febrifuge) went missing from the account. Other than this, some virtues are apparently misrendered (→ **427**), or misplaced (→ **435**): for example, the apophlegmatic powers of the plant (**451** = *DVH* 1259) should appear after, rather than before its value against hoarseness.

> **Literature**: CABBAGE (*Brassica oleracea* L.): *HP* i.3.4 (ῥάφανος), vii *Dur.Glos.*, 1–2 (καυλός); *MM* ii.120 (κράμβη ἥμερος); *NH* xx.78 ff. (*brassica*); *SM* xii.42 (κράμβη); *RM* ii.230; *OEH* 130 (*cawel, brassicam siluaticam*); *Dur.Glos.* 300 (*brassica. cavlic*), 301 (*caula. caul*); *DVH* 1201–1263 (*caulis, brassicca*); *LS* 32 (*corumb* [كُرُنب *kurunb*], *caulis*); *EPN* iv (*brassica. wudu-cerfille*), v (*caula, uel magudaris. caul*), vii (*hic caulus. uwle or thyme*); *Cl* s.22 (*strucium, caulis agrestis, wild caul*); *TH* 436 (*strucium*); *Pand.* 176 (_{AR}*combin, corumb*, _{GR}*cauben, brassica, lacana*, _{LA}*caulis*); *DVH(SME)* 16a.5 (*coul. brasssica*); *Alph.* 33 (*caulis non transplantatus, brasica idem*); *Sin.Bart.* 13 (*brasica, caulis nondum transplantatus, sed quandoque pro quolibet caule sumitur*); *AC* 175.29 (*caulus. wourte, cool*) ❧ *GH* 117 (CAULE, *coole wortes*); *Fu* 157 (ΚΡΑΜΒΗ 'Η 'ΗΜΕΡΟΣ, *brassica satiua, caulis*); *Tu* 1.253 (COLE, *kolwurt, krambe, brassica*); *DL* 397 (COLEWORTS, *cabbage cole*, κράμβη ἡμέραι, *brassicæ satiuæ, coles*); *Ge* 243 (COLEWOORTS, κράμβη, ἀμέθυστος, *caulis*).
>
> S (*SM, RM, Ge*) | C¹S¹ (*LS, Fu, Tu, DL*) | C²S² (*Cl, TH*) | F¹S¹ (*GH*)

427 hit²...428 clawynge. The value of cabbage against excoriations on the toes is not in the canonical version of the Latin poem, which reads instead (*DVH* 1217–1218):

> Hoc etiam morbis medicabitur articulorum,
> Hoc quoque syringas ait et luxata iuvare

Since it is hard to see any definite textual or paleographical rapport between the original *articulorum* and something along the lines of *d i g i t o r u m that could have elicited such a translation, nor it is clear how *syringas* or *luxata* could be rendered as "scratching", this is probably best put down as a case of interpolation or faulty transmission of the Latin text. Unfortunately, the apparatus criticus in Choulant's edition is silent to any major variant in those lines other than *DVH* 1218 *ait elixata* in two manuscript traditions (γ and δ), but this does not serve to explain the ME reading.

428 y-leide to in a plaster-wyse. This translates *DVH* 1219 *superpositum*. Emendation is based on a number of instances in MED: s.v. plāstrewīse, *adv.* where the word is treated as a noun preceded by a redundant preposition *in*. This is supported by two quotations from John Trevisa's translation of

Bartholomaeus's *De Proprietatibus Rerum*, and one from later in this same entry in *LH*, corresponding to **443–445**.

435 dede childe. The abortifacient quality does not belong here as it translates the second half of *DVH* 1233, and hence it should appear after the laxative powers of the species mentioned in **438**. Although (seemingly random) rearrangements of the original lines of the poem are regularly found in the ME text, it is possible that either the Latin scribe or its translator decided to relocate the passage in order to connect it to the cabbage's assumed quality as an emmenagogue, as gynecological conditions were frequently presented *en bloc* (see for example **340**, **1143** or **1674**).

449 þe evill of þe strechillis. This corresponds to *DVH* 1256 *uvam* [...] *iacentem*, and hence ‹strechillis› must refer to the uvula, although in **456** it translates *DVH* 1263 *uvae* [...] *morbos* metonimically (unless this is a copy mistake and a preceding *e v i l l   o f in the exemplar were unadvertedly skipped).

The word is very rarely found in the ME corpus: according to MED: *s.v.* strechel *n.*, it is only used in this herbal and London, BL, Add. 15236 (Hunt 1986–1987). The word is probably the same as "a strykylle; hostoriu*m*" and "A strylkell [prob. *s t r y k k e l l] for A buschell*e*" that are recorded in the *Catholicon Anglicum* (Herrtage 1881: 369) and from which PDE *strickle* naturally derives. The forms *strichell* (used in the herbal, cf. **1494**) and *stritchill* are found in the 1585 English rendering of Hadrianus Junius's *Nomenclator* (Stein 2006) to gloss *radius* and *hostorium*, respectively.

The spelling ‹strechillis› is particularly interesting insofar as it displays *-is* in the singular (cf. *uvam* and *uvae* [gen.] in the original), just like forms such of *streckles*, *strikeless*, *strickles(s)*, and *strickliss*, all of which are, according to EDD: *s.v.* strickle *n.*, used in the West Midlands.

The etymology provided in MED suggests connection with from the verb *strecchen* and the suffix *-el*, but derivation from OE *stricel* is easier and probably better. The sense of that word is "an implement for smoothing corn in a measure", but the same word was also used to indicate the nipples, sometimes under the name *tit-stricel* (BT: *s.v.*), the relation between both meanings being explained by the OE verb *strīcan* "strike". The peculiar form of the uvula, resembling one of those Indian clubs used in eurhythmics, or a drumstick, accounts easily for the use of the same root to designate this reality. This is confirmed by Gilbert the Englishman (*CM*: clxxvj), since the uvula is directly compared to a nipple: *Vua est membrum in modum mamille*.

458 earthnote. Judging from the Latin heading (which was deteriorated from an exemplary *CICLAMINUM due to minim misinterpretation and further reading the original cluster **cl** as *d), the chapter seems to deal with the properties of sow-bread (some *Cyclamen* L. spp.) according to the *AC* tradition. This is reassured by two copy mistakes ("cidamum" and "corhnote") that are very similar to those in S_1 and which suggest a common English exemplar. *AC* offers on the other hand a collection of ME synonyms that is missing here.

The pharmacographic evidence agrees with such identification but is not definitive. The two medical virtues offered in the entry (regenerative and trichogenous) were recorded already in *MM*, and either one or the other can be found in other treatises: the species is said to be regenerative in *Cl*, and trichogenous in *Grad.* and *LS* (*HAP* oppositely tells that the species is good "ad caput depilandum"). But then the *Cyclamen* was more universally commended as an excellent purgative, laxative and abortifacient, yet none of this is mentioned in the entry. It is strange as well that the bulb, which is the most valuable part of the plant according to the medical authorities, is never used as an ingredient.

On the other hand, the ME plant name and the physical description of the plant are very much against the notion that the plant could be a sow-bread. The readings *AC* 175.25 ⟨quyt flowres⟩ and *Sl*.6v/18 ⟨flores albas⟩ make better sense that ⟨wiþ flouris⟩ in the text, suggesting an exemplary *WHIT that must have been misread as *w i t h sometime during the textual transmission. Indeed some species of the *Cyclamen* family, for example *C. hederifolium* Aiton, frequently display a very light shade of pink which may qualify as whitish, if not purely white. The problem with the description provided in the ME and Latin texts is rather that the leaves of most sow-breads are distinctively cordate—several treatises, following *MM*, compare them to those of ivy, while others liken them to those of asarabacca—and could not be confused with the dissected filiform ones of fennel by any stretch of the imagination. The description provided suggests that the plant may be the one called βούνιον in Greek and identified as either the pig-nut (*Conopodium majus* (Gouan) Loret = *Bunium flexuosum* Stokes) or the earth-chestnut (*Bunium ferulaceum* Sm.), both of which were called "earthnut". See Moreno Olalla 2015: 56–58 for a more detailed explanation of the transmission of this entry and the confusion between the original La. *cyclamen* and the ME name. It seems that English pharmacography, from *OEH* onwards—in case OE *slite* refers to the ragged look of its leaves—identified La. *cyclamen* with the Apiaceae species called βούνιον in *MM*. Confusion of both is particularly clear in *Alph.*, where *panis* *porcinus* (i.e. sow-bread) was translated as *dilnote*, indicating a plant that looks like dill (ragged leaves, umbels) but has a tuber as well.

Literature: PIG-NUT (*Conopodium majus* (Gouan) Loret)/EARTH-CHESTNUT (*Bunium ferulaceum* Sm.): *MM* iv.123 (βούνιον); *NH* xx.21 (*napus* [...] *quod bunion vocant*); *SM* xi.852 (βούνιον, ἀρκτικόν); *RM* ii.201 ❦ Fu 46 (ΆΠΙΟΣ, ἴσχας, χαμαιβάλανον, *apios, raphanus syluestris*); Tu 1.238 (APIOS, *chamebalanos, ischas, carica, ernut, erthnut*); DL 416 (EARTH CHESTNUT, βολβοκάστανον, ἀγριοκάστανον); Ge 905 (EARTH NUT, *earth chestnut, kipper nut*, βολβοκάστανον, *balanocastanon, bunium Dioscoridis, apios, oenanthe*). ¶ SOW-BREAD (*Cyclamen hederifolium* Aiton): *HP* vii.9.4 (κυκλάμινος); *MM* ii.164; *NH* xxv.114 (*tuber terrae, cyclaminos*); *SM* xii.50; *RM* ii.232; *OEH* 18 (*herba orbicularis, slíte*); Grad. 379 (*cyclaminus*); Dur.Glos. 301 (*cyclaminos. eortheppel, slite, attorlathe*); LS 249 (*buchormarien* [بخّور مريم *baḫḫūr Maryam*], *ciclamen*); Cl c.1 (*ciclamen*); TH 87 (*ciclamen*); Pand. 113 (_{AR}*buthomarien, alcharincha, artanita*, _{GR}*lentopodion, adaminus*, _{LA}*panis porcinus*); Alph. 39 (*Ciclamen, ciclamum, citeranum, panis porcinus, malum terre.* _{AN}*dilnote*); AC 175.23 (*cidamum. corhnote, dilnote, slyte, haylwourth*) ❦ Fu 170 (ΚΥΚΛΑΜΙΝΟΣ, ἰχθυόθηρον, *rapum terræ, umbilicus terræ, tuber terræ, cyclamen, panis terræ, panis terræ, arthanita*); Tu 1.298 (SOWESBREDE, *ciclaminos, ciclaminus, rapum terrae, umbilicus terrae, panis porcinus, tuber terrae*); DL 238 (SOW-BREAD, κυκλάμινος, ἰχθυόθηρον, *cyclaminus, rapum terræ, tuber terræ, umbilicus terræ, orbicularis, palalia, malum terræ, rapum porcinum, panis porcinus, cyclamen, arthanita*); Ge 694 (SOWBREADE, κυκλάμινος, *tuber terræ, terræ rapum, orbicularis, palalia, rapum porcinum, terræ malum, cyclamen, panis porcinus, arthanita*).

C³S³ (*Grad., LS, Cl, TH,* Fu, DL, Ge)

461 feche a-wey. The passage is obviously nonsensical and appears to be corrupt: indeed *AC* 175.27 provides the much preferable reading "frete awey". Note that the coda ⟨and helpiþe renewe the quyck fleshe⟩ is not in any of the MSS of *AC* consulted by Brodin.

466 cardiake. The Latin and ME name ⟨cardiake⟩ suggest that the intended species here must be the motherwort (*Leonurus cardiaca* L.). Pharmacographically as well, the antiepileptic qualities of this species are also recorded in Fu₁₄₈ and can be put in connection with the spasmolytic and antiparalytic qualities allotted to the plant in Ge₅₆₉, but it is striking that the cardiac values, after which the species was named, are missing. Moreover, the description provided in the entry is against this identification, as the leaves of *Leonurus cardiaca* are not particularly similar to those of ⟨blynde-nettill⟩ (at least if this means dead nettle. i.e. some *Lamium* L. sp.), as already noted in André 1985: *s.v.* pycnocomon. Moreover, this plant has no known culinary value, which is in blatant contradicion with **469**. The reference to ⟨smalle coddis⟩ does not help the identification either for, while the motherwort displays schizocarps, they could be referred to as cods by stretching the term only.

The synonym ‹cilsper›, diversely misspelled ‹eylpere› and ‹caspere› in MSS from the *AC* textual tradition (from which the entry in S_1 derives), suggests otherwise. This word probably stems from an original *EILEPER, traced back in OED: *s.v.* † eileber *n.* to OE *ēalifer*. The same word seems to appear in Gerard's "Supplement or Appendix vnto the generall Table" of English plant names as "eileber is alliaria". To judge from its woodcut, Gerard's *Alliaria* refers to the garlic mustard (*Alliaria petiolata* (M.Bieb.) Cavara & Grande), the leaves of which are coarsely toothed and extremely similar to those of a *Lamium*, have a pungent smell and taste (similar to garlic as indicated by the modern binomial name), and displays long, thin siliquae that can easily be the ‹smalle coddis› which contain ‹litell sedis› (as the seeds are *ca.* 2.5–3mm long). The *Alliaria* was moreover a common ingredient in sauces, as suggested by such plant names as "beggarman's oatmeal", recorded in DEPN: 565, or "sauce-alone", mentioned by both Lyte and Gerard.

> **Literature**: GARLIC MUSTARD (*Alliaria petiolata* (M.Bieb.) Cavara & Grande): *HP* viii.1.4 (ἐρύσιμον); *MM* ii.158; *NH* xxii.158 (*irio, erysimon*); *SM* xi.877; *RM* ii.211; *LS* 347 (*huderegi* [تودرج *tūdrīğ*], *erisimon*); *Alph.* 58 (*eruca goratina*), 59 (*erismon*); *AC* 178.21 (*cardiaca. cardyake, caspere*) ❧ Fu 36 (ALLIARIA, *alliaris, pes asininus*); Tu 2.727 (SAUCEALONE, *alliaria, Jack of the hedge*); DL 458 (SAUCE ALONE, *Iacke by the hedge, alliaria, scordotis, pes asininus*); Ge 650 (SAUCE ALONE, *Jack by the hedge, alliaria, alliaris, rima Maria, pes asininus*). ¶ MOTHERWORT (*Leonurus cardiaca* L.): *MM* iv.174 (πυκνόκομον); *NH* xxvi.57, (*pycnocomon*); *SM* xii.110; *RM* ii.255 ❧ Fu 148 (CARDIACA); DL 92 (MOTHERWURT, *cardiaca, sideritis prima*); Ge 569 (MOTHER WOORT, *cardiaca, sideritis herculana*).
>
> C^2 (Tu)| C^2S^2 (Ge) | C^3S^3 (Fu) | [C^4S^4 (*LS*)]

472 croswort. Both the Latin and ME names were applied to a number of plants having four whorled leaves or petals. The plant cannot be corn spurrey (*Spergula arvensis* L.) as suggested in *Alph.*, since the flowers of this species display five petals, and they do not gather in groups around a single stem. The description given in the text is also against the possibility of its being *Cruciata laevipes* Opiz (= *Galium cruciata* (L.) Scop.), as usual in PDE or Brodin 1950: 271, since the flowers are said to be white, rather than yellow. Moreover, the leaves of *Cruciata* are too broad to be easily comparable to those of the cockle (at least if that means *Lolium temulentum* L.; see next note). The description of the leaves and flowers does fit on the other hand that of a white-petalled *Galium* species, such as the Northern bedstraw (*G. boreale* L.) or the common marsh-straw (*G. palustre* L.).

Pharmacographically, the vulnerary qualities of the species are mirrored in Ge (although the accompanying plate and the names "golden crossewoort" and "golden mugweet" make it clear that the species described there was actually *Cruciata laevipes*), Fu and DL (although they were in fact referring to *Gentiana cruciata* L.). The entry follows *AC*.

Literature: *Northern bedstraw/common marsh-straw (*Galium boreale* L./G. palustre* L.): *Alph.* 168 (*spergula major, herba cruciata*); *Sin.Bart.* 23 (*herba cruciata. croyse*); *AC* 190,24 (*herba cruriatica. croswourth, exan*) ✣ Fu 158 (cruciata); DL 241 (cruciasma, *dwarfe gentian, alisma, cruciata, gentiana minor*); Ge 964 (crossewoort, *golden mugweet, cruciata, cruciatis*).

CS ([Fu, DL, Ge])

472 somdell like to cokkyll. This fragment seems to be an addition in the *LH* tradition, as it is neither in any of the several MSS of *AC* used by Brodin in his edition nor in *Sl*.

477 comyn. According to the Latin and ME plant names the entry must deal with cumin (*Cuminum cyminum* L.), but the comparison of its leaves with those of coriander rather points to anise (*Pimpinella anisum* L.). Anise was referred to as "cuminum/ciminum dulce" in some late Medieval sources (see the *Literature* apparatus), and in many herbals (at least since Theophrastus) anise and cumin were treated as a group together with caraway and fennel (the so called four greater hot seeds, La. "quatuor semina calida majora" that were renowned for their carminative powers, Quincy 1727: 362).

In the medical literature both seeds were taken to be carminative (**480**), eupeptic and diuretic (**481**), cosmetic (**482**) and alexipharmic (**484**). *Cuminum* is extolled as antidysenteric (**483**) and anaphrodisiac (**483**; note that anise on the other hand is taken to be an aphrodisiac) in the literature, but the antihalitosic quality (**488**) is associated with *Pimpinella* only. This mixture of virtues from both species has a textual correlation, as this section is in fact a composite of three separate sources. Lines 437–441 (up to ⟨pisse⟩) were taken from the entry *ciminum* in *AC*, then some source akin to *DVH* is followed until ⟨bytyng⟩ (**484**), and finally a third source (as yet unidentified, but dealing with anise, rather than cumin) adds the recipe against bad breath. The presence of the last source can be also suspected through the reference to the temperament of the plant (**484**), an information which would as a rule appear early within the entry—and some other times end it.

Literature: Cumin (*Cuminum cyminum* L.): *HP* i.11.2 ($\kappa\acute{u}\mu\iota\nu o\nu$); *MM* iii.59 ($\kappa\acute{u}\mu\iota\nu o\nu$ $\H{\eta}\mu\epsilon\rho o\nu$); *NH* xx.159 (*cuminum*); *SM* xii.52 ($\kappa\acute{u}\mu\iota\nu o\nu$); *RM* ii.232; *Grad.* 374 (*cyminum*); *OEH* 155 (*cymen. quim(m)imum, quiminon*); *Dur.Glos.* 301 (*ciminum. cymen*); *DVH* 2111–

2124 (*cyminum*); *LS* 277 (*camum* [كمّون *kammūn*], *cyminum*); *EPN* ii (*ciminum. cymen*), iv (*cinnamomum. cymen*); v (*ciminum. cimen*), vii (*hoc siminum. comyne*); *Cl* c.20 (*ciminum. comyn*); *TH* 106 (*ciminum*); *Pand.* 127 (_{AR}*camin,* _{GR,LA}*ciminum*); *DVH(SME)* 37b.7 (*comyn*); *AC* 178.15 (*ciminum. comyn*) ✿ *GH* 101 (CIMINUM, *comyn*); Tu 1.295 (COMMYN, *kyminon*); *DL* 197 (COMIJN, κύμινον ἥμερον, *cuminum satiuum, cyminum*); Ge 907 (CUMIN, κύμινον ἥμερον, *cuminum, cyminum*). ¶ ANISE (*Pimpinella anisum* L.): → annys [**15**].

C²S² (*Cl, TH, GH*) | C³ (*SM*) | C³S³ (*DVH, Grad., LS,* DL, Ge)

490 confery. The entry describes the medical virtues of comfrey (*Symphytum officinale* L.) as presented in *AC*, although the virtue to stop nosebleed is found nowhere in that textual tradition and probably answers to a scribal addition. Although most medieval treatises made a threefold division between *Consolida maior, minor* and *media, LH* only refers to the former two (→ **522** about the *minor* species). The physical description provided here is too vague to be useful (the one in *AC* is much more informative), but pharmacographically it does fit the picture, as the species is said to be an excellent anticontusive (**491**), consolidative (**495**) and antepistactic (**495–497**).

Literature: COMFREY (*Symphytum officinale* L.): *MM* iv.10 (σύμφυτον ἄλλο); *NH* xxvi.45 (*symphytum*); *SM* xii.134 (σύμφυτον τὸ μέγα); *RM* ii.264; *OEH* 60 (*herba confirma. galluc*); Dur.Glos. 301 (*confirma. galluc*); *EPN* ii (*adriatica, vel malum terrae. galluc*), iv (*sinfitum. gallac*); vi (*cumfiria. cumfirie, galloc*), ix (*hec conseria. a wyld fr...*); *TH* 143 (*consolida maior*); *Pand.* 628 (_{GR}*simphitum, anagallicum,* _{AR}*picterion,* _{LA}*consolida*); Alph. 45 (*consolida maior. anagallicum, anangalla, anagallum, symphicum.* _{GA,AN}*comfille*); Sin.Bart. 16 (*consolida major. consin*); *AC* 180.1 (*consolida maior. dayessye, conforye*) ✿ *GH* 134 (CONSOLIDA MAIOR, *comfrey, more consoulde, analogicon, symphytum*); Fu 265 (ΣΥΜΦΥΤΟΝ ΜΕΓΑ, *symphytum, solidago, consolida maior*); Tu 2.584 (COMFREY, *symphiton alterum, consolida magna*); *DL* 103 (COMFREY, σύμφυτον μέγα, *symphytum magnum, solidago, consolida maior*); Ge 660 (COMFREY, *great consound, knit backe, blackwoort,* σύμφυτον, *symphytum maius, solidago, consolida maior, inula rustica, alus gallica, osteocollon*).

CH (*RM*) | CH³ (*SM*) | C²S² (Fu, DL)

499 cowslope. The ME name and the physical description provided in the entry seem to point to some *Primula* L. spp., either cowslip (*P. veris* L.) or oxlip (*P. elatior* (L.) Hill). The latter species seems a better possibility on account of the comparison drawn between the flowers of this species to those of ⟨prymrose⟩ (apparently, *P. vulgaris* Huds., → **1841**): the petals of oxlip, just like those of primrose, are whitish with a light yellow tinge at their base, while those of *P. veris* are as a rule bright yellow throughout. The Latin name supports this as it refers to the similarity of the blooms clustered around the scape to a bunch of keys, which is the well-known attribute of St. Peter (cf. the plant name *Peterwort* or *Himmelschüssel, S. Peters schlüssel* in Fu; Ge also equates oxlips—rather than cowslips—with *Herba S. Petri*, but DL thinks oppositely).

Textually the entry is a translation of the section *Ligusticum* in DVH (882–906), which apparently describes *Levisticum officinale* W.D.J.Koch and will be translated again later in the herbal (→ **1162**, with discussion). Both species, which are physically very different, were easily distinguished in texts from the Continent, assimilation of *Levisticum* and *Primula* being apparently a late Middle English affair (cf. *EPN* viii and ix, both dated in the 15th century, and → **1841**, with discussion). Still, confusions of *Primula veris/P. elatior* with other species seem to have been already current by the time the *Dur.Glos.* was composed, since the name *cūsloppe* was put in connection there with *hierebulbum*, even though this name is thought to have referred to meadow saffron (*Colchicum autumnale* L., cf. "greate wyrt. hieribulbum" in *OEH* 22; de Vriend 1984: 293), perhaps because both plants were taken to be excellent antiarthritics—as seen from synonyms such as *arthretica* (Ge) and *herba paralysis* (DL, Ge) applied to *Primula*.

Identification with *ligusticum* is borne out pharmacographically, as the plant is said to be carminative (**503** = DVH 887–888, again in **508** = DVH 894–899), eupeptic (**503** and again in **508** = DVH 888–889), deoppilant and diuretic (**505** = DVH 889–890), emmenagogue (**505** = DVH 890) and alexipharmic (**507** = DVH 891–893). The ophthalmic virtue attached to this species in DVH 900–906 is given in a very distorted way (→ **508**).

> **Literature**: OXLIP (*Primula elatior* (L.) Hill): *HP* ix.12.3 (φλόμος); *MM* iv.103 (φλόμος, φλομίς); *NH* xv.120 (*verbascum, phlomis*); *SM* xii.150; *RM* 270; *Dur.Glos.* 303 (*hierebulbum. cusloppe*); *EPN* ii (*brittannica. cusloppe*), viii, ix (*hoc ligustrum. a cowslowpe*); *TH* 230 (*herba paralisis, arthetica*); *Alph.* 78 (*herba sancti petri, herba paralesis. cousloppe*); *Sin.Bart.* 23 (*herba sancti petri, primula veris*); *AC* 192.9 (*herba petri. peter, cowsloppe*) ※ *GH* 211 (HERBA PARALISI, *cowslip, pagle, artetyke*); Fu 326 (ΦΛΟΜΟΣ, *verbascum, tapsus barbatus, candela regis, candelaria, lanaria*); Tu 2.767 (COWESLIPPE, *herba paralysis, oxislip, pagles*); DL 85 (PETIE-MULLEIN, *prime-roses, φλόμος, verbasculum, primula veris, herba paralysis, oxe lips*); Ge 635 (COWSLIPS, *pettie mullein, palsie woort, oxeslips, paigle, primula veris, arthetica, herba paralysis/S. Petri*). ¶ LOVAGE (*Levisticum officinale* W.D.J.Koch): → lovache [**1162**].
>
> S ([SM]) | CS ([Fu], Ge) | CS³ (DL)

508 he… 509 drinke. This is a faulty rendering of DVH 900–901: *hanc oculis Strabus potuque et odore nocivam / asserit*. The author *Strabus* mentioned by Macer Floridus is the Reichenau monk Walahfrid Strabo (*ca*. 808–849), since the passage appears to be a very free rendering to lines 230–233 of Strabo's poem *Hortulus*, where he described the plant *libysticum*:

> Hoc germen succo quamvis et odore gemellis
> Orbibus officere et tenebras inferre putetur,
> Semina saepe tamen quaesitis addere curis
> Parva solent, famamque aliena laude mereri.

The same passage proved problematic to the translator of the other account of this section included in *LH* (→ **1169**). Here it seems as if *oculis Strabus* in the original poem was misread as a syntactic unit and translated somehow into ‹shelowe body›. The sense of the phrase is not totally clear. MED: *s.v.* shalou(e a. assumes that it is a spelling variant of "shallow" and tentatively suggests the meaning "?thin, emaciated", quoting the fragment as evidence.

511 coluyr-fote. The Latin and ME names suggest that the plant described here must be a *Geranium* L. spp., probably the long-stalked cranesbill (*G. columbinum* L.) since it is opposed in the text to the soft-stalked *G. molle* L. (→ **1286**, with discussion). As is often the case with entries copied from *AC*, the physical description provided is unusually accurate and also points to a cranesbill. For all that it is worth, it might be relevant to mention here that a contemporary English source such as *Alph*. seems to describe *G. molle* in its entry for *pes colombinus*, as it mentions that its leaves are divided into seven lobes—the leaves of *G. columbinum* being usually dissected into just five parts.

On the other hand, the temperament does not agree with this identification, as *auctoritates* thought that *gerania* were cold, rather than hot. (*LS* did refer to *pes columbinus* a being hot and dry in the third degree, but the plant described there was not a *Geranium* but the alkanet, *Alkanna tinctoria* (L.) Tausch, a plant that does not fit the description provided in the entry.) Identification with a *Geranium* is pharmacographically uncertain as well. The species in the entry is praised as an ophthalmic (**514**), but *gerania* were used above all to cure swellings, particularly in the genital area (*MM, RM, GH,* DL, Ge); other virtues recorded in the literature include help against flatulence, phthisis, ear problems, opisthotonous, i.e. contorsion of the body into a bridging position (*NH*); bladder diseases, closing of wounds and ulcers, arthritis (Fu, DL, Ge); and ruptures (Ge). The entry in *LS* does mention apostemes in the eyes, but almost in passing among a large collection of virtues and hence seems unrelated to the ME entry.

Literature: LONG-STALKED CRANESBILL (*Geranium columbinum* L.): *MM* iii.116 (γεράνιον); *NH* xxvi.108 (*geranion*); *RM* ii.203; *LS* 269 (*hamenis* [أحمر *ḥumayra*], *pes columbinus, amomum*); *TH* 398 (*pes columbinus, sflectio*); *Pand.* 41 (GR*amomum,* LA*pes* *colombinus*, ₐᵣ*hameien*); *Alph.* 65 (*flectidos, pes columbinus*), 140 (*pes colombinus. clauerfot*); *Sin.Bart.* 40 (*spergula, pes columbinus*); *AC* p. 197.11 (*pes columbe. coluerfot, pes de columbe*) ✥ *GH* 361 (PES COLUMBINUS, *doues fote, ficene*); Fu 76 (ΓΕΡΑΝΙΟΝ, *geranium, rostrum ciconiœ, pes columbinus, amomum*); Tu 2.388 (PINK NEDLE, *cranes bill, geranium, starkis bill*); DL 34 (HERBE ROBERT, *pinke-needle, storkes-bill*, γεράνιον, *gruina, gruinalis... geranium alterum/columbinum, pes columbœ, doue-foote*); Ge 793 (CRANES BILL, *douesfoote, pigeons foote, pes columbinus, geranium alterum/ columbinum, pulmonia, gruina*).

FS (Fu, DL, Ge)

517 cvlrage. The Latin heading and the ME names suggest that the entry deals with some *Persicaria* L. spp. Note that ‹arsmeche›, taken as a hapax in MED: *s.v.*, is probably just a copy mistake for *a r s m e r t e , as seen from the other MSS of the *AC* textual tradition, to which this entry belongs. The entry mentions that there are two separate species but does not describe their differences. *AC* does provide such descriptions, indicating that one lives in hilly areas, has white leaves/petals and displays "a red sercle" along the stalk (surely the ochreae that sheathe the stipules) while the other lives in meadows and has a green stalk. *AC* also indicates the temperament. The two plants are traditionally taken to be the water-pepper (*P. hydropiper* (L.) Delarbre and the willow-weed (*Persicaria maculosa* Gray).

Pharmacographically, the species was used as antitumoral and antiinflammatory (*MM, SM, RM*, DL, Ge), detergent of wounds (Fu, DL, Ge), and antidysenteric (Fu), rather than an antiarthritic as stated in the entry (**519**).

Literature: WATER-PEPPER (*Persicaria hydropiper* (L.) Delarbre)/WILLOW-WEED (*P. maculosa* Gray): *MM* ii.161 (ὑδροπέπερι); *SM* xii.147; *RM* ii.268; *EPN* vi (*persicaria. saucheneie. cronesanke*); *TH* 387 (*persicaria, sanguinaria, sanguis sparsi*); *Pand.* 698 (*ydropiper, piper montanum, piperastrum, piper aque*); *Alph.* 46 (*currago, persicaria. arssmerte*); *Sin.Bart.* 33 (*persicaria minor. colerage*); *AC* 216.19 (*persiccaria. arsmert, keliage*) ✥ *GH* 353 (PERSICARIA, *arssmert, culrage*); Fu 241 (PERSICARIA), 325 (HYDROPIPER, ὑδροπέπερι); Tu 1.289 (ARSSMART, *culerage, crateogonum*); DL 453 (WATER PEPPER, *water pepperwurt, culrage*, ὑδροπέπερι, *hydropiper, piper aquaticum* | ARSESMART, *persicaria, ciderage*); Ge 360 (ARSMART, *water pepper, culrage*, ὑδροπέπερι, *hydropiper, piper aquaticum/aquatile*; *dead arsmart, peachwoort, plumbago, persicaria*).

C (*RM*, Tu) | CS (Ge [arsmart]) C³S³ (DL [water pepper]) |
FS (Fu, Ge [dead arsmart], DL [arsesmart])

522 daysye. The Latin headwort and the several ME synonyms suggest that the species here must be the daisy (*Bellis perennis* L.). As stated in the text (**530**), this was considered to be the *minor* species of comfrey (→ **490** about the *maior* counterpart). Identification is traditional as there is no physical description of the plant.

The entry was drawn from *AC* by blending data from the three different *consolidae* recorded in that tradition. The species is taken to be antitumoral (**524**), consolidative (**526**), analgesic, anti-inflammatory and anticontusive (**527**), but pharmacographically the bone-knitting properties were attached to the *maior* and *media* species only.

Literature: DAISY (*Bellis perennis* L.): *Dur.Glos.* 301 (*consolda. ban vyrt*); *EPN* ii, v (*consolda. dægesege*), vi (*consolida. consoude. daiseie*), viii (*hoc consolidum. a daysey*); *TH* 145 (*consolida minor, citasana, vincetoxicum*); *Pand.* 628 ($_{GR}$*simphitum, anagallicum,* $_{AR}$*picterion,* $_{LA}$*consolida*); *Alph.* 45 (*consolida minor, primula veris. waysegle, bonwort, brosewort*); *Sin.Bart.* 16 (*consolida minor. bonworte*); *AC* 180.12 (*consolida minor. þe lesse dayeseye, bryswort, bonwourtis*) ⚘ Fu 53 (BELLIS, *consolida minor, primula veris*); Tu 1.250 (DASEY, *bellis, consolida minor, primula veris*); *DL* 121 (DAISIES, *bellis, bellius, consolida minor, herba margarita, primula veris*); Ge 509 (LITTLE DAISIES, *bruisewoort, bellis minor, consolida minor, primula veris, herba margarita*).

CS (Fu) | FH (DL) | F²H² (Ge)

532 dauke. The Latin headword and the ME names suggest that the species here must be the carrot, particularly a wild variant (traditionally, *Daucus carota* L.). The synonym *bird's nest* is used in DL and Ge to refer to the third kind of *daucus*, the leaves of which are said to be similar to those of coriander, rather than hemlock (*Conium maculatum* L., → **872**).

Identification is borne out pharmacographically as well, as the plant was praised in most sources as a good antihydropic (**535**), alexipharmic (**535**), and deoppilant of the inner organs (**537**). *AC*, to which this entry belongs, offers a final virtue as a laxative, which is also frequently mentioned by medical *auctoritates*. The list of qualities for this species in *Grad.* is particularly close to the ME text and may have served as ultimate basis for the entry. It is worth mentioning that Fu also records similar qualities in the entry devoted to an akin species, parsnip (*Pastinaca sativa* L., → **1720**), where the plant is moreover called *Vogelnest*. This is not surprising since *pastinaca* was used to refer indiscriminately to either carrot and parsnip in several sources, as the noun was used to refer to several species, mainly Apiaceae having an edible taproot (see André 1985: *s.v.* pastināca).

Literature: WILD CARROT (*Daucus carota* L.): *HP* ix.15.5 (δαῦκος); *MM* iii.52 (σταφυλῖνος ἄγριος), iii 72 (δαῦκος); *NH* xx.30 (*staphylinus, pastinaca erratica*), xxv.110 (*daucus*); *SM* xi.862 (δαῦκος), xii 129 (σταφυλῖνος ἄγριος); *RM* ii.206 (δαῦκος); *Grad.* 369; *LS* 254 (*daucus*); *EPN* ii (*daucus. wealmora*), iii, v (*pastinaca. weal-more*), vii (*hic daucus. clap-wype*); *Cl* D.3 (*daucus. dawce*); *TH* 153 (*daucus*); Pand. 490 (*lezar* [جزر *ǧazar*], *daucus, bautia, pastinaca siluestris*); *Alph.* 47 (*daucus asininus, daucus agrestis*); *Sin.Bart.* 17 (*daucus, hujus duæ sunt species, agrestis et creticus.* [...] *daucus quandoque sumitur pro pastinaca*); *AC* 181.19 (*daucus asininus. bryddys neste, tauke*) ⚘ *GH* 143 (DAUCUS, *dawke*); Fu 85 (*ΔΑΥΚΟΣ, daucus*); Tu 2.490 (GARDEN/WILDE CAROT, σταφιλῖνος); DL 203 (DAUCUS, *wilde carrot*, δαύκος, *daucum, daucium*); Ge 873 (WILDE CARROT, *birds nest*, σταφυλῖνος ἄγριος, φίλτρον, *pastinaca syluestris tenuifolia, daucus*). ¶ PARSNIP (*Pastinaca sativa* L.) → pastyrnepe [**1720**].

CS (Fu) | C²S² (DL, Ge) | C³S² (*Grad.*) | C³S³ (*LS, Cl, TH, GH*)

539 dragancia femall. The extremely detailed description makes evident that the plant described here must be the same called δρακόντιον by Dioscorides and which have been identified as the dragons (*Dracunculus vulgaris* Schott), a species already analyzed earlier in the herbal (→ **38**, with discussion). This version reproduces the entry "dragansia femina" of the *AC* textual tradition. Brodin (1950: 219) argued that the distinction between "dragancia" and "dragancia femina" in this tradition—and by extension in *LH* as well—was an attempt to maintain the division between δρακοντία μεγάλη and δρακοντία μικρά, which seems likely. Such a distinction does appear in several Greek MSS and was kept in early editions (see Sprengel 1829–1830: i.307–310), but comparison of the entries has shown that in fact they both deal with the same species and hence the canonical edition (Wellmann 1906–1914: i.231–233) treats both as a single entry, maintaining the text of Sprengel's δρακοντία μικρά with some minor additions. The division is not recorded in the *Dioscorides Longobardus* (Stadler 1897a: 237).

Identification is also sustained pharmacographically, as the species is taken to be an acoustic (**545–546**), detergent (**547**), anticancerous and vulnerary (**549**), alexipharmic (**551**), ophthalmic (**552**), and aphrodisiac (**554**), all of which are virtues recorded in the preceding description of the species and in the usual medical literature since *MM*.

Literature: DRAGONS (*Dracunculus vulgaris* Schott): → addyrworte [**38**].

541 yelowe flour and a stalke. According to its *apparatus criticus*, no version of *AC* makes references to a flower here, and hence this must probably be taken as an innovation in *LH* or some direct ascendant not used by Brodin. Moreover, most MSS from the tradition (*HRBL*) offer ‹euen stok› (var. MS *R* ‹stalk›); only MS *X* and *LH* make reference to the colour yellow here (*X* reads ‹ȝelwe stalke›).

554 þis... drye. A copy mistake: *AC* 182.12 provides with a much better reading here: "þis herbe growith in dyrk placis and wete" (cf. *MM* ii.166.i φύεται ἐν συσκίοις ⟨τόποις⟩ περὶ φραγμοὺς καὶ αἱμασιάς "it grows in densely shaded places, around hedges and walls"), which suggests an exemplary *DYRK misread as *d r y e that the scribe of *LH* tried to emend. The sentence seems moreover to be displaced: it appears after ⟨yelowe⟩ (**544**) in the other MSS of the tradition.

556 dent de lyon. The Latin and ME names indicate that the entry must deal with dandelions, a name officially used to designate species of the genus *Taraxacum* F.H.Wigg. in general and *T. campylodes* G.E.Haglund in particular, but the word was surely stretched to include a number of akin genera within Cichorieae displaying a yellow flower such as catsears (*Hypochaeris* L. spp.), hawkbits (*Leontodon* L. spp.), or hawksbeards (*Crepis* L. spp.). In fact, for most Classical and medieval treatises dandelions may have been regarded as a kind of wild chicory (*Cichorium intybus* L., → **606**), and this is still seen from the inclusion in Fu of a plate for Hedypnois/Körlkraut within the entry devoted to σέρις (note yet that according to André 1985: *s.v.*, hedypnois is not a wild chicory; see also Ge, quoting *LS inter alia*). In any case, the description here and in its source, *AC* (which is slightly more detailed), is unfortunately too vague to allow a more accurate identification.

Identification with *Taraxacum* or any other Cichorieae is dubious, as all these plants were mostly praised as good stomachals and hepatics, rather than as febrifuges, as stated in the entry. Only Gerard mentioned a virtue against "hot burning feauers" but he did so in his chapter on "garden succorie" (i.e. endive, Ge$_{222}$), and then just in passing, in a list containing several other diseases.

Literature: DANDELIONS (*Taraxacum* F.H.Wigg. spp.): *HP* vii.7.1, 3 (ἀπάπη, ἀφάκη); *MM* ii.133,2 (χονδρίλη ἕτερα); *NH* xx.75 (*hedypnois*), xxi.89 (*aphaca*), xxii.91 (*condrion, condrille*); *SM* xii.156 (χονδρίλη); *RM* 273; *LS* 143 (*dundebe* [هندبا *hindibā*], *endiuia syluestris, taraxacon*); *Alph*. 49 (*dens leonis, capud monachi*. $_{GA}$*dent de lion,* $_{AN}$*doleroune*); *AC* 181.23 (*dens leonis. dendelyoun, lyonys toth*) ❀ Fu 262 (ΣΕΡΙΣ, *hedypnoïs, seris, intubus, aphaca, dens leonis, rostrum porcinum, taraxacon, altaraxacon*); Tu 2.403 (CYCORIE, *endive … intubus sylvestris, aphaca, hediopnis, dandelion*); DL 408 (CONDRILLA, *dandelion, gumme succorie*, κονδρίλλη ἕτερα, *dens leonis, rostrum porcinum*); Ge 228 (DANDELION, *dens leonis*).

F^{2}S^2 (Fu, DL, Ge)

560 lappa. The heading, an obvious scribal confusion with *l a p a c i u m, traditionally refers to *Arctium lappa* L., i.e. the greater burdock, which is quite a different species from the docks (see *NH* xxi.104). The opposite mistake is found in *Alph*. 94, 143, where *personacia* is given as a gloss for *Lappacium maius*, even though *personacia* is a Post-Classical Latin name for the burdock.

561 dokkys. The entry derives from the entry *Paratella* in *DVH* (1993–2014), as translated in the *DVH(NME)* tradition. Although the text gives no further description of any of them, the entry deals with the common medical qualities of four separate species (see next note). Identification with several species having a sharp taste that usually go under the names of *docks* and *sorrels* in English and belong to the genus *Rumex* L. is traditional, and sure on account of the virtues given here when compared with those in *MM* ii.114, § 2 for these species. Shared medical virtues include being a carminative (**563** = *DVH* 1997–1998), antipruritic (**564** = *DVH* 2000), antiodontalgic (**567** = *DVH* 2005), antidysenteric and antidiarrheic (**568** = *DVH* 2006), splenetic (**571** = *DVH* 2009), emmenagogue (**572** = *DVH* 2012) and lithontriptic (**572** = *DVH* 2012).

> **Literature**: Docks (*Rumex* L. spp.): *HP* vii.1.2 (λάπαθον); *MM* ii.114; *NH* xx.231–235 (*lapathum*); *SM* xii.56; *RM* ii.234; *OEH* 14 (*lapatium. docca*), 34 (*herba lapatium. wududocce*); *Dur.Glos.* 302 (*dilla. docc*), 303 (*lapatium. vude docce*); *DVH* 1993–2014 (*paratella*); *LS* 111 (*humadh* [حُمّاض *ḥummāḍ*], *acetosa*); *EPN* ii (*dilla, acrocorium. docce; cinoglossa, plantago, lapatium. wegbræde*) iv (*lappacium. docce; lappadium. lelopre; rodinaps. ompre, docce*), v (*dilla. docca*), viii, ix (*hec paradilla. a doke*); *Cl* L.8 (*lapacium acutum*); *TH* 254 (*lapatium*); *Pand*. 382 (LA*lapatium, pratella,* GR*lapaton, origma,* AR*hemason*); *DVH(NME)* 25iv.9 (*dockys*); *DVH(SME)* 22a.16 (*dokke. paradilla, lapacium*); *Alph*. 94 (*lappacium acutum, parella, paradella. reddokke*); *Sin.Bart*. 26 (*lapacium.* AN*dock*); *AC* 200.18 (*lapasium. rede dokke*), 214,16 (*paciens*) ⚭ *GH* 236 (LAPACIUM, *reed docke*); Fu 174 (ΛΑΠΑΘΟΝ, *rumex, lapatium*); Tu 2.549 (DOCKES, *rumex, lapathon*); DL 401 (DOCKS, *sorrell*, λάπαθον, *rumex, lapathum, lapatium*); Ge 310 (DOCKES, *lapathum, rumex, lapatium*).
>
> C/FS³ (DL, Ge) | CS (*DVH, GH*) | C³S³ (*Cl*) | F¹S¹ (*LS*, Tu) | F²S² (Fu)

561 iij kyndis. Although some authors made a threefold division (for example *GH* states that "there is lapaciu*m* docke that hath rough leues [...], there is another *þ*at hath rou*n*de leues [...] And there is another that is tame") and hence the MS reading has not been emended, this is probably a copy mistake, cf. *DVH* 1994 *illius species dicuntur quatuor esse*. The other MSS of the tradition, moreover, provide the expected number.

A fourfold division is traditional, as it is found already in Dioscorides and Pliny, but it is probably impossible to make sure correspondences between their names and descriptions, since variance among Classical, medieval and Renaissance authors is extremely large and complex. Besides the mistaken *lappacium maius* (→ **560**), for example, *Alph*. 94 recorded the following four species: *lappacium acutum, lappacium rotundum, lappacium aquaticum* and *lappacium ortolanum/ortense*. These may tentatively be identified as (*a*) *Rumex crispus* L. (the same as Dioscorides's ὀξυλάπαθον and Pliny's *oxylapathum*), (*b*) *Rumex obtusifolius* L., (*c*) *Rumex hydrolapathum* Huds. (Dioscorides's ἱππολάπαθον in *MM* ii.115 and Pliny's *hydrolapathum*), (*d*) *Rumex patientia* L. (Dioscorides's λάπαθον κηπευτόν, Pliny's *lapathum*). On the other hand, Fu distinguished between (*a*) *oxylapathum* (*mengelwurtz*), (*b*) *rhabarbarum monachorum* (*münch rhabarbarum*), (*c*) *bonus Henrichus* (*gûter Heinrich*), and (*d*) *oxalis* (*saur ampffer*). The corresponding woodcuts suggests that they correspond to *Rumex crispus* L., *Rumex patientia* L., *Chenopodium bonus-henricus* L., and *Rumex acetosa* L., respectively.

563 wyndis. *DVH* 1998 *per ructus* is missing here but diversely rendered in the other MSS as *B*25IV/11 ‹thorowe reftynge›, *W*.32r/9 ‹þrow ridyng*is*›, and *P*.273/1 ‹wiþ restyng›. The readings in *RH* look therefore like *lectiones faciliores* for *ÞROW RIFTYNG(E) (< ON *rypta, røpta*).

563 etyn ham colde. *DVH* 1999 *Sumptaque sicut olus*, cf. *B*.25IV/11 ‹ettynge als cale›, which indicates a faulty rendering of an original *ETYN ALS CALE (so *W*.32r/9–10) in Branch AS_1. Unfortunately for comparison purposes, this virtue is missing in *P*.

563 stroiþe. *DVH* 1999 *restringere*. Only *W*.32r/10 ‹strene› seems to maintain the correct sense of the Latin text. Both the readings in S_1 and *B*.25IV/11 ‹strenghe› answer to scribal emendations.

564 rewme. *DVH* 2000 *pruritus*. All three MSS from *RH* must have followed an exemplary reading that began with **r-** and contained at least three minims, diversely interpreted by each copyist: *W*.32r/11 ‹rym›, *P*.273/2 ‹reynes›. The Bodley version on the other hand reads ‹scurffe› (*B*.25IV/12). The forms of S_1 and particularly *P* are *lectiones faciliores*, while that of *B* can be interpreted in a number of ways. It may maintain a reading already present in Ω (which was altered by the scribe of *RH*), it may be a case of dialect translation, or else it could be taken as an inspired scribal conjecture based in the apparition later in the sentence of *SCABBE, i.e. the contagious eruption of minute pimples due to the burrowing into the skin of the itch mite (*Sarcoptes scabiei* var. *hominis* de Geer, 1778).

If the word reconstructed from *RH* is authorial, then there is a good chance that this was either *RUM, whence Early Modern English *room* "dandruff, scurf on the head", or else *RUU(E) (cf. MED: *s.v.* rŏve *n.* "[a] scabby condition of the skin"), which is perhaps etymologically related to PDE *dandruff*. Deciding which of the two is correct carries certain weight in the argument of the ultimate origin of *DVH(NME)*. *RUM (probably related, if not the same as OE *hrūm* "soot", see Holthausen 1974: *s.v.* hrūm) seems to have dialectally marked as a Somerset word to indicate dandruff (see EDD: *s.v.* room *n.*²), and therefore would suggest a SW Midlands origin for the text. On the other hand, *RUU(E) would indicate a Norse borrowing and hence point to a likely Northern origin for Ω, cf. OIc *hrufa* "the crust or scab of a boil or the like" (Cleasby and Vigfusson 1957: *s.v.*; see also de Vries 1962: *s.v.*). The Norse word is cognate of OE *hrēof* "scab" and, from the same Gmc. etymon, cf. also OE *hrēofla* "leper" and OIc *hrufla* "to scratch" which is akin in sense to La. *pruritus*.

566 swagiþ brenyngis. This corresponds to *DVH* 2003 *compescunt parotidasque*, which refers to mumps, but the sense is unclear here and the other MSS, all of which read like *B*.251v/13 ‹softys brynnynge› (also *W*.32r/13, *P*.273/4). The fragment is grammatically correct, but it is difficult to see how burnings can be softened (which surely explains the emendation in S_1). In fact, the very coupling of burnings and biles is somewhat unexpected: normally one recipe will cure related illnesses (in this same entry, cf. the pairs scurf and scabs, head- and toothache, disentery and lientery). The MSS readings are then *lectiones faciliores*. The word in Ω could have been *BRANKIS (DSL: branks, *n. pl.*²), a dialectal word that non-Scottish scribes would have easily misinterpreted into *brengis > *breningis. While the meaning "mumps" went unrecorded until the second half of the 18th century, the sense of the verb *brank* "to bridle, restrain (with a brank)" (see DSL: *s.vv.* brank *v.*¹, brankis, branks *n.*) was known in 15th-century ME, see *Alliterative Morte Arthure* 1861.

567 þe hede. This seems to correspond to *DVH* 2005 *uvas…tumidas*, that is staphyledema or swollen uvulas. All MSS of the tradition agree here, so the reading must have originated either in *Q* or Ω.

569 dokk…571 splene. Reference to wine as an ingredient is privative to S_1, cf. *DVH* 2008 *aceto*. It seems that the scribe perceived the copy mistake that he had just made and, rather than deleting the wrong fragment, simply added the correct reading immediately after. On the other hand the original sentence is much abridged: the other MSS renders the Latin text more accurately if only because they indicate how to use the mixture of dock and vinegar: cf. *B*.251v/16–17 ‹stampit and layd to þe splen þat is bolned it helpys› (and, with the usual minor variants, the parallel passages in *W*.32r/17–18 and *P*.273/8–10).

574 ditander. A difficult entry from an unknown source. The Latin heading and the ME name suggests that the plant treated here should be dittany of Crete (*Origanum dictamnus* L.). Identification is traditional and based on lexicological data only, since the entry provides no physical description, and there seems to be no pharmacographic support for it: none of the medical powers mentioned in the entry (anticephalalgic and purgative, **576**, or cardiac, **577**) are recorded in the usual literature, while on the other hand the entry fails to mention the foremost virtue of dittany: that of vulnerary and, above all, arrow-expeller, which is routinely recorded in almost all treatises on *materia medica* and the simples since Dioscorides (→ **1631**, which might deal with that species).

In Northern European sources, yet, the word *dictamnum* frequently referred to a very different species, the pepperwort (*Lepidium latifolium* L. (see Fischer 1929: 204, Daems 1993: 158–159, Harvey 1987: 3). This is clearly the species referred to as "diptanus" in *GH*, for the plant described there "groweth hyghe and hath leues moche lyke to strawberyes": *O. dictamnus* is not a high species by any standard (20–30 cm high on an average), whereas some *Lepidium* can reach up to two meters. The reference to strawberries may be a way to indicate that the leaves of both plants are slightly serrated. Renaissance English herbalists were well aware of this popular usage. William Turner stated that "some cal Lepidium also Dittany" (Stearn 1965: 176), which Tu_{422} then described to be "foulishly & unlearnedly", but "dittander" is given as a synonym for "pepperwoort" in Ge as a matter of course and DL quotes "dittander", "dittany" and "pepperwurt" as acceptable designations—although the last one is "more ryghtly".

As with *O. dictamnus*, identification with *Lepidium* is sustained by lexis only, since *auctoritates* generally commended that species as an emetic, mazolytic, anthelminthic, abortifacient and, above all, as the active ingredient for poultices against a number of internal diseases. Only the anthelminthic virtue may have been kept in the text, in case ‹venym humers to fle› (**576**) is a copy mistake for *v e n y m   w o r m e s   t o   f l e, which is quite likely. Although pharmacographic evidence is lacking, the fact that the plant is never told to be ingested, but ground, mixed with thick ingredients such as resin, and spread over the skin as an ointment may suggest that the entry deals with *Lepidium* rather than with *Origanum*, which was usually fed to the patient.

Literature: PEPPERWORT (*Lepidium latifolium* L.): MM ii.174 (λεπίδιον); NH xix.166 (*lepidium*); SM xii.58; RM ii.235; LS 362 (*seitaragi, hausab* [عضاب ،شِيترَج *šītarağ, 'uṣṣāb*]); EPN ii (*diptamnus, bibulcos. wilde næp*); Pand. 488 (*lepidum, gingion*, $_{AR}$*sceitaragi*); AC 181.6 (*diptanium. dytanye, ditandur*) ⚘ GH 145 (DIPTANUM, *dyptany*); Tu 2.422 (LEPIDIUM, *dittani, lepidium, peperwurt*); DL 452 (DITTANDER, *dittany, pepperwurt, piperitis, syluestris raphanus*); Ge 186 (HORSE RADISH, *dittander, ditany, pepperwoort, lepidium, raphanus syluestris, piperitis*). ¶ DITTANY OF CRETE (*Origanum dictamnus* L.): HP ix.16.1 (δίκταμνον); MM iii.32; NH xxv.92 (*dictamnum*); SM xi.863; RM ii.207;

Grad. 380; OEH 63 (*dictamnus*); LS 300 (*mescatremephir* [مشكطرامشير *maškaṭrāmašīr*], *dictamnum, diphthamum*); EPN vi (*diptannum. ditaundere*), viii (*hic ditamnus. detane*), ix (*hec ditanus. detany*); CI D.5 (*diptamum. ditayne*); TH 155 (*diptamus*); Pand. 215 (_{LA}*diptamum,* _{GR}*batin, diptamon,* _{AR}*sandenig*); Alph. 51 (*diptamnum* [...], *pulegium agreste* [...], *pilocella*); DVH(SME) 42a27 (*dittany*) ℘ Tu I.304 (DITTANI OF CANDY, *dictam(n)us, diptamus*); DL 191 (DICTAM, *dittanie of Candie,* δίκταμον, *dictamnum, pulegium siluestre, diptamum*); Ge 651 (DITTANIE, *wilde penniroiall, dittanie of Candie,* δίκταμνον, *dictamnum, pulegium siluestre, diptamnum*).

Lepidium: C⁴ (SM, RM) | C²S² (GH) | C³S³ (DL, Ge) | C⁴S⁴ (LS)
Origanum: CS (DL, Ge) | C²S² (TH) | C³S³ (Grad., CI, LS)

576 þe oþer of þe levis. The presence of ⟨oþer⟩ instead of a substance such as *j u i c e is unexpected. Assuming a mere copy mistake always remains a possibility but, since the anthelminthic virtue of the species is the second in the list, there is a chance that an original text *þ e o þ e r v i r t u e o f t h e e r b e : þ e l e v i s became corrupt in the transmission.

579 doworte. The (misspelt) Latin heading suggests that the species treated here must be some nightshade, a name loosely used to refer to some *Solanum* L. spp. and akin genera displaying big berries that were well known from its numbing powers. Comparison is drawn in the text between this species and ⟨hound-bery⟩, which is taken to be smaller in shape and probably stands for the black nightshade (*Solanum nigrum* L.). Since the latter plant usually went by such names as *morella minor* and *pety morell* (→ **1371, 1519**), it is likely that the species treated here is the *maior* counterpart (cf. the synonym ⟨more morell⟩ **580**), traditionally taken to be the deadly nightshade, *Atropa bella-donna* L. Such identification is reinforced in case that the synonyms ⟨doworte⟩ and ⟨dowech⟩ are scribal blunders for *d w a l e and *d u s c l e as suggested by the entry in *AC* which served as source, since—in opposition to *S. nigrum*— the name "dwale" applied to *Atropa* only, as demonstrated by Renaissance herbals. As for ⟨lesior⟩, this is not totally clear either: naturally, it might be yet another copy mistake, this time for *l e s s e r and thus correlative with the ⟨more⟩ that follows closely. But then the idea that a plant can be the lesser and the greater species at the same time does not seem to be too felicitous.

Identification with *Atropa* is borne out pharmacographically if we assume ⟨speke⟩ **584** to be a copy mistake for an original *s l e p e, as the plant was a strong narcotic. Note that, in opposition to what the author recommended, *auctoritates* agree that *Atropa* should best not be ingested as it contains extremely toxic alkaloids, particularly tropanes, that could prove deadly.

Literature: DEADLY NIGHTSHADE (*Atropa bella-donna* L.): HP ix.11.5 (στρύχνον); MM iv.72–73 (στρύχνον ὑπνωτικόν, σ. μανικόν); NH xxi.179 (*dorycnion, manicon*);

SM xii.145 (τρύχνον, στρύχνον); RM ii.263 (στρύχνον); Grad. 365 (strignum); OEH 76 (herba solata. solosece); Dur.Glos. 305 (solata. solesege); DVH 1918–1932 (maurella); LS 228 (hameb athahaleb [عنب الثعلب] 'inab aṯ-ṯa'lab], solatrum); EPN vi (morella. morele, atterlope), vii (hoc strigillum. morelle; hoc solatrum. morelle), ix (hec morella. morelle); Cl s.2 (solatrum, morella. morel); TH 418 (strignum); Pand. 315 (_AR_hameb, hupue phathahalep, _GR_strignum, cuculus, morella, _LA_solatrum, vua vulpis); DVH(SME) 35a.24 (morell. strignum, morella); Alph. 176 (strignus manicon, perisson, drion, furialis | solatrum mortale, solatrum nigrum, strignum maior, morella, uua lupina, solatrum uentaticum/montanum/ortolanum. _GA_morele, _AN_niththeschod, houndesberye); Sin.Bart. 41 (strignum. solatrum); AC 157.7 (solatrum nigrum. duscle, dwale, more morel) ⚘ GH 378 (SOLATRUM, petymorell, nyghtshade, lesse morell); Fu 264 (ΣΤΡΥΧΝΟΣ, τρύχνος, solanum, solatrum, cuculus, vua lupina, vua uulpis, morella); DL 318 (GREAT NIGHTSHADE, dwale, solanum lethale, solanum mortale, mandragoras Theophrasti), 319 (SOLANUM SOMNIFERUM, στρύχνος ὑπνωτικός, sleeping nightshade, halicacabon, dircion, apollinaris minor, viticana herba, opsago); Ge 269 (SLEEPING NIGHTSHADE, dwale, στρύχνος ὑπνωτικός, στρύχνος ὑπνώδης, solanum somniferum).

F (DVH) | F² (SM, RM) | F³ (DL₃₁₉) | F⁴ (Ge, DL₃₁₈) | F²S² (Grad., LS, Cl, TH, GH, Fu)

584 þis... 585 wodis. The place of the sentence within the entry is variable: according to Brodin's edition, in *AC* it appears just after the physical description of the plant, while in the Latin version of the text (*Sl.*19r/19; "*c*rescit in ortis & in quibu*s*dam *p*artibus in siluis & ca*m*pis") the passage appears at the very end, just like *LH*.

587 elenacampana. The Latin heading and the ME name indicate that this entry deals with the medical properties of the elecampane (*Inula helenium* L., → **899**, with discussion). The entry appears to be a conflation of the appropriate section in *AC* (up to ‹cogh› **594**: antigingivitic, **590**; lithontriptic and diuretic, **592**; abortifacient, **593**; antidiarrheic and antitussive, **594**), supplemented with a number of virtues translated from lines 1496–1502 in *DVH* (antisciatic, → **595**; antinephritic, **596**; antitussive and pulmonic, **598**; and against hernia, **599**). The last two recipes, as antiherpetic (**603**) and antiasthmatic (**604**), appear to derive from a third, unknown source. The value of the plant to relieve asthma is mentioned in many sources since Dioscorides. As for its powers against skin diseases, evidence is scarce other than the synonym "scabwo(o)rt" used in some English sources (*GH*, Ge; the latter source provides a recipe to make "an excellent ointment against the itche, scabs, manginesse, and such like", but it is nothing like the one here). Fu, quoting *NH* xx.38, states that "radicis vero decoctae succus tineas pellit", but Pliny's original text in fact reads "taenias" (i.e. tapeworms) and not *tineas.

Literature: ELECAMPANE (*Inula helenium* L.): → horshele [**899**].

595 þe tysain þat is þe evill of þe hede. This stands for *DVH* 1496: *radix trita fugat sciasim superaddita coxae*, which makes it evident that ‹tysain› is a *lectio facilior* (cf. La. *(p)tisana*, "barley-water") for *s c i a t i c a via the usual ML spelling *ciasim*. The mistake is repeated as ‹tysayne› in the retelling of the entry (→ **900**). We can only speculate as to why the author of *LH* decided to choose "head" instead of "hip" in his gloss both here and in the other instance of the word. Confusion with *tisik(e*, as tentatively suggested by MED: *s.v.* tisane *n.*, seems unconvincing, as phthisis was known to be a disease of the lungs (→ **937**); the sense "?headache" given there must thus be rejected. Perhaps *COXE in the Latin original was misread as *c a p *i t* e, since x—particularly when written in a cursive script—could be mistaken for **p**?

601 May buttyr. May butter was unsalted, purified butter made for medicinal use, cf. "[i]f during the month of May before you salt your butter you saue a lumpe thereof and put it into a vessell, and so set it into the sunne the space of that moneth, you shall finde it exceeding [...] medicinable for wounds" (*English Housewife* ii.iv.113 (1615); quoted from OED: *s.v.* May-butter *n.*).

606 endyue. The Latin heading and the English names indicate that the entry deals with the medical properties of the endive (*Cichorium intybus* L.), but the physical description provided in the text is against that notion. The editor of *AC* (the text that served as basis for this particular entry) suggested that the species may be some wild lettuce (*Lactuca virosa* L., *L. scariola* L.), but a plant such as the bristly ox-tongue (*Helminthotheca echioides* (L.) Holub) may make a better choice; reasons for this identification in Moreno Olalla 2015: 59–60.

Identification with some chicory is supported pharmacographically as well, as the species is deoppilant of the liver and the spleen (**611**), anticteric, antimalarial and antitumoral (**612**), and refrigerant (**614**).

Literature: *BRISTLY OX-TONGUE (*Helminthotheca echioides* (L.) Holub): *HP* vii.7.1 (κιχόρη); *MM* ii.132 (σέρις); *NH* xx.73 (*intubus*), xx.74 (*cichorium*); *SM* xii.119; *RM* 258; Grad. 353 (*endiuia*); *OEH* 31 (*herba lactuca siluatica. wudulectric*); *LS* 143 (*dundebe* [هندبا *hindibā*], *endiuia*); *EPN* vii (*hec endiva. endywe*); *Cl* E.1 (*endiuia, scariola. endiue*); *TH* 158 (*endivia, scariola*); *Pand.* 159 (LA*cicorea, sponsa solis, solisequia,* AR*hundebe,* GR*seris, intuba, gegucisi*); *Alph.* 57 (*endiuia, scariola.* GA,AN*endyue*); *Sin.Bart.* 27 (*lactuca silvestris. endivia*); *AC* 183.8 (*endiwe. endiwe, horsthystyl*) ⚜ *GH* 148 (ENDIUIA, *endyue, scoryole*); Fu 262 (ΣΕΡΙΣ, *seris, intubus, endiuia*); Tu 2.403 (CYCORIE, *endive, intubus, seris*); *DL* 404 (ENDIUE, *succory,* σέρις, πικρίς, *intuba*); Ge 219 (GARDEN SUCCORIE, σέρις, πικρίς, *hedypnois, intybum, cichorium, cicorea, endiuia, taraxacon, scariola, seriola*).

F¹H¹ (*LS*) | F¹S¹ (*SM, Grad., Cl, TH, GH*) | F²S² (Fu, DL, Ge)

612 jaundys. Jaundice, according to medieval medicine, was due to oppilations in the liver and the gallbladder. As a consequence, yellow bile was faultily digested and mixed into the blood-stream, spreading to the whole body and giving the patient a characteristically sallow skin. See *LS* iv.9 for details.

616 eufrase. The Latin heading, the English name and the physical description of the plant fit some eyebright (*Euphrasia* L. spp.). It is probably impossible to narrow down the exact species, but other than the type species (*E. officinalis* L.), likely candidates are the common eyebright (*E. nemorosa* (Pers.) Wallr.) and the English sticky eyebright (*E. anglica* Pugsley), both of which (particularly the latter) are frequently found in the SW of England where *AC*—which served as basis for the entry—was probably composed.

Identification with some type of eyebright is borne out pharmacographically, as the species is said to be an excellent ophthalmic (**620**).

> **Literature**: EYEBRIGHTS (*Euphrasia* L. spp.): *EPN* ix (*hec eufrasia. a heufrasy*); *TH* 175 (*eufragia, lummella*); *DVH(NME)* 256v.25 (*eufras*); *Alph.* 60 (*eupatorium, lilifagus, saluia agrestis, ambrosia*. $_{GA,AN}$*eufrasie*); *AC* 183.28 (*eufrax. eufrax*) ✤ *GH* 166 (EUFRAGIA, *eufrace, luminelle*); *Fu* 91 (EUPHRASIA, *ophthalmica, ocularia*); *Tu* 1.740 (EYEBRIGHTE, *eufragia, ophthalmica*); *DL* 30 (EIEBRIGHT, *euphrasia, ophthalmica, ocularis*, ὀφθαλμική, εὐφροσύνη, *euphrosyne*); *Ge* 536 (EIEBRIGHT, *euphrasia, euphrosyne, ocularis, ophthalmica*).
>
> CS (Fu, Ge) | C¹S¹ (DL)

622 erbe Christofyr male. The Latin heading can be applied to a number of separate species, very and particularly to the baneberry (*Actaea spicata* L.; this seems to be the species described in Ge). Stirling 1995–1998: *s.vv.* christophoriana, herba Christophori, herba Sancti Christophori mentions the ox-eye daisy (*Leucanthemum vulgare* (Vaill.) Lam.) as an alternative, while PNME: *s.v.* Herba Christophori further includes a couple of fleabanes (*Pulicaria dysenterica* (L.) Gaertn. and *P. vulgaris* Gaertn.), and the royal fern (*Osmunda regalis* L.) as further possibilities.

The physical description here and the fuller version provided in its source text, *AC*, where the flowers are said to be yellow (cf. also *Alph.*: "arnoglosse similis sed minora habet folia et albiora, florem habet croceum et durum"), preclude any possibility that the species is the baneberry, the daisy, or any fern. Brodin 1950: 227 prefers the yellow loosestrife (*Lysimachia vulgaris* L.) but offers no supporting evidence. Even so, comparison of the leaves of the plant with those of ‹crowesope þe lasse› (some *Saponaria* L.) or *arnoglossa* (*Plantago major* L.) seems to mean that they must be either ovate or elliptical and ribbed, rather than pinnate as those of the *Lysimachia* or the *Pulicaria*.

Fischer 1929: 261, drawing apparently from the *Gart der Gesuntheit*, mentions that the name *herba Christophori* was sometimes applied to the spiny starwort (*Pallenis spinosa* (L.) Cass. = *Asteriscus spinosus* (L.) Sch. Bip.). A Mediterranean species, the *Pallenis* fits the description as regards leaves, which are ovate, ribbed, whiter than those of a *Saponaria* as they are slightly pilose, and smaller as well. Further support for this identification may be found in the fact that another synonym for *herba St. Christophori* was *filius ante patrem* or *antipater*. This curious name, which refers to the fact that the flowers appear on the stems before the leaves, was applied to coltsfoot (*Tussilago farfara* L.), another yellow-flowered Asteraceae quite similar to the *Pallenis* but displaying cordate leaves. Burgess 1902: 71 similarly mentions that Otto Brunfels used that name to refer to a "Buphthalmum-like plant" that may well be the *Pallenis* (note that *Buphthalmum spinosus* was the Linnaean name for *Pallenis*; cf. *Pand.* "herba est faciens florem sicut butalmos"). Following Avicenna (*Pand.*: "Avicenna in secundo dicit quod [...] flos eius est similis croco hortulano"), other Renaissance herbalists (DL$_{53}$, Ge$_{131}$) applied the name *filius ante patrem* to the purple-flowered meadow saffron (*Colchicum autumnale* L.), which cannot possibly be the *Herba Christophori* in *LH*.

Pharmacographically, the plant is said to be antipestilential, antimanic (**626**) and antipleurodynic (**627**). Note that the last virtue must be an addition of *LH* as it is not recorded in the source text.

> **Literature**: *SPINY STARWORT (*Pallenis spinosa* (L.) Cass.): *OEH* 8 (*pes leonis, leonfot*); *TH* 275 (*leontopodion, oculus consulis*); *Pand.* 265 ($_{LA}$*filius ante patrem,* $_{AR}$*tarif,* $_{GR}$*gariofilon*); *Alph.* 78 (*herba Cristofori*); *Sin.Bart.* 44 (*Christoforia sive herba Christofori*); *AC* 190,28 (*herba Christofori masculus. Christofere þe male*) ⚕ Ge 829 (HERBE CHRISTOPHER, *christophoriana, S. Christophori herba, costus niger, aconitum bacciferum*).

630 erbe Waltir. The Latin heading and the ME name are generally taken to refer to sweet woodruff (*Galium odoratum* (L.) Scop.), but the physical description makes such identification unlikely (see Brodin 1950: 227–228 for a fuller discussion; the description of the plant in *Alph.* may on the other hand correspond to a *Galium*: "habet stipitem rectum aliquantulum et diuisionem foliorum per gradus diuisam, redolet ut muscum"). Based on the colour of the leaves, *WG* suggested that the species may be silverweed (*Potentilla anserina* L., hence its inclusion as a dubious possibility in MED: *s.v.* hĕrbe-wauter *n.* and PNME: *s.v.* Herba (Sancti) Walteri; → **2501**), but comparison of shape of their leaves with those of parsley is against that notion. Silverweed is moreover a perennial, not an annual species as suggested in the text—unless the passage refers to bloom times. The musky odour of the species according to *Alph.* and the shape of the leaf lead Whytlaw-Gray to suggest an alternative identification with moschatel (*Adoxa moschatellina* L.), but the rest of the description does not fit. It should be well noted that the entry expands on its source, *AC*, by adding information about the colour of the leaves and the lifespan of the plant: the original text only mentions the similarity of its leaves to those of parsley and the fact (missing in *LH*) that they are thick and tender. All things considered, it is therefore quite possible that the description here is a combination of two separate plants (one of them being *Gallium odoratum*), which turns identification of the exact species into a very thorny matter.

The species is antiseptic and vulnerary (**634**).

> **Literature**: *Sweet woodruff (*Galium odoratum* (L.) Scop.): *Alph.* 81 (*herba Walteri.* $_{GA}$*muge de bois*); *AC* 191.9 (*herbe Walterus. herbe water*); Tu 2.738 (wood rose, *wood rowell, cordialis, asperula, spergula odorata*).

636 erbe Robert. The Latin heading, the ME name and the physical description indicate that the species here must be herb Robert (*Geranium robertianum* L.). The description given here is, unusually for *LH*, more detailed than the one in the source text, *AC*. The same plant may have been repeated later in the treatise under a different name (→ **1286**).

Pharmacographically, the species is vulnerary (**638**) and anticancerous (**639**). Both virtues, the first one in particular (after all, the plant was taken to be the third type of Dioscorides's σιδηρῖτις—which in fact is generally identified as *Scrophularia lucida* L.), are abundantly mentioned in the Renaissance medical literature.

> **Literature**: Herb Robert (*Geranium robertianum* L.): *MM* iv.35 (σιδηρῖτις ἑτέρα, Ἡρακλεία); *NH* xxv.44 (*sideritis...cum teratur foedi odoris*); *EPN* vi (*herba Roberti. herbe Robert, chareville*); *Alph.* 81 (*herba Roberti*); *AC* 191.13 (*herba Robertus. herbe Robert*) ⚘ Fu 76 (ΓΕΡΑΝΙΟΝ, *rostrum ciconiæ...geranium tertii generis, herba Roberti, Robertiana*); Tu 2.388 (pink nedle, *cranes bill, geranium, starkis bill*); DL 34 (herbe Robert, *pinke-needle, storkes-bill*, γεράνιον, *geranium, gruina, gruinalis... the fourth kind of geranion, sideritis tertia, sideritis heraclea, Ruberta, herba Roberti*); Ge 794 (herbe Robert, *Ruberta, Roberti herba, Robertiana, Robertianum, sideritis 3. Dioscoridis*).
>
> S (Fu, DL) | F (Ge)

638 þe chafynge of a fox. Fu quaintly says that the taste and smell of herb Robert are unpleasant (*saporis & odoris iniucundi*), while Ge states rather more bluntly that its leaves are "of a most lothsome stinking smell". The odour of *Geranium robertianum* has been compared in fact to those of rams, bedbugs, and the urine of people who had eaten asparagus (Font Quer 2014: 434). Likening it to the strong scent of foxes is then quite apposite, but the problem remains of explaining the precise meaning of ‹chafynge›, for none of the senses provided in MED: *s.v.* chaufinge *ng.* is satisfactory. Since the word was created after the verb *chāfen* (OF *chaufer*) and hence derives ultimately from Latin **cal(e)fare, calefacere* "to make warm", the sense conveyed may have to do with the body temperature of the animal, which is synaesthetically connected to its natural musky scent. Alternatively, and probably even likelier, ‹chafynge› may refer to the fouler smell secreted by a fox when the animal is angry or feels threatened (Hepper and Wells 2015: 594; cf. the sense "to grow excited, become irritated" of the verb *to chafe*, which was already present in ME).

641 erbe benet. The Latin heading and the ME name indicate that the plant must be hemlock (*Conium maculatum* L.), but it is curious that the author compared the plant with itself, which apparently indicates that he took each plant name to be two sundry species. Perhaps this is due to the fact that the Latin designation was sometimes applied to other species, including valerian (*Valeriana officinalis* L.) and wood avens (*Geum urbanum* L.). Although the entry provides no physical description, identification with *Conium* is also positive on pharmacographic grounds: antimastitic **(642)**, antipodagric **(643)** and refrigerant **(644)**. The anaphrodisiac qualities of hemlock are missing here but do appear in the source text (*AC*). The virtues of hemlock according to *DVH* will be found later in the herbal (→ **872**, with discussion).

Literature: HEMLOCK (*Conium maculatum* L.): → hemloke **[872]**.

646 erbe Johann. The Latin heading, the ME name, and the physical description indicate that the species here must be St. John's wort (*Hypericum perforatum* L.). Although the plant was employed at least since *MM* for its medical virtues (diuretic, lithontriptic, vulnerary, febrifuge…), the entry offers none of these but attends to its powers as an exorcist only—as underlined by the Latin name as well. The entry follows *AC*, but is much more precise that its source text as regards when, where and how to carry out the exorcism **(650–654)**.

Literature: ST. JOHN'S WORT (*Hypericum perforatum* L.): *MM* iii.154 (ὑπερικόν); *NH* xxvi.85 (*hypericon*); *SM* xii.148; *RM* ii.269; *Grad.* 378; *OEH* 152 (*hypericon, corion*); *Dur. Glos.* 303 (*hypericon, corion*); *LS* 257 (*reiofricon* [هيوفاريقون *hyūfārīqūn*], *hypericon*); *EPN* vi (*ypis. herbe johan, velde-rude*); *TH* 237 (*ipericon, perforata, herba sancti Johannis, scopa regia*); *Pand.* 372 ($_{AR}$*infarion*, $_{GR}$*hypericon, biumi, atricum*, $_{LA}$*hypericon, scopa regia*); *Alph.* 78 (*herba sancti johannis, ypericon, scopa regea, triscalamus, herba perforata, fuga demonum.* $_{GA}$*herbe johan*; $_{AN}$*seynt jones uurt*); *Sin.Bart.* 23 (*herba sancti johannis, herba perforata. ypericon*); *AC* 192.4 (*herba Iohannis. herbe Jon*) ❦ Fu 321 ('ΥΠΕΡΙΚΟΝ, ἀνδρόσαιμον, χαμαιπίτυς, *hypericum, perforata, herba divi*

Ioannis, androsæmon, chamæpytis, fuga dæmonum); Tu 1.245 (GREAT SAINT JOHNES WURTE, *ascyron, ascaroides, hyperici*); DL 45 (S. IOHNS WURT, ὑπερικόν, *hypericum, perforata, fuga dæmonum*); Ge 432 (SAINT IOHNS WOORT, *S. Iohns grasse*, ὑπερικόν, *hypericum, perforata, fuga dæmonum*).

CS (*SM, RM,* Fu, Ge) | C³S³ (*Grad., LS,* DL)

647 more centaury. A probable copy mistake, cf. *AC* 192.5–6 "þis herbe haȝt lewys lyk to the lesse centorye". Brodin mentions no variant "more" in his apparatus (→ **335** on the identification for these species).

656 erbe moyntayne. An unknown plant taken from an unidentified source. The Latin heading ⟨herba Plenius⟩ reappears in the interpolation after the entry *Barba Jouis* (→ **1045**, where a physical description is provided that does not seem to tally with the one found here—unless some scribe mistake is assumed) but otherwise seems privative to this text. According to the description, which is unusually detailed, the plant in question is not a perennial species, and displays leaves that are thick, broad, large and palmate. Pharmacographically, the species is used in veterinary medicine to cure a ⟨montayne euyll⟩ that is equally unidentified and a hapax, according to MED: *s.v.*

The species described here might be the garden angelica (*Angelica archangelica* L.). This plant rises on a single stalk, and displays flowers in big umbels, which would explain the fragment ⟨þe levis loddeþ to-geder⟩ (but note that *lodden* is a hapax in MED, and hence the meaning "[t]o stick (together), cleave" is not necessarily obvious). The word ⟨flower⟩ was probably not used because the inflorescences of *Angelica* are frequently the same green colour as the real leaves and hence difficult to distinguish from one another to a rudimentary botanist. The leaves are divided into leaflets, usually five in number (see for example the plates of the plant in Fu and Ge). These are large and serrated, which may have triggered the comparison with those of ⟨kayre⟩, i.e. the rowan (*Sorbus aucuparia* L.), in **1046**, although this may refer to the inflorescences of both plants as well. As for the idea that the species is gone by July, this plant is known to die off about that time, after seeding just once (in fact it blooms early in May, but Renaissance authors placed its blooming in July and August). As further support of this identification, *Angelica* was popularly reputed as preservative against an ailment of cattle called "elf-shot", which produced skin-ulcers in cattle, as if arrowed by elves or goblins (Prior 1863: *s.v.* archangel). This could perhaps be the same disease called ⟨montayne euyll⟩ here.

Pharmacographically, some support for this identification can be put forth in case the powers of *Angelica* against "elf-shot" are connected with the value

Lelamour Herbal   295

of the species against "witchcraft and inchantments" that is mentioned in Fu and Ge.

Literature: *GARDEN ANGELICA (*Angelica archangelica* L.): Fu 43 (ANGELICA, *Sancti Spiritus radix*); Tu 2.728 (ANGELICA); DL 211 (ANGELICA); Ge 846 (ANGELICA).

C³S³ (Fu, Tu, DL, Ge)

663 ferne. As seen from the Latin heading and the ME name, the entry describes several ferns (phylum Pteridophytae): ⟨polypody⟩ and ⟨osmounde⟩ will be treated separately later in the treatise (→ **1899, 1613**), offering roughly the same medical virtues in both instances. The third species, ⟨euere-verrene⟩ (MS ⟨euere-verrewe⟩ < OE *eofor-fearn*), is traditionally taken to be the common polypody (*Polypodium vulgare* L.) on account of its growing near walls. Many medieval treatises describe its virtues together with another polypody growing on oaks (*Gymnocarpium dryopteris* (L.) Newman), and frequently employ the same name for both species. (To avoid duplication, in the Literature section I include those sources that mention walls as the natural habitat of the species or use "everfern" as ME synonym; the rest, some of which may apply here (the case of DL and Ge, probably also *LS*), will be found under ⟨polipody⟩ → **1899**.) The entry follows *AC*.

The species is said to be antipodagric and indurant of sinews (**671**), but *Polypodium*, just like the *Gymnocarpium*, is almost universally taken to be a laxative in the medical literature. Only Ge, quoting Mesue as source, mentions the value of the plant against "certaine kinde of *Arthritis*, or ache in the ioints" that causes that "the hands, the feete, and the ioints of the knees and elbowes do swell". I cannot find such virtue in *LS* where, on the other hand, the power to *strengthen* sinews is indeed included ("confert attritionibus neruorum", apparently a mistranslation of στρέμματα "sprains" in *MM* iv.186).

Literature: FERNS (Pteridophytae): *HP* i.10.5 (πτερίς); *MM* iv 184; *NH* xxvii.78 (*felix*); *SM* xii.109 (πτερίς, θηλύπτερις); *RM* ii.216 (θηλύπτερον), 255 (πτερίς); *OEH* 78 (*filix. fearn*); *Dur.Glos*. 302 (*filex. fearn*); *LS* 56 (*sarax* [سرخس *sarḫas*], *filix nigra*); *EPN* ii, iv, v (*filix. fearn*), vii (*hic felix, -cis. brakyn*), viii (*hec felix, -cis, media correpta. brakyne*); *TH* 184 (*filix, piterrigum*); *Pand*. 609 (ₐᵣ*saraex, saras*, ₉ᵣ*driopistri, pteris*, ₗₐ*filex, filix, kildaru, sarcos, siraes*); *Alph*. 64 (*felix, fillis, pateos*); *Sin.Bart*. 21 (*filix. ferne*); *AC* 187.2 (*filix. fern, brake*) ❀ *GH* 174 (FILEX, *ferne, pyterrigum*); Fu 226 (ΠΤΕΡΙΣ, πτέριον, *filix*); Tu 2.380 (BRAKE, *ferne, pteris, filix mascula | filix femina, thelipteris*); DL 290 (FERNE, *brake*, πτερίς, πτέριον, *filix mas* | θηλύπτερις, νυμφαία πτερίς, *filix fœmina, brake, common fern, female ferne*); Ge 968 (FERNE, πτέρις, βλῆτρον, *filix mas* | θηλυπτέρις, *filix fœmina, brake, female ferne, brake, lingua cervina*). ¶ COMMON POLYPODY (*Polypodium vulgare* L.): *HP* ix.13.6 (πολυπόδιον); *MM* iv.186; *NH* xxvi.58 (*polypodium, filicula*); *SM* xii.107; *RM* ii.253; *OEH* 85 (*herba radiola. eforfearn*); *Dur*.

Glos. 304 (*radiolum. eofer fearn, brun vyrt*); *EPN* iv (*felix minuta. eofor-fearn | felicina. eofor-fearn | radiolum. eofor-fearn*); *CI* P.12 (*polipodium*); *TH* 365 (*polipodium*); *Pand.* 216 (GR*dipteris, filicteron, saraxpteris,* AR*bisbeig, bisce,* LA*polipodium, filicica, filix arbor, pliricon*); *Alph.* 132 (*osmunda, filex siluestris. euerfarn, moreclam*); *Sin. Bart.* 32 (*osmunda. everferne*); ✿ *GH* 182 (FILEX MASCULUS, *osmunda, heferue*); Fu 223 (ΠΟΛΥΠΟΔΙΟΝ, *polypodium, filicula*); Tu 2.382 (POLYPODY, *vuallferne, okeferne, filicula, polipodium*); DL 292 (POLYPODIE, *wall ferne, oke ferne,* πολυπόδιον, *filicula, polypodium*); Ge 972 (POLYPODIE, *wall ferne, polypodie of the oke,* πολυπόδιον, *polypodium, filicula, parua filix*); → polypody [**1899**].

S (*SM, RM,* Fu, Ge) | S² (DL) | C³S² (*Grad., CI, TH*) | C³S³ (*LS, GH*)

673 filipendula. The Latin heading, the ME name and the physical description of the plant suggest that the entry deals with dropwort (*Filipendula vulgaris* Moench). It derives from *AC* but provides a poorer description of the species than its source text.

The species is praised as hepatic and splenetic (**678**), and lithontriptic (**678**). All of these virtues can be found in the medical literature, although the powers of the plant against ‹wekid wyndis› is directed to the stomach (i.e. as a carminative), rather than the to liver or spleen, as in Fu and DL.

Literature: DROPWORT (*Filipendula vulgaris* Moench): *HP* vi.8.1 (οἰνάνθη); *MM* iii.120; *NH* xxi.65 (*oenanthe*); *RM* ii.246; *CI* F.5 (*filipendula. fisalidos*); *TH* 180 (*fillipendula, fissalidos*); *Pand.* 264 (*filipendula, fisalidos, patrisciria, viscago, philantropos*); *Alph.* 66 (*filipendula, phisalidos, patrision, uiscago*); *Sin.Bart.* 21 (*filipendula, fisalidos*); *AC* 187.12 (*filipendula. filipendula, dropwortis, walwourt*) ✿ *GH* 170 (FILIPENDULA, *dropwort, fisalidos*); Fu 211 (ΟΙΝΑΝΘΗ, λεύκανθον, *oenanthe, filipendula, saxifraga rubea*); Tu 2.741 (FILIPENDULA); DL 31 (FILIPENDULA, *dropwort, red saxifrage, saxifraga rubea*); Ge 900 (DROPWOORT, *filipendula, saxifraga rubea, millefolium syluestre, molon*).

C³S³ (*CI, TH,* Fu, DL, Ge)

681 fvmyter. Although the Latin heading and the ME name point to fumary (*Fumaria officinalis* L.), the comparison made in the text with rue leaves suggests that the species that the author had in mind must have been a species akin species to a *Fumaria*, fumewort (*Corydalis solida* (L.) Clairv.). Some Renaissance herbalists (Ge for one) described the latter in the same chapter as fumary. The entry derives from *AC*, but the reference to the Thursdays in May is missing there.

Identification is also borne out pharmacographically, as the species is a stomachal and cardiac (**686**), deoppilant (**686**), anti-inflammatory (**688**), leprostatic (**689**), detergent and antiherpetic (**690**), diuretic and lithontriptic (**691**). The plant is also described as encephalic (**688**) and orectic (**692**), but these seems additions that are neither in the source text nor the usual medical literature.

> **Literature**: FUMEWORT (*Corydalis solida* (L.) Clairv.): *MM* iv.109 (καπνός); *NH* xxv.156 (*capnos*); *SM* xii.8 (κάπνιος); *RM* ii.220; *Grad.* 351 (*fumus terrę*); *LS* 71 (*scehiterig* [شهترج *šahtariǧ*], *fumus terræ*); *EPN* vi (*fumus terre. fumetere. cuntehoare*); *Cl* F.3 (*fumus terre*); *TH* 178 (*fumus terre*); *Pand.* 640 (_{AR}*steng, seterig*, _{GR}*capnos*, _{LA}*fumus terre*); *Alph.* 69 (*fumus terre, fumulus. fumetere*); *Sin.Bart.* 21 (*fistula bufonis, fumus terrae*), 22 (*fumus terrae. fumeter*); *AC* 186.5 (*fumus terre. fymter*) ✿ *GH* 169 (FUMUS TERRE, *fumyterre, fume, smoke of the earthe*); Fu 126 (ΚΑΠΝΟΣ, *fumaria, fumus terrę*); Tu 1.262 (FUMITORY, *capnos, fumaria, fumus terre*); *DL* 18 (FUMETERRE, καπνός, κάπνιον, καπνίτης, *fumaria, capnium, fumus terræ*); Ge 927 (FUMITORIE, καπνός, κάπνιον, καπνίτης, *fumaria, fumus terræ*).
>
> C¹S¹ (*LS*) | C¹S² (*Grad., Cl, TH, GH*) | C²S² (Fu, Tu, DL) | FS (Ge)

694 finell. The entry derives from the entry *Feniculum* in *DVH* (678–710), as translated in the *DVH(NME)* tradition. Identification with *Foeniculum vulgare* Mill. is traditional, and reassured by the common mention of the species as an alexipharmic and ophthalmic (**695** = *DVH* 680–685), galactogenous (**700** = *DVH* 694), antinephritic and diuretic (**701** = *DVH* 695–697), emmenagogue (**702** = *DVH* 697) and antacid (**704** = *DVH* 700). A few virtues, particularly those at the end of the entry (antiemetic **703** and rejuvenatory **707**, a well as remedy to phallalgia **705**) are included in *DVH* but not in Dioscorides.

> **Literature**: FENNEL (*Foeniculum vulgare* Mill.): *HP* i.11.2 (μάραθον); *MM* iii.70; *NH* viii.99 (*marathon*), xx.254 (*feniculum*); *SM* xii.67 (μάραθρον); *RM* ii.240; *Grad.* 364 (*marathri semen*); *DVH* 678–710 (*feniculum*); *OEH* 127 (*herba feniculus. finul*); *Dur.Glos.* 302 (*fumiclum. finul*); *LS* 314 (*raienigi* [رازيانج *rāzyāniǧ*], *fœniculus*); *EPN* ii (*feniculum. fynel*), iv (*fynuclum. finol*), v (*feniculum. fenol*), vi (*feniculum. fanuil. fenecel*), vii, viii (*hoc feniculum. fynkylle*), ix (*hoc feneculum. a ffenelle*); *Cl* F.7 (*feniculus. fenel*); *TH* 182 (*feniculus*); *Pand.* (_{LA}*feniculus*, _{GR}*maratron*, _{AR}*hazienis, haienegi, hakasinech*); *DVH(NME)* 247r.3 (*fynkell*); *DVH(SME)* 9b.4 (*fenell. maratrum*); *Alph.* 83 (*hues maratrum, feniculus idem. fenkele*), 106 (*maratrum, feniculum. fenicle*); *AC* 187.20 (*feniculus. fenkele*) ✿ *GH* 172 (FENICULUS, *hasiensis, hacasniech, fenell*); Fu 190 (ΜΑΡΑΘΡΟΝ, *fœniculum*); Tu 2.383 (FENEL, *feniculus, marathrom, fenkel*); *DL* 192 (FENELL, μάραθρον, μάλαθρον, *fœniculum*); Ge 877 (FENNELL, μάραθρον, *fœniculum*).
>
> C²S² (*Grad., DVH, Cl, TH, GH*) | C³S¹ (*SM, RM*, Fu, Tu, DL) | C³S³ (*LS*, Ge)

695 and inhansith lechery. The aphrodisiac property of fennel is missing from the canonical edition of the Latin poem, but several textual traditions (β, γ, η, λ and ζζ) do record it as *Et sic assumptum venerem stimulare videtur* [*fatetur* η]. The line seems to be due to an interpolation, as is the same as *DVH* 673 from the entry *Pulegium* that precedes *Feniculum*.

696 do on the ere or in the ere. The scribe must have realized that doing fennel *on* the ear would be less beneficial that putting it inside, hence the addition, which is missing in the other MSS. Perhaps the exemplar read *DOON, which was mistakenly split by the copyist?

697 in tysain laid to þe eryn. *DVH* 690 *renibus in ptisana*. Just like S_1, all MSS mention the ear, rather than the kidneys. Ears had been mentioned in the previous line of the poem (see previous note), so a misreading by the scribe of either Q or Ω is a likely explanation.

697 in tysain laid to þe eryn. *DVH* 691 *cum vino*. Either a reading *CUM MELLE in *Q* (not recorded in Choulant's apparatus) or else a mistranslation in Ω, for all MSS read alike here.

698 the attributis. *DVH* 692 *venenatis* [...] *morsibus*. S_1 reads together with *W* here, indicating that the *lectio facilior* stems from γ. *B* and *P* read correctly (*B*.247r/8 ‹att*er* bytte›, *P*.267/22 ‹adders bytyng›), suggesting that the reading in Ω must have been *ATT*I*R* BIT*I*S.

701 and lowsithe flouris in a woman. *DVH* 696 *menstrua sumpta resolvit*. The whole fragment is omitted in *B*, while the last three words are missing in *WP*, which is a probable indication of an addition in ΛS_1. The verb is different in each MS, cf. *W*.29v/16 ‹layses›, *P*.267/25 ‹slakeþ›. The reading in S_1, while a bit unexpected (*l ō s i t h seems more in keeping in a non-Northern text, see *OED*: *s.v.* loose *a.*), is etymologically defendable (< ON *lauss* "loose, free"; see Björkman 1900: 71).

706 swellinge for drinke. The Latin text does not state that fennel should be drunk, but rather laid on the swelling (*DVH* 704–705 *Ictu vel factos subito quoscunque tumores / appositum tantum iuncto sedabit aceto*), and hence the reference to drink is altogether missing in Bodley. All MSS in *RH* on the other hand record such idea: Pepys conjectures and reads *P*.268/3 ‹swellyng and drynk it› while, as usual, Wellcome is textually closest to S_1, cf. *W*.29v/20–21 ‹bolny*n*g of drynk*is*›. This may have been taken as a scribal addition in that branch, but the aphrodisiac virtue contained in the following line of the Latin version, where fennel must be drunk (*DVH* 706 *Semen cum vino bibitum veneris movet actus*), suggest that Ω probably offered a clipped or otherwise blotched version of the whole Latin passage that the scribes of each branch interpreted as best they could.

708 sacrefolium. A hapax, which could answer to an exemplary *S̃(R)FOLIUM in Λ that should in fact have been read *s *e m p e* r (Martin 1892: 134, André 1985: 234) but got wrongly expanded. Should this prove correct, it would add to the idea that the scribe of S_1 was more comfortable copying religious than with scientific texts (→ **149, 188, 282, 784, 1953**, for other possible instances of such trend).

709 full. According to the synonym that the scribe provided (actually not Latin, as stated in the text, but Old French: *j(o)ubarbe* < La. *Jouis barba*) this entry deals with the medical virtues of the houseleek, *Sempervivum tectorum* L. The same species will be treated again in the text following the *AC* textual tradition (→ **1031**, with discussion), but the Latin heading and the properties attached to the plant in either entry are completely different.

Identification with the houseleek, on the other hand, seems sure at least from a lexical basis. *Full* is given as a *hapax* in MED: *s.v.* ful *n.*2, and tentatively put in etymological connection with OF *fueil* < La. *folium* "leaf", but this is dubious since *folium* does not refer to any *Sempervivum* species in either Classical or medieval Latin. The name is perhaps just an aphaeretic form from OE *sinfulle* (wk. f.) that appears in several OE and eME works to translate La. *sempervivum* (see Literature). Dialectally, *full(en)* is markedly Northern, having been recorded in late 19th-century Northumberland (see EDD: *s.v.* fullen *n.*). Akin forms such as *f(o)uet* and *foose, fooze*, used in areas of the Scottish Lowlands (Galloway, Lanarkshire, Roxburgh; see EDD: *s.vv.*), confirm that this word was used in both sides of the Borders.

This entry reads together with *W* but is missing from the other members of *DVH(NME)*, which is extraordinary yet not a unique case (→ **1162** for another example). The entry seems to stem from the section *Acidula* in the Latin poem (apparently, *Rumex acetosa* L.; → **2262**).

    Literature: HOUSELEEK (*Sempervivum tectorum* L.): → jubarbe [**1031**].

713 fethirfoy. The Latin heading indicates that this must be one of the several plants praised as a febrifuge, but each ME synonym points to a different species: ⟨fethirfoy⟩ as a rule stands for feverfew (*Tanacetum parthenium* (L.) Sch.Bip.), while the hapax ⟨hersgall⟩ has been identified, probably correctly, as a by-form of *earthgall*, i.e. common centaury (*Centaurium erythraea* Rafn; Cockayne 1864–1866: iii.333). The white colour of the petals suggests that the species must be the former, since *Centaurium* displays pink flowers. The entry belongs to the *AC* textual tradition.

Identification with *Tanacetum* is on the other hand not well supported pharmacographically, since only the febrifuge powers of the species (**716**) are recorded in the literature. The antiherpetic qualities of the plant (**719**) are mentioned in some Renaissance herbals, but in connection with erysipelas (→ **877**), rather than impetigo (→ **319**). The other virtues are missing from the usual medical accounts: stomachal (**715**, mostly as antispasmodic (**717**) and calefacient (**717**)), alexipharmic (**718**), and vulnerary and consolidative (**719–722**). The antispasmodic and vulnerary qualities do appear in the lists of virtues of the chapters devoted to *Centaurium*, hence it is possible that the ME entry is a conflation.

    Literature: FEVERFEW (*Tanacetum parthenium* (L.) Sch.Bip.): *MM* iii.138 (παρθένιον); *NH* xxi.176 (*parthenium, leucanthes, amaracum, perdicium, muralis*); *SM* xi.823 (ἀμάρακον); *RM* ii.192; *Dur.Glos.* 302 (*febrefugia. smero vyrt*); *LS* 243 (*achuen* [أقوان *uqhwān*], *matricaria*); *EPN* ii (*febrefugia, vel febrifuga. fefer-fuge*), v (*febrefugia. feferfugia*), vi (*febrefugia. fewerfue. adrel-wurt*), vii (*hec febrifuga. fevyrfew*); *DVH(SME)* 42b.3 (*fetherfoy. febri-fuga*); *Alph.* 63 (*febrifuga. fetherfoye*); *Sin.Bart.* 20 (*febrifuga, centaurea minor*), 21 (*febrifuga, arbor sanctæ mariæ, matricaria*); *AC* 188.20 (*febrefuga. feuerfew*) ❡ *Fu* 221 (ΠΑΡΘΕΝΙΟΝ, ἀμάρακον, χαμαίμηλον, *parthenium, amaracum, solis oculus, millefolium, cotula fœtida*); *Tu* 2.489 (FEVERFEW, *parthenium, amaracus*); *DL* 15 (FEVERFEW, *whitewurt, S. Peters wurt*, παρθένιον, ἀμάρακον, *parthenium, amaracus, matricaria, amarella, marella*); *Ge* 526 (FEUERFEW, *fedderfewe*, παρθένιον, ἀμάρακον, *parthenium, matricaria, febrifuga*). ❡ COMMON CENTAURY (*Centaurium erythraea* Rafn): → centory [**335**].

C^3S^2 (*SM, RM, LS, Fu, DL, Ge*)

724 flour delice. The Latin heading refers to a number of *Iris* L. spp., a flowering genus much hybridized. Since the flowers of the species in the entry are blue, this must be the German flag (*I.* × *germanica* L.), by opposition to the yellow flag (*I. pseudacorus* L.), which has yellow flowers (the ⟨leuyr⟩ < OE *læfer* that is mentioned in the opening lines and is probably the same species called ⟨gladoyne⟩ later in the herbal, → **835**), and the Florentine iris (*I.* × *germanica* L. var. *florentina* (L.) Dykes), which displays white ones and will appear later in the herbal (→ **2097**, where it is spelt ⟨Safe⟩; cf. ⟨saue⟩ in **733**). The Latin names were loosely applied so the distinction between the species is sometimes blurry and as a consequence part of the Literature section applies to the other variants as well—and viceversa. The entry follows *AC*.

    The species is analgesic (**726**), antitussive (**727**), expectorant (**729**), alexipharmic and antispasmodic (**729**), oxytocic (**732**), and antihydropic (**734–739**) thanks to its laxative and emetic powers. References to dropsy are missing in the usual medical literature of the period, but several sources do mention the value of the species as a laxative, while some 19th-century pharmacopoeias indicate that the species, just like other *Iris* L. spp. is a good hydragogue (Redwood 1848: 495).

    Literature: GERMAN FLAG (*Iris* × *germanica* L.): *HP* iv.5.2 (ἶρις); *MM* i.1 (ἶρις Ἰλλυρική); *NH* xxi.140 (*iris rufa/candida*); *RM* ii.218; *Grad.* 358 (*iris*); *OEH* 158 (*iris*

Yllyrica); *DVH* 1456–1488 (*iris*); *EPN* ii (*pirus, gladiolus. læfer*), iii (*iris illyrica. hwatend*), iv (*scirpio. læfer*), v (*citsána. fana*), viii (*hec carex, -icis. a flege*), ix (*hic cucumer. a flage*); *CI* 1.4 (*iris*); *TH* 234 (*iris*); *DVH(SME)* 13a.13 (*gladene. iris*); *Alph*. 196 (*yris purpureum florem gerit, yreos album*); *Sin.Bart.* 25 (*yris purpureum florem in modum azuri gerit, yreos album* | *yris illirica, gladiolus hortensis*); *AC* 193.17 (*irus. flourdelys*) ✤ *GH* 215 (IRIS, *blewe flour delyce*); Fu 118 (*ΊΡΙΣ, iris, ireos*); Tu 2.404 (FLOUR DELYCE, *iris, irios*); DL 138 (FLOURE DE LUCE, *garden flags, iris germanica,* ἴρις, ἵερις, *consecratrix, radix naronica, lilialis, spatula*); Ge 45 (FLOWER DE-LUCE, ἴρις, ἵερις, *consecratrix, radix marica, radix naronica*).

C²S² (*DVH, CI, TH, GH*) | C²S³ (*Grad.,* Fu) | C³S³ (DL, Ge)

741 flax. The Latin heading and the ME names make it clear that the entry deals with flax (*Linum usitatissimum* L.), but from line → **745** onwards the text describes the properties of that species of dodder that parasites flax. The entry follows *AC*.

The species is medically described as laxative (**743**), a deoppilative power well recorded in the medical literature since *MM*. Its antipyrotic qualities (→ **743**), on the other hand, are unrecorded.

Literature: FLAX (*Linum usitatissimum* L.): *MM* ii.103 (λινόσπερμον); *NH* xix.7 ff. (*linum*); *SM* xii.62; *RM* ii.238; *LS* 21 (*bazarichichen* [بزر الكتان *bizr al-kittān*], *semen lini*); *EPN* iv (*elimos, lini semen. lin-sæd*); *TH* 277 (*linosa, semen lini*); *Pand*. 77 (ₐᵣ*bararichichene, bazarichichen,* ɢʀ,ʟₐ*semen lini*); *Alph*. 99 (*linelion, oleum quod fit de semine lini*); *Sin.Bart.* 28 (*linaria. wilde flax*); *AC* 201.3 (*linum. flax, lyne*) ✤ *GH* 256 (LINOSA, *lynesede*); Fu 177 (*ΛΙΝΟΝ, linum*); Tu 2.428 (FLAX, *line, lint, linon, linum*); DL 50 (FLAXE, *lyn,* λίνον, *linum*); Ge 444 (GARDEN FLAXE, *lyne,* λίνον, *linum*).

C¹ (*SM, RM, LS,* Fu, DL, Ge) | CH (*TH, GH*)

743 also… 745 brenynge. The antipyrotic powers of linseed are recorded in none of the MSS of *AC* compiled by its editor, hence the sentence is probably an addition due to some of the scribes of the $ΛS_1$ branch. This may be textually relevant. ⟨Paynter oyll⟩ is a synonym for linseed oil, used as a pigment binder in painting. This reference predates the earliest quotation in OED: *s.v.* painter *n.*¹ by almost ninety years (1545). The reference might arguably be used as evidence for the dating on the final formation the text, as oil painting was generally unknown in Western Europe until well into the 15th century. It would then impossible to believe that *LH* was composed in 1373, as stated in the *explicit*: the mention of linseed oil as a painting product would set the *terminus post quem* not earlier than the 1420s, when, according to Vasari's *Lives of the Artists*, Jan van Eyck (re)discovered the technique (de Vere 1912–1915: xi.265; Vasari mentions the year 1510, but naturally this cannot be correct as van Eyck died in 1441). Alternatively, this argument could be read so as to indicate the presence of at least two layers in the composition of the herbal: a first version, composed by John Lelamour in 1373, which in the 1460s was then supplemented with new entries, the one devoted to flax being one of them.

745 dodyr. Dodder, some of the several parasitic convolvulaceous *Cuscuta* L. spp., traditionally identified with *C. epilinum* Weihe.

The species is cholagogue (**746**), nephretic and thoracic (**747**), and analgesic (**748**). Other than its powers against yellow bile, the rest of the list is pharmacographically unknown: the species was commended as a rule as a deoppilant. According to the usual medical literature of the period, on the other hand, linseed was thought to be beneficial to the chest and the intestines, so perhaps this virtue belong to that species and should precede the treatment of dodder.

Literature: DODDER (*Cuscuta epilinum* Weihe): MM iv.177 (ἐπίθυμον); NH xxii.162 (orobanche. cynomorion), xxvi.55 (epithymum); SM xi.875; RM ii.210; Grad. 346 (cuscute); LS 39 (chasuhth [كَشُوثْ kašūṯ], cuscute, tima); EPN vi (cuscute. doder); Cl c.5 (cuscute); TH 91 (cuscute); Pand. 226 (AReasuch, GRhaborafa, LAcuscuta); Alph. 27, 146 (bruncus, cuscute, rasta lini, podagra lini. ANdoder), 46, 77 (podagra lini, rasta lini, grinicus, bruncus. ANdoder), 154 (rasta lini. ANdoder, haynde); Sin.Bart. 15, 17, 34 (cuscute, podagra lini. doder), 23 (grinicus, cuscute) ⚘ GH 85 (CUSCUTA, doder); Fu 130 (ΚΑΣΣΥΘΑ, cassutha, cuscuta, podagra lini); Tu 1.265 (DODER, casitas, cassutha, cuscuta, podagra lini); DL 288 (DODER, cuscuta, κασσύθα, podagra lini); Ge 462 (DODDER, cuscuta, podagra lini, cassutha, λινοδεσμόν).

CS (DL) | C¹S² (Grad., LS, Cl, TH, GH, Fu) | C²S² (Ge) | C³S³ (SM, RM)

750 fenygreke. The entry describes the medical properties of fenugreek (*Trigonella foenum-graecum* L.), as seen from the Latin heading, the ME name and the temperament.

The species is taken to be resolvent and antipodagric (**753**), ophthalmic (**756**), and hysteric (→ **756**–**757**), All of them, save its value as a collyrium, are to be found in the appropriate section in *NH*, from which the medical virtues of the entry were drawn. The direct source of the text, on the other hand, remains untraced.

Literature: FENUGREEK (*Trigonella foenum-graecum* L.): HP iv.4.10 (βούκερας); MM ii.102 (τῆλις); NH xxiv.184 (foenum graecum); SM xii.141; RM ii.266; Dur.Glos. 302 (fene grecio. vyle cerse); LS 174 (olba [حلبة ḥalba], fœnugræcum); EPN iii (seu britia. wille-cœrse), iv (fœnum græcum. wylle-cyrse); Cl F.8 (fenugrecum. femigreke); TH 183 (fenugrecum); Pand. 261 (LAfenugrecum, ARhalba, hulbe, alcula, GRbuceron, buthon, tilis); DVH(SME) 43a.8 (femygrek); Alph. 63 (fenugrecum); AC p. 156.1 (fenugrecum. fenucreke) ⚘ GH 173 (FENUGRECUM, fenigreke, setwall); Fu 307 (ΤΗΛΙΣ, κεραΐτις, αἰγόκερος, βούκερος, fœnumgræcum, siliqua, silicia, silicula); Tu 2.384 (FENEGREKE, fenum grecum, telis, keratitis, aigonkeros, boukeros, siliqua, silicia, silicula); DL 354

(FENUGREEKE, τῆλις, fœnum grœcum, siliqua); Ge 1026 (FENEGREEKE, τῆλις, carphos, fœnum grœcum, siliqua, silicia, silicula).

CS (Cl, GH) | C²S¹ (SM, RM, LS, Fu, DL, Ge)

751 þre spicis of maloue. Although Renaissance herbals made a threefold distinction within mallows (cf. "garden Mallowe", "wilde Mallowe" and "Marshe Mallowe" in Ge), in the Middle Ages only two species, garden and wild, were usually recognized (→ **1290, 2420**), cf. "duplex est maneries, domestica [...] et siluestris que maluauiscus et bismalua dicitur" in Cl. While a scribal mistake for an original *t w o (o) of course cannot be dismissed, the syntax of the sentence makes it equally possible that the source text offered some (abbreviated?) weight instead of ‹spicis›.

756 also...757 menstrue. According to the ME text, fenugreek seems to have some unclear virtue related to women's menses (either emmenagogue or antiemmenagogue), but there is no pharmacographic support for this. Already Dioscorides recorded some gynaecological application of the species, recommending it in a sitz-bath for swellings and oppilation (see next paragraph); in fact the passage is a faulty translation of NH xxiv.186: "farinam feni cum hordeo aut lini semine decoctam aqua mulsa contra vulvae cruciatus obiecit idem [Diocles] inposuitque imo ventri." It seems clear then that ‹menstrue› must be the ME translator's deduction to render La. *cruciatūs* ("torments", hence the medical sense "sharp pains") as the word was paired with *vulvae*.

A strikingly similar recipe is found in *DVH(SME)*: "A plastre of fenygrek and lyn-seed and flour wole destruye þe euel þat is clepid encaresma". The last word, diversely spelt ‹encasesma›, ‹encaresma› and ‹encatesma› in the several MSS of that tradition, is probably not an eye disease (*contra* Frisk 1949: 230) but a rendering of ἐγκάθισμα "sitz bath" that the translator mistook for some unknown illness.

759 garlek. The Latin heading, the ME name and the temperament make it clear that the entry deals with garlic (*Allium sativum* L.).

The arrangement of the virtues indicates that the ME section loosely translates the appropriate chapter in *DVH*. The species is said to be alexipharmic (**760** = *DVH* 163–164), herpetofuge (**761** = *DVH* 166), good against dog bites (**763** = *DVH* 165), anticontusive (**764** = *DVH* 170–171), anti-inflammatory (**764** = *DVH* 172 and again in **779** = *DVH* 191–192), mazolytic (**766** = *DVH* 173–174), pulmonic, anthydropic and dessicant (**770** = *DVH* 175–178), nephretic (→ **770**), anticteric (**772** = *DVH* 180–181), anticephalalgic (**773** = *DVH* 183–184), antiotalgic (→ **775**), antitussive (**775** = DVH 187), antiraucedo (**777** = DVH 188–189), and antitenesmus (**778** = DVH 190). The last two virtues diverge from the canonical Latin text but can be shown to answer to a garbled Latin exemplar (→ **780, 782**).

> **Literature**: GARLIC (*Allium sativum* L.): HP i.6.9 (σκόρδον); MM ii.152; NH xix.III (*allium*); SM xii.126; RM ii.260; Grad. 382; Dur.Glos. 299 (*allium. garlec*); DVH 161–195 (*scordeon, allium*); LS 321 (*chaom* [ثُوم *ṯūm*], *allium*); EPN ii (*allium. garleac*), iii (*alium. gar-leac*), iv (*allium. leac*), vi (*allium. ail. garlec*); vii (*hoc allium. garle*), ix (*hoc allium. garleke*); CI A.15 (*allium*); TH 18 (*allium*); Pand. 653 (_{AR}*taum*, _{GR}*scordum, scordeon,* _{LA}*allium*); DVH(SME) 3b.10 (*garlik*); Alph. 5 (*allium domesticum, tyriaca rusticorum. garleke*); Sin.Bart. 10 (*allium agreste. crawegarlek*); AC 165.27 (*alium. garlek, cherlys tryacle*) ❦ GH 18 (ALLIUM, *scordon, scordeon, thaum, garlyke*); Fu 281 (*ΣΚΟΡΟΔΟΝ, allium*); Tu 1.224 (GARLEKE, *skorodon*); DL 456 (GARLIKE, σκόροδον, *allium*); Ge 140 (GARLICK, *poore mens treacle, allium,* σκόροδον).
>
> C³S³ (LS) | C⁴S⁴ (SM, RM, Grad., DVH, CI, TH, GH, Fu, Tu, DL, Ge)

770 frentekill men and for þe fallynge evill. DVH 179 *idem nefreticis elixum sumere iussit*. The reference to epilepsy is apparently a scribal addition, but the variant *phreneticis* that would explain the ME reading is recorded in the Basel 1527 edition of the poem (siglum δδ).

775 the hede. The source text indicates that this recipe is good for earache (cf. DVH 185–186: *anseris huic adipem iungas tepidumque dolenti / infundas auri, praeclare subvenit illi*); the translation was surely contaminated by the preceding virtue in the text.

780 wormes in þe wombe. The anthelminthic powers of garlic are mentioned at the beginning, rather than the end, of the Latin chapter (DVH 167–168) but then misplacement of virtues within the entries seems to have been not infrequent in the MS that served as exemplar to translate Macer Floridus's poem. The translation of original *mulsa* as ‹swete mylke› is also unexpected and is probably to be read as a translator's quirk (→ **837**).

782 evill eyre of pestlens. Even though the assumed antipestilential powers of garlic are not in the canonical version of Macer's poem, the passage looks like a garbled rendering of DVH 193–195, where garlic is said to make any water drinkable, cf. the reference to having garlic for breakfast, which parallels DVH 195 *mane ieiuno sumpserit ore*.

784 gromyll. Both the Latin heading and the ME name are common to the several species of *Lithospermum* L. generally called gromwells or stoneseeds, and particularly field gromwell (*L. arvense* L.) and common gromwell (*L. officinale* L.). The physical description provided suggests that the plant is the latter, as the nutlets of this species are white and smooth (hence the comparison with a pearl); *L. arvense* on the other hand has wrinkled grey or brownish ones. The source text, *AC*, used the heading *granum solis* to refer to the *arvense* species, and *granium* to indicate the *officinale*.

Pharmacographically, the species is lithontriptic (**786**) and diuretic (**787**), which is naturally in agreement with the usual medical literature since its stony nutlets were associated with the vesical calculi following the doctrine of the signatures.

Literature: COMMON GROMWELL (*Lithospermum officinale* L.): *HP* iii.13.3 (λιθόσπερμον); *MM* iii.141; *NH* xxvii.98 (*lithospermum*); *RM* ii.238; *OEH* 180 (*herba litosperimon. sunnancorn*); *LS* 67 (*kulb* [قلب *qulb*], *milium solis*); *EPN* vii (*hec gensta. gromylle*); *Cl* G.8 (*granum solis. gromel*); *TH* 207 (*granum solis*); *Pand.* 194 ($_{AR}$*culb, cuulb, cuulbi, culibi, calibi,* $_{GR}$*calib, lithospermon eraclion, halistos bathangliscos, astorchos, lapideum semen, hachala, calebum,* $_{LA}$*milium solis*); *Alph.* 72 (*granum solis, milium solis, cauda porcina. gromel*), 99 (*lithosmon. granum solis, milium solis. gromel*), 117 (*milium solis, granum solis, cauda pecorina. gromel*); *Sin.Bart.* 23 (*granum solis, milium solis. gromil*), 30 (*milium solis, palma christi. gromil*); *AC* 189.15 (*granium. gromelye, lytyl wale*), 190.9 (*granum solis. wylde gromelye*) ℥ Fu 185 (*ΛΙΘΟΣΠΕΡΜΟΝ, lithospermum, milium solis*); Tu 2.429 (GRUMMEL, *graymile, lithospermon, milium solis*); *DL* 207 (GROMELL, *gremell,* λιθόσπερμον, γοργόνιον, *lithospermum, milium soler, milium solis*); *Ge* 486 (GROMELL, *pearle plant, lichwale,* λιθόσπερμον, *gorgonium, aegonichon, leontion, diosporon, diospyron, heracleos, milium soler, milium solis*).

$$CS\ (Fu)\ |\ C^1S^1\ (LS)\ |\ C^2S^2\ (DL, Ge)\ |\ C^3S^3\ (Cl, TH)$$

784 mount syon. There is no ME evidence of a phytonym by that name, but in Classical pharmacopoeia there was σίον/*sium* (*MM* ii.127, *NH* xxii.84), traditionally identified as *Berula erecta* (Huds.) Coville. That species does not look like a *Lithospermum* but, just like that species, it was praised also as a lithontriptic and diuretic; perhaps that is the missing link between both species. On the authority of *Ps.Dios.*, where the synonym ἀναγαλλὶς ἔνυδρος is given, the plant might equally be a *Veronica* L. spp., perhaps marsh speedwell (*V. scutellata* L.) which has small white flowers similar to those of gromwell. Whatever the actual plant meant here, the alteration is suggestive yet again of a religious background for the scribe (→ **149, 188, 1953** and perhaps also **282, 708** for other instances), as the plant name may have been (wrongly) assimilated to Mount Zion, the hill in Jerusalem where the City of David was built (*2Sam* v:7–9) and the Ark of the Covenant was placed (*2Sam* vi:12). Textually, note that the comparison is not found in the source text but seemingly answers to an independent scribal addition.

789 galynga. The Latin heading and the ME name generally refers to galingale (*Alpinia galanga* (L.) Willd.; part of the Literature surely refers to that species), but this plant was probably unknown in Britain at the time. Moreover, the description provided in the entry, where the plant is compared to some wild grass, does not fit that species. The plant therefore must be rather the English galingale (*Cyperus longus* L.).

The entry follows the brief chapter in *DVH* closely: just like in the source text, the plant is phlegmagogue and carminative (**791** = *DVH* 2125–2127), eupeptic and antihalitosic (**791** = *DVH* 2128–2129), nephretic and aphrodisiac (→ **793**).

> **Literature**: ENGLISH GALINGALE (*Cyperus longus* L.): MM i.4 (κύπερος); NH xxi.115 (*cyperus*); SM xii.34; RM ii.233; Grad. 372 (*galanga*); DVH 2125–2130; LS 192 (*saherade* [سعد *suʻd*], *cyperus*), 322 (*rhulungen* [خولنجان *ḫūlangān*], *galanga*); CI G.3 (*galanga*); TH 202 (*galanga*); Pand. 297 (_{AR}*gulungen*, _{GR,LA}*galanga*), 608 (_{AR}*sapurios, sahade*, _{GR}*erisceptron*, _{LA}*ciperus*); DVH(NME) 257v.21 (*galinga*); DVH(SME) 37b.25 (*galingale*); Alph. 70 (*galanga, ciperus babilonicus. galyngale*); Sin.Bart. 15 (*ciperus babilonicus, galanga*); AC 190.3 (*ganyngale*) ⚜ GH 104 (CYPERUS), 187 (GALANGA, *galingale*); Fu 171 (ΚΥΠΕΡΟΣ, *cyperus*); Tu 1.300 (ENGLYSHE GOLANGAL, *cipe(i)rus*); DL 250 (ENGLISH GALANGALL, κύπερος, *cyperus, aspalathum, erisisceptrum, iuncus quadratus, iuncus angulosus, triangularis*); Ge 28 (ENGLISH GALINGALE, *cyperus, iuncus quadratus, iuncus angulosus, triangularis, aspalathum, erisis, cypresse*).
>
> CS (SM, RM, Fu) | C²S² (GH, Ge) | C³S³ (Grad., LS, CI, TH, DL)

792 helyth þe reynes. A faulty translation of *DVH* 2130 *augmentat sumptum veneris renumque calorem*, unless ⟨helyth⟩ is a copy mistake for an original *h e t i t h.

794 gryniswelly. This entry translates lines *DVH* 1664–1689, which deals with the plant called *senecio*. A different translation of the same Latin text has already been given (→ **824**); this particular entry derives from its rendering in *DVH(NME)*. Identification of the plant name with the groundsel, *Senecio vulgaris* L., is traditional and supported as well by the shared qualities attributed to the species in the literature: against orchitis (**797** = *DVH* 1669–1671), indurant and as vulnerary (**797** = *DVH* 1672–1673), and antiodontalgic (→ **800**). The warnings against using its root or drinking it will be also found in the Classical medical literature. Only its virtue against the sicknesses in the uterus is missing in the accounts by Pliny or Dioscorides (→ **799**).

> **Literature**: COMMON GROUNDSEL (*Senecio vulgaris* L.): HP vii.7.1 (ἠριγέρων); MM iv.96; NH xxv.167 (*erigeron, senecio*); SM xi.884; OEH 77 (*herba senecio. grundeswylige*); RM 215; Dur.Glos. 303 (*idrogias. grundes svilige*), 305 (*senecio. grunde svilige*); DVH 1664–1689 (*senecio*); EPN ii (*sintea, senecion. grundeswelge*), iv

(*senecio. grund-swylige, syr*), v (*sinitia. grunde-swelige*), vi (*iregerontis. cenesuns, grundeswilie*), vii (*hec sintecula. synthon*), viii (*hoc sinicium. tasylle*); *Pand.* 242 (_{GR}*erigion, erigeron, sedum senition, entricomon, senation,* _{AR}*xhuseaz achantidan,* _{LA}*cardo benedictus*); *DVH(NME)* 255r.9 (*griniswall*); *DVH(SME)* 32a.13 (*groundeswely. senecion, yrigeon*); *Alph.* 34 (*cardo benedictus, carducellus, cressiones, senecio, senechion. gowndeswilie*), 39 (*cressiones, cardo benedictus, senicio. growndeswylie*), 165 (*senecio, senecium, cardo benedictus, carducellus terestris, benedicta. groundeswile*); *Sin.Bart.* 39 (*senecio, carduus benedictus. grounswili*); *AC* p. 203.18 (*senacion. growndswthele*) ⚜ *GH* 409 (SENACIO, *grownswell, senechon sellechon*); Fu 109 ('ΗΡΙΓΕΡΩΝ, *senetio*); Tu 2.565 (GROUNDSELL, *senecio, erigeron, groundiswil*); DL 409 (GROUNDSWELL, ἠριγέρων, *senecio, herbulum, erechtites*); Ge 216 (GROUNDSELL, ἠριγέρων, *senecio, herbutum*).

Æ (*SM, RM,* Fu, Ge) | F (*DVH,* DL) | C³H³ (*LS*)

794 non medicyne. The text has been emended after *W.*38r/1 translating *DVH* 1668 *In medicinali radix non ponitur usu.* Cf. as well ‹no medicine› (**828**) in the other rendering of this entry.

795 and rykkylles. Incense was not an ingredient against orchitis in the original recipe (*DVH* 1669–1671), but it was asked for in the next virtue, against soft tendons and wounds (*DVH* 1672–1673). It looks as if the ME translator simplified the original Latin text because the presence of incense was the only innovation in comparison with the previous recipe (cf. *DVH* 1672 *addito thus istis* [i.e. the flowers with the leaves and the wine]). Curiously, the translator of the alternative version of this entry did likewise, cf. **828–831**.

796 in maner of a plaster. The syntax of the original reading was nonsensical and has been rearranged after *BW*.

799 stampe...800 matrice. This virtue is recorded in neither the Classical nor the medieval pharmacopeia. The reference to grinding and the use of salt as an ingredient, yet, makes it clear that the passage translates *DVH* 1683–1684, which describes the value of the plant against hardened scrofulous sores (*DVH* 1684 *duras* [...] *strumas*). Virtually the same recipe is given in the other version of this entry (**831–833**), and this makes mistranslation unlikely here. It rather suggests the existence of a textual family of *DVH*, perhaps a strictly English one (and hence not recorded in Choulant's apparatus), where there was a faulty passage or an interpolation. The MHG version, for example, translates correctly: "Daz krůt gestosen mit salze swendit di drůse, di scrofule heisent" (Schnell/Crossgrove 2003: 362).

Note that a number of lines preceding this virtue are missing in *DVH(NME)*: viz, *DVH* 1676–1678 against jaundice and *DVH* 1678–1682 against illnesses in several internal organs. These are also missing in the other version of the entry, which reinforces the idea of a common textual family for the Latin exemplar in both ME translations.

800 Plenius seiþ. This translates *DVH* 1685–1689. The ME version, in any case, has been abridged almost to the point of distortion, for the original passage in Pliny (*NH* xxv.167) reads as follows:

> hanc si ferro circumscriptam effodiat aliquis tangatque ea dentem et alternis ter despuat ac reponat in eundem locum ita, ut vivat herba, aiunt dentem eum postea non doliturum.

801 with-oute eny yryn. Emended after *W*.38r/7 ⟨wi*th*outyn yryn⟩, which translates *DVH* 1685 *sine ferro*.

804 gencyan. Although the hot quality provided in the entry is correct according to the *auctoritates*, as is the commonplace mention of the bitter taste of its root, identification of *genciana/gencyan* with some Gentianaceae species (PNME: *s.v.* gentiana suggests identification with *Gentiana amarella* (L.) Börner, but it may also be *G. lutea* L./*G. purpurea* L.) is difficult on pharmacological grounds, since just a few of the properties mentioned here are represented in the appropriate literature. The only common ground between the entry in *LH* and Classical and medieval pharmacological accounts of *gentiana* seems to be the shared power of the species as stomachal, hepatic and splenetic (**805**), antipleurodinic (**808**), and diuretic and alexipharmic (**810**; cf. *MM*, *Grad.*, *LS*; cf. also the entry in *AC*). Its value against nervous attrition is also recorded in *LS*. Other virtues in the medical literature of the period, particularly its abortifacient and vulnerary powers, are not mentioned here. On the other hand, neither the claimed properties of *gencyan* as an antiasthmatic (→ **806**), antitussive and anthydropic (**807**), nor its value against hoarseness and halitosis (**809**) are is found in the literature.

The entry follows the *DVH(NME)* tradition. *Genciane* is one of the five entries from this tradition that are not included in the canonical version of *DVH*. Besides *gencyan*, other two of these five plants are recorded in *LH*: *lawreoll* (→ **1149**) and *myllefoly* (→ **1376**; see Moreno Olalla 2018 for further details).

Literature: GENTIAN (*Gentiana amarella* (L.) Börner): *MM* iii.3 (γεντιανή); *NH* xxv.71 (*gentiana*); *SM* xi.856; *RM* ii.203; *Grad.* 367; *OEH* 17 (*herba gentiana. feldwyrt*); *Dur.Glos.* 302 (*gentiana. eorth nutu, feldvyrt*); *LS* 253 (*gentiana*); *EPN* ii (*anadonia. feldwyrd*), iv (*gentiana. feld-wyrt*), v (*avadonia. felt-wyrt*); *Cl* G.2 (*gentiana*); *TH* 201 (*gentiana, alungalica*); *Pand.* 280 ($_{LA}$*gentiana,* $_{GR}$*narcar,* $_{AR}$*sentiana*); *DVH(NME)* 257r.25 (*genciane*); *DVH(SME)* 40b.20 (*baldemoyne*); *Alph.* 4, 75 (*allogallica, basilicus. genciane*), 18 (*basilica, herba gentiana*), 37 (*centaurea maior, marta*); *Sin.Bart.*

22 (*genciana, baldemoyne, careswete*); *AC* 189.26 (*genciana, gencian, feldworth, baldemoyne*) ❦ *GH* 86 (GENCIANA, *felwort, baldymony*); Fu 74 (ΓΕΝΤΙΑΝΗ, *gentiana*); Tu 2.387 (GENTIAN, *gentiane*); DL 240 (FELWORTE, *gentian*, γεντιανή, νάρκη, χειρόνιον, *gentiana, aloë gallica, narce, chironion, basilica, cymilanis*); Ge 352 (GENTIAN, *felwoort gentian, bitterwoort, baldmoyne, baldmoney, gentiana*).

C (Ge) | CS (Fu, Tu) | C³S³ (*Grad., LS, Cl, TH, GH*, DL)

806 ciaticus. All four MSS from *DVH(NME)* offer the same word here but, since the word is paired with the antitussive qualities of the species, there is some chance that it be a copy mistake instead of *ASTHMATICUS.

812 germandir. This is a composite entry. The physical description (up to ‹medis› **816**) and the first two recipes are taken from the entry in *AC*; from that point onwards the text derives from *DVH* 1903–1917, which describes the medical virtues of the wall germander (*Teucrium chamaedrys* L.), a plant treated elsewhere in the herbal (→ **344**, with discussion).

The physical description of the plant provided in the text, though brief, is certainly not that of a germander, for this species does not display any kind of pods. Brodin has suggested (1950: 242) that the reference of the sound that the seed makes when ripe points to a *Rhinanthus* L. spp., probably the hayrattle, *R. minor* L. (so Brodin) or the yellow rattle, *R. crista-galli* L. (so tentatively PNME: *s.v.* camedreos). The seeds of the *Rhinanthus* are flat and golden brown (the ‹sede like to a peny› mentioned in the text), and kept inside a big globular capsule that rattles if shaken when it is ripe. While not strictly alike morphologically, *Teucrium* and *Rhinanthus* present a number of similarities: similar height, opposite leaves (scalloped in the case of the germander and serrated in the case of the hayrattle) and flowers gathered in racemes from the leaf axils. Most importantly, though the flowers are of different colour (the germander's is blue, while the hayrattle's is yellow), they both display a noticeable protruding adaxial lip of corolla that resembles a hanging lower lip.

Although the several *Rhinanthus* seem to have been best called *med(e)-ratel(e)* in ME and distinguished from the germander (cf. *AC* p. 200.20–21: "Qvercula maior is an herbe þat me clepuþ germandre or horsechire þis herbe hath leues lich to medratele bot hij buþ more sharp at þe ende"), the confusion between both genera appears in a number of ME lexicographical works, including *Alph.* (see PNME for details), and is still maintained in Fu.

Literature: *RATTLES (*Rhinanthus* L. spp.): *AC* p. 200.20 (*quercula maior. germandre, horsechire*). ¶ WALL GERMANDER (*Teucrium chamaedrys* L.): → colombyne [**344**].

824 growndswelow. This entry translates *DVH* 1664–1689, which describes the medical properties of common groundsel, *Senecio vulgaris* L., as copied from *DVH(SME)*. The same species was already treated in an entry copied from *DVH(NME)* (→ **794**, with discussion). Other than the addition of a synonym and the physical description, the entry contains roughly the same collection of virtues.

    Literature: GROUNDSEL (*Senecio vulgaris* L.): → gryniswelly [**794**].

824 swython. A copy mistake for *s(i)NICHON. FEW (*s.v.* senecio *n.*) records foms such as *sęrãšõ, snichon* or *šnišõ* in Norman (together with alterations such as *cherenchoun* or *fumechon*), and *selechion, senechiun* or *senenchon* in Francien. See also MED: *s.v.* seneciŏun *n.*; the entry swithon *n.* there should hence be merged with seneciŏun.

826 Plenius saith. The original Latin text, which is translated faultily, was quoted above (→ **800**). Besides the fact that Pliny stated that a line should be traced round the plant with an iron tool (rather than *sine ferro*, as stated in *DVH* 1685), there is no reference in any of the two ME renderings to the spitting that is required after each of the three strokes on the tooth (*DVH* 1687 *unaquaque spuens vice*), nor to the fact that the plant must be replaced into its original place in the orchard and remain alive after the whole procedure is completed (*DVH* 1687–1688 *postque reponat eodem, / quo fuit orta, loco, sic rursum vivat ut herba*). It is also important to note that the passage is placed in different positions within each of the two entries: as the first virtue here, but as the last one in the translation from *DVH(NME)* just like in the canonical Latin edition.

835 gladoyne. Although the Latin heading was as a rule applied to both gladioli (*Gladiolus* L. spp., particularly *G. italicus* Mill.) and the gladdon (*Iris pseudacorus* L.), the ME synonym suggests that this must be the latter. Identification must in any case remain traditional as the entry provides no physical description: in fact three types of *Iris* were customarily distinguished according to the colour of their flowers, the gladdon being the one displaying yellow ones (cf. the synonym *yellow flag*). The other two species are treated elsewhere in the herbal: the one having blue petals in → **724** (with discussion; a great deal of the literature there surely applies here as well, and viceversa), the white species in → **2097**. The entry is a loose translation of the chapter *Iris* in *DVH* (which was meant to cover all irises to judge from its opening lines: *iri dat florum nomen color ipse suorum: / coelestis similes sunt nempe coloribus iris*, *DVH* 1456–1457), but a substantial number of virtues quoted there are not recorded in the English version, and at least one of them seems mistranslated (→ **840**). In fact there is evidence that the original Latin MS must have been badly corrupt, the second half of the chapter in particular being missing almost in its entirety (→ 841).

Literature: GLADDON (*Iris pseudacorus* L.): *MM* i.2 (ἄκορον); *NH* xxv.157 (*acoron*); *SM* xi.819; *RM* ii.190; *Grad.* 355 (*acorus*); *OEH* 80 (*herba gladiolum. glædene*); *Dur. Glos.* 302 (*gladiolum. gladene*); *DVH* 1456–1488 (*iris*); *LS* 259 (*uaeg* [ζ, *wağğ*], *acorus, spatella*); *EPN* ii (*gladiolus. glædene | pirus, gladiolus. læfer*), iii, iv (*scilla. glædene*), iv (*scilla, gladiola. glædene | scirpio. læfer*), v (*citsána. fana*), viii (*hec carex, -icis. a flege*), ix (*hic cucumer. a flage*); *Cl* A.16 (*acorus*); *TH* 19 (*acorus*); *Pand.* 290 (*glaspatella, affrodisia, venerea, piper apium*, GR*acorus*, LA*spatella, gladiolus*, AR*laeg, hulhegi, naeg, hugoc, zueg*); *Alph.* 71–72 (*gladiolus.* GA*glaiol*, AN*leure*); *Sin.Bart.* 9 (*accorus est species yris cujus radices sunt rubræ et gerit florem croceum*), 22 (*gladiolus. accorus idem*), 25 (*yris purpureum florem in modum azuri gerit, yreos album*); *AC* 190.14 (*gladiolus. gladene*) ⚭ *GH* 19 (ACORUS, *affrodisyus, veneramy, sigenciana, mutica, gladon*); *Fu* 4 (ἈΚΟΠΟΝ, *acorum, aphrodisia, uenerea, piper apium*); *Tu* 2.404 (FLOUR DELYCE, *iris, irios... gladdon, swerdling*); *DL* 143 (YELLOW WILD IREOS, *yellow floure de lice, wild flags, water flags, lauers, pseudoiris lutea, iris lutea, acoron, pseudoacorus*); *Ge* 45 (FLOWER DE-LUCE, *iris palustris lutea, pseudoacorus, acorus palustris. water flags, bastard flower de-luce, water flower de-luce*).

C^2S^2 (*Grad., DVH, Cl, TH, GH*) | C^3S^3 (*SM, RM, LS,* Fu, DL, Ge [dry]) | C^4S^4 (Ge [fresh])

837 swete mylke. The passage obviously translates *DVH* 1469 (*cum mulsa bibitus choleram depellit iniquam*) but, as seen from the gloss in the parallel passage in *DVH(SME)* ("Mulsa is a drinke mad of hony and water, VIII parties water and þe IX hony", 13a.26–27), La. *mulsa* means "hydromel" rather than "sweet milk". That mistranslation is not exceptional but rather seems to have been the rule for the translator of *DVH* (→ 780).

840 þe narthe. This word means "constriction, congestion" and is frequently used in the treatise to translate La. *asthmaticus* (→ 72), but the corresponding Latin line reads *spleneticis et contractis et frigore laesis* (*DVH* 1472). A variant *a s t h m a t i c i s is not recorded in Choulant, so one is led to assume that the exemplary Latin MS must have offered a very botched rendering of the first word or else missed it altogether, and therefore ⟨narthe⟩ translates *contractis* metonymically. Yet it is striking that *laesis* should be rendered precisely ⟨shronke⟩ instead of *h i t , h u r t , s t r i c k e n or the like, which are more accurate translations—and then the evidence of Choulant's apparatus can hardly be deemed conclusive.

841 also…842 blode. The vulnerary virtue of the gladdon is the only one from the second half of the Latin entry that was translated, and then faultily (cf. *DVH* 1482–1483 *commixtus melli desiccat vulnera pulvis, / carneque nuda replet, si sit superadditus, ossa*). It seems very probable that *DVH* 1473–1488 were severely maimed in the original Latin and these lines formed the only passage which the scribe could make some sense of, by joining together some scattered words belonging to sundry virtues. In opposition to the English version, the original recipe does not mention roots, but *radicibus* does appear earlier in the Latin text (*DVH* 1479), when dealing with the emmenagogue powers of the species.

844 garofull. The entry describes the medical powers of wood avens (*Geum urbanum* L.), a plant already treated elsewhere in the herbal under a different name (→ **30**, with discussion). Identification is confirmed textually, as the entry translates the brief parallel chapter in *DVH* 2141–2146. Pharmacographically, the species is described as stomachal and eupeptic (→ **845**), and aphrodisiac (**847** = *DVH* 2144–2145, though the sense in the ME text could also suggest that the plant will make a man's penis larger), but misses the last line of the Latin original, where the species was praised as an anamnestic (the word ‹confortith› **847** is a remnant of this virtue, cf. *DVH* 2146 *confortat*), and as a hepatic.

Literature: WOOD AVENS (*Geum urbanum* L.): → avance [**30**].

845 all thingis wiþ-in a man. Rather than being beneficial to the internal organs, as suggested by the ME text, the Latin original actually states that the plant is good not only for the stomach (and the liver) but also for whatever is inside it: *iecur et stomachum corroborat haustum, / et ferme cunctis valet interioribus ipsum* (*DVH* 2142–2143).

849 holyhok. As seen from the Latin heading and the ME names, the entry is a description of the medical qualities of the marshmallow (*Althaea officinialis* L.) according to *AC*. A wholly different and more complete rendering of the pharmacological powers of this species is given later in the treatise (→ **2420**). This version only mentions its value as antipodagric (**851**) and carminative (**853**). The digestive powers of the species are well recorded by medical *auctoritates* but there is no evidence in the usual pharmacographic literature of its value against podagra.

Literature: MARSHMALLOW (*Althaea officinialis* L.): *HP* ix.15.5 (ἀλθαία); *MM* iii.146; *NH* xx.29 (*ibiscum*), 229 (*althaea*); *SM* ix.867 (ἐβίσκος); *RM* ii.190 (ἀλθαία); *OEH* 39 (*herba hibiscus. merscmealwe*); *Dur.Glos.* 299 (*althea. merc mealeve*); *DVH* 366–394 (*althaea*); *LS* 76 (*chitini* [خطمي *ḥiṭmy*], *altea*); *EPN* ii (*altea, eviscus. seo-mint*), iii (*ibiscum. biscep-wyrt*), iv (*althea. mersc-mealewe | althea. sæ-minte*), vi (*althea. ymalue. holihoc*), vii (*hec altea. wyld malle*);*Cl* M.4 (*malua siluestris, bismalua. holy hoke*); *TH* 291 (*malva*); *Pand.* 33 (LA*altea, malua hispanica, malua agrestis, maluauiscus, hibiscus, euiscus,* AR*eriscoscos, shobozetitan, rosasamen,* GR*molochia agria*); *DVH(NME)* 250r.5 (*wymalle*); *DVH(SME)* 13b.19 (*vyldemalwe, holy hocke, wylde* *malowe. altea, euisca*); Alph. 4 (*altea, bismalua, alta malua, ibiscus. holyhokke*), 29 (*caulus Sti. Kutberti. malua*), 61 (*euiscus, altea. Seynt Cutbertscole*), 110 (*alua siluestris, malua uiscus, altea.* ₐₙ*merch⟨e⟩-malue, bismalua, caulis Sancti Cutberti, alta malva,* ₐₙ*Seynt Cutbertscole*); Sin.Bart. 10 (*altea. holihocke*); AC 164.27 (*altea. holy-hok, wylde malwe*) ❀ GH 40 (ALTEA, *malowe, eiuscas, moloche agrie, molochin, spreophilon, ligemos, ribiscus, oblacius, harulus*), 270 (MALUAUISCUS, *wilde malowe*); Fu 5 (*'ΑΛΘΑΙΑ, althæa, ebiscus, ibiscus, bismalua, maluauiscus, euiscus*); Tu 1.227 (MARRISHE MALLOWE, *althea, hibiscus, eniscus, (bis) malva, malvavisens, water mallow*); DL 418 (MARRISH MALLOW, *white mallow, ἀλθαία, hibiscus, anadendron, aristalthæa, bismalua, maluauiscum*); Ge 787 (MARSHE MALLOWE, *moorish mallowe, white mallowe, ἀλθαία, ἰβίσκος, bismalua, maluauiscus, malua ibiscus*).

$$\text{CH (Ge)} \mid \text{C}^2\text{H}^2 \text{ (GH}_{270}\text{)} \mid \text{CS}^1 \text{ (DL)} \mid \text{C}^1\text{S}^1 \text{ (LS, Fu [flower])} \mid$$
$$\text{C}^2\text{S}^2 \text{ (GH}_{40}\text{, Fu [root])} \mid \text{F}^2\text{H}^2 \text{ (Cl, TH)}$$

856 houndfynell. The ME synonyms and the comparison made with camomile suggest that the entry describes the medical properties of the stinking camomile (*Anthemis cotula* L.) according to AC. The Latin heading and the comparison could also refer to the feverfew (→ **713**; a section of the Literature there, particularly the Classical *auctoritates*, may apply here): the plant was regarded as another camomile by some early authors (→ **366**) and this seems to have led to confusion in later compilers (Fu for one, where *A. cotula* is described in association with the virtues of the sweet-smelling camomiles).

Identification with *Anthemis* is textually secure but not borne out pharmacographically. The species is said to be anticancerous (**857**), antihemorrhoidal and antitonsillitic (**859**), and good against muteness (**860**), but none of them is recorded in the chapters devoted to camomiles or feverfew of the usual medical literature. Renaissance authors such as Dodoens and Gerard thought that the species was of no medical use, although they referred to its value against gynaecological disorders, "seeing all stinking things are good against those diseases"—as Gerard quaintly puts it.

Literature: STINKING CAMOMILE (*Anthemis cotula* L.): EPN ii (*caluna. mægþa; herba putida. mægða*), vii (*amarusa. donfynkylle*), viii (*hec cimnicia. hundfynkylle*); Alph. 7–8 (*amaracus, amarascus, maiorana, persa sansucus, colimbrum. maiorane, unde versus fetet amarusca, redolet similis camamilla*), 64 (*fetida. amarusca*), 112 (*mesandus, amarusca. maythe*), 116 (*merzandus, mersandus, amaracus*); Sin.Bart. 10 (*amarusca, ameroke. maythe*), 19 (*emeroc. hounde fenel*); AC 165.7 (*amarusca. mawth, doggis fenkel, maydewode*) ❀ Fu 221 (*ΠΑΡΘΕΝΙΟΝ, ἀμάρακον, χαμαίμηλον, parthenium, amaracum, solis oculus, millefolium, cotula fœtida*); DL 132 (WILDE OR COMMON CAMOMILL, *cotula fœtida, cauta, camomilla fœtida, κυνάνθεμις, κυνοβοτανή, dogs cammomill, mathers, mayweed, stinking cammomill, dog fenell*); Ge 617 (MAIEWEEDE, *wilde cammomill, stinking mathes, cotula fœtida, κυνάνθεμις*).

CS (DL, Ge)

857 the pipis of the em rodys. MED: *s.v.* pīpe *n.*¹, § 2.a takes this as a hapax and offers the meaning "hemorrhoidal veins", but this is probably misguided. The actual sense must be fistula, i.e. "a long, sinuous pipe-like ulcer with a narrow orifice" (OED: *s.v.*), as suggested by **1747**, where ⟨pipe⟩ translates *DVH* 219 *syringia*.

863 horsmynte. The (misspelt) Latin heading generally refers to either costmary (*Tanacetum balsamitoides* Sch.Bip.) or some wild mint (*Mentha* L. spp.; → **1318**); the English synonyms naturally point towards the latter possibility. Identification of the exact species is probably impossible since a physical description is lacking; traditional candidates are horsemint (*M. longifolia* (L.) L. = *M. sylvestris* L.) and water-mint (*M. aquatica* L.). The author of *LH* may have intended to cover both species but it is intriguing to see that the source text (*AC*) does not mention ⟨medemynt⟩ in the list of synonyms, and neither does the parallel chapter in Ge, the first woodcut of which is clearly a drawing of *M. aquatica*. Moreover, the literature, *EPN* and *Alph*. in particular, seems to suggest (albeit dimly) that the Latin names *balsamita* and, above all, *sisymbrium* were applied to *M. aquatica*, while *mentastrum* was used to refer to *M. longifolia* (about which, → **1454**). This is supported also by the following statement in Fu:

> Sisymbrij duo sunt genera. Vnum quod simpliciter Sisymbriu*m* dicitur: hoc seplasiarij Balsamita*m*, ut manuscriptus etiam testatur herbarius, uulgus autem Mentha*m* aquaticam, Germani Fischmüntz, Wassermüntz, oder Bachmüntz uocant.

The species is taken to be stomachal and digestive (**865**), purgative and eloquent (**866**), calefacient and carminative (→ **867**), and oxytocic (**869**), but only the medical virtue for the stomach is regularly recorded in the usual pharmacographic literature of the period.

> **Literature**: WATER-MINT (*Mentha aquatica* L.): *HP* ii.1.3 (σισύμβριον); *MM* iii.41; *NH* xx.247 (*sisymbrium*); *SM* xii.124; *RM* ii.259; *Grad.* 359; *OEH* 92 (*herba mentastrus. horsminte*), 107 (*brocminte. sisimbrium*); *Dur.Glos.* 300 (*balsemita. balsemite*), 305 (*sisimbrius. broc minte*); *LS* 288 (*nahanaha* [نعنا *na'na'*], *menta*); *EPN* ii (*sisimbrium. balsminte*), iv (*mentarium. feld-minte*), iv (*sisymbrium. broc-minte*), vi (*mentastrum. mentastre. hors-mynte* | *silimbrium. balsamitis. broc-minten*); *Cl* s.18 (*sisimbrium*); *TH* 446 (*sisimbrium*); *Pand.* 631 (*sisimbrium, absinthium ponticum, menta aquatica, balsamita,* ᴀʀ*culudes,* ɢʀ*cardaninon*); *Alph.*. 19 (*balsamita, salmentica, sisimbrium, menta aquatica, mentastrum. horsminte*), 118 (*mentastrum, menta siluatica*), 169 (*sisimbrium, balsamita, menta aquatica, menstrastrum, calamentum agreste. horsminte*); *Sin.Bart.* 12 (*balsamita, menta aquatica. horsminte*), 29 (*mentastrum, menta agrestis*); *AC* 170.11 (*balsamita, horsmynte, watermynte*) ❦ *GH* 404 (SISIMBRIUM); Fu 275 (ΣΙΣΥΜΒΡΙΟΝ, *sisymbrium, corona Veneris, balsamita mentha aquatica*); Tu 2.449 (MINT ... *sisymbrium, wild mynte*); *DL* 174 (MINT, σισύμβριον, *sisymbrium, damegeron*,

Lelamour Herbal 315

scimbron, brooke mint, white water mint); Ge 555 (HORSE MINT, water mint, brooke mint, horse mint, σισύμβριον, sisymbrium).

C¹S¹ (*RM* [green]) | C¹S³ (Fu)| C²S² (*RM* [dry], *Grad.*, DL [green]) | C³S³ (*SM, LS, Cl, TH, GH*, DL [dry], Ge)

867 leþer woundis. This is a scribal mistake for *leþer wyndis (a usual collocation in the text, cf. **127, 480, 790–791, 999, 1071, 1083**), parallel to "wycked wyndys" in the source text (*AC* 170.20).

872 hemloke. The (mispelt) Latin heading and the ME name indicate that the entry is an account of the medical properties of hemlock (*Conium maculatum* L.). The entry follows *DVH*, dropping as per usual all the historical and literary references included by Macer Floridus in the opening lines. The same species had already been treated earlier in the text following another textual tradition (→ **641**).

Pharmacographically, the species is antiherpetic (**877** = *DVH* 2044), antimastitic and galactophygus (**879** = *DVH* 2045–2048), anaphrodisiac and antispermatorrheic (**882** = *DVH* 2049–2050), antipodagric and and refrigerant (**883** = *DVH* 2051–2055). The use of hot wine as an antidote against hemlock poisoning is also mentioned, albeit the original text was somewhat modified (see next note). On the other hand, the scribe must have have misread the lines of the poem where hemlock is commended as an ophthalmic (→ **874**).

Literature: HEMLOCK (*Conium maculatum* L.): *HP* i.5.3 (κώνειον); *MM* iv.78; *NH* xxv.151 (*cicuta*); *SM* xii.55; *RM* ii.233; *Grad.* 376; *Dur.Glos.* 301 (*cicata. heomlic, vude vistle*); *DVH* 2029–2055 (*cicuta*); *LS* 337 (*sucaram* [شُوكَران *šūkarān*], *cicuta*); *EPN* ii (*cicuta. hemlic*), iv (*septiphilos. hymelic | cicuta. hymelic | cicuta, wode-þisele*), vi (*herba benedicta. herbe beneit. hemeluc*), vii (*hic tipus. homelok*), viii (*hec secuta. a humloke*), ix (*hec secuta. a humlok*); *Cl* c.22 (*cicuta. hemlok*); *TH* 107 (*cicuta*); *Pand.* 644 (ARsuccaram, GRconisa, tenela, conium, LAcicuta); *DVH(SME)* 22b.25 (*hemelok*); *Alph.* 39 (*cicuta, celena, incubus, coniza, conium, herba benedicta. hemelok, hornwistel*), 86 (*incubus nomen est morbi, et nomen demonis, et inde succubus id quod sicuta*); *AC* 174.3 (*cicuta. humlok, herbe benet*) ⚜ *GH* 102 (CICUTA, *hemlocke*); Fu 153 (ΚΩΝΕΙΟΝ, *cicuta*); Tu 1.275 (HEMLOKE, *cicuta, koneiou*); DL 322 (HEMLOCKE, κώνειον, *cicuta, harmel*); Ge 903 (HOMLOCKS, *herbe bennet, kexe*, κώνειον, *cicuta*).

F (*DVH*) | F⁴ (*SM, RM*, Fu, DL, Ge) | F³S³ (*LS*) | C³S³ (*Grad., Cl, TH, GH*)

872 þe…874 wyne. This passage seems to correspond to *DVH* 2037–2038 (*hac sumpta si quis morti sit proximus herba / forte merum tepidum bibat evadetque periclum*), but the ME author included a reference to parsnips (*Pastinaca sativa* L., although it could also refer to wild carrots, *Daucus carota* L. subsp. *carota*) that is not in the original Latin text. The scribal addition is of a fully practical nature, as hemlock, parsnips and carrots belong to the same subfamily of Apiaceae (Apioideae) and their taproots (and, in the case of *Daucus*, also their leaves) can be easily mistaken.

874 stampe...877 ham. The original passage (*DVH* 2041–2043) was evidently unclear to the scribe: the original Latin does not mention anything about a sore head: rather, it states that the green leaves should be rubbed against the forehead (*frons* [...] *operta, DVH* 2042). The exemplar must thus have offered *FOREHEDE, which the scribe misread, or else it was faultily written, an idea reinforced by the presence of ⟨blether⟩, which looks like a *literatim* rendering that the scribe prudently chose not to emend. The Latin in fact reads *aestivas* [...] *epiphoras* (*DVH* 2041), i.e. morbidly watery eyes during summer. Therefore ⟨blether⟩ must stand for such ME words as *blēr, blēred*, or *blērī* (see MED: *s.vv.*). The unexpected presence of **th** may arguably indicate an exemplary *Y, mistaken as *þ by the scribe. The intended fragment was thus probably something along the lines of *b l e r (e)   e y (e) n (e) or else *b l e r y   e y (e) n (e).

877 a sekenys callid þe holy fire and in latyn herpeta. In all but the more technical textbooks of the time the Latin term *ignis sacer* was employed as a mere functional synonym of *herpes*, a medically blurry designation that covered most cutaneous diseases characterized by a burning sensation and skin marks due to corrosion, from ergotism and erysipelas to herpes zoster and anthrax (an overview of the development of the terminology since Classical Antiquity and the different classifications of herpes during the Middle Ages will be found in Demaitre 2013: 91–95); Other designations in *LH* for apparently the same illness include ⟨fu de inferne⟩ (**1375**), and ⟨vretyng evyll⟩ (**1749**). Neither *Grad.* nor *LS* devoted a chapter to herpes, even though the authors mentioned the disease frequently in their works. Gilbert the Englishman did include two short chapters on herpes in Book III of *CM*, just after the section on serpigo and impetigo, but never cared to analyze its etiology: he just provided remedies for *herpes milium* and *herpes cingulum*. He moreover mentioned *sacer ignis* as a synonym for *herisipilas*, describing it as a variant of lupus in the chapter devoted to the latter disease (Bk VII). The disease was thought there to be caused by an accumulation of burnt yellow bile (*colera incensa combusta*).

884 horeworte. The ME synonyms (including ⟨chauuede⟩, which is not in MED and predates OED's first quotation, Turner's 1548 *Names of Herbes*, by almost a century) and the brief physical description suggests that the entry describes the medical properties of either the common cudweed, *Filago* *germanica* (L.) Huds., or the akin broadleaf cottonrose (*F. pyramidata* L. = *Gnaphalium germanicum* L.). The source for the section remains untraced.

From a medical perspective, the species is said to be antidysenteric (**887**), anticancerous and vulnerary (**888**). This is in accordance with the usual pharmacographic literature of the period, where the species was indeed praised as a remedy to stop the emission of blood (note that the German synonym in Fu is *heydnisch Wundkraut*). Ge is exceptional since the several species analyzed in the parallel section *Cotton-weede* are said to be antiphtheriac, anthelminthic, antitussive, etc.

> **Literature**: CUDWEED (*Filago germanica* (L.) Huds.)/COTTONROSE (*F. pyramidata* L.): *MM* iii.117 (γναφάλλιον); *NH* xxvii.88 (*gnaphalium, chamaezelon*); *SM* xi.861 (γναφάλιον); *RM* ii.205; *EPN* viii (*hec filago, quedam herba*); *Alph.* 66 (*filago*); *Sin.Bart.* 21 (*filago. chauvet*); *AC* 189.6 (*filago. flodwourt*) ⚜ Fu 278 (SARRACENICA SOLIDAGO, *cartafilago, filago, ceratophylax, herba fortis*); Tu 1.267 (CUDWEED, *chafweede, centunculus, gnaphalion, cartaphilago*), 2.391 (COTTENWEDE, *gnaphalium*); DL 63 (GNAPHALION, *small-cotton, pety-coton, small bombace, cudiweed, chafeweed, cartaphilago,* γναφάλιον, *centunculus, centuncularis, tucularis, albinum, gelafo, anaphalis, anaxiton, hires, tomentitia, bombax humilis,*); Ge 515 (COTTON WEEDE, *cudweede, chaffe weede, petie cotton,* γναφάλιον, *chamæxylon, tormentitia, cotonaria, centunculus, centuncularis, albinum, bombax humilis, filago, herba impia*).

S (Fu, DL, Ge)

886 cowe of a colour. The passage is probably corrupt. Since it is inserted in a remedy to stop the flow of blood, an original reading *COWE OF A RED(E) COLOUR seems likely.

893 heyhofe. The Latin heading, ME synonym and the physical description provided indicate that the entry is devoted to ground ivy (*Glechoma hederacea* L.). The entry seems to follow *AC*, but the version of the text edited by Brodin does not include any medical property. Brodin 1950: 153 includes a fragment from MS R that contains the beginning of a recipe where the species is used together with pork grease to make an ointment but a parallel passage is missing here. According to *Sl.*8v/24 that ointment would be against herpes (‹*contra* arsuras›), while in the appropriate section in *NH* there is a reference to using it with lard to heal burns ("folia [medetur] ambustis cum axungia"). The leaves of the species are moreover compared in the source text with those of ‹catmynte›, i.e. catnip (*Nepeta cataria* L.), rather than ‹calamynte› (*Calamintha nepeta* (L.) Savi; → **383**); note that there is evidence that both species were confused by the scribe throughout the herbal (→ **1504**). Besides, the flower of the plant in the source text is said to be red, rather than blue. All in all, then, the entry in *LH* appears either to derive from a better branch of the *AC* textual tradition than the one used by Brodin for his edition, or else it was substantially (and successfully) emended by some scribe during the transmission of the text.

The species is said to be emollient (**895**), antipleurodynic (**897**), and antiodontalgic (**897**). None of these virtues are recorded in the usual medical literature of the period: Classical authors commended the plant as antisciatic and anticteric, while Renaissance authors thought it to be also diuretic and antipestilential (so Fu); vulnerary, ophthalmic, purgative and analgesic (Ge); and above all, acoustic (Fu, DL, Ge). According to the *auctoritas* consulted, the species is both emmenagogue (so Fu) and antiemmenagogue (Ge). There are also some veterinary uses, particularly for horses (Fu, Ge).

> **Literature**: GROUND IVY (*Glechoma hederacea* L.): *MM* iv.125 (χαμαίκισσος); *NH* xxiv.82 (*cissos erythranos, chamaecisson*); *SM* xii.153; *RM* ii.271; *OEH* 100 (*hedera terrestris/nigra. eorðyfig*); *Dur.Glos.* 303 (*hedera nigra. eorth-ifig*); *EPN* iv *(hedera nigra. eorð-ifig)*, vi (*hedera nigra. iere. oerþ-ivi*), ix (*hic papillus. a heyoffe*); *TH* 172 (*edera...terrestris*); *Pand.* 122 (ᴳᴿ*camecissos*, ᴸᴬ*infima hedera, terrena hedera*); *Alph.* 52 (*edera terrestris, paulina. alehoue*); *Sin.Bart.* 18 (*edera nigra/edera terrestris. hayhof*); *AC* 184.15 (*edera terrestris. orpyn, heyhoue*) ❦ Fu 325 (ΧΑΜΑΙΚΙΣΣΟΣ, γῆς στέφανος, *hedera terrestris, terræ corona*); DL 281 (GROUND IUIE, *hedera terrestris, corona terræ*, χαμαίκισσος, ἐλατίνη); Ge 705 (GROUND IUIE, *alehoofe, gill creepe by the ground, tunehoofe, cats foote, hedera terrestris, corona terræ*, χαμαίκισσος).
>
> CS (Fu, DL, Ge)

899 horshele. This entry renders *DVH* 1489–1502 as translated in *DVH(NME)*. Identification with elecampane (*Inula helenium* L., → **587** for another account of the same species; a synonym for the species is misapplied in → **1616**) is sure on etymological (see OED: *s.v.* † horseheal *n.*) and pharmacographic grounds. Not only its supposed purgative and antitussive powers, but also its antisciatic (→ **900**), nephretic (→ **901**) and against apnea (**903**) are routinely recorded in the medieval pharmacopeia. On the other hand, a block of virtues contained in *DVH* 1493–1494 (including its usefulness as an emmenagogue, diuretic and abortifacient) is missing from this account.

> **Literature**: ELECAMPANE (*Inula helenium* L.): *MM* i.28 (ἑλένιον); *NH* xx.38 (*inula*), xxi.59 (*helenium*); *SM* xi.873; *RM* ii.209; *Grad.* 367 (*enula*); *OEH* 97 (*sperewyrt. hinnula campana*); *Dur.Glos.* 303 (*hinnula campana. spere-vyrt*); *DVH* 1489–1502 (*enula, elua*); *LS* 328 (*iasim* [راسن, *rāsin*], *enula*); *EPN* iv (*beribalbum. greate wyrt*; *innule campane. spere-wyrt*), vi (*elna enula. ialne, gret-wurt* | *enula. alne. hors-elne* | *hinnula campana. spere-wurt*), viii (*hec elenacampana. horshalle*); *Cl* E.2 (*enula campana*); *TH* 160 (*enula*); *Pand.* 237 (ᴳᴿ*ellenium*, ᴬᴿ*rasin, ilsaran*, ᴸᴬ*enula campana*); *DVH(NME)* 247v.14 (*hersheline*); *DVH(SME)* 12a.12 (*horsehelne. henula, elena*); *Alph.* 53 (*elena campana uel enula, ortolana et campana differunt, ortolana maior, elena campana*

minor, scabiosa maior idem. ₐₙ*horshelne*); *Sin.Bart.* 19 (*enula campana. similis est majori titimallo*); *AC* 182.25 (*elena campana. elena campana, horshillere*) 🙠 *GH* 150 (ENULA CAMPANA, *elfe docke, scabwort, horshele, canne*); Fu 89 (*ἘΛΕΝΙΟΝ, elenium, inula, enula campana*); Tu 2.403 (ELECAMPANE, *innula, helenion, alecampane, enula campana*); DL 242 (ELECAMPANE, *scabwort, horseheele,* ἑλένιον, *inula, enula, enula campana, panaces chironion, panaces centaurion*); Ge 648 (ELECAMPANE, *scabwoort, horseheale,* ἑλένιον, *inula, enula, enula campana, helenium*).

CH (Fu [green], DL [green]) | C²H¹ (*DVH*) | C³H¹ (*Grad., GH*) | C³H³ (*LS, Cl, TH*) | CS (*SM, RM,* Fu [dry]) | C³S² (DL [dry]) | C³S³ (Ge [dry])

900 tysayne that is þe evill of þe hede. As stated in → **595**, ⟨tysayne⟩ is a *lectio facilior* standing for *DVH* 1496 *sciasim*, i.e. sciatica (→ **338**). The copy error stems from a form *TYASIN already in Ω, since all the MSS from this tradition provide some version of this word. The explanation as to which part of the body is grieved by *TYASYN, on the other hand, is different according to the text: *B*.247v/16 ⟨on the Ee⟩ and *P*.275/1 ⟨of ey3e⟩ suggest an ophthalmic disease, while *W*.33v/2 reads exactly like *S*₁. The reconstructed form in Ω must have looked like *THEYE 'thigh' (→ **309**), probably translating *DVH* 1496 *coxae*, and which was read as **th'eye* by some scribes, and as **th'(h)eyd* by others. For the implications of this as regards the textual history of the tradition, see Moreno Olalla 2017: 675–676.

901 newe-frantikes þat is þe evill of þe reynes. This renders *DVH* 1498 *Mire nefreticis renes involvere prodest* quite correctly, but there seems to be no nephretic virtue attached to this species in the medieval pharmacopeia. Since there is as yet no detailed *Quellenforschung* on *DVH*, it is difficult to be sure as to why this illness is mentioned in the Latin poem, but it might be a faulty rendering of a phrase similar to the *attritioni neruorum* that appears in *LS*, misread as **nevrorum*, then conected to the root **nefr-*.

905 henbane. Henbane, common name for several *Hyoscyamus* L. spp. The author of *DVH* made a threefold division between them according to the colour of the seed, following *MM* and other medical writers: white (*H. albus* L.), red, or rather golden (cf. *DVH* 1936 *subrufum, H. aureus* L.), and black (*H. niger* L.); *NH* included a fourth species ("unum nigro semine, floribus paene purpureis, spinosum calice, nascitur in Galatia"), identified as *H. reticulatus* L. (André 1956: *s.v.* altercum). The entry stems from *DVH(NME)*, and ultimately from *DVH* 1933–1961.

Identification is sure on pharmacographic grounds, as the plant is praised as an anti-inflammatory, particularly against those inflammations derived from gout, or in the testicles and women's breast (**909** = *DVH* 1941–1942; **914** = *DVH*

1958), antirheumatic (**912** = DVH 1949; → **1712**), antiodontalgic (→ **910**) and vulnerary (**914** = DVH 1954–1955). The virtue of henbane as an vermifuge if instilled in the ears (**910** = DVH 1943), which is frequently recorded in medieval and Renaissance pharmacopeia, seems to be missing in MM and NH while, on the other hand, the soporific value of this species (poisonous if overdosed) is not mentioned in the ME text.

 Literature: HENBANES (*Hyoscyamus* L. spp.): MM iv.68 (ὑοσκύαμος); NH xxv.35 (*hyoscyamus*); SM xii.147; RM ii.269; Grad. 384; OEH 5 (*herba sinphoniaca. belone, hennebelle*); Dur.Glos. 303 (*iusquiamus, simphoniaca. hennebal*); DVH 1933–1961 (*iusquiamus, caniculata*); LS 330 (*bengi* [༜ *bang*], *iusquiamus*); EPN ii (*simphoniaca. henne-belle*), iv (*symphoniaca. beolone*), v (*simphoniaca. henne-belle*), vi (*jusquiamus. chenille. hennebonne*), ix (*hic jusquianus. a hennebane*); Cl 1.1 (*iusquiamus. henban*); TH 231 (*iusquiamus*); Pand. 93 (_AR_*beng, elfozium,* _GR_*simphoniaca,* _LA_*iusquiamus*); DVH(NME) 256r.22 (*henbane*); DVH(SME) 35b.7 (*hennebane. iusquamus, caniclata*); Alph. 84 (*iusquiamus, caniculata, simphonica, cassilago, dens caballinus. henbane, hennedwole*); Sin.Bart. 26 (*iusquiamus. henebon*); AC 192.12 (*iusquiamus. henbane*) ⚕ GH 212 (JUSQUIAMUS, *cassilago, symphoniaca, henbane*); Fu 322 (ΥΟΣΚΥΑΜΟΣ, *hyoscyamus, apollinaris, altercum, jusquiamus*); Tu 1.226 (HENBANE, *altercum, apollinaris, fabasuilla, iusquiamus, hyosciamos*); DL 321 (HENBANE, ὑοσκύαμος, ἀπολλενάρις, *hyoscyamus, apollinaris, faba suilla, dioscyamos, Iouis faba, fabulonia, symphoniaca, calicularis, remenia, faba lupina, mania, fabulum, altercum, altercangenum, deus caballinus, herba pinula, canicularis, caniculata*); Ge 282 (HENBANE, ὑοσκύαμος, *apollinaris, faba suilla, altercum, faba Iouis, zoroastes, insana alterculum, symphoniaca, calicularis, remenia, fabulonia, faba lupina, dens caballinus, milimandrum, cassilago, herba pinula, iusquiamus, hyoscyamus*).

 F (*DVH*, Fu) | F³ (*SM*, RM, Tu, DL [white]) | F⁴ (DL [yellow, black], Ge) | F⁴H⁴ (*Grad.*) | F³S² (*Cl*, TH, GH) | F³S³ (*LS*)

910 þe hede-ake. This renders DVH 1944 *illarumque* [...] *dolores*, referring to the ears that had just been mentioned. There is no reference in Choulant's apparatus to the expected variant *c a p i t i s q u e . Immediately after this, the Bodley version provides the translation of DVH 1945–1947, which is missing in WS_1: cf. B.256v/1–2 ‹& seythe it in aysell & wesch thy mouthe þer-with & it abatis toghwerke›. This suggests a homoioteleuton somewhere in the transmission (*w e r k e ... w e r k e). Unfortunately the whole entry is missing in P so it is impossible to know whether the error derives from γ or was already present in RH.

914 washe…915 helith. This seems to stand for DVH 1954–1955, which refer to hemoptysis (instead of the more general references to effusion of blood in MM) and hence should have appeared before the references to swollen testicles and breasts. Both Bodley and Wellcome offer a different quality here:

B.256v/5 ⟨it is gude in plaster to hott guttys⟩, which is given last in S_1 (**917**). The vulnerary qualities of the species were oppositely copied at the end of the entry in those MSS.

915 take... 917 goute. A probable *lectio facilior* in AS_1 (cf. *B*.256v/6–7 ⟨hyngand in clusters⟩, also *W*.38r/22) which also explains the lack of concordance between ⟨berys⟩ and ⟨hit⟩—unless the pronoun is taken to refer back to ⟨morell⟩ and ⟨clostris⟩ was taken by the copyist to mean "convents", which is quite doubtful.

916 hit growis. This fragment is not found in the canonical Latin entry of *DVH* and may be an interpolation from another entry. It was recorded in all ME versions of *DVH(NME)* (although its exact place within the entry varies, see the preceding note).

919 hertwort. The entry, which derives from *AC* but misses the information provided there about its habitat, appears to be a revisitation of the virtues of the bugle (*Ajuga reptans* L., → **223**), but is mixed with some information usually connected with the European birthwort (*Aristolochia clematitis* L., → **67**). For example, the heart-shaped leaves are a known feature of the latter, but the blue flower and the short stalk surely refer to the *Ajuga*, since the *Aristolochia* displays recognizable tubular pale-yellow flowers that resemble a birth canal. From a pharmacographic point of view the plant is said to be a good remedy against sores (**920**), and hence points again to the bugle, a well-known vulnerary—the birthwort being the mazolytic plant *par excellence* and also a good alexipharmic since Classical times. The synonyms ⟨edebreune⟩ (surely a copy mistake for original *WODEBROUNE) and ⟨silfehale⟩ similarly point to the bugle (the names make reference to the dark hue of its leaves and its vulnerary qualities), while ⟨hertwort⟩ is of course another reference to the shape of birthwort leaves. As for the Latin heading, as a rule ⟨fraxinus⟩ means the ash-tree (*Fraxinus excelsior* L.) but is given in several ME synonyma as the equivalent of both the heartwort and wood-brown (see PNME: *s.v.*; also Ge_{1289}).

    Literature: BUGLE (*Ajuga reptans* L.): → browne bugill [**223**]. ¶ BIRTHWORT (*Aristolochia clematitis* L.): → astrologie [**67**].

920 sharpe. The comparison is odd, so probably a word such as *s h a p p e *n* (< OE *scapen*), less likely *s h a p p e d , was intended: just like many other Aristolochiaceae, *A. clematitis* L. displays large cordate leaves. Note that only two of the four MSS of the *AC* tradition used by Brodin in his edition (*H* and *R*) offer the expected reading ⟨y-schaped⟩. The other two MSS, *X* and *L*, read together with S_1.

923 hertis-tonge. The Latin headword, and the ME synonyms point to the hart's-tongue fern (*Asplenium scolopendrium* L.). The entry follows the *AC* textual tradition, but misses most of the physical description given there, as well as the reference to its habitat. On the other hand, the anticolic virtue given here is missing in the source text. Both *LH* and the Stockholm copy of *AC* miss the sentence about the species temperament—which is diversely taken to be hot and dry (MS *R*) or hot and wet (MSS *B, L* and probably also *H*) in the other MSS from the tradition. *Sl*.12r/9 reads ⟨ca*lida* & hu*mida* ij° grado⟩

According to the text, the species is anti-inflammatory (**925**), antidiarrheic (**925**), antitussive (→ **926**) and anticolic (**928**). Only the antidiarrheic virtue of the species is usually recorded in the Classical and medieval pharmacopoeia.

> **Literature**: HART'S-TONGUE FERN (*Asplenium scolopendrium* L.): *MM* iii.107 (φυλλῖτις); *SM* xii.152; *RM* ii.270; *OEH* 57 (*teuerion. brunewyrt*); *Dur.Glos.* 305 (*splemon. brun vyrt*); *LS* 193 (*scolopendrion*); *EPN* ix (*hec seniglossa. hertes-tunge*); *Pand.* 48 (_{GR}*aplenon, aplinium, splemon, scolopendrion,* _{AR,LA}*ceterach*); *Alph.* 80 (*herba cerui, scolopendria, lingua ceruina.* _{GA}*cerflange.* _{AN}*hertestonge*), 103 (*lingua cerui, herba scripta, splenetica*); *Sin.Bart.* 27 (*lingua cervina, scolopendria*), 38 (*solopendria, lingua cervina, spleneon*); *AC* 195.8 (*lyngua cerui. hertystungge*) ⚜ *GH* 422 (SCOLOPENDRIA, *ceruilingua, tispenidion, trimon, locitas, figicis, herba panaie, hertes tongue*); *Fu* III ('ΗΜΙΩΝΙΤΙΣ, ἁπλίνιον, *teucrion, scolopendria, lingua ceruina, asplenon*); *Tu* 2.500 (HARTIS TUNGE, *phyllitis, lingua cervina, scolopendria*); *DL* 293 (STONE HARTS-TONGUE, φυλλίτις, *scolopendria, lingua ceruina*); *Ge* 976 (HARTS TOONG, φυλλίτις, *lingua ceruina, scolopendria, radiolus*).
>
> CS (DL, Ge) | C^{1}S^2 (Fu) | C^{2}S^2 (*LS*)

926 þe cow. The MS reading ⟨sow⟩ makes no sense in the context, and has been emended in the light of ⟨cow3e⟩ in *AC*. There is some internal evidence suggesting that the exemplar might have actually read *COW(E), → **947**.

930 houndystonge. The Latin headword, ME synonym, and the brief physical description suggest that the entry describes the medical properties of hound's-tongue (*Cynoglossum officinale* L.) according to *AC*, but misses most of the description given there.

The species is said to be antitussive and anti-inflammatory (**931**), and maturative (**933**), but none of these are recorded in the usual pharmacgrachical literature. The plant, according to *NH*, is febrifuge and antimalarial, and according to Renaissance authors it serves as a good antidysenteric, vulnerary, antiherpetic and antihemorrhoidal. Ge adds antialopecic qualities as well.

> **Literature**: HOUND'S-TONGUE (*Cynoglossum officinale* L.): *MM* iv.127 (βούγλωσσον); *NH* xxv.81 (*cynoglossos*); *OEH* 42 (*herba buglossa, bubula. glofwyrt, hundes tunge*); *Dur.Glos.* 301 (*canis lingua. hundes tunga* | *cynoglossa. ribbe*); *EPN* ii (*cinoglossa,*

plantago, lapatium. wegbræde), iii (*cinoglossa. ribbe*), iv (*cynoglossa. rybbe* | *canis lingua. hundes tunge*), vi (*lingua canis. chen-lange. hundes-tunge*); *TH* 281 (*lingua canis, cinoglossa, lingua bona*); *Pand.* 499 (_LA_*lingua canis,* _GR_*cinoglossa*); *Alph.* 39 (*cinoglossa, lingua canis. houndestonge*), 104 (*lingua canis. houndestonge, hareflex*); *Sin.Bart.* 15 (*cinoglossa, lingua canis*); *AC* 196.28 (*lingua canis. houndistungge*) ⚶ *GH* 259 (CYNOGLOSSA, *houndestongue*); Fu 154 (*ΚΥΝΟΓΛΩΣΣΟΝ, lingua canina*); Tu 1.299 (DOGGIS TONGE, *cynoglossum*); *DL* 9 (DOGS TONGUE, *hounds tongue, κυνόγλωσσον, cynoglossum, lingua canis*); Ge 659 (HOUNDES TOONG, *hounds pisse, κυνόγλωσσον, lingua canis, cynoglossos*).

FS (DL, Ge) | F²S² (Fu) | C²H³ (*GH*)

935 horehounde. The Latin headword, the ME synonyms and the description point to the white horehound (*Marrubium vulgare* L.). Textually, the entry is a composite of the appropriate chapters in *DVH* and another source (from ‹Also› **947** onwards) which is akin to *AC* but frequently condenses the information or deviates from it.

Therapeutically and as regards that section of the chapter drawn from Macer Floridus' text, the species is said to be antiphthisic and antiasthmatic (→ **937**), oxytocic and mazolytic (**940** = *DVH* 1444), anti-inflammatory and antiseptic (**941** = *DVH* 1445–1446), antipleurodynic (**942** = *DVH* 1447), ophthalmic and antiotalgic (**944** = *DVH* 1449–1453). On the other hand the anticteric virtue (*DVH* 1451) is missing. All of them are routinely found in the usual medical textbooks since *MM*, as is the suggestion that horehound is to be avoided in renal and bladder treatments (**946**). The section taken from *AC* on the other hand supports the idea that the species is antispasmodic (**945**, again in **958**), antitussive (→ **947**), stomachal (**950**), febrifuge and alexipharmic (**952**), antiherpetic (→ **953**), emollient (**954**), and prophylactic (**961**), but many of these virtues are not found in the Classical or Renaissance pharmacography. Only its purported value against spasms, coughing and snake bites, all of which can be traced back to *NH*, are usually recorded in (post-)medieval medical works.

Literature: WHITE HOREHOUND (*Marrubium vulgare* L.): *HP* vi.2.5 (πράσιον); *MM* iii.105; *NH* xx.241 (*marrubium*); *SM* xii.107; *RM* ii.254; *Grad.* 361 (*prassium*); *OEH* 46 (*herba prassion. harehune*); *Dur.Glos.* 303 (*marrubium. harhune*); *DVH* 1450–1468 (*marrubium, prassion*); *LS* 198 (*farasio* [فراسيون *farāsyūn*], *prasium*); *EPN* ii (*marrubium, vel prassium. harhune*), iii (*marrubium. hune*), iv (*marrubium. hare-hune* | *prassion. hune*), v (*marrubium. har-hune*), vi (*marrubium. maruil. horehune*); *Cl* M.14 (*marubium, prassium. horehound*); *TH* 570 (*marubium*); *Pand.* 252 (_AR_*farasion, fraxion, marmacur,* _GR_*philoflores,* _LA_*prassium*), 521 (_LA_*marrubiastrum, marrubium nigrum, marrubium siluestre,* _GR_*bublocte,* _AR_*marmacur*); *DVH(SME)* 29b.13 (*horhoune. marubium. prassion*); *Alph.* 111 (*marrubium nigrum, prassium.*

horhoncie, houndesuede), 138 (*prassium duplex est, album et nigrum | prassium aut filofores*); *Sin.Bart.* 29 (*marubium, prassium. horehoune*); *AC* 205.12 (*marubium. marube, horrowne, houndbene*) ❦ *GH* 283 (MARRUBIUM, *prassion, horehounde*); Fu 224 (ΠΡΑΣΙΟΝ, *marrubium*); [Tu 1.249 (STYNKYNGE HOREHOUNDE, *ballote, megaprasion, melanprasion, marrubium magnum/nigrum, blake horehounde*);] DL 182 (HOREHOUND, πράσιον, *marrubium, prassium*); Ge 561 (HOREHOUND, πράσιον, *marrubium, prassium, melittena, labeonia, ulceraria*).

C^2S^2 (*DVH, LS*) | C^2S^3 (*SM, RM, Grad.*, Fu, DL, Ge) | C^3S^3 (*Cl, TH, GH*)

937 the tisike and þe narthe. The passage is an abridgement of *DVH* 1440–1443 that drops the reference to cough:

Seminis aut eius phthisicos mire iuvat hausta,
Pectoris haec varios compescit potio morbos,
Et melius prodest, illi si iungitur iris;
Asthmaticos sic sumpta iuvat tussimque repellit.

Phthisis, according to medieval medicine, was the consequence of an accumulation of superfluous humours drawn from the several body members into the lungs (*LS* ii.26). As for ‹narthe›, it renders *asthmaticos* in the original. Asthma was assumed to be due to the clogging of alveoli by thick and sticky humours (*ex humore grosso, viscoso, adhærente meatibus paruis in pulmone*; *LS* ii.24).

947 also…949 hole. The passage seems corrupt as the text alternatively refers to a man and to some female beast, even though none of the MSS used by Brodin in his edition suggests that the recipe provided is anything but a solution to a severe case of cough. It is likely that the word "cough" was spelt *COW(E) in the exemplar (as suggested by readings such as ‹kuow› and ‹kowe› in MS *R*) and this must have misguided the copyist. Further support for this assumption will be found in the entry devoted to hart's-tongue fern, which was also drawn from *AC* (→ **926**).

953 tetterys. This word was used as a synonym for scab (→ **413**), and particularly in burning varieties such as ringworm, cf. Boorde's *Breuiary of Helthe* (1547, f. 120v):

In Englysshe it [herpes] is named a tetter, and some doth name it lupus or lupie bycause a wolfe hath oftymes suche impedimentes, it dothe crepe and corode and eateth the skyn and waxeth broder and broder (f. 74v) . . . [T]his sicknes or disease named serpigo is a burnynge skabbe, and doth ronne in the skyn infectynge it more or lesse, and it is named in Englyshe a tetter.

963 horshoue. While all the synonyms provided (other than the mysterious *diuee*) and the reference to the distinctly different colour of the adaxial and abaxial surfaces of the leaf clearly point to the coltsfoot, *Tussilago farfara*

L., the medical qualities correspond to those attached to a different species, the purslane (*Portulaca oleracea* L.), a species treated other two times (→ **976**, and particularly **1868**, with discussion). Note on the other hand how the antitussive value of the *Tussilago*, routinely recorded in Classical, medieval and Renaissance pharmacopeia and which apparently served to give the plant its name in the Classical languages (cf. βήξ, βηχός, and *tussis* "cough"—although this may be a calque from Greek, see Chantraine 1999: s.v.), is oddly missing from this account. The entry follows *AC*.

Emendation from MS ⟨horsho*n*⟩ is well sustained by *horse-hoof* in several sources ("hors huoue" in Trevisa, "horshoue" in Thornton, "horse houe" in Turner, etc.). Both MED: s.v. hors-hǫve *n*. and PNME: s.v. pes pulli missed the tilde over the final letter and read "horsho" here, and note that ⟨horshoo⟩ is used in **984** to refer to the purslane, which probably was instrumental in the confusion between the species.

Literature: COLTSFOOT (*Tussilago farfara* L.): MM iii.112 (βήχιον); NH xxvi.30 (bechion, tussilago); SM xi.850 (βηχίον); RM ii.201; EPN ii (*caballopodia, ungula caballi. colt-græig*); DVH(SME) 28a.1 (*purslane, fole-foot. adragmis*); Alph. 140 (*pes pulli, herba terrestris,* ᴳₐ*pee de polayn, pe de clyual,* ₐɴ*donnhoue, wowell, feldhoue*); Sin.Bart. 34 (*pes pulli. purcelan*); AC 215.18 (*pes pulli agrestus. folys foot, pes pully*) ⚜ GH 474 (UNGULA CABALLINA, *lytell clote*); Fu 50 (BHXION, *tussilago, farfaria, ungula caballina*); Tu 2.592 (HORSE HOVE, *bulfoote, tussilago, bechion*); DL 16 (FOLEFOOTE, *horsehoofe, coltsfoot, bull foote,* βήχιον, χαμαιλεύκη, *tussilago, farfara, ungula caballina*); Ge 666 (COLTES FOOTE, *horse foote, fole foote, horse hoofe, bulfoote,* βήχιον, *tussilago, farfara, ungula caballina, pata equina*). ¶ PURSLANE (*Portulaca oleracea* L.) → portulake [**1868**].

H (DL [green]) | S (DL [dry]) | CH (*RM*) | CS (Fu [dry], Ge [dry]) | FS (Fu [green], Ge [green])

963 this...964 oþer. *DVH* does not provide a physical description of the purslane. Choulant indicates in a long footnote (1832: 59) that a passage at the beginning of this entry (*DVH* 750–754) is very corrupt, so MSS differed greatly in their readings. The canonical version states the temperament of the species as being cold in the second degree and moist in the third (→ **1868**) and then goes on to explain that purslane is a good medicine against the burning fever called *causon* (Gk καύσων), if pounded while still green and rubbed on the stomach, or else if its juice is drunk.

One of the main differences is the order in which the virtues are copied. Some traditions (ββ, γγ, ζζ) offer the febrifuge quality first, then the antidysenteric one follows, while some other (κκ) reverses this arrangement.

Other (δδ, εε) miss the reference to fever altogether and abridge the whole passage so as to convey that the plant is good to the stomach.

The ME translator must have conjectured and associated *DVH* 753 *viridis* with the colour of the leaves. → **976** for a similar scribal solution to the same problem but in a different tradition.

967 stone. Emendation is supported by the parallel reading in *AC* 215.25: "it wele hele a man of þe ston". This passage corresponds to *DVH* 762, which deals with diseases of the bladder.

970 hayreff. The Latin headword and the physical description (particularly the reference to the hooked prickles on the fruit that will hang on clothes or animal fur, whence the Gk name φιλάνθρωπος) suggest that the entry deals with cleavers (*Galium aparine* L.). The first two ME synonyms support that identification but the inclusion of ‹aron› is striking, for as a rule this refers to a very different species, cuckoo-pint (*Arum maculatum* L.; → **2195** for another instance where a synonym for this species is misapplied, and also **1018**). The synonym appears to be an addition in *LH*, as it is not recorded in the source text (*AC*, but note that this particular chapter was drawn from the Laud MS and an apparatus criticus is lacking; it may be that some other MS not collated by Brodin does mention *aron*).

Medically, the species is commended as a hemostatic (**972**), which is in accordance with *NH* and with the Renaissance pharmacographers drawing from it but missing in *MM* and the medieval works. The text also includes a value for husbandry, since the species is taken to be a fattener of poultry (**973**; it is curious then that Ge should mention that women made the species into a pottage with mutton and oatmeal "to cause lanknesse, and keepe them from fatnes").

Literature: CLEAVERS (*Galium aparine* L.): *HP* vii.8.1 (ἀπαρίνη); *MM* iii.90; *NH* xxvii.32 (*aparine*); *SM* xi.834; *RM* ii.195; *Grad.* 351 (*rubea*); *OEH* 174 (*philantropos. menlufigende*); *Dur.Glos.* 299 (*apparine. cliue*); *EPN* iv (*appasina. clife*), viii (*hec uticella. haryffe*), ix (*hic papillus. a hayoffe*); *Cl* R.6 (*rubea*); *TH* 406 (*rubea*); *Pand.* 62 (*aspergula, spargula, rubea minor*), 381 (*lappa minor, sanction, fagasmon, aparine, philantropos, bardana*); *Alph.* 157 (*rubea minor. renele, cliuer, tongebledes*); *Sin.Bart.* 37 (*rubea minor. hayrive*); *AC* p. 201,8 (*rvbea minor. clyuere, hayroue*) ⚜ Fu 14 (ΑΠΑΡΙΝΗ, ὀμφαλόκαρπος, φιλάνθρωπος, aparine, aspergula); Tu 1.238 (GOOSHARETH, *clyuer, aparine, philantropos, omphalo carpos*); DL 387 (GOOSE-GRASSE, *cliuer, gooseshare, ἀπαρίνη, φιλάνθρωπος, ὀμφαλόκαρπος, aparine*); Ge 963 (GOOSE-GRASSE, *clyuers, gooseshare, clauer, ἀπαρίνη, lappa minor, lappago, philanthropos, philadelphos*).

C (Fu, DL) | CS (*SM, RM*, Ge) |C¹S¹ (*Grad.*) | C²S² (*Cl, TH*)

973 yf hit be broke small. The sentence is incomplete, cf. *AC* 201.11–12 "if þis herbe be broke smale among hure ‹met›".

976 helow. An account of the pharmacological virtues of the purslane, *Portulaca oleracea* L., according to *DVH* 748–764 as rendered in the *DVH(NME)* tradition. Versions of substantially the same entry are found twice in the ME herbal (→ **963**, where the virtues are attached to a wholly different species, and especially **1868**). According to MED: *s.v.* helow *n.*, the word is a hapax with an untraced etymology; it may be a garbled version of an exemplary *WOWELL (reasons for this hypothesis in Moreno Olalla 2013b: 946, fn. 27).

The entry is missing in *P*, while the Northern MSS of the tradition add *B*.254r/7 ‹is a greyne gresse›, *W*.37v/19 ‹of þe gryne gres› after the ME name (→ **963**); the Bodley version offers moreover a synonym *B*.254r/6 ‹dethtonge›. In fact, while a common origin with *B* is clear, the syntax and the wording of the first lines in *W* and, particularly, S_1 (up to **979–980** ‹swagith ham›) have been substantially reworked.

 Literature: PURSLANE (*Portulaca oleracea* L.): → portulake [**1868**].

981 wiþ white saltt. This corresponds to *DVH* 761 *cum vino et cum sale*. Bodley offers the correct *B*.254r/11 ‹*with* wyne & saltt›. The sentence is missing in *W*.

982 Plenius saithe. While the medicinal powers of purslane against an aching bladder are regularly recorded in Classical (*MM*), medieval (*LS*) and Renaissance pharmacopeia (Fu), Pliny never actually mentions it in connection with this species. The passage is best explained as a misinterpretation in *Ω*: the ME translator took *DVH* 762–764 to form a syntactic unit, but this cannot be the case since *DVH* 762 *vesicaeque* links that line with the previous virtue about the purgative virtues of the species. The reference in any case was already inaccurate in *DVH*, for *NH* xxv.162 compares purslane to "aizoi" (the houseleek, as suggested by the literature in → **709**), rather than "acidulae" (i.e. the sourdock, → **1879**).

984 and... horshoo. This fragment, missing in the Northern versions of the entry (*W*.37v/26 just reads ‹þat is dry & cald›), must be an addition in the $\varLambda S_1$ branch. *Horshoo* usually refers to *Hippocrepis comosa* L. (PDE *horseshoe vetch*), but this is a post-medieval word (OED: *s.v.* horseshoe *n.* records the first instance of this word in 1706). Its appearance here is surely due to a reading or copy mistake for *h o r s - h o u e , translating ML *ungula cavalli/caballina*. While this is a name for *Tussilago farfara*, it was sometimes confused with *Portulaca*, as seen also in the synonymy given in *DVH(SME)* and part of the Literature quoted at → **963**.

986 isope. The Latin headword and the ME name refer to hyssop (*Hyssopus officinalis* L.). From ‹Also› 994 onwards the entry follows the appropriate chapter in *DVH*, but the source of the preceding lines remains untraced. Whatever the original text might have been, the reference to hyssop being hot and dry in the second degree must be regarded as a mere copy mistake, since all medical *auctoritates* since Galen concur in attributing a more acute temperament—bar Ge, which does not mention that information but is unlikely to differ from the other authors in this point.

Medically, the untraced section of the entry states that the species is abortifacient (**987**), tonic and ophthalmic (**988**), hepatic (or splenetic, → **989**), anthydropic (**990**), antiaphthic (**993**). Of these, the tonic, ophthalmic and anthydropic are in *MM*, as is the antiaphthic virtue if one takes the English version as a loose rendering of the Dioscoridean account of the species's powers against toothache (note for example the common reference to vinegar, σὺν ὄξει/‹with aysell›, in both texts). Concerning the section drawn from *DVH*, the species is claimed to be antiraucedo and pulmonic (→ **995**), antitussive and antiphthisic (**996** = *DVH* 1510–1512), laxative, phlegmagogue and carminative (**999** = *DVH* 1513–1517), anti-inflammatory (**1000**–**1001** = *DVH* 1534–1524), antiodontalgic (**1001** = *DVH* 1525–1526), and antiotalgic (or so it seems, → **1003**). The virtues contained in *DVH* 1518–1524 (tonic and anthydropic) and 1527–1531 (acoustic, and anticteric) are yet missing. The combination of two separate textual traditions probably explains that some properties are repeated in both halves: pulmonic (**990** and → **995**), anthelminthic (**989** and **995** = *DVH* 1509), antiasthmatic (**992** and **1000**, apparently related to *DVH* 1510–1511 but not in Choulant's canonical edition). Note as well that the tonic and anthydropic virtues of *DVH* 1518–1522 are missing in the section from Macer Floridus's work but are included in the section of the text drawn from an uncertain treatise. It is hence possible that the source for this section ultimately came from *DVH* as well—although both ideas are routinely included in the usual pharmacographic literature since *MM* iii.25,2 (περιποιεῖ δὲ καὶ εὔχροιαν. καταπλάσσεται δὲ μετὰ σύκου καὶ νίτρου πρὸς σπλῆνα καὶ ὕδρωπα, "it achieves even fresh and healthy looks. It is used as a plaster with fig and soda for the spleen and for edemata").

Literature: HYSSOP (*Hyssopus officinalis* L.): *MM* iii.25 (ὕσσωπος); *NH* xxv.136 (*hysopum*); *SM* xii.149; *RM* ii.269; *Grad.* 370; *DVH* 1503–1531 (*ysopum*); *LS* 260 (*cyfæ* [زُوفَا *zūfā*], *hysopus sicca*); *EPN* ii (*cedria. hissæp*), vi (*ysopus. ysope*), vii (*hic ysopus. ysoppe*), viii (*hic isopus. ysope*), ix (*hic isopus. isopp*); *Cl* 1.2 (*isopus. isope*); *TH* 232 (*isopus*); *DVH(NME)* 251r.24 (*ysope*); *DVH(SME)* 12b.13 (*isope*); *Alph.* 87 (*iria maior et minor galielni, ysopus*), 197 (*ysopus. ysope*); *Sin.Bart.* 25 (*ysopus agrestis, satureia*);

AC 192.28 (*isopus. ysope*) ⚭ GH 213 (ISOPUS, *ysope, asoe oneal*); Fu 324 (ΎΣΣΩΠΟΣ, *hyssopus*); Tu 2.399 (HYSOP); DL 162 (HYSSOPE, *hyssopus*); Ge 463 (HYSSOPE, *hyssopus*).

C³S³ (*SM, RM, Grad., DVH, LS, CI, TH, GH,* Fu, DL)

989 the lyuer. A hepatic virtue is not recorded for this species in the usual medical literature, but its position within the entry, near the reference to dropsy, suggests that this passage originally dealt with the spleen and hence derives ultimately from *MM* iii.25, § 2 (see quotation above). As for the reference to lungs that immediately follows, → **995**.

995 þe mylt. While splenetic qualities have been attached to this species at least since *MM* (→ **989**), reference to the spleen is unexpected here in light of the parallel line in the Latin poem, which reads *Et prodest cunctis pulmonum sumpta querelis* (*DVH* 1508). No MSS in Choulant's apparatus criticus offers a reading *l i e n u m or *s p l e n u m that would account for the ME translation, but a faulty Latin exemplar might have triggered the misreading: note the common presence of letters **p**, **l** and **n** in both *splenum* and *pulmonum*.

1002 also… 1004 ham. An obscure passage that could have been mangled already in the original Latin exemplar: several of the MSS used by Choulant for his edition miss the last two lines of the chapter and there are major variants in the *apparatus*. The main problem with the ME text is ascertaining the sense of ⟨hosyng⟩. The possibility that this is etymologically related to ME *hōse* < OE *hās* "hoarse" should be discarded for a number of reasons, both linguistic and extra-linguistic. Linguistically, that explanation renders unnecessary the presence of the tag ⟨of one-is⟩ unless a word such as * v o i s e is added, but then "voice" is only implied, never actually mentioned, in the references to hoarseness in the text (see **807** and **995**; naturally turns of phrase such as "X clears/opens the voice" in **777** or **2087** do not belong here). Moreover, it would not be easy to explain the antecedent of the pronoun ⟨ham⟩ that appears later on as there is no noun in the plural in the sentence (of course an assumed *v o i s e would not qualify here as it is in the singular and does not refer to any organ that can become swollen). Textually, while there is a reference to hoarseness in the corresponding Latin chapter, this is found at the beginning of the entry (*DVH* 1507) and was duly translated at the expected place in the ME version (cf. **995** ⟨for hosnes⟩). A second possibility is that the passage is a translation of *DVH* 1528–1529, where ⟨yf hit be sod and y-laide⟩ neatly renders *elixum appositum*. Would this prove correct, then ⟨hosyng of one-is⟩ must represent *livores* [var. *humores* in several early editions] … *omnes*, yet this could not account for the tag ⟨of one-is⟩ but would offer an equation ME

⟨hosyng⟩ = La. *livores/humores* that is equally hard to explain—even more so since, just like *voice, skin spots nor humours can hardly become swollen. Perhaps ⟨swellyng of ham⟩ is in fact connected to *DVH* 1530–1531, which deals with earache, and that *h o s y n g   o f   o n e - i s   e r i s was originally intended, perhaps from an exemplary reading such as *(H)AKYNG OF ONE-IS ERIS translating *DVH* 1530 *auriculae ... gravem ... dolorem*.

1006 ivy. The Latin heading, and the ME name point to ivy (*Hedera helix* L.). Although some English sources (particularly the early ones, see *EPN* for details) seem to have used the Latin heading to refer to some *Lonicera* L. spp. (probably the woodbine, *L. periclymenum* L., or else ground ivy, *Glechoma hederacea* L.), the reference to black berries makes those identifications impossible as the berries of the woodbine are red and ground ivy of course displays no berries at all.

The species is said to be anti-inflammatory (**1009**), anticephalalgic (**1011**) and good against sunstroke (**1012**), and lithontriptic (**1016**). While the anticephalalgic virtue of this species is recorded in most sources, its usefulness against swellings and insolation is not found in the usual pharmacographic literature. References to ivy as a good stone breaker seem to appear in English sources only (*GH*, Ge).

The text closely follows *AC*, but the last virtue against the stone is apparently missing in that tradition.

Literature: IVY (*Hedera helix* L.): *HP* i.3.2 (κίττος); *MM* ii.179 (κίσσος); *NH* xvi.144 (*hedera*); *SM* xii.29; *RM* ii.225; *OEH* 121 (*herba hedera crysocantes. ifig*); *Dur.Glos.* 303 (*hedera. ifig*); *LS* 41 (*lebleb, acsin/athin* [ﻟﺒﻼب، أﻗﻄﯿﻦ *lablāb, aqṭin*], *volubilis minor, cussus*); *EPN* ii (*hedera nigra. wudebinde*), iii (*eder. ifig*), iv (*hedera nigra. eorð-ifig*), vi (*hedera nigra. iere. oerþ-ivi*), vii (*hec edera. iwyn*); *TH* 172 (*edera nigra*); *Pand.* 165 (GRcissos, LAhedera), 366 (ARieblech, GRcussus, LAvolubilis); *Alph.* 4 (*allacium. edera*), 52 (*edera arborea. yuy*); *Sin.Bart.* 18 (*edera arborea. yvi*); *AC* 184.3 (*edera. iwy*) ❦ *GH* 163 (EDERA MAGNA, *edera arborea, cissomelle, yuy*); *Fu* 159 (ΚΙΣΣΟΣ, *hedera, dyonisia*); *DL* 280 (IUIE, κίσσος, *hedera nigra, dyonisia, hedera arborea, hedera muralis*); *Ge* 707 (IUIE, κίττος, *hedera attollens, hedera assurgens. hedera excelsa, hedera arborea, hedera muralis*).

C¹S¹ (*LS*) | F³S³ (*SM*)

1006 he hathe to him an herbe that is callid bryony. The sentence makes little sense unless the author intended to say that bryony (*Bryonia cretica* subsp. *dioica* (Jacq.) Tutin) grows near ivy, which is an unlikely possibility. Comparison with the source text indicates that in fact the passage is faulty here and the exemplar must have read something like *HE HAÞ LEVYS LIKE AN HERBE THAT IS CALLID BRYONY, cf. "it haȝt lewys lik an herbe men clepe bryan" (*AC* 153.4–5). Part of the same fragment (from "ha3t" to "he*r*be") is missing in MS B of that tradition, and this could indicate a common faulty exemplar for both MSS.

1018 ive. Comparison with the source text, *AC*, shows that the chapter combines information from the beginning of the entries *Iua* (up to ‹downe› **1020**) and *Iarus* that must have followed in the original version of the herbal. The mistake was not made by Lelamour but was already in the copy of *AC* that he used as an exemplar, as evident from the fact that at least ten MSS of that tradition share that feature (Brodin 1950: 104–105 used this as Token 5 to separate the MSS of that tradition into two main branches).

While the ‹knobbys of þe rotis› (**1022**) surely mean the tubers of many aroids and hence support the idea that the virtues given in the entry refer in fact to the plant *Iarus* (the cuckoo-pint, *Arum maculatum* L., as seen from the accurate physical description in *AC*), identification of the species meant in the first part of the entry is unclear. The synonyms ‹ive› and ‹herbe yue› can mean ground pine (*Ajuga chamaepitys* L.), but ‹hertishorne› and the comparison drawn between the leaves of the plant and the antlers of a hart is regularly found in connection with buck-horn's plantain (*Plantago coronopus* L.) and swine's cress (*Lepidium coronopus* (L.) Al-Shehbaz). As for the Latin headword, it refers to danewort (*Sambucus ebulus* L.), in case it is the same misspelling of *ostriago* that can also be found in *EPN* vi. The confusion may lie on a mistake in some synonyma between *c(h)ameacte (χαμαιάκτη, the usual Greek name for the *Sambucus*) and *cardamine, *cardamum or even *c(h)amedafne (χαμαιδάφνη, usually the Alexandrian laurel, *Danae racemosa* (L.) Moench, but applied to some crowfoot or buttercup (*Ranunculus* L. spp.) in several English sources, cf. *Dur.Glos.* and PNME: *s.v.* camedaphne, whence it might have been loosely attached to the equally bitter *Lepidium*).

Always bearing into account that the virtues in this entry must refer in principle to the cuckoo-pint and not to the plantain/cress, in the entry the species is said to be laxative (**1022**), cosmetic (**1024**), dietetic (**1026**) and antidysenteric (**1027**). None of this matches the literature on these species. According to Classical pharmacopoeia, *coronopus* was used against the coeliac disease, while the Renaissance authors commended it as a good lithontriptic and antihematuric (DL), ophthalmic and febrifuge (Ge). As for *Arum*, Greeks and Romans thought it good for the same diseases as the dragons (→ **38**), besides being a good antipodagric, while medieval pharmacopoeia also praised it as an ophthalmic, antiherpetic and lithontriptic (*Grad.*), expectorant and febrifuge (see for instance *Cl*).

Literature: BUCK-HORN'S PLANTAIN (*Plantago coronopus* L.)/SWINE'S CRESS (*Lepidium coronopus* (L.) Al-Shehbaz): *HP* vii.8.3 (κορωνόπους); *MM* ii.130; *NH* xxii.48 (*coronopus*); *SM* xii.40; *RM* ii.230; *Dur.Glos.* 301 (*chamedafne. leoth vyrt, hreafnes fot*); *EPN* vi (*iva. ive | ostragium. herbyve. lipe-wurt*); *TH* 136 (*cornucervino, scornamontone*); *Alph.* 46 (*cornu seruinum. erbeyue*), 208 (*coronopus. mala cytonia*); *Sin.Bart.* 17 (*cornu cervi. herbive*); *AC* 193.21 (*iua. herbe jue*) ❀ Fu 169 (ΚΟΡΩΝΟΠΟΥΣ, ἄστριον, *pes cornicis, sanguinaria, stellæ, ceruinum cornu*); Tu 1.288 (HERBE IVE, *coronopus, silago*); DL 66 (BUCKHORNE PLANTAINE, *coronop plantaine, herbe iue, crowfoote plantaine, buckhorne, harts horne plantaine, conu ceruinum, herba stellæ, stellaria*), Ge 346 (BUCKHORNE PLANTAINE, *harts horne, herbe iuie, herbe Eue, cornu ceruinum, herba stella, stellaria, harenaria, sanguinaria*, κορωνόπους). ¶ CUCKOO-PINT (*Arum maculatum* L.): *HP* vii.12.2 (ἄρον); *MM* ii.167; *NH* xxiv.142–148 (*aron*); *SM* xi.839; *RM* ii.196; Grad. 350 (*aros*); LS 43 (*sara* [ەارص *ṣāra*], *aron, iarus*); *Cl* A.34 (*Aaron, iarus*); Pand. 1 (GR*Aaron,* AR*siricantica,* LA*barba Aaron, iarus, serpentaria minor, luf, minor Aaron*); *Alph.* 5 (*alcon, [i]arus, pes uituli,* GA*[i]arouse,* AN*cokkowespitte*), 21, 75 (*iarus, gigarus, barba aron, alcon, pes uituli, rasga,* GA*iaruse,* AN*cokkowespitte*), 158 (*saturion, iarus, leporina,* GA*iarouse,* AN*kukkowspitte*); *Sin.Bart.* 1, 12 (*barba Aaron, iarus, pes vituli, zekesterse*); *AC* p. 165.2 (*iarus*) ❀ GH 214 (*jarus, cuckowe pyntyll*); Fu 22 (ΆΡΟΝ, ἀρίσαρον, *arum, aris, iarus, pes uituli, serpentaria minor, sacerdotis uirile*); Tu 1.242 (ARON, *cockow pynt, rampe, arum,pes vituli, serpentaria minor*); DL 232 (ARON, *calfes-foote, cockowpint, priests pintell, rampe, wake Robin,* ἄρον, *arum, iaron, barba aron, pes vituli*); Ge 684 (COCKOW PINT, *wake Robin, cockow pintle, priests pintle, aron, calfes foote, rampe, starch-wort, arum,* ἄρον, *iarus, barba aron, pes vituli*). ¶ DANEWORT (*Sambucus ebulus* L.): → walworte [**2385**].

Plantago/Lepidium: S (Fu) | FS (DL, Ge)
Arum: C¹S¹ (SM, RM, LS, DL[Italian], Ge) | C¹S² (Grad.) | C³S³ (GH, Fu, Tu, DL[English])

1031 jubarbe. The Latin headword, English synonyms and physical description suggest that the entry describes the houseleek (*Sempervivum tectorum* L.), a species already treated in the treatise (→ **709**); an akin—arguably the same—plant is described in → **2151** and maybe in → **2262** as well. Identification is borne out on pharmacographic grounds as well: the species is maturative (**1036**), antipyrotic (**1039**), refrigerant (**1040**), anti-inflammatory (**1041, 1043**), and consolidative (**1044**). All except the last virtue are regularly found in the usual medical literature since *MM*.

Textually, the entry derives from *AC* but there are a number of differences between both texts. In Brodin's text, the antipyrotic quality of the species follows rather than precedes the refrigerant virtue. *AC* similarly refers to the temperament ("colde & moyste", just like *LS*) but this information is missing in *LH*. Moreover, the final part of the entry (from ‹Also› **1041** onwards) looks like an interpolation from another source.

Literature: Houseleek (*Sempervivum tectorum* L.): *HP* vii.15.2 (ἀείζῳον); *MM* iv.89 (ἀείζῳον τὸ μικρόν); *NH* xxv.160–161 (*sedum, aizoum*); *SM* xi.815 (ἀείζῳον); *RM* ii.188; *Grad*. 374 (*semperuiua*); *OEH* 125 (*herba semperuiuus. sinfulle*); *Dur.Glos*. 305 (*semperuimus. sinfulle*); *LS* 340 (*beiahalalem* [حيّ العالم] *ḥayy al-'ālam*], *semperuiua*); *EPN* iii (*eptafolium. sinfulle*; *parullus. sinfulle*), iv (*sempervivum. sinfulle*), vi (*Jovis barba. jubarbe. singrene* | *aizon. sinfulle*), ix (*hoc jurbarium. a silfgrene*); *Cl* s.10 (*semperuiua, barba iouis. senigrene*); *TH* 421 (*semperviva*); *Pand*. 61 (_{AR}*ascukodos, sceha*, _{LA}*sticados citrinum, barba Iouis*); *DVH(NME)* [MS *W*] 37b16 (*fulle*); *DVH(SME)* 27b.22 (*iubarbe, senegrene, lesse sorell*); *Alph*. 18 (*ayzon, semperuiua*. _{GA}*iubarbe*, _{AN}*syngrene*), 20 (*barba Jovis, Iouis barba, sticados citrinum, themolus, semperuiua. syngrene, erewort, houslek*), 80 (*hynnula campana, semperuiua. syngrene*), 167 (*semperuiua, sticados citrinum, herba auricularis, Iouis barba. syngrene*), 175 (*scicados. ayzon, semperuiua, temolus, herba auricularis, polium marinum, barba Iouis, sperma Iouis, Iouis barba. erew‹o›rt, housleke, sinegrene*); *AC* p. 204.3 (*semperuiua. sengrene, housleke, rubarbe*)

🙰 *GH* 381 (SEMPER UIUA, *howsleke, selfe grene, jombarde, abzo, centros, engini*); Fu 10 (ʾΑΕΙΖΩΟΝ, *sedum, semperuiuum, Iouis barba*); Tu 2.563 (HOUSLEKE, *sempervivum, sedum magnum, aeizoon mega, singren, aygrene*); DL 79 (HOUSELEEKE, *sengreene*, ἀείζωον, *sedum, semperuiuum, vitalis*); Ge 411 (HOUSLEEKE, *sengreene, aygreene, Iupiters eie, bullocks eie, Iupiters beard, Iouis barba*).

F³H³ (*LS*) | F³S¹ (*SM, RM, Grad., Cl, GH,* Fu, Ge) | F³S³ (DL)

1034 sede coryandyr. The MS reading is mistaken since a red variety of coriander seems to exist neither in Nature nor in the medical literature of the period, and in fact the obviously correct "sed coryaundre" is given in the source text (*AC* p. 204.8). The collocation is included in MED: *s.v.* red *a*.) quoting this passage as sole illustration of the sense 10*b*, and refers to the entry *coriaundre* for specific identification (but there identification of the mysterious red species is missing).

1044 jubarbe. The main scribe left a blank here, which Hand A₃ later mistook for a gap between virtues and filled with the customary pilcrow. The emendation, based on the internal logic of the entry, is pharmacographically dubious for no consolidative virtue seems to have been attached to this species in the usual medical literature.

1045 herba Plenius. This short entry does not start a new paragraph as is the rule in the herbal but was copied as a coda immediately at the end of the preceding section. Its textual pedigree is untraced. About the possible species treated here, → **656**. The physical description provided would fit nicely that of *Angelica archangelica* L. if ‹verne› (La. *filix*) was in fact a misrepresentation or mistranslation of *f i n e l (La. *feniculum*).

Literature: *Garden angelica (*Angelica archangelica* L.): → herbe moyntayne [656].

1049 kalketrap. A problematic entry from an untraced source. The Latin headword generally refers to the Celtic spikenard (*Valeriana celtica* L.; André 1985: *s.v.* spīca) or else to adder's tongue (*Ophioglossum vulgatum* L.; PNME: *s.v.*). According to DL$_{299}$ and Ge$_{1374}$, old herbalists also applied that name (but falsely) to some moss of the *Lycopodium* genus (cf. *Alph.* 174: "Spica celtica similis est musco"). As for the English name, it refers to the military device to slow down the advance of enemy troops but was loosely used for several thorny plants or species with prickly seeds as well. The exact species is unclear: it is traditionally identified with the buckthorn (*Rhamnus cathartica* L.) or else the bramble (*Rubus plicatus* Weihe & Nees = *R. fruticosus* L.), which were called *calcatrippe, calcatræppe* in OE, but sea holly (*Eryngium maritimum* L.) and star thistle (*Centaurea calcitrapa* L.) make better candidates for the ME word. Although the word "caltrops" is not in the entry of Ge, it is crossreferenced to star thistle in the English table and DL does mention it as a synonym; in *AC* the word is apparently used to refer to restharrow (*Ononis spinosa* subsp. *procurrens* (Wallr.) Briq. = *Ononis repens* L., → **1054**). Whatever the exact species meant, the confusion with *Valeriana* appears to have originated in some English source where *saliunca*, the original (Ligurian) name of Celtic spikenard (cf. *MM*: ἡ δὲ Κελτικὴ νάρδος γεννᾶται μὲν ἐν ταῖς κατὰ Λιγυρίαν Ἄλπεσιν, ἐπιχωρίως ὠνομασμένη σαλιούγκα, "[t]he Celtic spikenard grows in the Alps, around Liguria. The locals call it *saliunca*"), was misapplied to other species: wild poppy (*EPN* ii, *Sin.Bart.*), caltrops (*Alph.* and *Sin.Bart.*, also the *Promptorium Parvulorum*) or willow (*EPN* vii, in case ‹wyne› is a copy mistake for *w y l u e , in which case the scribe surely took the headword to be the same as La. *salix*, stem *salic-*).

Identification is again dubious on pharmacographic grounds, but all in all the evidence points towards *Valeriana* rather than *Eryngium* or *Centaurea*. As seen below, all candidates are either hot, rather than cold, and/or dry instead of moist; it is a bit intriguing nonetheless to discover that the degrees of *celtica* and *spica nardi* in *Grad.* coincide with those mentioned for ‹kalketrap› in the text. Concerning virtues, the species is said to be laxative (**1050**), and good for the nails (**1051**). Only the first one is usually recorded in the literature in connection with *Valeriana*, and then applied to the stomach rather than the intestine, as suggested in the ME text.

Literature: CELTIC SPIKENARD (*Valeriana celtica* L.): *MM* i.8 (κελτικὴ νάρδος); *NH* xiv.107 (*nardus celticus*); *SM* xii.85; *RM* ii.245; *Grad.* 348 (*celtica*); *DVH* 2200–2203 (*spica*); *LS* 52 (*sumbel* [سنبل *sumbul*], *spica ... celtica*); *EPN* ii (*saliunca. wilde popig*), vi (*saliunca. gauntelée. foxes-glove*), vii (*saliunca. wyne*); *Cl* c.34 (*celtica*); *TH* 417 (*spica*); *Alph.* 36 (*celtica, fascigallicum*), 123 (*nardus indica, spica celtica*), 159 (*saliunca.*

kalketreppe), 232 (*senacis, spica celtica*); *Sin.Bart.* 31 (*nardus celtica, spica celtica*), 37 (*saliunca, wilde popi vel spica celtica*) ꧂ Ge 919 (MOUNTAINE SETWALL, *nardus, spikenard*). ¶ CALTROPS (*Eryngium maritimum* L., *Centaurea calcitrapa* L., etc.): *HP* vi.1.3. (ἠρύγγιον); *MM* iii.21; *NH* xxii.18–22 (*erynge*); *SM* xi.884; *RM* ii.215; *OEH* 173 (*eringius*); *Dur.Glos.* 302 (*ermigio. hind berge*); *EPN* iv (*heraclea. calcitrippe*), vi (*tribulus marinus. calketrappe, sea-þistel*); *LS* 96 (*astaraticon, centum capita, iringi*); *TH* 474 (*seccachul, iringi, calcatrippa, cardanelli*); *Pand.* 63 (₍ₐᵣ₎*astariticon, astaruticon, secacul,* ₍ɢʀ₎*biomon,* ₍ʟₐ₎*centuncapita, yringus*); *Alph.* 32, 87 (*iringi, iringion, nux agrestis, secacul, cardobanis*), 85 (*icerdatel, iringe*), 160 (*sanatilis, yringus,* ₍ₐɴ₎*yringus*), 213 (*eryngium, centum capi[ta]*); *Sin.Bart.* 25 (*yringus. saliunca*) ꧂ Fu 111 (ʜᴘʏʀʀɪᴏɴ, *eryngium, iringus, centumcapita*); *Tu* 1.311 (SEA HOLLY; *eringium, se hulver, see holly*); *DL* 373 (SEA-HOLLY, ἐρύγγινον, *eryngium marinum, erynge, iringus, hundred headed thistle, centum capita*), 374 (STARRE THISTLE, *caltrop, carduus stellatus, stellaria, calcitrapa*); Ge 999 (SEA HOLLIE, *sea holme, sea huluer,* ἐρύγγινον, *eryngium marinum, erynge, centum capita*), 1003 (STAR THISTLE, *carduus stellatus, stellaria*).

Valeriana: C (*SM, RM,* Ge) | C¹S¹ (*DVH, Cl, LS*) | C¹S² (*Grad., TH*)
Eryngium: CS (*SM, RM,* Fu, DL, Ge) | C¹H¹ (*LS*)
Centaurea: C (DL, Ge)

1052 a-boue þe nayles. Given the position of the quick, i.e. the ungual bed, in relation to the nails, a reading such as *vndir þe nayles was surely expected here.

1054 kammok. The Latin headword, the English name and the physical description indicate that this section of the herbal deals with restharrow (*Ononis spinosa* subsp. *procurrens* (Wallr.) Briq. = *Ononis repens* L.). The entry, which is atelous, was drawn from *AC*. Concerning the medical virtue attached to this species, → **1059**.

Literature: RESTHARROW (*Ononis spinosa* subsp. *procurrens* (Wallr.) Briq.): *HP* vi.1.3 (ὀνώνις); *MM* iii.18 (ἀνωνίς, ὀνωνίς); *NH* xxi.91 (*anonis*), 98 (*tribulus, anonis*), xxvii.29 (*anonis, ononis*); *RM* ii.195; *OEH* 96 (*herba peucedana. cammoc*); *Dur.Glos.* 304 (*peucedanum. cammoc*); *EPN* ii (*tribulus. þorn*), iii (*tribulus. bræmbel-brær*), iv (*tribulus. gorst* | *peucedanum. cammoce*), vii (*hec tribulus. brame*); *Alph.* 25, 156 (*bulmago, resta bovis, retinens boves.* ₍ɢₐ₎*restebeof,* ₍ₐɴ₎*cammok, yseneherde*), 153 (*raphanus romeus, resta bouis, bulmago. cammok, resteboef*); *Sin.Bart.* 36 (*resta bouis.* ₍ₐɴ₎*cammoc*); *AC* p. 201.26 (*reta bouis. cammok, whynne, calketrap*) ꧂ Fu 18 (ἈΝΩΝΙΣ, ὠνωνίς, *anonis, ononis, resta bouis, remora aratri, acutell*); *Tu* 1.236 (PETY WHINE, *grounde whyne, lytle whyne, ononis, anonis, resta bovis, remora aratri, acutella*); *DL* 481 (CAMMOCKE, *rest harrow, petie whin, whym, ground furze,* ἀνωνίς, ὀνωνίς, *anonis, ononis, arresta bouis, resta bouis, remora aratri, acutella*); Ge 1141 (CAMMOCK FURZE, *rest harrow, petie whinne,* ἀνωνίς, ὀνωνίς, *anonis, ononis, arresta bouis, remora aratri, acutella*).

C (*RM*) | C³ (Fu, Tu, Ge) | CS³ (DL)

1059 sleeþ a man. The entry in the MS is obviously defective as it presents no medical qualities attached to it. The emendation is taken from the Harley version of *AC* (Brodin 1950: 201), but seems unsatisfactory as poisoning a man being described as a medical virtue strikes as quite odd. Unfortunately, the editor of *AC* chose not to provide an apparatus criticus for those entries drawn from MSS other than the Stockholm version and hence it is difficult to ascertain the sense of the original English passage. The parallel section in the Latin translation of the herbal states that the plant was used as antidiarrheic and antidysenteric: ⟨Eius v*irtus* es*t* pulu*is* fac*tu*s et cu*m* vi*n*o & mell*e* bib*itus* lient*eriam* & discent*eriam* constipat⟩ (*Sl*.17v/3–4; the reference to powder, which is missing in *LH*, does appear in *AC*). This is helpful but it is also in blatant contradiction with the usual pharmacographic evidence, which praise it as a diuretic, lithontriptic and antiodontalgic. The Renaissance authors, drawing from *NH*, also commended it as a good vulnerary and antiepileptic.

1061 kerwell. This is a composite entry: the first half (up to the antidinic value of the plant in **1068**) translates the chapter *Cerefolium* of *DVH* as given in the *DVH(NME)* tradition and thus is virtually a twin entry of **1105–1111**. The second part was copied from the entry *Apium risus* in *AC*.

According to PNME, the Latin phytonym *Apium risus* can refer to the celery-leaved crowfoot (*Ranunculus sceleratus* L.; this, together with *R. sardous* Crantz, is the sole possibility given in André 1985: s.v. apium), lovage (*Levisticum officinale* W.D.J.Koch), smallage (*Apium graveolens* L.) and wild chervil (*Anthriscus sylvestris* (L.) Hoffm.), which is given as unsure since it is only recorded twice in Hunt's corpus: and an early 15th-century synonyma contained in London, British Library, Royal 12 E 1, ff. 69r–107v (referenced there as C1) and S_1 (= C42). The ME synonym of course points to the latter possibility, and fortunately *AC* 159.22–24 provides a description of the plant that the scribe of ΛS_1 did not include but which reinforces the idea that the species intended here is certainly the chervil:

> þis he*r*be hatȝ smale lewys lyke to þe lewys of emeloke. *and* þis he*r*be is good in sauo*ur and* it hatȝ a quyte flo*ur* and long seed lyke to otyn.

Note in particular the reference to the white flower (that of the *Ranunculus* is distinctively yellow) and the comparison of the elongated seed of chervil (with its noticeable central ridge) with oats, in opposition to the globular and ribbed schizocarps of the *Apium* and *Levisticum* species. The pinnated leaves shared by the hemlock and the chervil also serve to discard the lovage.

Identification with the chervil is also sure on textual grounds (→ **1105** for details, and note that the species will be treated for a third time in **2137**).

The source for the first part of the entry was the same exemplar from where the scribe draw the second entry kerwell (**1105–1111**), as evinced by the pharmacological virtues that are missing from both accounts and two common errors, *maudeslamy(l)ke* and *glottis* instead of *m a l d e f l a u n k e and *g l e t t i s (→ **1106, 1107**). The sole difference, besides the expected modicum of spelling variants, is a slight syntactic modification in the last sentence (→ **1111**).

> **Literature**: WILD CHERVIL (*Anthriscus sylvestris* (L.) Hoffm.): *NH* xix.170 (*caerefolium*); *Grad.* 379; *OEH* 106 (*herba cerefolia. cerfille*); *Dur.Glos.* 301 (*cerefolium. cerfille, hynne leac*); *DVH,* 928–946 (*cerefolium*); *EPN* ii (*cerefolium. cærfille*), iii (*cerefolium. cerville*), iv (*cerefolium. enne-leac | cerefolium. cerfelle*), vi (*cerefolium. cerfoil. villen | herba Roberti. herbe Robert. chareville*); *Cl* A.36 (*apium cerfolium*); *TH* 125 (*cerfollium*); *Pand.* 47 (*cerofolium*); *DVH(NME)* 248r.9 (*haruall*); *DVH(SME)* 21b.28 (*cerfoile*); *AC* 159.21 (*apium risus. cerfoylle, chirefelle*) ⚘ *GH* 119 (CERIFOLIUM, *cheruell*); Fu 78 (ΓΙΓΓΙΔΙΟΝ, *chærefolium*); Tu 2.389 (GINGIDION, *cerefolium, chervell*), 2.735 (chervell,); DL 439 (CHERUILL, *chærophyllum, cerefolium*); Ge 882 (CHERUILL, *cerefolium, chærephyllum*).
>
> [S² (Fu)] | C¹ (Tu) | CS (*DVH*, Ge, DL) | C²S² (*TH*, *GH*) | C³S² (*Cl*)

1063 helith. The sentence, which is verbless, translates *DVH* 932 *Cum mulsa bibitum pituitae noxia solvit*. Emendation to *helith*, rather than a more accurate translation of *solvit* (for example, *delivereth*, *lousith*…), is due to ⟨helyt⟩ **1107** in the parallel entry.

1078 kokkyll. The Latin headword suggests that the entry refers to darnel (*Lolium temulentum* L.), even though the English name points to corn cockle (*Agrostemma githago* L., another weed frequently found in wheat and rye fields) and the physical description is rather that of black cumin (*Nigella sativa* L.). This could help explain the reference to the two kinds of ⟨kokkyll⟩, which is not found in other textual traditions. While *lolium* and *nigella* were confused in some sources (cf. *DVH* 2015–2016, where *lolium* is said to be Greek for Latin *nigella*, or the confusion that reigns in the synonyma), other texts made the distinction (for instance, *LS*, *Cl*, or *Pand.*). Perhaps Lelamour tried to make the best of his Latin original, which he knew was misguided, by acknowledging the existence of two separate species going under the same name.

Textually, the section is a composite that uses *DVH* as basis: the physical description of the plant and its value in bread-making were taken from the entry on black cumin that is included as *spuria Macri* in several MSS, while the virtues from line **1089** onwards can be easily traced back to Macer's chapter on darnel. But then there is a longish interpolation in the middle of the entry, taken from the description of *Nigella* in *AC* (**1082–1087**) and a third unidentified source (**1087–1088**). The latter part of the entry will be copied again later in the herbal (→ **2538**).

Identification with darnel is also borne out medically, as the plant is said to be anticancerous and vulnerary (**1082**, **1090** = *DVH* 2017–2018), oxytocic (**1086** = *DVH* 2027–2028), leprostatic (**1087** = *DVH* 2019), anti-inflammatory (**1092** = *DVH* 2020–2024) and antisciatic (**1095** = *DVH* 2025–2026). The value of the species as stomachal and hepatic (**1083**), carminative (**1083**), diuretic and ophthalmic (**1084**), and galactogenous and resolvent (**1088**) are, as stated above, taken from the entries on *Nigella* in other medical treatises.

Literature: DARNEL (*Lolium temulentum* L.): *HP* i.5.2 (αἶρα); *MM* ii.100; *NH* xxii.160 (*lolium*); *SM* xi.816; *RM* ii.189; *Grad.* 361; *Dur.Glos.* 303 (*lolium. coccel, ate*); *DVH* 2015–2028 (*lollium*); *LS* 70 (*sceilem* [شايلم *šaylim*], *lolium*); *EPN* iv (*lolium. ate*), vi (*zizania. neele. cockel*), ix (*hoc lollium/hoc git. kokylle*); *Cl* N.4 (*nigella. þe sed of cocul*); *TH* 336 (*nigella*); *Pand.* 674 (_L*aueccia*, _{GR}*ysofracius*, _{AR}*lachinis, lechurios, lolium, sceilem, sirim*); *DVH(NME)* 25IV.18 (*nettell*); *DVH(SME)* 22b.10 (*kockul. lolium, nigella*); *Alph.* 105, 125, 198 (*lollium, zizannia, nigella. kokkel*); *Sin.Bart.* 28, 44 (*zizannia, lollium. cokel*), 31 (*nigella, zizania, cocle*); *AC* 200.1 (*lolium. cockkyl, popy, wyldsauagre*) ❦ *GH* 245 [bis] (LOLIUM, *cockle*); *Fu* 43 (ΑΙΡΑ, θύαρος, ζιζάνιον, *lolium*); *Tu* 2.431 (DARNEL, *lolium*); *DL* 336 (IURAY, *darnell, ray*, αἶρα, θύαρος, *lolium, zizania*); *Ge* 71 (DARNELL, *iuray, raye*, αἶρα, *zizania, sceylen*). ¶ BLACK CUMIN (*Nigella sativa* L.): → wylde sanagrene [**2538**].

CS (*SM*) | C¹S² (*LS*) | C²S² (*Grad.*) | C³S² (Fu, Tu, DL) | C³S³ (*RM, Cl, TH*)

1079 foure hornys tawarde þe walkyne. *MED*: *s.v.* horn *n.*¹ includes the collocation *flour horne*, which is glossed as "a petal" on the evidence of *LH*. This is a ghost word taken from *WG*. In fact the horns are the styles of each of the carpels that form the capsule of the fruit of a *Nigella*. These carpels are always odd in number (three to seven, but usually five), hence ‹foure› cannot be correct, even though the same number appears in source text.

1085 subiugacioun. An evident *lectio facilior* instead of *SUBFUMIGACIOUN, i.e. the "fumes or vapours generated by burning herbs, incense" (OED: *s.v.* suffumigation *n.*); the parallel passage in *AC* 200.15 reads "subimigac*iou*n" here (Brodin's ‹subimigacou*n*› is surely a transcription error), but other MSS of the tradition offer the expected reading. *MED*: *s.v.* subjugācio̞n *n.* quotes this excerpt with a sense "[t]he positioning of something underneath someone", which is obviously misguided.

1098 knotwort. A species of dubious identification. The Latin headword refers to myrtle (*Myrtus communis* L.), while the English name *knotwort* is given in *MED*: *s.v.* knotte n., § 6 as a designation for the knotgrass (*Polygonum aviculare* L.; → **2156**). There are considerations yet that suggest the convenience of rejecting both candidates. First, the physical description provided in the entry matches neither. The plant is compared there to a ‹whityngtree› (probably the guelder rose, *Viburnum opulus* L. or else the wayfaring tree, *V. lantana* L.), which would indicate that ‹knotwort› displays white flowers and small red drupes.

A more satisfactory identification of the species is butcher's broom (*Ruscus aculeatus* L.). It has red berries and white flowers (although, unlike *Viburnum*, these are not arranged in corymbs), and is frequently found in woods near other trees (for example, holm oaks; Font Quer 2014: 941). *Ruscus* was regarded moreover as a kind of wild and/or small myrtle by early authors (cf. the several names used in *MM* or *NH*, whence also the synonyms in DL or Ge), and this would explain the Latin headword.

From a medical perspective, though, identification with *Ruscus* is problematic, since ‹knotwort› is taken in the entry to have consolidative powers (**1100**), but such virtue is attached to butcher's broom in neither the usual Classical or Renaissance pharmacopoea: only Nicholas Culpeper, in *The English Physitian*, recorded such quality in connection with *Ruscus* (Culpeper 1652: 21). It may be worth mentioning here, nonetheless, that bone-knitting has been one of the several powers regularly attached to *Myrtus communis* since Classical times, so it stands to reason that some medieval scholar might have associated the virtue of the cultivated species to its wild counterpart. On the other hand, the knitting of broken bones is frequently found in connection with *Polygonum* in any medical description at the time (although not, curiously, in *LH*, → **2156**), so perhaps the physical description of one species got mixed with the virtues of another.

The final problem remains of explaining the English synonyms ‹gasar› and ‹knotwort›. As for the first name, Friar Henry Daniel glossed the Latin plant name *gazara* as *nodula maior* and *herba/arbor nodalis*, and praised it for its bone-knitting qualities (Harvey 1987: 4, 10). Harvey identified La. *gazara* with *Ruscus* but quoted this very passage in *LH* as main support, so it is much more prudent to assume that *gazara* and ‹gasar› are actually plant names referring to *Polygonum*—as suggested by usage of Latin *nōdālis* "knotty, having knots" in the synonyms, cf. πολυγόνατον, lit. "full of joints/knots", and of course English *knotwort*. As for ‹knotwort›, at least two explanations are possible. The first and surely safest course is to take this as a copy mistake instead of *k n i t w o r t, referring of course to the consolidative quality of the species. This may or may not be the same species referred under that name in one medical recipe (Henslow 1899: 66, taken by MED: *s.v.* knit-wort *n.* to be a type of comfrey, *Symphytum officinale* L., after the gloss in Henslow 1899: 212–213 but without actual support for this, textual or otherwise). The second possibility is to reconstruct an exemplary reading *KNOHOLN (cf. OE *cnēowholen*) or else *KNOHOLUER (OE *cnēow* + OI *hulfr*), which was emended or somehow miscopied by the scribe. (Naturally, ⟨o⟩-spellings in *KNO- (surely representing *knō-*) instead of *KNE- could in turn be evidence of a South-Western origin; Jordan 1974: § 84).

 Literature: *BUTCHER'S BROOM (*Ruscus aculeatus* L.): MM iv.144 (μυρσίνη ἀγρία); NH xxiii.165 (*myrtus silvestris, oxymyrsine, chamaemyrcine, ruscus*); OEH 59 (*herba uictoriola. cneowholen*); Dur.Glos. 305 (*ruscus. cneopholen* | *uictoriale. cneopholen*); LS 278 (*cubebe* [ڊڊ *kabāba*], *myrta agria, myrtus siluestris*); EPN ii (*sinpatus. cneowhole* | *crispa, victoriola. smering-wyrt*), iii (*ruscus, cneo-holen, fyres*), iv (*ruscus. cneowholen* | *victoriala. cneowholen*); TH 84 (*bruscus*); Alph. 118–119 (*mirta agrestis, exmursine, mircacante*) ❦ Tu 2.551 (KNEHOLME, *buchers browme, petigre, ruscus, myrsine agria, myrtus sylvestris, bruscus*); DL 484 (KNEEHOLME, *kneehull, butchers broome, petigree, wilde myrtell*, μυρσίνη ἀγρία, ὀξυμυρσίνη, μυρτάκανθα, μυάκανθα, *ruscus, myrtus syluestris, scopa regia*); Ge 759 (KNEEHOLME, *butchers broome, kneehulme, kneehuluer, petigree*, ὀξυμυρσίνη, *myrtus syluestris, ruscus, bruscus, scopa regia*).

¶ *KNOTGRASS (*Polygonum aviculare* L.): → sparowe-tonge [**2156**].

CS (Ge) | C²S¹ (DL) | C³S³ (LS, TH)

1105 kerwell. An account of the virtues of chervil (*Anthriscus cerefolium* (L.) Hoffm.), according to the *DVH(NME)* translation. This is the second of the three renderings of the species (→ **1061** with discussion, and **2137**). Identification is traditional and reinforced not only by textual comparison, but pharmacologically as well: cf. its virtue against cancer and pain in the side (**1106** = *DVH* 929–930), against slimy matter (**1107** = *DVH* 932), swellings (**1109** = *DVH* 937–939) and diarrhea and vomit (**1110** = *DVH* 940–941). The perceived anthelminthic, diuretic and emmenagogue powers of the chervil (*DVH* 934–936, 942–943) are missing from this account.

 Literature: WILD CHERVIL (*Anthriscus cerefolium* (L.) Hoffm.): → kerwell [**1061**].

1106 mal de flaunke. Emended after *B*.248/10 in light of *DVH* 930 *lateris* [...] *dolorem* (cf. also "þe ach of þe side" in *DVH(SME)* 21b.30). MSS from the *RH* branch are gibberish here: *W*.36r/16 ⟨maudeflamyki*s*⟩ (suggesting a *MAUDEFLAUNKIS in γ, whence also the reading ⟨maudeslamylke⟩ in S_1) and *P*.282/18 ⟨mannes lamyngi*s*⟩. A very similar spelling had been used in **1063**.

1107 glettis boundyn in þe mouthe. Emended after *W*.36r/16, rather than singular *B*.248r/10, *P*.282/19 ⟨glete⟩, in light of *DVH* 932 *pituitae noxia*. La. *pituita* means "mucus, catarrh, phlegm" (OLD: *s.v.*), and in medieval usage was apparently used to refer to the sudden discharge of slimy matter into the nasal and oral cavities. Note that the same spelling was also used in **1064**.

1111 akynge. DVH 944 *vertigo*. Apparently a stylistic decision to avoid repetition of the word *hede* (cf. B.248r/13 ⟨hede warke⟩, P.282/24 ⟨hed ache⟩) that had just been mentioned in the sentence. The modification may have been already present in γ (cf. W.36r/20 ⟨werk*is*⟩), yet note ⟨akyng of þe hede⟩ in **1068**, which in all likelihood was taken from the same exemplar.

1112 lekys. The entry describes the medical properties of the leek (*Allium porrum* L.) as given in the *DVH(NME)* translation of *DVH* 507–548. Identification is sure on textual and pharmacological grounds: cf. its value as anthemoptyic, hemostatic and antiepistactic (→ **1112** = *DVH* 509–517) an emmenagogue and fertility booster (**1118** = *DVH* 518–519), antitussive and phlegmagogue (**1125** = *DVH* 521–525), laxative (**1127**, **1135** = *DVH* 526–529, 548), alexipharmic (**1127** = *DVH* 530–531), consolidative and vulnerary (→ **1132**, **1133**), etc.

> **Literature**: LEEK (*Allium porrum* L.): HP vii.1.2 (πράσον); MM ii.149 (πράσον κεφαλωτόν); NH xx.44 (*porrum*); RM ii.254; Dur.Glos. 299 (*ambila. lec*); DVH 507–548 (*porrum*); LS 351 (*curat* [كُلُّ *karrāṯ*], *porrum*); EPN ii (*porrus. por-leac*), iii (*ambila. leac*), iv (*anbila. leac*), v (*allium. leac*), vi (*porius. poret. lek*), viii (*hoc porrum. a leke*), ix (*hoc porrum. a leke*); TH 399 (*porrus*); Pand. 198 (_AR_*curat*, _LA_*porrum*); DVH(NME) 245r.1 (**lekys*); DVH(SME) 8a.15 (*leeke*); Alph. 148 (*porrus. poret*); Sin.Bart. 35 (*prassus, porrus*); AC 215.28 (*porrum. lek*) ❧ GH 368 (PORRUM, *leke*); Fu 243 (ΠΡΑΣΟΝ, *porrum*); Tu 2.523 (LEKE, *porrum*, πρασον,); DL 460 (LEEKS, πράσον, *porrum*); Ge 138 (LEEKES, πράσον, *porrum*).
>
> CS (Ge) | C²S² (Fu, Tu) | C³S³ (TH, GH, DL) | C⁴S⁴ (LS)

1112 Ypocras byddith. The passage renders *DVH* 507–517 faultily, for there is no recipe against hemoptysis in the *Corpus Hippocraticum* that involves leeks. What the Latin poem states is, first, that Hippocrates adviced to use leeks for many illnesses (508–509); second, that the plant is good against hemoptysis, if taken with a number of ingredients (510–515); and third, its value against nose bleeding.

The closest one can get to a Hippocratic recipe against blood effusion that contains leeks as an ingredient is probably a passage from *De mulierum affectibus* 192 (Littré 1853: 372), but the differences are probably too big for the Greek text to be the actual source of Macer: νάρθηκα ξύσας, ὅσον ὀξύβαφον, καὶ πράσου χυλὸν, ἐν οἴνῳ λευκῷ κεκρημένῳ, τοῦτο καὶ ἐκ ῥινῶν αἷμα ῥέον παύει, "as much as one *oxýbaphon* [⅛ of a pint] of grated giant fennel [*Ferula communis* L.] and leek juice mixed with white wine will stop blood running down the nose".

The other MSS of the *RH* tradition describe Hippocrates as *W*.30r/3 ⟨þe michil mast*er* of medicy*n*⟩ (and similarly *P*.268/17), in keeping with *DVH* 508 *medicinae maximus auctor*.

1116 If… 1118 akynge. The hemostatic virtue of leeks must be an interpolation in the *ΛS*₁ branch, as it is neither in *DVH* (it should appear between lines 517 and 518), nor in *W* or *P*. The fragment may be a translation of *NH* xx.44–45 ("inlitis foliis sanantur vari et ambusta et epinyctides—ita vocatur ulcus quae et syce, in angulo oculi perpetuo umore manans; quidam eodem nomine appellant pusulas liventes ac noctibus inquietantes—et alia ulcera cum melle tritis").

1118 a… 1119 with-in. The corresponding Latin text deals with woman sterility due to a contracted uterus (*DVH* 518 *contractas vulvas*), which may be a reference to vaginism. The source of the passage is apparently *NH* xx.44 ("item ex abortu profluvia poto sueo cum lacte mulieris"). The text of *RH* may have been faulty, for the passage was skipped in *P* while the reconstructed reading for γ looks as having suffered some scribal redaction: perhaps ⟨brenynge⟩ stands for an original *BROKYN, since Choulant records a variant *confractas vulvas* in some witnesses.

1119 wiþ þe fyrst medicyne. This is missing in the other MSS of the tradition, and is probably a scribal conjecture for *OFTEN SITHIS (cf. *B*.30r/8 ⟨oft sithis⟩).

1122 and… 1124 hame. This must be a copy mistake for *ÞAM OFT that translates *DVH* 519 *persaepe*, cf. *B*.245r/1 ⟨þame oft⟩, and similarly in *W*.30r/12 and *P*.269/1–2.

1123 þere-off. A copy mistake for an exemplary *CONSAYUE, as seen both from *DVH* 519 *fecundas* and from *B*.245r/1 ⟨co*n*sayue⟩ (similarly in *W* and *P*).

1124 contayne. The syntax of the exemplar must have been a bit faulty here, so the scribe had to conjecture again, distorting the sense of the passage, which appears to be complete only in Pepys, cf. *P*.268/28–269/2 ⟨and ȝif ony humours comeþ to þe hed it schal spurge it. women þat eteþ he*m* ofte it doþ hem conseyue⟩. The whole passage is a clumsy rendering of *DVH* 521 (containing the reference to humours from the head) followed by *DVH* 519 (on fertility), suggesting that *Q* may have been scrambled here. The Wellcome version dropped the reference to humours from the head altogether.

1124 helith hame. This fragment is missing in *W* and *P*, while *B* and *S*₁ read differently, cf. *B*.245r/1 ⟨helys þe lym⟩. According to its relative position within the entry, this must stand for *DVH* 520 *Ulcera cum melle tritum iuvat appositumque*. The word *ulcus* is frequently found in many medical texts, including *DVH*, so it is very dubious that a competent translator would fail to recognize it. Perhaps *Q* read *MEMBRA here (although the variant is unrecorded in Choulant's apparatus), which was translated as *LI(*M*)M*IS* in *Ω*, whence ‹hame› in *ΛS*₁ (note the confusable shafts of **l** and **h**, and the cluster of minims in the same place).

1129 a catte. This stands for *DVH* 537 *caprae*. The error was present in *RH* and was transmitted to all MSS of this branch (in opposition to the correct *B*.245r/6 ‹gaytt*is*›). The original word in *Ω* must have been therefore *GATTIS.

1132 knetith veynes. The passage stems from *DVH* 545 *fracturas solidat*, as seen also by *W*.30r/20–21 ‹brokyn thing it knytt*is*›. Emendation to ‹veynes› in *S*₁ is probably due to an exemplary *BAINES, confusion between **b** and **v** being common in Anglicana scripts, but it is likely that *Ω* was messy, and hence was dropped in *B* and *P*.

1133 grynde hit with salt. As stated in the previous note, *Ω* must have been faulty here, for none of the MSS provide a full correct translation of the corresponding Latin text (*DVH* 546 *vulnusque recens citu cum sale claudit*). *B* and *P* managed to keep the word *GRENE standing for *recens* and which the scribes of *W* and *S*₁ mistook for some verb that was probably already missing in *γ* (note *W*.30r/21 ‹geue›). *B*.245r/9 on the one hand offers ‹wound› for La. *vulnus* that is missing from the renderings of the text in *NH*, yet substituted ‹asell› for *SALT that does appear in the other MSS. The original verb *claudit* is probably maintained only in *P*.269/9 as ‹stopeþ›, which all in all provides the fullest and more faithfull version of what must have once read something like *GRENE WOUND WITH SALT IT STOPPIS.

1136 lylly. An account of the medical qualities of some *Lilium* L. spp. (probably the white lily, *L. candidum* L., which is the one usually described and depicted in the literature), drawn from the *DVH(NME)* textual tradition. Identification is positive both textually and on account of the assumed pharmacological properties: against hard nerves and burnt members (*DVH* 817–818), against snake bites (**1138** = *DVH* 819), as a hair-restorer (**1141** = *DVH* 824–825), emmenagogue (**1143**, and again on **1148** = *DVH* 828, 840), vulnerary (**1145** = *DVH* 834–836), and against several skin problems in the face (**1146** = *DVH* 837–838).

> **Literature**: LILY (*Lilium candidum* L.) HP vi.6.8 (κρίνον); MM iii.102; NH xxi.22 (*lilium*); SM xii.45; RM ii.231; OEH 109 (*herba lilium. lilie*); Dur.Glos. 303 (*lilium. lilie*); DVH 808–842 (*lilium*); LS 189 (*susen* [سوسن *sūsan*], *lilium*); EPN ii (*lilium. lilie*), v (*lilium. lilige*), vi (*argentea. argentine. lilie*), vii (*hoc lilium. lylle*), viii (*hoc lilium. a lylye*), ix (*hoc lilium. a lylly*); CI L.4 (*lilium. lily*); TH 250 (*lilium*); Pand. 493 (ₗₐ*lilium*,

$_{AR}$*ansea, alscoscan,* $_{GR}$*licina, kirion, krinon*); *DVH(NME)* 248v.21 (*lelye*); *DVH(SME)* 11a.11 (*lilie. liliuus*); *Alph.* 98 (*lilium, elixemum, limphea*); *AC* 195.15 (*lylium. lilie*) ✣ *GH* 232 (LILLIUM, *lylly*); Fu 136 (ΚΡΙΝΟΝ, *lilium album, Iunonis rosa*); Tu 2.427 (LILY, *lilium, krinon, lirion*); DL 144 (WHITE LILLY, κρίνον, λείριον, καλλείριον, κρινάνθεμον, κρινώνια, *lilium album, rosa Iunonis*); Ge 146 (WHITE LILLIES, κρινώνια, *lilium album, rosa Iunonis*).

Æ (*SM, RM,* Fu) | CH (*TH, GH*) | C¹H¹ (*CI*) | C²S¹ (Ge, DL) | C²S² (*LS*)

1140 schepis talowe. *DVH* 824 *pingui porcino.* So in all MSS of the tradition: *B.*249r/1–2 ‹scheype talgh›, *W.*33v/23 ‹schep talow›.

1144 veynes. This reference is neither in *DVH* 830 nor in the other witnesses.

1146 sursanouris. Only S_1 reads *DVH* 835 *cicatricem* correctly: the other versions provide *lectiones faciliores*: Bodley mentions the unexpected "gluttons" (*B.*249r/6 ‹surfato*urs*›) and Wellcome "sour tastes" (*W.*34r/2 ‹sour sauo*urs*›).

1147 flewme and frantiklys. ‹flewme› apparently translates *DVH* 838 *lichenas*, i.e. a type of eczema characterized by chronic itching and scratching, and which results in a leathery skin. *WG* misread ‹frantiklys› word as *frantikkys*, which caused the inclusion of a ghost spelling *frantik* in MED: *s.v.* ferntikel *n. & a.*

1149 lawreoll. This is one of the few entries from *DVH(NME)* that are not in the canonical version of *DVH*. The ME name is traditionally identified with the spurge laurel (*Daphne laureola* L.) and this is reassured by the purgative and emetic virtues (**1150**), which are described at some length. The text also offers a final cosmetic virtue (**1161**) which is not generally recorded in the literature for this species. Virtually the same text will be repeated under a different headword later in the treatise (→ **2217**).

> **Literature**: SPURGE LAUREL (*Daphne laureola* L.): MM iv.146 (δαφνοιδές); NH xv.132 (*daphnoides*); SM xi.863 (δάφνη ἡ πόα); RM ii.206; Grad. 380 (*lacterides*); OEH 113 (*herba lactyrida. giþcorn*); Dur.Glos. 303 (*lactirias, lactirida. gyth corn, lib corn*); LS 324 (*gaur* [ﮕﺎﺭ *gār*], *laurus daphnides*); EPN iv (*lacyride. lib-corn*), viii (*hec loriala. loryalle*); CI L.15 (*laureola. laureole*); TH 265 (*laureola*); Pand. 202 ($_{GR}$*dasnoides,* $_{AR}$*species gare alexandrie, mezereon,* $_{LA}$*laureola*); *DVH(NME)* 257r.14 (*spurge*); *DVH(SME)* 41a.12 (*laureole*); *Alph.* 4 (*alipiados, anglica, herba catholica, laureola.* $_{GA,AN}$*lauriole*), 95 (*lepidon, gingelide*); AC 201.15 (*lauriola. lauryol*) ✣ GH 244 (LAUREOLA, *rybwort, messeron, laurell terrestre, mustilage, vsilien, alipiados*); Fu 83 (ΔΑΦΝΟΙΔΕΣ, *daphnoides, laureola*); Tu 1.302 (LAWRELL, *lowry, lorell, daphnoides, laureola*); DL 265 (LAURIELL, *lowry,* δαφνοιδές, *daphnoides, laureola*); Ge 1218 (SPURGE LAURELL, *lauriell, lowry,* δαφνοιδές, χαμαιδαφνή, πέπλιον, *daphnoides, laureola*); → spurge [**2217**].

C (*SM, RM*) | CS (*TH,* Fu, Ge) | C³S³ (*LS, CI,* DL)

Lelamour Herbal 345

1149 don. Although the reading in the MS has been kept as the sentence may be understood to mean "they are used to make men…", the variant *B*.257r/14 ⟨dowtus⟩ and *P*.280/23 ⟨douteous⟩ makes better sense and is surely authorial. The Pepys version is the only one that records what might have been the passage in Ω, including the correlation *e i t h e r … o r : *P*.280/23–25 ⟨þo beþ douteous for to vsyn for eiþer þei delyueren aboue or be-neþe or þey *p*erische þe bewayles⟩. *W*.35v/15 also reads ⟨don⟩, which suggests that *DON was already present in γ. The whole plant is poisonous to humans (its caustic sap can cause skin rashes on contact) and hence small quantities of the seed or leaves were used as emetic. An adjective warning the reader of its danger would then not come amiss. Note moreover the parallel reading *B*.257r/19–20 ⟨noȝt so dowt*us* ne so violent⟩ (and similarly in *W* and *P*) for ⟨mighty⟩ **1156**, where an implicit comparison is drawn between the power of the leaves, which had been treated at the beginning of the entry, and that of the seed of the species.

1153 iij peny-wight. The text in S_1 is obviously incomplete. Even though the dose to be given to weak men is stated in Bodley and (faultily) Wellcome, only the Pepys version provides a complete passage here: ⟨iij peny-weyȝte⟩ (*P*.280/28–281/1). The spelling for *pennyweight* used in the edition is the one more frequently found in the Sloane version. The other rendering of this entry simply reads ⟨lasse⟩ here (**2220**).

1154 lase. Emended (after *P*.281/2 ⟨lasse⟩) from original ⟨late⟩, rather than *lite* (cf. *W*.35v/20 ⟨litil⟩), since the latter word does not convey the sense "weaker" required here that opposes to ⟨harde⟩ appearing earlier in the passage (on the other hand, see MED: *s.v.* lēs(se *a*. § 6.a).

1162 lovache. Analysis of the ME text indicates the Latin source for this entry is the chapter *ligusticum* in *DVH* 882–906 as translated in *DVH(NME)*. The species is traditionally taken to be the lovage (*Levisticum officinale* W.D.J.Koch). Identification is sure on account of the pharmacological properties: carminative, anticolic and peptic (**1164** = *DVH* 887–888, and again at → **1169** = *DVH* 894–899), deoppilant (**1166** = *DVH* 889), diuretic and emmenagogue (**1166** = *DVH* 890). The same section of the Latin poem served as basis for another entry in the herbal (→ **499**). The lines of the poem dealing with the ophthalmic value of the species (*DVH* 900–906) seem to have been distorted (→ **1169**), while the alexipharmic qualities are given rather as vulnerary (**1167** = *DVH* 891–893).

Other than S_1, this entry is only kept in *W*, but the general style of the translation (lack of a Latin heading, short and to-the-point sentences, purposely omitting the complexion and the introductory etymological matter that is given in the opening lines, and providing no ME synonyms) suggests that the text may have been present already in Ω but got lost both in B and P (→ **709** for another instance of this).

Literature: LOVAGE (*Levisticum officinale* W.D.J.Koch): *MM* iii.51 (λιγυστικόν); *NH* xix.165 (*ligusticum, panaces*); *RM* ii.236; *Grad.* 379; *Dur.Glos.* 303 (*lubestica. luuestice*); *DVH* 882–906 (*ligusticum*); *EPN* ii, iv (*lubestica. lufestice*), v (*libestica. lufestice*), vi (*levisticum. luvesche, luvestiche*); *Cl* L.16 (*leuisticus, louach*); *TH* 266 (*levisticus*); *Pand.* 492 (*ligustici, panaces*); *DVH(NME)* 37r.24 (*louache*); *DVH(SME)* 26b.25 (*wodebynde. caprifolium, ligusticum*); *Alph.* 95 (*leuiticus. louache*), 98 (*leuisticus. keisim*), 102 (*ligusticus*); *AC* 195.1 (*leuticulum. loueache*) ⚭ *GH* 245 (LEUISTICUM, *louage*); Fu 290 (ΣΜΥΡΝΙΟΝ, *smyrnion, leuisticum*); DL 211 (LOUAGE, λιγυστικόν, λιβυστικόν, *ligusticum, panaces, siler montanum, leuisticum*); Ge 855 (COMMON LOUAGE, *leuisticum, ligusticum, siler montanum*).

C (*RM*) | C²S² (*Cl, TH*) | C³S³ (*DVH, GH,* Fu, Ge, DL)

1168 the foundement that is callid colyk. Emendation of MS ⟨coly⟩ is sure on account of *DVH* 894–897, where the anticolic powers of lovage are described. The reference to ⟨foundeme*nt*⟩ (i.e. the anus) is difficult to explain unless it is a case of metonymy, an unexpected copy mistake instead of *s e k e n y s , or else there is some missing portion from the exemplar—although there seems to be no parallel passage in the Latin poem that would fit the sense.

1169 Plenius saithe. The reference to "all medicines" indicates that this passage must correspond to *DVH* 898–899 (cf. *omnibus antidotis*), which deals with the peptic, rather than the laxative virtue of the species suggested by the word ⟨solibyll⟩. There is no reference to Pliny in those lines but there is one to Walahfrid Strabo just after those lines (*DVH* 900), where he is quoted warning against the use of the species for eye diseases. It seems likely that the word *antidotis* on line 901 misled the translator into thinking that the fragment dealt with the same virtue as the preceding lines, perhaps because the Latin original was unclear or defective. The passage was faultily rendered in the other translation of the entry as well (→ **508**).

1172 lauandyr. The Latin headword, English synonym and the reference to the ⟨nobyll sauo*ur*⟩, i.e. pleasant scent, of the plant (**1173**) make identification with some lavender (*Lavandula* L. spp.) virtually sure. Traditional candidates are Portuguese lavender (*L. latifolia* Medik.), French lavender (*L. stoechas* L.) and, above all, English lavender (*L. angustifolia* Mill.). There are reasons to prefer this identification over the former two. First of all, this is the species depicted in DL and Ge, *L. stoechas*—traditionally taken to be the species described by the Classical and Arabic pharmacographers—being described in a separate chapter. Medically as well, the species described in the entry is said to be a good antiparalytic (**1173**), a virtue that Renaissance authors associated with *L. angustifolia* but not with *L. stoechas*.

Concerning the textual ascription of the section, the antiparalytic virtue is found in the appropriate entry of *AC* using similar words, but the physical description given there is missing in *LH* and oppositely the reference to the good smell that the plant imparts to clothes is apparently not recorded in that textual tradition and may be a scribal addition. The temperament of the species is missing in the manuscript used by Brodin as base text but given in part of the family (MSS RB, according to his *apparatus*), and in *Sl*.

Literature: ENGLISH LAVENDER (*Lavendula angustifolia* Mill.): *MM* iii.26 (στοιχάς); *NH* xxvii.131 (*stoechas*); *RM* ii.262; *Grad.* 350 (*stichas*); *OEH* 169 (*stecas*); *Dur.Glos.* 303 (*lauendula. lauendre*); *LS* 17 (*stichados*); *EPN* vi (*lavendula. lavendre*), viii (*hec lavendula. lavandyre*); *Alph.* 93 (*lavendula. lauendre*); *AC* 198.16 (*lauandula. lauandre*) ✣ Fu 341 (ΨΕΥΔΟΝΑΡΔΟΣ, *pseudonardus, spica, lauandula*); Tu 2.745 (LAVANDER, *stichados, lavandula*); DL 189 (LAUENDER, *spike, lauandula, pseudonardus, hirculus, rosmarinus coronarium, casia, cneorus albus*); Ge 467 (LAUANDER SPIKE, *lauandula, spica, casia*).

C^1S^1 (*Grad., LS*) | C^2S^2 (Fu, Tu, DL) | C^3S^3 (Ge)

1175 lavandyr coton. The English name and the physical description suggest that this brief entry, of untraced pedigree, must treat either lavender cotton (*Santolina chamaecyparissus* L.) or sea wormwood (*Artemisia maritima* L.). Comparison of the virtues of the species described here with those given in the usual pharmacographic literature points to the latter possibility: *Artemisia*, although not exactly an antiphtheiriac as stated in the ME text (**1178**), was used to kill moths and other house pests, and praised as an anthelminthic as well. The assumed value of the plant to ward off pestilence (**1177**) is on the other hand missing from the usual medical accounts.

Literature: SEA WORMWOOD (*Artemisia maritima* L.): *HP* i.12.1 (ἀψίνθιον); *MM* iii.23,5 (ἀψίνθιον θαλάσσιον, σέριφον); *NH* xxvii.53 (*absinthium marinum, seriphum*); *SM* xii.119; *RM* ii.258; *LS* 319 (*schea* [شيح *šīḥ*], *sandonicum, absinthium marinum*); *Pand.* 5 (*absinthium, sceha*) ✣ Fu 1 (ΑΨΙΝΘΙΟΝ, *absinthium marinum, seriphium*); Tu.1.217 (WORMODE ... *absinthium maritimum, seryphum, sea wormwod*); DL 4 (WORMEWOOD, *sea-wormewood*, ἀψίνθιον θαλάσσιον, σέριφον, *seriphium, absynthium marinum*); Ge 940 (SEA WORMWOOD, *garden cypresse*, ἀψίνθιον θαλάσσιον, *absinthium marinum, seriphium, santonicum*).

CS (Fu, Tu, Ge) | C^2S^1 (*RM*) | C^2S^3 (*SM, LS*, DL)

1180 lasse sper-wort. The Latin headword and the English synonyms (both of them faultily spelt in the MS, see below) suggest that the species in this section is the lesser spearwort (*Ranunculus flammula* L.), but identification is traditional as there is no physical description to support it. Other Ranunculaceae are described later in the herbal (→ **1851, 1907**; part of the literature there may apply here as well), as is the *maior* counterpart of this plant (→ **2175**).

The plant is praised as a vulnerary, but this is not found in the literature, where the dangers of using it are frequently stressed. Even so, it seems likely that the ⟨wound⟩ mentioned in the text is in fact a way to refer to blisters or warts, for this species burns the skin and makes them to fall away.

The text derives from *AC*, where the same spelling ⟨famula⟩ (likely to be a *lectio facilior*, cf. La. *famula* "female servant") is also found instead of exemplary *FLAM(M)ULA. The same mistake is repeated in **2174**.

Literature: LESSER SPEARWORT (*Ranunculus flammula* L.): MM ii.175 (βατράχιον); NH xxv.172 (*ranunculus*); SM xi.849 (βατράχιον); RM ii.200; Cl F.1 (*flammula*); TH 176 (*flammula*); Alph. 23 (*borith, lanceolata aquatica,* ₐₙ*sperewort*), 63, 214 (*flammula*); Sin.Bart. 21 (*flammula, sperwort*); AC 189.10 (*famula minor. lesse sperewourth*) ⚜ GH 167 (FLAMMULA, *serewort*); Fu 57 (BATPAXION, *batrachium, ranunculus, scelerata, pes corui, flammula, agreste apium, apiastrum*); Tu 2.542 (crowfoot, kingeux, gollande, βατραχιον ... *the second kind, lanceola, spere worte*); DL 305 (SPEREWURT, *banewurt, flammula*); Ge 813 (SPEAREWOORT, *banewoort, speare crowfoote, flammula, ranunculus flammeus, cordus ranunculus,* πλατύφυλλος, *platyphyllos, ranunculus longifolius*).

CS (*SM, RM*, Fu) | C⁴S⁴ (*Cl, TH, Sin.Bart., GH*, DL, Ge)

1183 longe de beffe. The Latin heading *Lingua bouis* and the ME synonyms refer generally to the alkanet, which is as a rule identified with *Anchusa officinalis* L. Since this is a Mediterranean species, in England and the North of Europe the name was probably applied to a slightly different species, *A. arvensis* (L.) M.Bieb. (so PNME: *s.vv.* lingua bovina, buglossa).

Pharmacographically the virtues assumed in the text for the plant do not match the ones assumed for *Anchusa* in the usual medical literature (where it was used for skin diseases and as an abortifacient → **214**), but rather fit those of borage (*Borago officinalis* L.). This is not surprising since it is evident that many species from genera *Alkanna, Borago, Anchusa,* and *Echium* were not always well distinguished in Classical, medieval and Renaissance treatises but lumped together, totally or partially, under the common name *borago* and/or *buglossa* (still given as in single section as late as Culpeper 1652: 18). In other sources (for example, *GH*) they appear under two separate entries containing roughly the same virtues. In *LH* the same species is apparently treated three times in the herbal, each of them drawn from a different textual tradition (→ 205, 214). The present version was copied from AC, which is an incomplete retelling of the appropriate chapter in DVH, but does include a sentence on the antisciatic and antiasthmatic powers of the plant that is not in Brodin's edited version. Moreover, it provides the correct temperament (AC mistakenly states that the plant is "hot & drye").

The species is anamnestic (1184), anticholeric and cardiac (1185), pulmonic (1186), antisciatic (1188), and exhilarant (1190), all of which are routinely found in the medical literature on *Borago*; its antiasthmatic powers (1188) are on the other hand not recorded.

Literature: ALKANET (*Anchusa officinalis* L./*A. arvensis* (L.) M.Bieb): MM iv.127 (βούγλωσσον); NH xxv.81 (*buglossos*); SM xi.852; RM ii.201; OEH 42 (*herba buglossa... bubula. glofwyrt, hundes tonge*); Dur.Glos. 303 (*lingua bobule. oxan tunge*); DVH 1127–1138 (*buglossa*); LS 83 (*lisen althaur* [لسان الثور *lisān aṯ-ṯaūr*], *lingua bovis*); EPN iv (*blugosse. foxes glofa*), vi (*buglosa. bugle.wude brune*), viii (*hec blugossa. oxtunge*), ix (*hec buglossa. langue-de-befe*); TH 72 (*buglossa, lingua bovina*); Pand. 498 (ʟᴀ*lingua bouis, buglosa*, ᴀʀ*sedenalchaur*, ɢʀ*aleptofilon, siluestris bugo*); DVH(NME) 254r.21 (*bugill*); DVH(SME) 28b.16 (*langedeboef, oxetunge*); Alph. 24 (*buglossa, lingua bouis*. ɢᴀ*lange de beof,* ᴀɴ*oxtunge*), 124 (*lingua bouis. buglossa*); Sin.Bart. 13 (*lingua bouis. buglossa*); AC 196.8 (*lingua bouis. langdebef, oxtungge*) ⚭ GH 68 (ʙᴜɢʟᴏssᴀ, *buglose, lingua bubela, wylde bourache*); Tu 1.233 (ᴀɴᴄʜᴜsᴀ ... *orchanet, rede bugloshe*); DL 6 (ʙᴜɢʟᴏssᴇ, *common langue de beufe, oxe-tongue, buglossa, lingua bouis*); Ge 656 (ᴀʟᴋᴀɴᴇᴛ, *wilde buglosse, orchanet,* ἄγχουσα, *anchusa, fucus herba, onocleia, buglossa hispanica*). ¶ Borage (*Borago officinalis* L.): → borage [214].

CH (SM, RM, Fu, DL) | C¹H¹ (LS, TH) | CS (AC)

1192 lvpyne. The Latin headword, ME name and the physical description make it sure that the entry describes the medical properties of the lupin (*Lupinus albus* L.). Identification is also borne out pharmacographically: the species is said to be anthelminthic (1195), anthydropic (1198), detergent (1201), and anti-inflammatory (1204), but misses the deoppilant virtue given in AC, the source text.

Literature: Lupin (*Lupinus albus* L.): HP i.3.6 (θέρμος); MM ii.109; NH xxii.154 (*lupinus*); SM xi.885; RM ii.215; Grad. 352; OEH 112 (*lupinum montanum*); LS 74 (*tarinus* [ترمس *turmus*], *lupinus*); Cl L.11 (*lupinus. a frensch ben*); TH 260 (*lupinus*); Pand. 651 (ᴀʀ*tarmus, termes, tarmos,* ʟᴀ*lupinus*); DVH(SME) 43b.3 (*lupinus*); Alph. 106 (*lupinus, faba egiptiaca*); Sin.Bart. 28 (*lupinus, faba egiptiaca*); AC 197.9 (*lippinis. lyppynys*) ⚭ GH 240 (ʟᴜᴘɪɴɪ, *lupyns*); Fu 115 (ΘΕΡΜΟΣ ΗΜΕΡΟΣ, *lupinus satiuus*); Tu 2.434 (ʟᴜᴘɪɴᴇs, *thermos*); DL 344 (ʟᴜᴘɪɴᴇs, θέρμος, *lupinus*); Ge 1042 (ʟᴜᴘɪɴᴇ, *figbeane*, θέρμος ἥμερος, *lupinus satiuus*).

CS (Fu) | C¹S¹ (Grad., LS) | C²S² (DL) | C³S³ (Cl, TH)

1207 letuse. The Latin headword and ME name make identification with lettuce (*Lactuca* L. spp., and *L. sativa* L. in particular) virtually secure. This is also reinforced by the medical powers assumed for this species, all of which are included in the usual pharmacographic literature: refrigerant (**1209**), hematogenous and galactogenous (**1210**) febrifuge (**1211**), deoppilant (**1212**), soporific (**1215**, **1216**, **1219**), anti-inflammatory (**1218**), and antigonorrheic (**1221**). The assumed damage to the sight if lettuce is consumed in great quantity (**1222**) is similarly found in several Classical and medieval texts since *MM* (αὐταὶ δὲ συνεχῶς ἐσθιόμεναι ἀμβλυωπίας εἰσὶ ποιητικαί, "[a] steady diet of lettuce causes dim-sightedness").

The origin of this entry is a treatise very close to *AC*, although the wording is somewhat different and *LH* missed the physical description of the species that is usually recorded in the section copied from that source.

Literature: LETTUCE (*Lactuca sativa* L.): *HP* vii.2.4 (θρίδαξ); *MM* ii.136; *NH* xix.125 (*lactuca*); *RM* ii.216; *OEH* 31 (*herba lactuca siluatica. wudulectric*), 114 (*herba lactuca leporina. lactuca*); *Dur.Glos.* 303 (*lactuca siluatica. vude lectric* | *lactuca leporina. lactuca*); *DVH* 765–775 (*lactuca*); *LS* 239 (*cherbas* [خس *ḥass*], *lactuca*); *EPN* iv (*lactuca. leahtric*), vi (*lactuca. letue. slep-wurt*), vii, viii (*hec lactuca. letys*), ix (*hec letusa. letuse*); *CI* L.10 (*lactuca. letuse*); *TH* 257 (*lactuca*); *Pand.* 355 (ARh*lra*, GR*tragma*, LA*lactuca*); *DVH(SME)* 10a.12 (*letuse*); *Alph.* 93 (*lactuca domestica/agrestis, endiuia agrestis*. GA,AN*endyue* | *lactuca domestica. latewes*); *Sin.Bart.* 26 (*lactuca agrestis, scariola*), 27 (*lactuca silvestris, endivia*); *AC* 199.15 (*lactuca siluatica. þe wyld letuse*), ꝏ *GH* 238 (LACTUCA, *letuse*); *Fu* 112 (ΘΡΙΔΑΞ, *lactuca*); *Tu* 2.409 (LETTES, *lactuca, thridax*); *DL* 411 (LETUCE, θρίδαξ ἥμερος, *lactuca satiua*); *Ge* 238 (LETTUCE, θριδακίνη, ἐυνούχιον, *lactuca*).

FH (*DVH, CI, TH,* Ge) | F²H² (*LS, DL*) | F³H³ (*Fu*) | F⁴H⁴ (*GH*)

1224 longwort. According to the Latin headword, the entry translates the chapters in *DVH* on the black and the white hellebore (*Helleborus niger* L. and *Veratrum album* L., respectively), a species treated several times in the herbal (→ **1851** and **2385**). As stated in the text, *Veratrum* is a strong emetic, while *Helleborus* is a laxative. The ML name *Elleborus* was used by default to refer to the white species, which is a much more potent purgative (cf. *Sin.Bart.* 18, *Alph.* 53 "Elleborus quando simpliciter ponitur albus intelligitur"), so in the Literature section of this entry the *Veratrum* is mainly attended to (→ **1851** for *H. niger*).

While ‹longwort› and ‹elebyr› refer to hellebores, ‹piletir of Spayne› refers to a different plant, traditionally identified as *Anacyclus pyrethrum* (L.) Lag., a native of North Africa, "plante jamais décrite dont seule la racine était utilisée" (André 1956: s.v. pyrethrum). Its inclusion here must answer to the strong purgative qualities of this plant, as seen in the entry πύρεθρον in *MM* iii.73, which likened it to the two well-known European purgatives. Identification of this plant as a type of *Elleborus* is not privative of *LH*, but is found in other English texts such as *AC* and *GH* as well.

The ME text misses a substantial number of lines of the Latin poem, as it leaps from *DVH* 1785 to *DVH* 1850. Many of these lines consist on a discussion on which patients should be given this strong emetic (*DVH* 1807–1832), and therefore the fragment was plausibly dropped on purpose. There are yet several important medical virtues there as well, ones that the ME translator would have normally included in his rendering without a second thought: among others and in the part of the entry devoted to the white species, the species is said to be emetic, antidinic, antiepileptic, anthydropic, antitussive, and febrifuge; and alexipharmic, antiaphthic, exhilarant and anticephalalgic in the section devoted to the black counterpart. All in all, the gap is better explained as due to a missing number of lines in the Latin exemplar. Even with this handicap, identification of the species is sure on textual and pharmacological grounds, cf. its quality as an abortifacient (**1229** = *DVH* 1779), sternutatory and apophlegmatic (**1230** = *DVH* 1780–1781), rodenticide (**1232** = *DVH* 1784), ophthalmic (**1233** = *DVH* 1782–1783; this virtue is misplaced, as it should have appeared before rather than after the virtue as a pesticide), muscicide (**1234** = *DVH* 1785), acoustic (**1234** = *DVH* 1850–1851), cosmetic and leprostatic (**1236** = *DVH* 1852–1853) and antiodontalgic (**1237** = *DVH* 1854–1855).

> **Literature**: BLACK & WHITE HELLEBORES (*Helleborus niger* L., *Veratrum album* L.): *HP* ix.10.1 (ἐλλέβορος λευκός); *MM* iv.148 (ἐλλέβορος λευκός); *NH* xxv.48 (*helleborus candidus, veratrum album*); *SM* xi.874 (ἐλλέβορος); *RM* ii.210; *Grad.* 371 (*elleborus albus, elleborum nigrum*); *OEH* 140 (*herba elleborus albus. tunsingwyrt*); *Dur.Glos.* 302 (*elleborus. vede berige, thung | elleborus albus. tunsing vyrt*); *DVH* 1774–1832 (*elleborus albus*); *LS* 323 (*cherbachen* [خربقان *ḥarbaqān*], *hellebori*); *EPN* ii (*elleborum, veratrum. wode-þistel*), vi (*elleborum album. alebre blonc | eleborum. ellebre. lung-wurt*); *CI* E.8 (*elleborus albus. peletre of Spayne*); *TH* 167 (*elleborus*); *Pand.* 236 (GR*elleborus, elleborelentum, elleboron, verucaria, polirizon,* AR*cherbachen,* LA*velatrum*); *DVH(NME)* 255v.1 (*walworthe*); *DVH(SME)* 33a.19 (*ellebore*); *Alph.* 52 (*elleborus albus, yeratrum, adorasta*), 189 (*vellatrum, elleborus albus. clofthounk*); *Sin.Bart.* 18 (*elleborus albus*); *AC* 184.20 (*elebourrus. longwourt, pelethre of spanye*) ❧ *GH* 157 (ELEBORUS ALBUS, *lyngwort, peleter of Spayne*); *Fu* 104 (ʼΕΛΛΕΒΟΡΟΣ ΛΕΥΚΟΣ, *elleborus candidus, veratrum album, elleborus albus*); *Tu* 2.593 (VERATRUM, *helleborus, white/ black hellebore*); *DL* 251 (WHITE ELLEBOR, *niesewurt, lingwort*, ἐλλέβορος λευκός, *veratrum album, helleborus albus, pignatoxaris, sanguis Herculis*); *Ge* 356 (NEESING ROOTE, *neesewort, white hellebor, lingwoort*, ἐλλέβορος λευκός, *veratrum album, helleborus albus, sanguis herculeus*). → pedelyon [**1851**].
>
> C³s³ (*SM, RM, Grad., DVH, LS, CI, TH, GH, Fu, DL, Ge*)

1231 rattys and myse floure. The passage is nonsensical, being probably due to a homoioteleuton, but a plausible emendation is unclear. The expected reading should offer one or more words conveying the idea of "thick pap, porridge", as seen from the original Latin sentence *pultibus admixtus mures pulvis necat eius* (*DVH* 1784). Latin *puls* was translated as ‹grewyll› (**1856**) and ‹grewell› (**2391**) in the other two renderings of the same line, and similarly in *AC* 184.29 ("a lytyl growel"), but emendation to *g r e w e l l would leave the word ‹floure›, which looks original, unexplained. Linguistically, and leaving aside the semantic differences between *gruel* and *flour*, the analysis of the whole treatise suggests that the scribe of *LH* used *of*-constructions with the latter word, cf. ‹flour of whete› (**1378**), ‹flour of barly› (**1577**). Hence an emendation *w h e t e / b e r e f l o u r e, while naturally possible, would be perhaps unadvisable too. The near-synonym *meal*, on the other hand, is found both in synthetic and analytic constructions, cf. ‹bere mele› (**301**) and ‹barly mele› (**425, 756, 1789**, ‹barly mell› **2115–2116**) next to ‹mele of lupyne› (**1195–1196, 1199**, ‹mell of lupyn› **1202, 1203–1204**), ‹mele of whete› (**1856**).

1239 colour and flewme. Although he reference to the virtue of hellebores as cholagogue and phlegmagogue is surely a translation of *DVH* 1841 (*educit choleras varias et flegma per alvum*), the choice of words indicates that the passage was drawn from *AC*, although the virtue is attached to *Veratrum album* there: "Also it p*u*rgyt þe colo*u*r of sau*n*fle" (184.24–25; *saunfle* means "salty phlegm").

1241 levirwort. The Latin headword, ME name and physical description point to a liverwort (some species of Marchantiophyta, traditionally identified as *Marchantia polymorpha* L.). Identification is also supported pharmacographically, as the species is praised as a hepatic (**1243**) and vulnerary (**1245**). Both of these are repeated in the usual medical literature. References to the value of the species as febrifuge (**1245**) and consolidative (**1246**), on the other hand, are not normally found in those text, although the former was usually attached to all cold herbs as a matter of course.

The text is a somewhat abridged version of the same chapter in AC, but misses the more detailed physical description given there; on the other hand, neither the bone-knitting qualities of the species nor the temperament are found in the source.

Literature: LIVERWORT (*Marchantia polymorpha* L.): *MM* iv.53 (λειχήν); *NH* xxvi.22 (*lichen*); *SM* xii.57; *RM* ii.234; *LS* 113 (*hazez alsacher* [حزاز الصخر *ḥazāz aṣ-ṣaḥar*], *epatica*); *Cl* E.5 (*epatica. liuerworte*); *TH* 164 (*epatica*); *Pand.* 70 (ₐᵣ*azemalsacher, azezalsacher,* ₗₐ*epatica*); *Alph.* 57 (*epatica, empatica. liureuurt*); *Sin.Bart.* 19 (*epatica.*

liverwort); AC 185.11 (*esparica. leuere-wourt*) ⚜ GH 154 (EPATICA, *lyuerwort, epatyke*); Fu 178 (*ΛΕΙΧΗΝ, lichen, hepatica*); Tu 2.424 (LYVERWURT, *lichen, bryon, hepatica*); DL 297 (STONE LIUERWOORT, λειχήν, *lichen, hepatica*); Ge 1375 (LIUERWOORT, λειχην, βρύον, *lichen, muscus, hepatica petræa*).

FS (*SM, RM*, Fu, DL, Ge) | F¹S¹ (*LS, TH, GH*) | F³S³ (*Cl*)

1248 lycorys. The Latin headword, the ME name and the virtues allotted to the plant—antitussive (**1249**) and adipsic (**1251**)—make identification with liquorice (*Glycyrrhiza glabra* L.) virtually sure. The entry follows the AC textual tradition quite closely.

Literature: LIQUORICE (*Glycyrrhiza glabra* L.): HP ix.13.2 (γλυκεῖα σκυθική); MM iii.5 (γλυκύρριζα); NH xxii.24 (*glycyrrhiza*); SM 858; RM ii.205 (γλυκύριζον); Grad. 347 (*liquiritia*); OEH 145 (*herba glycyrida*); LS 147 (*sus* [سوس *sūs*], *liquiritia*); EPN vii (*hec licoricia. licorys*); Cl L.2 (*liquiricia*); TH 248 (*liquiritia*); Pand. 501 (_LA_*liquiritia*, _GR_*glicoriçaslis*); DVH(SME) 41a.25 (*liquorice*); Alph. 99 (*liquiricia, gliconia, glicoricia. licoris*); Sin.Bart. 28 (*liquiricia, glicoricia*); AC 201.23 (*licoricia. licoris*) ⚜ GH 229 (LIQUIRICIA, *lycoryce*); Fu 70 (*ΓΛΥΚΥΡΡΙΖΑ*, ἄδιψον, *dulcis radix, liquiritia, scithica radix*); Tu 2.392 (LYCORES, *glycyrrhiza, radix dulcis*); DL 498 (LIQUORISE, γλυκύρριζα, *dulcis radix, liquiritia*); Ge 1119 (LICORICE, γλυκύρριζα, *dulcis radix, liquiritia, scythica herba*).

F¹H¹ (*LS*) | CH (*SM, RM*, Grad., *Cl, TH, GH*, Fu, DL, Ge)

1253 lvnary. The ME name is usually applied to moonwort (*Botrychium lunaria* (L.) Sw.) but the physical description strongly points to Italian starwort (*Aster amellus* L.): just like the species in the text, *Aster* bears purple ligules—hence the references to the colour of corn cockle (*Agrostemma githago* L.) and foxgloves (some *Digitalis* L. spp.)—around yellow disk flowers, i.e. the ‹yelowe flourys and rounde›, and a reddish stalk. The suggested habitat for the plant is correct, as is the Latin headword. Naturally, the imaginative references to the ‹merke of the mone› in the leaves and a behaviour for this species parallel to the moon (shining at night, having waning and waxing phases) are to be read as examples of medieval fantasies.

Identification with *Aster* is also borne out pharmacographically, as the species is said to be an antiepileptic (**1262**), which is one of the several virtues usually attached to this species in the medical literature.

Literature: ITALIAN STARWORT (*Aster amellus* L.): MM iv.119 (ἀστήρ ἀττικός); NH xxvii.36 (*aster, bubonion*); SM xi.841; RM ii.198; OEH 61 (*herba asterion*); LS 96 (*astarticon*); Pand. 64 (_GR_*asterion, aster acticus, bubonium*, _LA_*inguirialis, stellaria*); AC 166.9 (*astertoum. lunarie*) ⚜ Fu 47 ('*ΑΣΤΗΡ ΑΤΤΙΚΟΣ*, βουβώνιον, *aster atticus, inguinalis*); DL 27 (STERREWURT, *sharewurt*, ἀστήρ ἀττικός, βουβώνιον, *aster atticus*, *inguinalis, flos amellus, stellaria)*; Ge 391 (STARRE WOORT, *sharewoort*, ἀστήρ ἀττικός, βουβώνιον, *aster atticus, bubonium, inguinalis, asterion, astericon, hyophthalmon*).

FS (*SM, RM*, Fu, DL, Ge) | F¹S¹ (*LS*)

1260 bayis. The emendation restores the exemplary reading, as demonstrated by *AC* 166.24 "bayis". The unexpected turning of *-is in the exemplar into ‹-ith› is relevant to the history of the transmission of *LH*, see Moreno Olalla 2011: 61 for details.

1265 magiron. Although the plant names used in the entry make identification not immediately evident and a physical description of the species is never provided, comparison of the text with its source (*AC*) indicates that the plant in this chapter must be sweet marjoram (*Origanum majorana* L. = *Majorana hortensis* Moench; identification of this plant in PNME: *s.v.* majorana with *O. vulgare* L., i.e. oregano, is probably misguided, see already Fischer 1929: 277). The name was spelt in a diversity of ways: both the Latin headword and the ME name are apparently hapax legomena and may derive ultimately from Middle Latin spellings such as *magitana, magorana, margerona*, etc. (see Stirling 1995–1998: *s.v.* maiorana, and Renaissance spellings like those of *GH* or Ge); an accurate reconstruction of the exemplary reading is hence probably useless.

Identification with sweet marjoram is supported by medical literature, but just partially. The species is said to be sternutatory and hence, good for the brain (**1266**), stomachal (**1267**), and orectic (**1268**). All of these are found in *GH*, but the rest of the pharmacographers included only its sneezing powers.

Literature: SWEET MARJORAM (*Origanum majorana* L.): *HP* vi.7.4 (ἀμάρακος); *MM* iii.39 (σάμψουχον); *NH* xxi.61 (*amaracus, sampsucus*); *SM* xi.823 (ἀμάρακον), xii.118 (σάμψυχον); *RM* ii.192 (ἀμάρακον), ii.257 (σάμψουχον); *Grad.* 371 (*sansucus*); *OEH* 168 (*herba samsuchon. ellen*); *Dur.Glos.* 305 (*samsuchon. ellen uel cinges-vyrt*); *LS* 286 (*merzenius* [مرزنجوش *marzangūš*], *maiorana*); *EPN* iv (*samsuhthon. cyninges wyrt*); *Cl* M.21 (*maiorana*); *TH* 313 (*maiorana*); *Pand.* 532 (ARmercenius, GResbrium, *amatrum, amaricum*, LAmaiorana, *sansucus*); *Alph.* 7 (*amaracus. amarascus, maiorana, persa sansucus, colimbrum*. GA,ANmaiorane), 107 (*maiorana, esbrium, sansucus persa*); *Sin.Bart.* 29 (*majorana, persa samsucus*); *AC* 208.23 (*maiorona. maioron*) ⚜ *GH* 290 (MAIORANA, *margeryn gentyll, sausucus*); Fu 258 (ΣΑΜΨΥΧΟΝ, ἀμάρακον, *maiorana, amaracus*); Tu 2.228 (MARIERUM GENTLE, *samsychos, amarokos, amaracus, maiorana*); DL 168 (MARJEROM, *majorana, amaracus*, σάμψυχον, ἀμάρακον); Ge 538 (MARIEROME, *maiorana, amaracus, sampsychum*).

C²S² (*GH, Cl, TH*, Ge) | C³S² (*SM*₈₂₃, *RM*₁₉₂, Tu) | C³S³ (*SM*₁₈₈, *RM*₂₅₇, *Grad., LS*, Fu, DL)

1271 madyr. The Latin headword and the ME names suggest that this entry describes the medical virtues of madder (*Rubia tinctorum* L.). The physical description is limited to the colour of the roots, which is indeed the source of the red dye. The plant name ⟨rede mader⟩ was unexpectedly used to refer to a birthwort (*Aristologia longa* L.) elsewhere in the herbal (→ **67**). The entry follows *AC*.

Pharmacographically, the species is detergent and deoppilant (**1272**), vulnerary and prophylactic (**1273**), stomachal and hepatic (**1275**), consolidative (**1276**), cosmetic (**1278**), anthelminthic (**1279**), and abortifacient (**1283**). Other than the beneficial effects on the stomach and liver, these powers are not supported by the Classical evidence, but most of them are recorded in medieval and Renaissance treatises (DL in particular mentions all of them save the value of the species as a cosmetic and anthelminthic).

Literature: MADDER (*Rubia tinctorum* L.): *HP* ix.13.6 (ἐρευθέδανον); *MM* iii.143 (ἐρυθρόδανον); *NH* xxiv.94 (*erythrodanum, ereuthodanum, rubia*); *SM* xi.878; *RM* ii.211; *Grad.* 351 (*rubea*); *OEH* 51 (*herba gryas. mædere*); *Dur.Glos.* 303 (*gryas. medere*); *LS* 60 (*paue* [ꝩfuwwa], *rubea tinctorum*); *EPN* ii (*vermiculi. mæddre | rubia. mæddre*), iv (*anchorum. mædere | veneria. mædere*), vii (*hec scandix. madyr*), viii (*hec sandax. maddyre*), ix (*hec ffallax. madyr*); *CI* R.6 (*rvbea maior. mader*); *TH* 406 (*rubea*); *Pand.* 243 (GR*eritrodanum, entradanon, eritron,* AR*faue, eira,* LA*rubea tinctorum*); *Alph.* 59 (*eritridanum, eritrodanum, rubea maior. mader*), 155 (*rubea maior.* GA*wadde,* AN*mader*); *Sin.Bart.* 37 (*rubia major. mader*); *AC* p. 201.1 (*rvbea maior. reed mader, warance*) ꝥ *GH* 367 (RUBEA, *madder*); *Fu* 107 (ἘΡΥΘΡΟΔΑΝΟΝ, *rubia tinctorum*); *Tu* 2.546 (MADDER, *rubia, erithrodanon*); *DL* 386 (MADDER, ἐρυθρόδανον, *rubia tinctorum*); *Ge* 960 (MADDER, ἐρυθρόδανον, *rubia tinctorum, rubeia, thapson, herba rubia*).

S (DL) | CS (Ge) | C¹S¹ (*Grad., LS*) | C²S² (*CI, TH, GH*) | C²S³ (Fu)

1286 maworte. A brief and obscure entry. ⟨Spicarius⟩ is a hapax and looks like a copy mistake, while ⟨maworte⟩ has been explained in a number of ways. MED: *s.v.* mat-wort *n.*, quoting the source for this entry (*AC*) as evidence, defined it as a "rough-leaved plant, probably of the Borage family" and tentatively identified it with madwort (*Asperugo procumbens* L.) on account of the spelling "matwo*u*rth" used in the edition. But madwort displays small blue flowers, green stalks, and lanceolate leaves which can hardly be confused with those of ⟨coluyrfote⟩ (unless this is not *Geranium columbinum* L., → **511**). Moreover, it is unclear whether the word "matwo*u*rth" in *AC* is really exemplary, since other MSS from that tradition (at least B and L, according to the *apparatus criticus*) read ⟨maworte⟩ just like *LH* does. Alianore Whytlaw-Gray, in her glossary, assumed a copy mistake for *m a y w o r t e and suggested identification with crosswort (*Cruciata laevipes* Opiz = *Galium cruciata* (L.) Scop.), perhaps taking ⟨spicarius⟩ as an error for *s p e r g u l a (cf. *Alph.* 168: "spergula major, herba cruciata idem"). This identification is misguided as well, since the species described in the text looks nothing like *Cruciata*, but was accepted by MED: *s.v.* mai n.¹, § e nonetheless. The editor of *AC* was inclined to think that "matwo*urth*" was in fact herb Robert (*Geranium robertianum* L.; Brodin 1950: 247–248), and indeed the physical description fits a *Geranium* perfectly. The fact that the flowers of herb Robert were indeed compared to those of mallow (see below) also supports Brodin's idea. On the other hand, *AC* already included a chapter on herb Robert (→ **636**); while not impossible, it is odd that a species that was lexically so identifiable both in Latin and English would be reprised under different designations.

The internal opposition between ‹maworte› and ‹coluyrfote› made in this entry and also in lines **511**–**513** above suggests that the former plant has petals of a darker shade of violet and a softer stalk than the latter. The description applies well to bloody cranesbill (*Geranium sanguineum* L.) which, according to Fu, "ramos habet tenues, lanuginosos, folia laciniata, tenuia, flores in summo purpureos". Ge further compares the plant to mallows: "it hath many, flexible branches creeping vpon the grounde: the leaues are much like vnto doues foote in forme, but cut euen to the middle rib: the flowers are like those of the wilde mallowe, and of the same bignesse, of a perfect bright purple colour".

The task remains of explaining the Latin and ME names. ‹Spicarius› must be connected to spergula (cf. *Sin.Bart.* 40: "Spergula, i. pes colombinus"), and the several spellings recorded in PNME (*sparagus, spargia, spergula*) indicate confusion with crosswort and asparagus, but it is hard to go any further. As regards ME ‹maworte›, emendation to either *m a t w o r t, *m a d w o r t or *m a y w o r t is difficult from a textual point of view. The word as stands in *LH* must represent an original reading, as it is used also in **511** to compare it to ‹coluyr-fote› and at least in two copies of *AC*, and this greatly reduces the possibility that the reading is a clerical error. It is moreover recorded under several headwords of PNME (*s.vv.* malva crispa, pes columbe, sparagus), sometimes with the spelling *mas(e)wort* (which may be an confusion with *m a s e w e which apparently refers to the primrose, *Primula veris* L.; vid. MED: *s.v.*, where it is recorded as a hapax).

Linguistically, the safest course all in all is to take the word as a compound of *maw* "mallow" (< OF *mauve*, earlier *malve* < La. *malva*). Both scientific and popular synonymy make it clear that several *Geranium* L. spp. were confused or at least likened with *Malva* L. spp., obviously due to the similar colour and shape of their flowers. Comparison between the two families, particularly herb Robert and common mallow, were routinely repeated in herbals since the times of Dioscorides (φύλλα μολόχῃ ἐμφερῆ, "leaves resembling those of the mallow" *MM* iii.116). Caspar Bahuin grouped a number of cranesbills (but not *G. sanguineum*) under the heading *Geranium malvæ folio* (Bauhin 1623: 318), and the botanist Nicolaas Laurens Burman suggested the binomen *G. malvaceum* to refer to *G. columbinum* in his study of cranesbills (Burman 1759: 24). As for vernacular names, Spanish *malva* is applied dialectally to *G. molle*, while *G. rotundifolium* is called *mauvin, mauvette* in areas of France and *petito malbo* in Languedoc (all of these meaning "little mallow"), *malva selvadega* ("wild mallow") in Brescia, and *malobran* (Breton for "raven's mallow" in the Île de Sein (drawn from Rolland 1896–1914: III.315–316). Concerning ME evidence, cf. PNME: *s.vv.* malva crispa, crispa malva, muscata (cf. muskmallow, *Malva moschata* L.).

Identification with some *Geranium* is unsupported by the medical literature. Species from this family were generally praised for their hemostatic and vulnerary values, but the species described here is taken to be a deoppilant (**1287**).

> **Literature**: *BLOODY CRANESBILL (Geranium sanguineum L.): AC 157.2 (spragus. matwourth)* ⚜ Fu 76 (ΓΕΡΑΝΙΟΝ, *geranium, rostrum ciconiæ ... geranium sexti generis*); Tu 2.388 (PINK NEDLE, *cranes bill, geranium*); DL 34 (HERBE ROBERT, *pinke-needle, storkes-bill*, γεράνιον, *gruina, gruinalis ... the sixth kind of geranion, sanguine roote, bloud roote, geranium hæmatodes*); Ge 799 (DIUERS WILDE CRANES BILS, *geranium sanguinarium, hæmathodes*); → coluyr-fote [**511**], → erbe Robert [**636**].

1290 maloys. The Latin heading and the ME names are traditionally identified with the common mallow (*Malva sylvestris* L.). Two types of mallows were usually distinguished in the literature of the period (→ **2420** for other species). The entry seems to derive from *AC*, but misses the physical description provided there and adds a virtue at the end of the entry.

The species is said to be maturative (**1293, 1295**), emollient of the liver and the spleen (**1296**), laxative (**1297**), and hematogogue (**1299**). The first three virtues are pharmacographically recognizable, as mallows were, above all and since *MM*, regarded as an excellent softener: the Greeks connected its name, probably by folk etymology, with μαλάσσω "to soften, to make supple" (Cocco 1955, although the idea was already in Ge$_{786}$, Chantraine 1999: *s.v.* μαλάχη *n.*; see also the corresponding entry in Frisk 1960). The powers of the plant to draw blood from a wound is on the other hand neither in the source text, nor in the usual literature.

> **Literature**: COMMON MALLOW (*Malva sylvestris* L.): *HP* vii.7.2 (μαλάχη); *MM* ii.118 (μολόχη); *NH* xx.222 (*malva*); *SM* xii.66 (μαλάχη); *RM* ii.239; *Grad.* 364; *OEH* 41 (*herba malfa erratica. hocleaf*); *Dur.Glos.* 303 (*malua. hoc leaf | malua erratica. hoc leaf,*

geormen leaf); *DVH* 1962–1992 (*malua*); *LS* 149 (*chubeze* [خبازة *ḥubbāza*], *malua*); *EPN* ii (*malua. malwe, geormen-letic*), iii (*malva. hoc leaf*), iv (*malva. mealewe | malva herratice. geormen-leaf*), v (*malfa. hoc-leaf*), vi (*malca. malue. hoc*), vii (*hec malva. malle*), viii (*hec malva- a maloo*), ix (*hec malvia. a hok*); *Cl* M.4 (*malua. hokkus*); *TH* 291 (*malva*); *Pand.* 33 (_{LA}*altea, malua hispanica, malua agrestis, maluauiscus, hibiscus, euiscus,* _{AR}*eristostos, shobozetitam, rosasamen,* _{GR}*molochia agria*); *DVH(NME)* 256v.8 (*malues*); *DVH(SME)* 36a.6 (*hocke. malua*); *Alph.* III (*malua siriaca, molochia, malua domestica siue ortolana.* _{GA}*mauue,* _{AN}*malewe*); *Sin.Bart.* 24 (*herba siriaca. malve*); *AC* 205.1 (*malua. malwe, hockys*) ☙ *GH* 269 (MALUA, *malowes*); *Fu* 192 (ΜΑΛΑΧΗ, *malua*); *Tu* 2.435 (MALLOW, *maw, malua, malachi*); *DL* 416 (MALLOWES, *hockes*, μαλάχη, ἄνθεμα, διάδεμα, *malua*); *Ge* 782 (GARDEN MALLOW, *hollihocke*, μαλάχη, *rosa ultramarina, rosa hyemalis*), 784 (WILDE MALLOWE, *malua sylvestris, osiriaca*, ἄκοπος).

CH (Fu, DL, Ge) | F¹H¹ (*LS*) | F²H¹ (*Grad.*) | F²H² (*Cl, TH*) | F³H³ (*GH*)

1290 Plenius…1291 for-bedith. This reference is found neither in *NH*, nor any other Classical, medieval or Renaissance medical treatise that I know of. It is not in the source text either, so the recommendation was probably interpolated from another entry.

1301 maydenhere. Both the Latin headword and the ME name suggest that the entry is devoted to some of the plants called maidenhair; since the text compares its leaves to those of a fern, the species is probably maidenhair spleenwort (*Asplenium trichomanes* L.), rather than maidenhair fern (*Adiantum capillus-veneris* L.), the leaves of which are usually compared to those of coriander (cf. the synonym *coriandrum putei* in Literature). The reference to ‹smale black here› in the middle of the leaves must be therefore either the middle vein of the fronds, or (less likely) the sori on their underside. That again points to *Asplenium*: the sori of *Adiantum* are set on the edge of the underside, and its fronds do not have a middle vein. Textually, the section derives from *AC*.

Pharmacographically, the species is taken to be an excellent lithontriptic (**1303**) and alexipharmic (**1304**). Both virtues are attached to *Adiantum* in many treatises since *MM*, but then, according to pharmacographers since Classical times, *Asplenium* enjoyed the same medical powers.

Literature: MAIDENHAIR SPLEENWORT (*Asplenium trichomanes* L.): *HP* vii.14.1 (τριχομανές); *MM* iv.135; *NH* xxvii.138 (*trichomanes*); *SM* xii.144; *RM* ii.188; *Grad.* 349 (*capillus Ueneris*); *LS* 3 (*berscegnascen* [برسياوشان *barsyāwšān*], *capillus Veneris, coriandrum putei, capillus algol, capillus porcinus*); *Cl* C.14 (*capillus veneris. maydenher*); *TH* 40 (*adianthos*); *Pand.* 95 (_{AR}*berscegasten, persice, capillus algel, capillus algil,* _{LA}*coriandrum putei, capillus porcinus, capillus Veneris,* _{GR}*adianton*); *Alph.* 29 (*capillus Ueneris. maydenher*); *Sin.Bart.* 14 (*capillus Veneris, adiantos*); *AC* 176.18 (*capillis uirginis. maydenheer, waterwourth*) ☙ *GH* 95 (CAPILLI VENERIS, *mayden here*); Fu 28 (ʹΑΔΙΑΝΤΟΝ, πολύτριχον, καλλίτριχον, ἐβνότριχον, *cincinnalis, terrę capillus, supercilium terrę, capillus Veneris*); Tu 2.591 (ENGLISH MAYDENS HEARE, *trichomanes, calliphyllon, politrichon, cellitrichon, capillum veneris*); DL 297 (ENGLISH *or* COMMON MAIDEN HAIRE, τριχομανὲς, *fidicula capillaris, trichomanes, polytrichon*); Ge 984 (ENGLISH *or* COMMON MAIDEN HAIRE, τριχόμανες, *filicula, capillaris, callitrichon, polytrichum*).

ÆS (*SM, RM, Grad.*, *LS*, Fu, DL, Ge) | C¹H¹ (*TH*) | CS (*GH*) | FS (*CI*)

1306 morre y-bitt. According to medieval folk-lore (cf. Tu as well), the devil bit off the root of several plants so that humans could not benefit from the many medical virtues originally instilled inside them. The species is traditionally identified with either devil's-bit scabious (*Succisa pratensis* Moench) or autumnal hawkbit (*Scorzoneroides autumnalis* (L.) Moench). The physical description provided in the entry, where the plant is compared to a yellow-flowered dandelion, clearly points to the latter species (cf. the Linnaean synonym *Leontodon autumnalis*). It is possible that the medical powers of *Succisa pratensis* were described later in the treatise as well (→ **2206**).

The entry has particular textual interest insofar as, while stemming from *AC*, it still maintains what must have been the exemplary ME name, in opposition to the unexpected derivations ‹more herbyw›, ‹more herbe yue› and other forms that are recorded in the MSS collated by Brodin for his edition.

Hawkbits were praised as excellent ophthalmics, but the species described here is febrifuge and antimalarial (**1309**), and vulnerary (**1310**). Even so, helping against the fever is attached to virtually any cold plant (→ **1438**), and the vulnerary powers are included in the Classical treatises.

Literature: AUTUMNAL HAWKBIT (*Scorzoneroides autumnalis* (L.) Moench): *NH* xx.60 (*hieracium*); TH 318 (*morsus diaboli, sucusa*); Alph. 120 (*morsus diaboli. deuelesbite*); AC 202.27 (*morsus diaboli. forbete, more herbyw*) ⚜ GH 295 (MORSUS DIABOLI, *remcope, deuylles bytte*); Fu 119 (ʹΙΕΡΑΚΙΟΝ, σογχίτης, *hieraceum, lactuca syluatica*); Tu 2.748 (DEVILS BITE, *morsus diaboli, succisa*); DL 407 (HAUKWEED, ἱεράκιον, σογχίτες, *accipitrina, lactuca syluatica, picris, thridax agria … the second lesser kind, morsus diaboli, deuils-bit*); Ge 232 (HAUKEWEEDE, *hieracium*, ἱεράκιον, *accipitrina, yellowe haukeweede, yellow Diuels bit, morsus diaboli*).

CS (Fu, DL, Ge)

1312 mercury. The Latin headword applies both to some *Mercurialis* L. sp. (traditionally identified either as annual mercury, *M. annua* L., or dog's mercury, *M. perennis* L.) and allgood (also known as English mercury and good King Henry, *Chenopodium bonus-henricus* L.). The two English synonyms and the physical description, where the plant's spike is compared to that of a beet suggest that the species intended must be the latter (after all, both *Beta* and *Chenopodium* are Amaranthaceae). The entry is a somewhat abridged rendering of a similar entry in *AC*.

Most entries recorded in the Literature belong in fact to *Mercurialis* (according to Guigues 1905a: 18, *LS* means either *Chenopodium bonus-henricus*, or *C. capitatum* (L.) Asch., even though in fact the Arabic name normally refers to Guernsey pigweed, *Amaranthus blitum* L.), but it seems that in medieval England the name could be applied as well to an amaranth-like species such as a *Chenopodium* (compare Gk ἀμάραντος "unfading" with the gloss "mercurialis, everlesten" included as one of the *freides herbes* in a 13th-century botanical trilinguale = *EPN* vi). Ge provides an explanation of the mixing of *Mercurialis* and *Chenopodium*:

> [*Chenopodium*] is taken for a kinde of Mercurie, but vnproperly, for that it hath no participation with Mercurie, either in forme or qualitie, except yee wil call euery herbe Mercurie which hath power to loose the bellie.

As seen from the preceding quotation, mercuries were deemed to be good laxatives and indeed the species here is said to be detergent of the stomach (**1313**), while its value as ophthalmic (**1316**) is included in *GH* but missing elsewhere. The anthelminthic powers of the species if warm juice is instilled into the ear (**1316**) look like a compromise between the antiseptic qualities mentioned in sources such as Ge, where it value against maggots is stressed, and the antiotalgic virtue recorded in *GH*.

Literature: ALLGOOD (*Chenopodium bonus-henricus* L.): *MM* iv.189 (λινόζωστις); *NH* xxv.38 (*linozostis, hermupoa, mercurialis*); *SM* xii.63; *RM* ii.238; *OEH* 84 (*herba mercurialis. cedelc*); *Dur.Glos.* 304 (*mercurialis. cedele, merce*); *LS* 232 (*bachala iemenia* [بقلة اليمانية] *baqla al-yamānya*], *holus iamenum*); *EPN* iv (*mercurialis. cedelc, cyrlic*), vi (*mercurialis. everlesten. mercurial*); *Cl* L.6 (*linochites, mercurialis. mercurie*); *TH* 253 (*linochis, lichitis, parcenotidos, mercurialis*); *Pand*. 500 (GR*linostosis, linoçotis, partemon,* AR*alileb,* LA*mercurialis*); *Alph*. 101 (*linozotis, linochides, mercurialis, thalphi*), 116 (*mercurialis, linozostis, lenochides, calfu,* GA*mercurie,* AN*scandany*); *Sin.Bart*. 28 (*linochides, mercurialis*); *AC* 203.3 (*mercurialis. mercurie, papwourtʒ, smerewourt*) ⚘ *GH* 235 (MERCURIALIS, *mercury, linotis, alguras, pallemon, agiliotes, altancus*); *Fu* 179 (*ΛΙΝΟΖΩΣΤΙΣ, ἑρμοῦ βοτάνιον, ἑρμοῦ πόα, mercurialis*); *Tu* 2.452 (MERCURY, *mercurialis, ermou batanion, linozostis*); *DL* 403 (ALGOOD, *good Henry, mercurie, tota bona, χρυσολάχανος*); Ge 259 (ENGLISH MERCURIE, *all good, good Henry, good king Harry pes anserinus, tota bona*).

CH (*Cl, TH, GH*) | CS (DL, Ge) | C¹S¹ (*Pand.*, Fu) | F²H² (*LS*)

1318 mynte. The entry describes the medical properties of some species of mint (*Mentha* L. spp.), which is undescribed but probably stands for the spearmint (*M. spicata* L.), as this is the plant usually referred to in botanical literature when not followed by an adjective (see André 1985: *s.v.* menta). The healing virtues of mints are analyzed several times in the text (→ **863, 1454**). Identification with some *Mentha* is traditional and corroborated by textual and pharmacological evidence: cf. its virtues as a peptic and stomachal (*DVH* 1570–1571), anthelminthic (**1319** = *DVH* 1572), against diseases in the testicles (**1320** = *DVH* 1573–1574) and the ear (**1322** = *DVH* 1576), as a galactogogue (**1321** = *DVH* 1575) and contraceptive (**1325** = *DVH* 1581–1582). The well-known effects of the essential oil of mints on breath (**1323** = *DVH* 1577) and the preservative value of the species (→ **1325**) are also included. The following virtues of the species are missing from the ME account: antiemetic (*DVH* 1571), parturifacient (*DVH* 1578), and anthemoptyic (*DVH* 1580).

    Literature: MINTS (*Mentha* L. spp.): *HP* vii.7.1 (ἡδύοσμον); *MM* iii.34; *NH* xix.159 (*menta, mintha*); *SM* xi.882; *RM* ii.214; *Grad.* 359; *OEH* 122 (*herba menta. minte*); *Dur. Glos.* 304 (*menta. minte*); *DVH* 1569–1584 (*mentha*); *LS* 288 (*nahanaha* [نعنع na'na'], *menta*); *EPN* ii, v (*menta. minte*), iv (*mentha. minte*), vi (*menta. mente. minten*), viii (*hec minta. mynt*), ix (*hec mentica. a mynte*); *Cl* M.6 (*menta. mynt*); *TH* 295 (*menta*); *Pand.* 212, 531 (LA*mentha,* GR*ediosmon,* AR*nachama, dichanacha*); *DVH(NME)* 247v.2 (*myntte*); *DVH(SME)* 21a.20 (*mynte*); *Alph.* 85 (*idiosmum, menta*), 115 (*menta domestica uel ortholana. mynte*); *AC* 204.3 (*menta. mynte*) ❀ *GH* 273 (MENTA, *mynte*); *Fu* 110 (ΉΔΥΟΣΜΟΣ, μίνθη, *menta*); *Tu* 2.449 (MINT); *DL* 174 (MINT, ἡδύοσμος, μίνθη, *mentha*); *Ge* 551 (MINT, ἡδύοσμος, μινθὴ, *mentha*).

    C³ (*SM, RM*) | C²S² (*Grad., DVH, LS, Cl, TH, GH,* DL) | C³S² (Fu, Tu) | C³S³ (Ge)

1322 frote. Emended in light of *B*.247/6 ⟨frote⟩ (and *W*.29v/26 and *P*.268/11), ultimately from *DVH* 1577 *fricatae*.

1325 washe... 1326 festerynge. This passage corresponds to *DVH* 1583–1584, where Macer provides a recipe to avoid the rotting (S_1 ⟨fretynge⟩ seems a scribal mistake for *f e s t e r y n g e that substituted the original *ROTYNGE, cf. *W*.30r/2, *P*.268/16 ⟨rotyng⟩) of a product called *caseolus*. The word, which literally means "small cheeses", was surely unknown to the ME translator, who obviously conjectured on the assumption that "rotting" referred to the ulceration of a wound. The recipe is missing in *B*, but its inclusion in *DVH* suggests that these lines were already in *Ω*.

1327 mostarde. Mustard, common name for several Cruciferae of strong pungent flavour, from the genuses *Brassica* L. and *Sinapis* L. The intended species is probably the black mustard (*Brassica nigra* (L.) K.Koch; → **2506** for an akin species). The entry belongs to the *DVH(NME)* textual tradition.

    Identification with the mustard is traditional and reassured by the textual and pharmacological evidence: mustard is though to be apophlegmatic (**1327**, again in **1333** = *DVH* 1142, 1157); caustic (**1328** = *DVH* 1143, again in

1155); psychostimulant (**1329** = *DVH* 1145) purgative, lithontriptic, diuretic and emmenagogue (**1329–1330** = *DVH* 1146); alexipharmic (against snakes, **1332** = *DVH* 1152–1153, but also against toadstools, *DVH* 1154, which is missing here); ophthalmic (**1333**, and again in **1346** = *DVH* 1157, 1182); antitussive and antiphthisic (**1334** = *DVH* 1159), antisciatic (→ **1335**); splenetic and antihepatitic (**1336** = *DVH* 1162, → **1346** as well); antilumbalgic and anti-inflammatory (**1347** = *DVH* 1185); antiepileptic and antilethargic (**1350** = *DVH* 1191–1195); leprostatic, antiscrofulous and antiscabious (**1353** = *DVH* 1189–1190; but see note). The supposed antiodontalgic, trichogenous and febrifuge virtues of mustard (*DVH* 1186–1187, 1196–1197, 1199–1200) are missing from the account (yet → **1353**). The value of the species against hiccups (*DVH* 1151) is missing in S_1 but recorded in other MSS, cf. *B*.245v/3 ⟨abat*is* 3yskynge⟩.

Literature: BLACK MUSTARD (*Brassica nigra* (L.) K.Koch): *HP* vii.1.2 (νᾶπυ); *MM* ii.154 (σίνηπι); *NH* xx.236 (*sinapi*); *SM* xii.85 (νᾶπυ); *RM* ii.244; *Grad.* 386 (*sinapis*); *DVH* 1139–1200 (*sinapi*); *LS* 363 (*cardel* [خَردَل *ḥardal*], *sinapi*); *CI* s.15 (*sinapis. sineuey*); *TH* 427 (*sinapis*); *Pand.* 153 (ARchardel, GR,LAsinapis); *DVH(NME)* 245r.25 (*mustarde*); *Alph.* 122 (*napeum, napei semen sinapis | naper semen napis*), 172 (*sinaphe. mustard*); *Sin.Bart.* 31 (*napi, semen sinapis*), 39 (*sinapis*) ※ *GH* 387 (SEMEN NAPEI, *musterde sede, seneuey*); *Fu* 203 (ΝΑΠΥ, σίνηπι, *sinapi*); *Tu* 2.571 (MUSTARDE, *napi, sinepi, sinapi*); *DL* 443 (SENUY, *mustard*, σίνηπι, *sinapi*); *Ge* 189 (MUSTARD, *senuie*, νάπυ, *sinapi*).

C⁴S⁴ (*SM, RM, Grad., DVH, LS, CI, TH, GH, Fu, Ge, DL*)

1330 the wombe. An exemplary *STONE must have been substituted in γ, cf. *W*.30v/1 ⟨wa*m*be⟩ on the one hand, and *DVH* 1146 *lapidem, B*.245v/2 ⟨stone⟩ and *P*.269/14 ⟨ston⟩ on the other.

1335 hit... 1336 grewe. A chaotic rendering of *DVH* 1160–1161. The Bodley version is accurate: *B*.245v/5–6 ⟨it draws outt thorow a bledder on euyll þai call tyasyme⟩. The transmission from Ω to *RH* must have been faulty here since all MSS from that branch render the passage in an imperfect manner (cf. *W*.30v/6–8 ⟨it draw it oute þrow þe blede & euils þat is callid tiasi*n* in gru⟩) or with substantial scribal redaction (*P*.269/20–21 ⟨þe olde aches of þe reynes drawyþ out þorw þe bladdere and relesiþ⟩).

1339 the maistrys comaundiþ. *DVH* 1166 *iubeat Menemachus*. As with → **180**, the name of this physician is distorted in most Latin traditions, which probably explains the paraphrase. Both S_1 and *P* refers to "masters" in the plural, cf. *P*.269/24–25 ⟨mayst*er*yes comaunded⟩, surely due to influence from the preceding ⟨lechis⟩.

1342 and². ...1343 saide. The ME text distorts the sense of the Latin passage (*DVH* 1177–1178), for Macer actually warned the readers to use sinapisms sparsely (*raro*) and only with such grievances that are very noxious and have been suffered for a long time (*morbis ... magnis ... inveteratis*). Bodley provides an almost complete rendering of the Latin passage, omitting only a translation of *magnis* (*B*.245v/10 ‹all ald euyllis›), while the scribe of Pepys also dropped the adjective *all* (*P*.270/1 ‹old euyl›). This suggests that Ω may have read *ALL ALD EUILLIS. Since S_1 and *W* read together here, it is probable that the scribe of γ misread *ALL ALD as *a l l a l l, assumed a dittography in the original, and (mis)emended the text. Alternatively, it is also possible that the scribe of *RH* simplified the original *ALL ALD into *ALD, which was kept unchanged in πP but misread in γ.

1343 Plenius biddith. This passage, which renders *DVH* 1179–1783, derives ultimately from *NH* xx.240:

> semen ac radix, cum inmaduere musto, conteruntur manusque plenae mensura sorbentur ad confirmandas fauces, stomachum, oculos, caput sensusque omnes, mulierum etiam lassitudines, saluberrimo genere medicinae.

Both Pliny and Macer Floridus state that the mixture of must and mustard seeds and roots will make a very healthy beverage. It seems that the reference to this medicinal draught in the poem as *vinum* (*DVH* 1181) may have confused the ME translator, who associated it with the *musto* that preceded and assumed an opposition between both concepts.

1344 stampe. This reading, shared with Bodley, corresponds to *DVH* 1180 *mergi*. Only Wellcome reads correctly here, cf. *W*.30v/15 ‹step›. Just like S_1 and *B*, *P*.270/3 ‹ley› looks like a scribal conjecture.

1346 for þe splene. There is no reference to the spleen in the Latin passage, and in fact this is not recorded in the other MSS of the tradition. It is yet interesting to note that the fragment translates *DVH* 1182 *faucibus*. It stands to reason then that the reading in S_1 is the remnant of some word in Ω, which was discarded by the other scribes, but which the scribe of ΛS_1 strove to keep even though he did not know the word and had to conjecture. Among the several ME synonyms for throat, jaw or neck, maybe the best possibility is *SWELUE (etymologically related to *swallow*, cf. OE *swelg* "abyss"), followed by *SWIR(E) (< OE *swēora*) and *STROUPE (< ON *strjúpi*).

1348 ale and borys grece. *DVH* 1189 *adipi ... vetusto*, diversely rendered as *B*.245v/14 ‹ald gattis greyse›, *P*.270/7 ‹old cattes grece›. Only *W*.30v/19 translates correctly ‹ald galt smere›, which demonstrates that the reading in Ω must have been *ALD GALTIS SMERE (see Moreno Olalla 2017: 690 for reasons supporting an authorial *SMERE over *GRECE). The actual spelling in *W* was initially ‹als galt›, which was emended by the main scribe. This probably indicates that the final letterform in γ must have been a badly drawn Anglicana **d** with a loop, so as to be confusable both with a diamond-shaped final **s** (which the Wellcome scribe turned as a matter of course into a final sigma) and reversed **e**, whence S_1 ⟨ale⟩.

According to the poem, this plaster should be used to clean scrofula (*DVH* 1190 *scrophas disperget*), while it should be drunk in order to strengthen veins in the neck, cf. **1353**.

1350 the levys and þe stalke y-brent. A scribal misrendering of *DVH* 1191 *illius fumus*. The other MSS of the tradition read correctly here: *B*.245v/15 ⟨þe reyke of þe bryntt greyse⟩ (and similarly *W*.30v/20–21), *P*.270/8–9 ⟨þe smeche of þe grece y-brent⟩. *A* may have been faulty here or else the scribe was unsure about some word in the text (probably *REIK) and conjectured.

1352 þe litarge. Lethargy was an illness characterized by unnatural stupor or drowsiness, which could be fatal sometimes (Norri 1992: 347). According to medieval medicine, lethargy was produced by an accumulation of putrid phlegm in apostemes around the hind part of the brain. Some physicians, such as Gilbert the Englishman (*CM* 107v) or Serapion the Younger (*LS* i.17), stated that lethargy was a sickness that induced forgetfulness (cf. Gk $ληθαργία < λήθαργος$ "forgetful"), together with acute fever and debilitation of the senses (hence the patient's continuous sleepiness) due to the corruption of phlegm. The Classical evidence suggests that the name could refer to some comatose form of malaria or, more broadly, any neurological disease accompanied by coma (Rackham/Jones 1938–1963: vi.70).

1353 helpiþ þe lepir. The ingredients were actually to be used in a recipe to make hair grow again (*DVH* 1196–1197): the recipe to clean off leprosy was a simple mix of mustard seed and sour wine (*DVH* 1198). The translator mistakenly crammed everything into a single recipe. The reference to ⟨evill scroffe and scabbe⟩ suggests that this must correspond to *DVH* 1189–1190, which is misplaced: it should have appeared before the recipe against epilepsy, unless ⟨evill scroffe and scabbe⟩ refer to alopecia (but then these terms actually refer to eczema → **413**) and the passage then renders *DVH* 1196–1197.

1355 medewort. Although there are other, less likely possibilities, the ME name *medewort* usually corresponds to common balm (*Melissa officinalis* L.; see MED: *s.v.* mēd(e-wort *n*. for details). Comparison of the text with *DVH* yet indicates that the entry is in fact a blending of lines 1395–1423, which correspond to the first half of the chapter *Aristolochia*, and the whole entry for *Barrocus* (*DVH* 1641–1663), which does describe the medical powers of balm.

Note that several virtues from *Melissa* were treated elsewhere in the text (→ **267**). The ME entry derives from the *DVH(NME)* tradition. The merging of both chapters cannot answer to a faulty exemplar but must have been done on purpose by the scribe of either Ω or *Q*, since the heading is followed immediately by the virtues of the birthwort, then by those of the balm, but the reason for such decision is not clear.

The usual three *Aristolochia* species had been already treated in the herbal (→ **67**, with discussion on the separate species and their complexion). In opposition to that version of the text (cf. ‹and þe crampe›, **76**), the carminative virtue recorded in *DVH* 1414 and which should appear after ‹feue*r*› **1361** is missing in all MSS from the *RH* branch due to a homoioteleuton *h e l p i s ... h e l p i s, but is kept in *B*.252v/11 as ‹it helpys þe senowys þat er drawne to-geder›. The collection of virtues contained between *DVH* 1406–1411 (antiasthmatic, vulnerary, calefacient and antipleuritic) is missing altogether from the whole tradition (the last two are also missing from the other rendering of the species), as is the value of birthwort smoke as a demonifuge and exhilarant (*DVH* 1421–1422; cf. on the other hand **77–78**).

Identification of the second half of the entry with *Melissa* is sure on textual and pharmacographic grounds, including the reference to the attraction that bees feel for its white flowers whence the plant got its name (*DVH* 1642–1647; cf. Gk. μέλισσα "bee"). Hence also the supposed value of the plant against insect bites (**1366** = *DVH* 1648–1650) and, by extension, against other swellings in the body like those caused in the joints (**1367** = *DVH* 1658) and also dogbites (**1368** = *DVH* 1660). The assumed disinfectant powers of the plant (**1367** = *DVH* 1658) probably derive from here as well. The antiodontalgic and ophthalmic qualities of the species (**1369** = *DVH* 1661–1663) are also included, but a large number of lines (*DVH* 1651–1657), including the value of the plant as a antiparotiditic, antidysenteric and anticoeliac, antiasthmatic and anthemoptyic, went untranslated. The language of such lines is not particularly obscure and the illnesses were regularly attended to by the translator in other entries from the same source, so it is likely that *Q* was faulty here.

> Literature: COMMON BALM (*Melissa officinalis* L.): *MM* iii.104 (μελισσόφυλλον); *NH* xxi.149 (*melissophyllum*); *SM* xii.71; *RM* ii.241; *DVH* 1641–1663 (*Barrocus*); *LS* 23 (*bederangie* [بادرنجويه *bādaringūya*], *mellissa*); *EPN* ii (*malletina. mede-wyrt*) vi (*regina. reine. med-wurt*); *Cl* M.22 (*mellissa, herba citraria. medewort*); *TH* 314 (*melissa, citraria*); *Pand.* 86 (_AR_*bedarungie, bederambia, cirungemil, marulmahor,* _GR_*melisophillos, mellisophillum,* _LA_*citraria, mellissa*); *DVH(NME)* 252v.5 (*modworthe*); *DVH(SME)* 31b.12 (*honysokel*); *Alph.* 115 (*mellissa, apiasia, mellilempnias, suringula, citrago, citraria, melago, herba est pigmentaria. bonrefair, bouruurt, beuurt, beruurt,*

medwor), 156 (*reginela, remede. medewort*), 177 (*scrophularia. medwort*); Sin.Bart. 29 (*melissa, herba pigmentaria. medewort secundum quosdam*); AC 208.16 (*mellisa. bawme, pentarie*) ✥ GH 291 (MELLISSA, *bawme*); Fu 189 (ΜΕΛΙΣΣΟΦΥΛΛΟΝ, μελίφυλλον, *apiastrum, citrago, melissa*); Tu 1.239 (APIASTRUM, *baume, meli(sso)phillon, citrage, melissa*); DL 184 (BAWME, μελισσόφυλλον, μελίφυλλον, *apiastrum, melitæna, citrago, melissa*); Ge 560 (BAWME, *balme*, μελισσόφυλλον, *melittis, melissa apiastrum, citrago, melissophyllon, meliphyllon*). ¶ BIRTHWORT (*Aristolochia* L. sp.) → astrologie [67].

C^1S^1 (*LS*) | C^2S^1 (Fu) | C^2S^2 (*Cl, TH, GH*, Ge, DL)

1356–1357 wysillis bytt. *DVH* 1402 *pestiferos morsus* was diversely translated in the several witnesses of the tradition: *W.*35r/5 ⟨wesils bite⟩ agrees with S_1, while Bodley and Pepys read together as *B.*252v/7 ⟨woluys bytte⟩, *P.*278/27 ⟨wolues bytyng⟩. A variation of this alternation is recorded in → **1965**.

1357 brekiþ... 1358 to-geder. The Latin text (*DVH* 1404) records the properties of the plant as a mazolytic. The passage is confusing in *W, P*, and particularly in S_1, due to the different syntax used in the version, and it is quite clear that it must have been garbled already in *RH*. Only Bodley makes complete sense: *B.*252v/7–8 ⟨brekis þe chyld hame þa*t* is longe stekkytt if be w*ith* pep*er* & myrr*e* dronkyne⟩.

Comparison between Macer Floridus's text and the ME variants suggests that the words ⟨hame⟩ "membrane" in Bodley (cf. ⟨hayme⟩ **1656** < OE *hama*; the sense "placenta" is not included in MED: *s.v.* hāme *n.*1) and *WOMAN in *RH* stand for *DVH* 1404 *secundas*. The appearance of **m** in the words used in all MSS suggests that the reading in Bodley is authorial and that of *RH* a conjecture based on the immediate presence of *CHILD/*BARNE. A reconstructed *RIME "membrane, pellicle" is also theoretically possible (see MED: *s.v.* rīm(e *n.*2), but the first letter in Ω probably contained a loop (a feature common to Anglicana **h** and **w**), and this speaks against this possibility.

The Latin passage, moreover, is inaccurately translated: according to the poem, the species must be drunk with wine (*DVH hocque modo*, referring back to *cum vino ... hausta* in previous lines) if it is to expel the placenta. The beverage with pepper and myrrh actually belongs to the next virtue (*DVH* 1405–1406), which describes the qualities of the species as an emmenagogue after a woman has delivered a child.

1364 þe fester. This refers to a fistula, nor to a festering wound, cf. *DVH* 1423 *fistula*. The confusion is shared by all MSS from the tradition.

1368 wiþ stale ale. A copy mistake instead of the expected *s a l t (e), cf. *B.*252v/17 ⟨saltt⟩ (and similarly *W* and *P*), and *DVH* 1659 *sale*.

1369 Plenius saiþe. This is an abridgement of *DVH* 1662–1663, the other MSS from the tradition giving a more accurate version of the original text, cf. *B*.252v/18–20 ‹þe juys & hony & anoyntt þin [*corr*. þim] eyne þer-*with* & it clenc*is* þe eyne & amendys þ*i* seight›. The use of honey is in accordance with the original Latin text (*NH* xxi.151): "caligines oculorum suco cum melle inungui eximium habetur".

1371 morell. The entry corresponds with the chapter on *maurella/strignum* in *DVH* 1918–1932, as translated in the *DVH(NME)* tradition. Identification with the black nightshade (*Solanum nigrum* L.) is traditional and supported by the textual and pharmacographic evidence, as demonstrated by its assumed properties as antiotalgic and anticephalalgic, antipruritic and antimetrorrhagic (**1373** = *DVH* 1926–1927) and antiherpetic (**1375** = *DVH* 1928–1932). The powers the species against eye-fistulas (*DVH* 1922) and as an antiparotiditic (*DVH* 1924–1925) are yet missing from this version. The species is treated again under a synonym (→ **1519**), but only the antiotalgic virtue is common to both texts.

> Literature: BLACK NIGHTSHADE (*Solanum nigrum* L.): *HP* vii.7.2 (στρύχνον); *MM* iv.70 (στρύχνον κηπαῖον); *NH* xxi.177 (*trychnum, strychnon*); *SM* xii.145 (τρύχνον); *RM* ii.263 (στρύχνον); *Grad.* 365 (*strignum*); *OEH* 76 (*herba solata. solosece*); *Dur.Glos.* 305 (*solata. solesege*); *DVH* 1918–1932 (*maurella, strigum*); *LS* 228 (*hameb athahaleb* [عنب الثعلب *inab aṯ-ṯaʿlab*]*, solatrum*); *EPN* ii (*solsequium, heliotropium. solsece, sigelhwerfe*), vi (*labrusca. hundes-berien | morella. morele. atterloþe*), vii (*hoc strigillum/ solatrum, morelle*), ix (*hec morella. morelle*); *Cl* s.2 (*solatrum, morella. morel*); *TH* 418 (*strignum, morella, solatrum*); *Pand.* 315 (ₐᵣ*hameb, hupue phathahalep*, ᴳᴿ*strignum, cuculus, morella,* ₗₐ*solatrum, vua vulpis*); *DVH(NME)* 256r.17 (*morele*); *DVH(SME)* 35a.24 (*morell. strignum. morella*); *Alph.* 119 (*morella, solatrum ortolanum, solatrum mortale, strignum, uua lupina. nichtheschode, houndesberie*); *Sin.Bart.* 30 (*morella, maurella, solatrum, uva lupina, strignum*); *AC* 202.18 (*morella. morel, houndys berye*) ⚜ *GH* 378 (SOLATRUM, *petymorell, nyghtshade, lesse morell*); *Fu* 264 (STRYCNOS, στρύχνος, τρύχνος, *solanum, solatrum, cuculus, vua lupina, vua uulpis, morella*); *Tu* 2.577 (NIGHTESHAD, *petemorell, strichnos, solanum, solatrum*); *DL* 317 (NIGHTSHADE, *petimorel, morel*, στρύχνος κηπαῖος, τρύχνος, *solanum hortense, solatrum, morella, vua lupina, vua vulpis*); *Ge* 267 (NIGHTSHADE, στρύχνος, *solanum hortense, solatrum, morella, vua lupina, vua vulpis, strumum, cucubalus*).
>
> F (*DVH*) | FS (*SM*, Fu) | F²S² (*RM, Grad., LS, Cl, TH, GH, DL, Ge*)

1371 þe juis... hede-ake. The text seems to have been corrupt or else unclear to the translator of *Q*, as this passage mixes two different properties: *DVH* 1920–1921 describes how the juice of this plant can ease the pain of the ears if instilled, while *DVH* 1923 informs the reader that the same plaster mentioned in the previous line—but not translated—as a solution against aegilops (i.e. a fistula or ulcer in the inner corner of the eye, → **378**) is also profitable against headache.

1374 blankett and þe scome of siluer. The original readings ‹blay› and ‹setine› in S_1, which stand for *DVH* 1931 *cerussam* and *argenti spumam* respectively, have been emended in light of *B*.256r/20 ‹blankett & þe scome of syluer›. The text of *RH* must have been already corrupt, since both *W* and *P* are also faulty here (although, contrary to S_1, the scribes of these two MSS managed to keep *SCOME): Pepys dropped the reference to white lead altogether, while Wellcome offers ‹glayer›, which suggests that γ may have read something similar to *BLAYER. The different spellings in each MS can be used as evidence that **b** must have been looped and hence confusable with the lower bowl of a diamond-shaped **g** in γ, particularly if its lower loop rested on the baseline.

This is not the sole translation mistake in the passage, since ‹oyle and rosyn› rendering *DVH* 1931 *oleumque rosatum* is common to all MSS from *RH*. Bodley translates the fragment correctly as ‹oyll roset›. More generally, the whole passage misrepresents the original antiherpetic recipe in the poem (*DVH* 1928), which is merely a poultice of the crushed leaves of the plant and *polentam*, that is pearl barley or porridge. The admixture of such chemical components as white lead or litharge and oil of roses served, so the poem says, as a way to render the resulting cataplasm stronger and better (*DVH* 1932 *fortius et melius*).

1375 the fu de inferne. A skin disease, probably a type of corroding herpes, that slavishly renders *DVH* 1929 *sacer ignis* (→ **877, 1749** for other designations of the same illness).

1376 myllefoly. Identification with the yarrow (*Achillea millefolium* L.) is traditional and fits the physical description provided in the text, but it is not sustained by classical pharmacopea other than by its epistactic value in desoppilations of the head (**1380**; cf. the synonym *noseblod*, i.e. "nosebleed", in *AC* 202.9–10). Although effusion of blood is referred to in connection with the nose and the bowels, the vulnerary qualities of this species are not mentioned in the ME text, even though they were much commended by Classical and Post-classical *auctoritates* (*MM, SM, RM* and all the Renaissance herbals; the plant got its Greek name from its widespread usage among soldiers, cf. στρατός "army"). The antidysenteric virtue (**1379**) is also recorded in DL.

The entry stems from *DVH(NME)*, being one of the few species that are not included in the canonical version of the Latin poem.

Literature: YARROW (*Achillea millefolium* L.): *MM* iv.102 (στρατιώτης χιλιόφυλλος); *NH* xxiv.152 (*myriophyllon, milifolium*); *SM* xii.131 (στρατιώτης); *RM* ii.262; *OEH* 90 (*herba milefolium. gearwe*); Dur.Glos. 304 (*millefolium. gearve*); EPN ii (*millefolium, myrifilon, centifolia. gæruwe*), iv (*millefolium. gearewe*), v (*millefolium. gearwe*), vi (*millefolium. milfoil*), vii (*hoc milifolium. mylfoile*), viii (*hoc millefolium. ʒarow*); TH 320 (*millefolium, ambroxia, ventus apium, formicularis*); Pand. 538 (_{GR}*minofilos,* _{LA}*millefolium*); DVH(NME) 257r.8 (*ʒarowe*); Alph. 118 (*millefolium maius, supercilium ueneris, centifolium, uenter apis*); Sin.Bart. 9 (*achilles. millefolium*), 30 (*millefolium, supercilium veneris*); AC 202.9 (*millefolie. millefoly, noseblod, ʒarwe*) ⚘ GH 297 (MILLEFOLIUM, *yarow, myllefoyle, carpenters grasse*); Fu 277 (ΣΤΡΑΤΙΩΤΗΣ ὁ χιλιόφυλλος, *stratiotes millefolia, millefolium*); DL 103 (YARROW, *milfoyle, nosebleede*, ἀχίλλεια, *achillea, myriophyllon, myriomorphos, chiliophyllon, stratioticon, heracleon, chrysitis, supercilium Veneris, acron syluaticum, militaris, diodela, millefolium*); Ge 915 (YELLOW YARROW, *milfoile, nose bleede*, στρατιώτης χιλιόφυλλος).

F (Ge) | S (Fu, DL) | FH (SM, RM)

1376 and²... 1377 yarowe. An obviously botched attempt by the scribe of $ΛS_1$ to solve the problem caused by his earlier substitution of the original *ʒAR(O)W(E) in the heading into his own dialect's ⟨myllefoly⟩. The text in the other MSS, the scribes of which did not redact the original text as heavily, makes better sense. The passage in Wellcome stands surely closest to $Ω$: *W*.31r/27 ⟨& for þi it is cald mylefule [*var.* myldfule]⟩, while in Pepys the original sentence was rephrased into *P*.271/15–16 ⟨and manye clepiþ it millefoyl⟩. Bodley is faulty here as the last word went missing: *B*.257r/9 ⟨& for þi it is callid⟩; but its use of ⟨ʒarowe⟩ at the head of the sentence is sure proof that the missing word must have been also *m i l e f o i l .

1378 and makiþ forthe to ete. Comparison with the other MSS from *RH* suggests that the passage in S_1, which makes little sense, was redacted: cf. *W*.31r/28–31v/1 ⟨and mak it in a cr*u*sel & gif it to ete⟩. Other than some dialectal choices, *P*.271/17–18 reads exactly alike but uses ⟨gobettes⟩ (*g o b l e t t e s was probably intended) instead of *crusel* "crucible". The corresponding reading in *B*.257r/10 ⟨bake it i*n* cak*is*⟩ makes much better sense. While one would be at some pains to explain the exact purpose of cooking the pap in a crucible instead of simply using a kitchen pot, or why the thickish mixture should be eaten, rather than drunk, in a goblet, there is nothing particularly remarkable in baking cakes out of a dough made of juices and flour.

Reconstructing the reading in $Ω$ without a supporting Latin text is not an easy task, but I think that *MAK IT IN A TORTELET(E) is likely to be behind these readings. *TORTELET(E) is a word used in cookery with the sense of "a small meat, cheese, or fruit dumpling or rissole", and in heraldry to refer to "a device resembling a small round cake or loaf of bread" (MED: *s.v.* tŏurtelet *n.*). While the scribe of Bodley translated the infrequent word into the near-synonym *cake* and slightly adjusted the verb into ⟨bak⟩, the scribe of *RH* seems to have copied the fragment verbatim but for some reason (perhaps because it was at the end of the line?) split the word into *t o r t e l + *e t e, which explains the presence of *to ete* in all MSS from that branch but not in *B*. The scribe of *W* misread *TORTEL into *cr*u*tel, hardly a cause for wonder as the change **c** *pro* **t** and viceversa is universal, then conjectured into ⟨cr*u*sel⟩. The scribe of S_1 similarly conjectured, but this time turning final **l** into **h**, which is again frequent, and/or **f** instead of **t** (both of them are barred letters). The scribe of *P*, just like *W*, transformed original **t** into **c**, and then into **g** (there are other instances of this behaviour in this MS, cf. next note for the opposite case), mistook the brevigraph for -*or*- (º) as a mere superscript **o**, then swapped final **tel** into **let**, and conjectured as his companions had also done. Alternatively, the split of the word may have happened only in γ, while in *P* *TORTELET(E) was simply read as *g o t e l e t (e) according to the preceding explanation, and was then emended (a change **be** pro **te** is also easy to account for). But then the appearance of the coda ⟨ʒif it to ete⟩ in that MS would be more difficult to explain.

1382 delyuereth... 1383 dropesy. There are three different versions of this passage, and none of them seems completely accurate. S_1 and *W* agree here, other than the natural alternation between ⟨javndys⟩ and ⟨golsouth⟩. Pepys does not mention jaundice, but rather reads *P*.271/21 ⟨cold cowʒe⟩ and offers moreover ⟨mekeþ⟩ in the following line, instead of *MAKYS as the other MSS from *RH*. As for Bodley, the passage there is very short, and only reads *B*.257r/13 ⟨it swag*is* bolnynge⟩.

It seems clear that *make* asks syntactically for an adverbial complement such as *s o f t (e) after the object ⟨gall⟩, or else a complement clause that would turn *make* into a causative, for example *t o   b e   s o f t (e). Since nothing of the sort appears in S_1, *W* or *P*, we would need to assume a missing fragment already in *RH*. On the other hand a form *MEKIS in Ω, after the reading in Pepys, can be taken as a slavish translation of Latin *mitigo*, which would be applied to internal organs such as the gall-bladder with the sense "soften" (see MED: *s.v.* mēken *v.*, § 1.c).

The reason behind the different disease mentioned in each MS (jaundice and cough) is less evident, but an explanation can also be ventured. If Ω read *GOLSO(U)ʒ(T), then the scribe of Pepys may have interpreted *c o l s o (u) g h (t), which was assumed as a matter of course to mean *cold cough*, hence ⟨cold cowʒe⟩. (See previous note for another example of confusion between **c** and **g**.)

1385 mogwort. The Latin and ME names indicate that the entry describes the medical virtues of mugwort (*Artemisia vulgaris* L.). A very popular species pharmacographically, the entry is a composite of several sources, not all of them identified. A continuous block of lines (**1399–1405**) clearly follows *AC*, but misses the physical description provided there. Other virtues (roughly **1387–1393**, perhaps also **1405–1409**) are arranged in a way reminiscent of *DVH*, but again missing a few ideas mentioned there. Some are included in *CI* (for example its value as conceptive or antihemorrhoidal), while there are a few privative to *LH*.

Artemisia was taken since Antiquity to be an excellent remedy against feminine diseases and, more generally, those related to the internal organs (particularly the abdomen) and the genitals. Indeed the plant is described in the entry as being a conceptive (**1387**), emmenagogue (**1388**), abortifacient (**1390, 1396**), hysteric (**1391**), anticteric and cosmetic (**1393**), antihemorrhoidal (**1395**), diuretic and lithontriptic (**1398**), anticolic (**1405**), stomachal, cordial and splanchnic (**1409**). Mugwort is moreover taken to be corroborant (**1400**), exorcist (**1402**), antipruritic (**1403**), analgesic (**1404**), alexipharmic (**1407**), febrifuge (**1411**), antispasmodic (**1412**) and prognostic (**1413**). Some of them, namely the corroborant and alexipharmic properties are included in medical treatises. The antispasmodic virtue is in Ge, who also hinted its usage against the supernatural but never explained in full as they were "things vnwoorthie of my recording or your reuiewing".

> **Literature**: MUGWORT (*Artemisia vulgaris* L.): MM iii.113 (ἀρτεμισία); NH xxv.73 (*artemisia, parthenis*); *SM* xi.839; *RM* ii.197; *OEH* 11 (*herba artemesia. mucgwyrt*); *Dur.Glos.* 300 (*artemesia. mugvyrt*); *DVH* 1–30 (*arthemesia*); *LS* 319 (*schea* [شيح *šīḥ*], *sandonicum, absinthium marinum*); *EPN* ii (*atemisia, matrum herba. mug-wyrt*), iv (*artemisia. mug-wyrt* | *gagantes. mug-wyrt*), v (*artemessia, mug-wyrt*), vi (*artemisie. mug-wrt. merherbarum*), viii (*hec artemesia. mugwortt*); *CI* A.24 (*arthemisia, mater herbarum. muggeword*); *TH* 30 (*artemisia, mater herbarum*); *Pand.* 58 ($_{LA}$*archemisia, mater herbarum, matricaria,* $_{GR}$*tageles,* $_{AR}$*berengesif, leptafilos*); *DVH(NME)* 244r.25 (*mugworthe*); *DVH(SME)* 1a.1 (*mogworte, moderwort. arthemesia*); *Alph.* 13 (*archemesia, matricaria, matricalis, mater herbarum.* $_{GA}$*armoyse,* $_{AN}$*mugwort, mugwed*), 106 (*la miere de herbes*); *Sin.Bart.* 11 (*arthemesia, armoyse. muggewede*), 20 (*ermoyse. muggewede. arthemesia*); *AC* 161.9 (*arthemesia. mugwourth*) ❀ *GH* 29 (ARTHEMISIA, *mugwort, moderwort, regina, terator, ephelia, patermon, apolyses, succosa, lyopas, vtropium, cereste, encacista, tronissis, bubastes, obstancepon, emoromy, gomosestus, phylaterion, ferula*); *Fu* 13 (ἈΡΤΕΜΙΣΙΑ, *artemisia*); *Tu* 1.243 (MUGWURT, *artemisia*); *DL* 13 (MUGWORT, *artemisia, mater herbarum*); *Ge* 945 (MUGWOORT, ἀρτεμισία, παρθένις, *artemisia, parthenion, mater herbarum*).
>
> CS (Tu, DL) | C²S¹ (SM, RM, Fu) | C²S² (Ge) | C³S³ (TH, GH) | C⁴S⁴ (CI)

1402 stampe the gres. While the MS reading may stand if ⟨gres⟩ is taken to be an instance of the verb "to grease, lubricate" in the imperative, the sense of the sentence is awkward at best. From a syntactic point of view, moreover, the sentence would not be in keeping with the normal usage of the scribe, since the expected direct object of those two transitive verbs would be missing.

1416 mandrake. All available evidence from the entry (Latin headword, ME name and physical description) points to mandrake (*Mandragora* L. spp.). As usual during the period, a male and a female mandrake are distinguished, which are traditionally identified with *M. officinarum* L. and *M. autumnalis* L., respectively. The comparison of their leaves with those of beets and lettuces, respectively, can be found already in *MM*, where the female species is actually called θριδακία (cf. Gk θρίδαξ "lettuce"). The entry was drawn and very much abridged from *AC*.

According to the text, mandrakes are soporific (**1419**), antiherpetic (**1426**), antidysenteric (**1428**), both conceptive and anticonceptive, depending on the woman's mood (**1430–1432**), anti-inflammatory (**1433, 1440**), alexipharmic (**1433**), anticephalalgic (**1434**), and febrifuge (**1438**). Most of these are routinely mentioned in the usual medical literature since *MM*, but the assumed powers of mandrake to help women get pregnant (→ **1428**) and against fever (→ **1438**) are more sparsely found.

> **Literature**: MANDRAKES (*Mandragora* L. spp.): *HP* vi.2.9 (μανδράγορας); *MM* iv.75; *NH* xxv.147 (*mandragora*); *SM* xii.67 (μανδραγόρας); *RM* ii.240; *OEH* 132 (*mandragora*); *LS* 333 (*iabora* [يبروح *yabrūḥ*], *mandragora*); *EPN* ii (*mandragora, eorð-æppel*), v (*mandragora*), ix (*hec mandragora: a mandrak*); *Cl* M.9 (*mandragora. mandrak*); *TH* 300 (*mandragora*); *Pand.* 484 (_AR_*leborac, lufaha, joborohahah, jabroth,* _GR_*antimon, circeon, morion,* _LA_*mandragora*); *Alph.* 109 (*mandragora*); *Sin.Bart.* 11 (*apolinaris, mandragora*), 29 (*mandragora*); *AC* 206.15 (*mandragora, mandrake*) ❀ *GH* 278 (MANDRAGORA, *mandrake, antimon, androporeos*); *Fu* 200 (ΜΑΝΔΡΑΓΟΡΑΣ, κιρκαία, ἀνθρωπόμορφος, *canina malus, terrestris malus, mandragora*); *Tu* 2.437 (MANDRAGE, *mandragoras*); *DL* 312 (MANDRAKE, *mandrage,* μανδράγορας, *mandragoras, autimalum, anthropomorphos*); *Ge* 280 (MANDRAKE, *mandrage, mandragon,* μανδραγορας, κιρκαία, ἀντίμηλον, *anthropomorphos, morion, terra malum, terrestre malum, canina malus*).
>
> F³ (*SM, RM,* Tu, Ge) | FS (*Cl, TH, GH*) | F³S³ (*LS,* Fu) | F⁴S⁴ (DL)

1428 Placeus saiþ. ⟨Placeus⟩, i.e. Platearius, is the surname of a renowned saga of physicians from the Medical School of Salerno (Hamilton 1906: 377). In this passage it must refer to Matthaeus Platearius (†1161), as shown by the following passage from *Cl*:

> Quidam dicunt feminam formatam esse ad formam mulieris, masculum ad formam viri, quod falsum est. Natura enim formam humanam herbis nunquam attribuit. Quidam autem opinantur formam talem, vt a rusticis accepimus.

The idea that mandrakes help fertility is in fact nowhere to be found in Platearius's Latin text, but was probably sewn into the same sentence by the author of *AC* (who also quoted Dioscorides to impart more authority, cf *AC* 207.19 ff.: "Also dyacolydes seyth *and* placens bothe *and* legyn þat ʒef þis herbe be takyn in due tyme or in Resonable manere..."). The notion was current in popular medicine but was mentioned also by some Renaissance scholars (Tu for one, who put in connection with the cleansing properties of the species). It derives from a passage in the story of Joseph (Gen. 30:14–16): Rachel, who was barren, asked her older sister Leah to give her some of Reuben's mandrakes. This was later interpreted as an indication that the plant could help barren women conceive, even though this is never stated in the Biblical passage (see the commentary in *Ge*, who seems to have doubted that the Hebrew text in fact referred to mandrakes at all): rather, it seems that the mandrakes were thought to be aphrodisiac, as suggested by the Hebrew etymology (דוּדָאִים *dūḏā'īm*, properly meaning "love-exciting (plant)", related to דּוֹד *dōḏ* "beloved"; Klein 1987: *s.v.* דּוּדָא, דּוּדָי *n*. Cf. also Song 7:13, where the Beloved is lured into love by the smell of mandrakes and "all manner of pleasant fruits").

1438 manys poucys. Since the mandrake is a very cold herb, it was taken as a good febrifuge almost as a matter of course, but the virtue is not normally mentioned in the pharmacographic literature of the period. It is found just in *CI* (and *GH*, whose author drew extensively from it), whence the passage in *AC–LH* must have originated: cf. "[s]i vero pulsus inungatur febrilem calorem reprimit". It is clear from here that the MS reading ⟨pomys⟩ translates La. *pulsus*. The spelling in the archetype, probably *POUS(E), must have been miscopied early in the transmission: besides ⟨pomys⟩, variants from MSS belonging to the *AC* tradition include ⟨pous⟩, ⟨bous⟩, and ⟨pownse⟩. The reading in the Bodley version of that herbal, ⟨powrys⟩, is particularly close to that of *LH* and suggests an exemplary cluster *u c (in a plural form *POUSES > *POUCYS) that was misread as **m** by the scribe of *LH* (or its exemplar's) and as *u r, copied as **wr** in MS *B*. This may in turn be construed as an indication of a careless Formata exemplar that was common to both MSS, where *u and *n were confusable and *c could be misread by separate copyists as the third minim of an **m** or as a short-shouldered **r**. The MS reading ⟨pomys⟩ in → **2293**, on the other hand, seems to refer to the pores in the skin.

1443 moleyne. The ME synonyms indicate that the chapter must describe the medical qualities of great mullein (*Verbascum thapsus* L.). The textual pedigree of the entry has not been traced.

The species is commended as an antihemorrhoidal (**1446**). Besides being used to make wicks (as seen by such synonyms as *lucernaris, luminaria, candela regis*, or English *taperwort*), *Verbascum* was mainly known as a pulmonic (in particular an excellent antitussive) in Classical antiquity. But some medieval and early Renaissance sources do mention its powers to alleviate the pain of piles, for example *CI* and *GH*. (*Pand.*, where the species is recommended against the same if fomented in wine, pretended to have borrowed the idea to Pliny, but this is apparently not recorded in *NH*). The recipes indicated in those sources are in any case different from that in *LH*.

> **Literature**: GREAT MULLEIN (*Verbascum thapsus* L.): *HP* ix.12.3 (φλόμος); *MM* iv.103; *NH* xxv.120 (*verbascum*); *SM* xii.150; *RM* ii.270; *OEH* 73 (*herba uerbascum. feltwyrt*); *Dur.Glos.* 305 (*verbascum. felt vyrt*); *EPN* ii (*fromos, lucernaris, insana, lucubros. candel-wyrt*), v (*avadonia. felt-wyrt*); vi (*tapsus barbatus. moleine. softe*); *CI* T.7 (*tapsus barbassus, flosmus, ponfiligos*); *TH* 494 (*tassus verbassus, flosmon, bladone, argimon*); *Pand.* 268 (_GR_*flommos, flosmus,* _AR_*busuri,* _LA_*tapsus barbassus*); *DVH(SME)* 30a.10 (*softe, moleyn. asarum, uulgago*); *Alph.* 68 (*flosmus, filtrum, tapsus barbatus maior, herb luminaria, pantifilagos. feltwort, cattestayl*), 80 (*herba luminaria, flosmus, tapsus barbatus maior, filtrum. cattestail, feldwort*); *Sin.Bart.* 14 (*cauda equi, tapsus barbastus*), 23 (*herba luminaria, tapsus barbastus*), 41 (*tapsus barbastus, flosmus*) ⚜ *GH* 450 (TAPSUS BARBATUS, *hareberde, hyghtapper, moleyne, flosmon, blandone, agymon*); *Fu* 326 (ΦΛΟΜΟΣ, *verbascum, tapsus barbatus, candela regis, candelaria, lanaria*); *Tu* 2.595 (MOLLEN, *hickis taper, longwurt, verbascus, phlomos*); *DL* 83 (MVLLEIN, *hygtaper, wullein, torches, longwort*, φλόμος, *verbascum, lychnitis, pyenitis, candela regis, candelaria, lunaria, tapsus barbatus*); *Ge* 629 (MULLEIN, *woolen, higtaper, torches, bullockes longwoort, hares beard*, φλόμος, *tapsus barbatus, candela regis, candelaria, lanaria, verbascum*).
>
> S (*SM, RM*, Fu, DL, Ge) | FS (*CI, TH, GH*)

1448 melilote. The ME names applied to a number of several species displaying three leaflets, traditionally identified as belonging to the genera *Melilotus* Mill., *Trifolium* L. or *Medicago* L. Classical and medieval medical scholars thought of *mel(l)ilotum* as single yellow-flowered species but, as seen from the entry, some authors distinguished a number of them. Since the entry provides neither a physical description nor a Latin headword and there are many possible candidates, it is useless to try and pinpoint the exact species. In any case, there seems to be no black-leaved melilot, and probably the author meant some species with deep purple flowers such as lucerne (*Medicago sativa* L.)., or else hopclover (*Medicago lupulina* L.), which is connected to black colour in many languages, even though its flowers are yellow, due to the dark colour of its ripe seeds: cf. "black medick" in English, "maglys du" in Welsh, "trèfle noir" in French, "mielga negra" in Spanish or "luzerna preta" in Portuguese.

The text derives from *AC*, but misses the second half of the entry as given in the Stockholm version, which served as base text to Brodin's edition. The missing fragment refers to the exorcist powers of the plant and may have been an addition by the copyist of the MS, for it is not recorded in other copies of the herbal collated by the editor. Note moreover that the source text does not mention a black, but rather a red species.

Pharmacographically, all three species are ophthalmic (**1450**), which is in accordance with the Classical, medieval and Renaissance evidence, where it is praised moreover as an anti-inflammatory and mollificative. The sweet smell of the plants is also recognized in the literature, where it was connected to good digestion.

> Literature: MELILOTS (*Melilotus* Mill. spp./*Trifolium* L. spp./*Medicago* L. spp.): HP vii.15.3 (μελίλωτος); MM iii.40; NH xxi.151 (*melilotos*); SM xii.70; RM ii.241; Grad. 349 (*melilotum*); OEH 183 (*herba milotis*); LS 18 (*alchilel melich* [اكليل الملك] *iklīl al-malik*], *corona regia*); EPN ii (*ligustrum. hunisuge*), iv (*ligustrum. hunisuce*), vi (*ligustrum. triffoil. hunisuccles* | *trifolium. trifoil. wite clovere*), vii (*hoc ligustrum, idem* | *hoc trifolium. hart-claver*), viii (*hoc ligustrum. a primerose* | *hoc ligustrum. a cowslowpe*), ix (*hoc ligustrum. a cowyslepe*); Cl M.3 (*mellilotum, corona regia. hony souk*); TH 290 (*mellilotum*); Pand. 27 (ARalilelmeliche, alchelilamech, alchilelmelich, GRmellilotum, LAcorona regia); DVH(SME) 31b.12 (*honysokel, mellisophiles. baracum, dorocus*); Alph. 110 (*matris silua, periclimenon, mellilotum secundum quosdam, corna regia, caprifolium. honysocle, wodebynde*), 115 (*mellilotum, eius flos uocatur corona regia*); Sin.Bart. 30 (*mellilotum, trifolium aquaticum*); AC 203.17 (*melilotum. mellito, honysukkle, iij lewyd gres, mel siluestre*) ⚜ GH 268 (MELLILOTUM, *mellilot, kynges crowne*); Fu 199 (ΜΕΛΙΛΩΤΟΣ, *melilotus, sertula campana, corona regia*); Tu 2.567 (*Italian* MELILOTE, *sert(ul)a campana, melilotos*); DL 357 (MELILOT, μελιλωτος, *melilotus, stertula campana*); Ge 1033 (MELILOT, *plaister clauer, harts clauer, melilotus, trifolium odoratum, trifolium equinum, sertula campana, corona regia*).
>
> CS (Fu, DL) | C¹S¹ (*Grad., LS, Cl, TH, Pand., GH*, Ge)

1454 mynte. The ME name naturally indicates some species of mint (*Mentha* L. spp., → **863, 1318**), but the Latin headword and its synonyms, collected both in the Literature section and Rolland 1896–1914: VII.77–79 point towards costmary (*Tanacetum balsamitoides* Sch.Bip. = *Chrysanthemum balsamita* L.). Cf. the entry *menta* in *Cl* as well, where the *romana* variety is equated with *costum vulgare*:

> Est et menta que longiora et acutiora et latiora habet folia, et hec menta romana

vel saracenica dicit*ur* .i. costu*m* vulgare et hec magis diuretica est q*uam* alie, quod perpenditur eius acumine vel amaritudine.

On the other hand, costmary does not grow ‹in bankys of watrys› and, while the synonym ‹white mynte› could apply to that species due to the colour of its stalk and leaves, ‹horse-mynte› does not fit. The use of "horse" in connection with plants normally serves to qualify a larger, coarser version of another species, be it in taste or to the touch (OED: *s.v.* horse *n.*, § 28.c), and *Tanacetum* has a bitter savour, as seen from the above quotation, but ‹stronge› in **1455** is rather suggestive of some *Mentha* having a very potent (sweet) taste, cf. ‹stronge of sauour› in **864**. Taking the entry to describe a mint was the sensible stance taken by the editor of *AC*, whence this entry derives.

Even though as a rule all mints are water lovers, the species living in damp places would be water mint (*M. aquatica* L.). But then this species was called *mentastrum* or *balsamita* (as seen in **862**) rather than *menta romana* or *sarracenica*, and it is not particularly white either. Application of *Menta romana* to spearmint (*M. spicata* L.) appears to be a strictly Renaissance development (cf. DL, Ge, and Stirling 1995–1998: *s.v.* mentha, quoting Bauhin) and hence should be discarded too, all the more so since it does not match the description provided either. All in all, the best candidate is horsemint (*M. longifolia* (L.) L.), which has a stronger taste than other mints and hoary stalk and leaves, although it does not grow in expansions of water. In keeping with the description provided in *Cl* for *menta romana*, horsemint has quite long, broad and almost acuminate leaves.

Medically, the species is taken to be anthelminthic (**1456–1458, 1460**) and eupeptic (**1459**). These virtues are not critical to decide the exact species, as both apply to mints generally (→ **1318**). Even so, *Cl* does mention worm-killing as the one of the main virtues of *menta romana*, including the idea of instilling the juice into the ear: "[s]ucc*us* etia*m* ei*us* [mentae romanae] dat*ur* lu*m*bricos interficit. Aurib*us* istillat*us* v*er*mes necat".

Literature: HORSEMINT (*Mentha longifolia* (L.) L.): *Cl* M.6 (*menta ... romana/ saracenica, costum vulgare*); *TH* 296 (*menta romana/saracenica*); *Alph.* 116 (*menta romana/saracena*); *Sin.Bart.* 24 (*herba Sanctæ Mariæ, febrifuga, athanasia*), 29 (*menta romana, herba Sanctæ Mariæ*); *AC* 204.20 (*menta romana. wylde mynte*) ⚘ *GH* 274 (MENTA ROMANA, *whyt mynte, mynte romayne, sarazyne*); *Tu* 2.449 (MINT, *garden mynte, spere mynte*); DL 174 (MINTS, *the third kind, menta sarracenica, menta romana, speare mint, common garden mint, baulme mint*); Ge 551 (MINTS, *the third* [*kind*], *mentha sarracenica/romana, saluia romana, herba Sanctæ Mariæ, speare mint, common garden/ladies/browne/macrell mint*); → horsmynte [**863**].

C^2S^2 (*Cl, TH, GH*, DL, Ge)

1462 mistilte. The Latin heading suggests that the entry deals with the fern osmund (→ **1613**), but the first ME synonym and the idea that the plant grows on oaks make it evident that the entry is in fact devoted to mistletoe (*Viscum album* L.). ⟨Osmunda⟩ is probably a clerical mistake for an original *osimum, as demonstrated from the source text (*AC*). The Latin word regularly refers to basil, *Ocimum basilicum* L., but the plant name was misapplied to *Viscus* in many English sources since Anglo-Saxon times (see Literature below, Bierbaumer 1975–1979: III.172, and PNME: *s.v.* for details).

The second synonym provided in the entry might arguably be a *lectio facilior* for *a r b u t e , i.e. the strawberry tree (*Arbutus unedo* L.): indeed du Fresne 1938: *s.v.* arbustus records the exact same mistake in a French glossary and it is evident that arbutus posed problems to medieval scribes, who spelt it *albatrum*, *arbitrum*, etc. (a fuller, but surely not comprehensive, list in Stirling 1995–1998: s.v.). La. *arbustum* refers to the trees about which the vines are trained (see for instance *NH* xviii.242), so the idea of having one species living upon another, as it were, could have easily triggered comparison with mistletoe, which parasites trees.

Identification with *Viscum* is yet not borne out by the usual medical literature of the period. The species is antiepileptic (**1464**), anticephalalgic (**1465**) and febrifuge (**1466**; not in the source text); although DL records the first virtue (almost in passing and lending little credit to it), mistletoe was praised mainly as an emollient and maturative.

Literature: MISTLETOE (*Viscum album* L.): *HP* iii.7.6 (ἰξία); *MM* iii.89 (ἰξός); *NH* xxiv.11 (*viscum*); *SM* xi.888; *RM* ii.217; *OEH* 119 (*herba ocimus. mistel*); *Dur.Glos.* 304 (*ocimus. mistel* | *uiscus. mistelta*); *LS* 167 (*dababch, dibach* [دِبق *dibq*], *viscus*); *EPN* ii (*viscarago. mistiltan*); *Pand.* 199 (ARdabalch, GRhele, hisos, LAviscus); *Alph.* 191 (*viscus.* GAwy de chene, ANmistel); *Sin.Bart.* 43 (*viscus*); *AC* 211.27 (*osinum. mistilto*) ❦ Fu 123 ('ΙΞΟΣ, *viscum*); Tu 2.598 (MISSEL, *misselto tree, ixos, viscum*); DL 538 (MISSEL, *misselto, ἰξός, viscum, viscus quercinus*); Ge 1168 (MISSELTOE, *mistletoe, viscum,* ἴξὸs, ἴξια).

CS (*SM, RM,* Fu, DL, Ge) | C²S² (*LS*)

1468 mowsere. Judging from the Latin headword, ME name and physical description, the plant must be some kind of hawkweed having stolons (cf. ⟨growith lowe by the grownde⟩), traditionally identified with *Pilosella officinarum* Vaill. = *Hieracium pilosella* L., although the name was applied to several species, the blue-flowered forget-me-nots (*Myosotis* L. spp.) in particular. The pedigree of the entry has not been traced.

The species is lithontriptic (**1470**), diuretic (**1472**), prognostic in case of wounded people (**1474**), and antitonsillitic (**1475**). The prognostic powers of the species are mentioned in *Alph.* and *GH*, but the other are missing from the usual pharmacographic literature.

Literature: MOUSE-EAR HAWKWEED (*Pilosella officinarum* Vaill.): *MM* ii.183 (μυὸς ὦτα); *NH* xxvii.105 (*myosota, myosotis*); *SM* xi.823 (ἀλσίνη), xii.80 (μυὸς ὠτίς); *RM* ii.191, 243; *EPN* vi (*pilosella. peluselle. mus-ere*); *TH* 390 (*pilosella*); *Pand.* 42 ($_{GR}$*anagallus, mioschays,* $_{AR}$*xantala, ippia,* $_{LA}$*auricula muris*); *Alph.* 17 (*auricula muris, pilosella. moushere, langbeue*), 117 (*mirion, auricula muris. mousher*), 144 (*pilocella.* $_{GA}$*pelosee, peluette,* $_{AN}$*langheue, moushere*); *Sin.Bart.* 12 (*auriculus muris, pilocella*), 30 (*murion, auricula muris*), 33 (*pelvette. mouser*); *AC* 166.29 (*auricula muris. moushere*) ⚜ *GH* 356 (PILOCELLA, *mows eare*); *Fu* 7 (ΆΛΣΙΝΗ, *auricula muris, morsus gallinæ*); *Tu* 2.755 (MOUSE EARE, *pilosella, auricula muris*); *DL* 40 (MOVSE-EAR, μυὸς ὦτα, *auricula muris*); *Ge* 512 (MOUSEARE, *pilosella, auricula muris*).

FH (*SM*, Fu) | CS (Tu, Ge) | S (DL)

1477 nettyll. Although there is no physical description, the Latin headword, ME name and hot temperament indicate that the entry probably describes the medical properties of nettles (*Urtica* L. spp.), and especially its *species typica*, the stinging nettle (*U. dioica* L.) and the small nettle (*U. urens* L.). The ‹rede nettill› (**1497**) probably refers to the red deadnettle (*Lamium purpureum* L.). The pedigree of the entry is untraced; whatever the source, and just like *GH*, influence from *DVH* seems clear in the general arrangement of the virtues, although *LH* includes several qualities that are not found in Macer Floridus's text.

The species is deemed to be antitussive (**1478**), hysteric (**1480, 1498**), vulnerary and antirabic (**1481**), anticancerous (**1483**), regenerative (**1484**), desiccant (**1484**), splenetic and antipodagric (**1485**), analgesic (**1486**), both hematogogue and hemostatic (**1488**), antilumbalgic and diuretic (**1491**), antiepileptic (**1492**), laxative (**1493**), antiuvulitic (**1494**), diaphoretic (**1495**), antialopecic (**1496**), eloquent (**1497**), and anaphrodisiac (**1501**). Virtually all of these qualities are found in the pharmacographic literature of the period, particularly those related with a soluble body, but medical *auctoritates* since Dioscorides thought that the plant was aphrodisiac, in keeping with hot herbs.

Literature: NETTLES (*Urtica* L. spp.): *HP* vii.7.2 (ἀκαλύφη); *MM* iv.93 (ἀκαλήφη); *NH* xxii.31 (*urtica*); *SM* xi.817 (ἀκαλύφη); *RM* ii.189 (ἀκαλήφη); *OEH* 178 (*herba urtica. netele*); *DVH* 115–160 (*urtica, acalife*); *LS* 150 (*hvniure, vraith latu* [قريص .أنجرة‎ *angura, qurrayṣ*], *vrtica*); *EPN* ii, iv (*urtica. netle*), v (*urtica. netel*), vii (*hec urtica. nettylle*), viii, ix (*hec urtica. a netylle*); *TH* 509 (*urtica*); *Pand.* 360 ($_{AR}$*huiure, varik flatum, sarich,* $_{GR}$*ygnidalis, alcalifex,* $_{LA}$*vrtica*); *DVH(SME)* 3a.1 (*nettle. acaliphe. vrtica*); *Alph.* 1 (*achalaphe, ygia, acanturie, acantum, urtica purgens*), 193 (*urtica greca, crekischenetche*) ⚜ *GH* 465 (VRTICA, *apalife, achantis, vrgiba, osminon, nettle*); *Fu* 37

('ΑΚΑΛΥΦΗ, κνίδη, vrtica); Tu 2.605 (NETTELL, urtica, acalyphe, knide); DL 89 (NETTLE, ἀκαλύφη, κνίδη, vrtica); Ge 569 (STINGING NETTLE, ἀκαλύφη, κνὶδη, vrtica).

CS (Fu, DL) | C¹S¹ (Ge) | C²S² (LS)

1504 nepte ryall. The synonym *catt-mynte* and the reference to the attraction that the plant has on cats indicate that the species intended must be the catnip (*Nepeta cataria* L.). Identification with the catnip is yet not borne out on examination of the textual and pharmacological evidence, if only because the species seems to have been never treated in Classical pharmacopea. Closer reading of the contents of the ME text indicates that it is actually a translation of the chapter *nepeta* in *DVH*, which is traditionally taken to record the medical qualities of the lesser calamint (*Clinopodium nepeta* (L.) Kuntze = *Calamintha nepeta* (L.) Savi), as seen by its purported value as a diaphoretic (**1505** = *DVH* 595–596), calefacient and febrifuge (**1507** = *DVH* 597–599), leprostatic (**1513** = *DVH* 604–608), alexipharmic (**1512** = *DVH* 609–610), anthelminthic (**1513** = *DVH* 611–613), anticteric and antiasthmatic (**1514** = *DVH* 615–616), herpetofuge (**1515** = *DVH* 623) and antisingultus (**1517** = *DVH* 624). A number of properties of the species are missing from the ME account, namely as an antisciatic (*DVH* 600–602), emmenagogue (*DVH* 603), abortifacient (*DVH* 614), hepatic and antipleuretic (*DVH* 617–618), detergent (*DVH* 619–621), stomachal (*DVH* 622) and anaphrodisiac (*DVH* 625). Confusion between *Nepeta cataria* and *Clinopodium nepeta* was apparently usual among apothecaries, cf. Ge$_{554}$, in his description of the former: "[i]t is named of the Apothecaries *Nepeta*; but *Nepeta* is properly called [...] wilde Penie royall."

The text follows the same tradition as *AC*, but as usual lacks the physical description provided there. Another translation of the same entry will be found below (→ **1526**); for another entry which seems to deal with the same, or an akin, species, → **383**.

Literature: LESSER CALAMINT (*Clinopodium nepeta* (L.) Kuntze): MM iii.35 (καλαμίνθη [...] ταύτην Ῥωμαῖοι νεπέταν καλοῦσιν); NH xx.158 (*nepeta*); SM xii.4 (καλαμίνθη); RM ii.219; Grad. 376 (*calamenthum*); OEH 115 (*herba nepitamon. nepte*); Dur.Glos. 304 (*nereta. sea minte*); DVH 592–625 (*nepeta*); LS 301 (*calamentum*); EPN ii (*nepita. næpte*), iv (*nereta. sæ-minte*), vi (*nepta. nepte. kattes-minte*); CI c.9 (*calamentum*); TH 95 (*calamentum*); Pand. 120 ($_{AR}$*calamentum*, $_{GR}$*calamitatis*, $_{LA}$*nepita, menta non odorifera*); DVH(NME) 246v.18 (*nep*); DVH(SME) 8b.24 (*nepis. calamentum*); Alph. 125 (*nepta, calamentum maius, hasta regia. catwort*); Sin.Bart. 31 (*nepta | nepita dicitur calamentum minus*); AC 209.25 (*nepta. nepte, cattys mynte*) ✽ GH 90 (CALAMENTUM, *calamynt, nelpyte*); Fu 164 (ΚΑΛΑΜΙΝΘΗ, *calamintha, calamentum ... alterum generum, nepeta, syluestre pulegium*); Tu 1.259 (CALAMYNTE, *the third kind ... nepita, nepe, catmynt*); DL 177 (CALAMINT, *the third kind, catmint, nep*, καλαμίνθη, *calamintha,* *calamentum, mentastrum, nepita*); Ge 553 (NEP, *cat mint, herba cataria, herba catti, nepeta*), 556 (MOUNTAINE MINT, *calamint, καλαμίνθη, mentastrum, montana calamintha, calamentum*).

C³S³ (*SM, RM, Grad., DVH, LS, CI, TH, GH,* Fu, Tu, DL, Ge)

1519 nyght-shade. The Latin headword and ME synonyms suggest that the plant treated here is black nightshade (*Solanum nigrum* L.). While this section derives from *AC*, the same species had been already treated in an earlier entry following the appropriate chapter in *DVH* (→ **1371**, with discussion; → **579** for another plant, deadly nightshade (*Atropa bella-donna* L.) that is more toxic than the *Solanum*, was hence taken as its greater counterpart, and is referred to as ‹dwale› in the text). The detailed physical description provided here supports identification with *Solanum*, the berries of which grow ‹in clustris› (i.e. gathered into bunches) as opposed to those of ‹dwale›/*Atropa*, which grow individually.

The species is described in the entry as calefacient (→ **1522**), antiotalgic (**1523**), and antihemorrhoidal (**1524**), but only the assumed powers of the plant against earache are found in the medical literature of the period (it is already in *MM*).

Literature: BLACK NIGHTSHADE (*Solanum nigrum* L.): → morell [**1371**].

1521 Our Lady day. Lady Day refers as a rule to March 25th, the Annunciation of the Virgin (Butler 2003: i.705–708) but in the Middle Ages the name could be loosely applied to the other two main Marian festivities of the devotional calendar: the Assumption and the Nativity, on August 15th and September 8th respectively (Butler 2003: iii.331–334, 506–507). Even though Pope Pius IX defined it as a Catholic dogma only in 1854, the Immaculate Conception of the Virgin (December 8th) might be included in the list as well since the feast was known already in some Anglo-Saxon calendars and was popular in Europe at least since the 13th century (Butler 2003: iv.520). The immediate reference to harvests in the text makes it plain in any case that the holiday intended is the Virgin's birthday, and indeed the berries of the nightshade come to maturity by that date, cf. Ge: "[i]t flowreth in sommer, and oftentimes till autumne be well spent; and then the fruite commeth to ripenesse."

1522 enchafe. Comparison of the ME entry with the probable passage in the pharmacographic works of the period suggests that the original fragment must have praised the plant as a deoppilant of the liver and spleen, cf. "[c]o*n*tra oppilationem splenis et epatis" in *Cl*. The MS reading ‹enchase› makes little sense here if it represents a form of ME *enchācen* "to pursue, put to flight"

Lelamour Herbal 381

(< OF *enchacier*; FEW: *s.v.* *captiare). The word has therefore been emended into *enchafe*, *faute de mieux* and because the clerical error s instead of an exemplary *f is paleographically defendable, even though—as stated by the author of the treatise himself—the nightshade is a cold species and hence could hardly be expected to warm any organ of the body.

1526 nepis. The Latin heading suggests that the species must be some *Brassica* L. spp., traditionally identified as *B. rapa* (L.) L. (subspecies of this plant include the turnip and the rape). Comparison with the Latin original indicates yet that the entry corresponds with the entry *nepeta* in DVH 592–625, which is traditionally identified with the lesser calamint (*Clinopodium nepeta* (L.) Kuntze). This repeats most of the virtues already provided in a previous section (→ **1504**, with discussion), and it is likely that a third entry in the herbal describes the same, or an akin species (→ **383**).

This version of the Latin chapter was copied from the *DVH(NME)* tradition, but other than S_1 the entry is recorded in *B* only (→ **1694** for another example), where the species is similarly spelt ‹nep›. Usage of *neep* to refer to *B. napa* is mainly restricted to the northern dialects, but there are some references to its use also in some southern counties, including Hereford (see for example the quotation from Thomas Blount's *Glossographia* in OED: *s.v.* neep *n.*). The confusion between *nep* and *nepte* is actually not infrequent in texts of the period: it happened also in *DVH(SME)* as well, but the translator of this text was able to identify *nepis* with *calamentum*, which served to avoid any possible confusion. The scribe of AS_1 mistakenly attached *nepis* to the plant that usually bore that name, surely resorting to his own knowledge, since entries from *DVH(NME)* did not originally display Latin headings.

This account is silent as to the qualities of the plant as a calefacient and febrifuge (*DVH* 597–599), emmenagogue (→ **1528**), anticteric, antiasthmatic, hepatic and antipleurodynic (*DVH* 615–618), and anaphrodisiac (*DVH* 625), but does record some other virtues that went unrecorded in the version drawn from *AC*: antisciatic (**1528** = *DVH* 600–603), abortifacient (**1534** = *DVH* 614), stomachal (**1535** = *DVH* 622) and detergent (**1537** = *DVH* 619–621).

Literature: Lesser calamint (*Clinopodium nepeta* (L.) Kuntze): → nepte ryall [**1504**].

1528 accese of flourys. Although *prima facie* this might look as a translation of *DVH* 603 (if a slightly peculiar one, since menses do not normally have accesses), the reading *B*.246v/19 ‹axys of þe feuer› that translates *DVH* 597–599 indicates that this is in fact a scribal mistake. Note that a febrifuge property here is moreover in keeping with the relative position of the sentence within the entry: the emmenagogue virtue of the plant would have been expected after the reference to pain in the kidneys (which stands for *DVH* 600 *sciasim*), and so it does in Bodley, which does record it, cf. *B*.246v/20–21 ‹it gerys make flowrys›.

1529 vmeris...elefanciasys. Apparently, a copy mistake. *DVH* 604 reads *est leprae species elephantiasisque vocatur*, so perhaps the unexpected ‹splene› is only an unfortunate misreading of *SPECIES by the ME translator. As for ‹delle›, this seems to be some heavily distorted rendering of an exemplary *LEPIR, as suggested by *B*.246v/21 ‹lepre› and the reference to elephantiasis (a type of hypertrophic fibrosis in the lower legs, where swelling is accompanied by plaques similar to warts). The Bodley version has severely abridged the whole passage, dispensing altogether with the Latin passage where the elephant was compared to the disease (*DVH* 605–606).

1537 sleyth. A copy mistake for Ω *FLEES, cf. *DVH* 623 *effugat* and *B*.247r/3 ‹flees›.

1539 notemyge. The Latin headword and the ME name indicate that the entry describes the medical properties of the spice nutmeg, i.e. the seed of the tree *Myristica fragrans* Houtt. from the Moluccas. The text follows *AC* closely.

In accordance with the usual pharmacographic literature of the period, the spice is stomachal (→ **1542**), encephalic and psychostimulant (**1545**), antihalitosic (**1546**), carminative (**1547**), and hepatic (**1548**).

> **Literature**: NUTMEG (*Myristica fragrans* Houtt.): *Grad.* 355 (*nux moscata*); *LS* 161 (*ieumbaue, iumbague* [جوز بَوّا ǧūz bawwā'], *nux muscata*); *Cl* N.5 (*nux muscata. notemyggis*); *TH* 331 (*nux muscata*); *Pand.* 561 (L_Anux miristica, _ARjeumbaue); *DVH(SME)* 41b.11 (*notemuge*); *Alph.* 124 (*nux muscata, centrum galli, nux mirifica*); *Sin.Bart.* 32 (*nux mirifica, nux muscata*); *AC* p. 188.1 (*nux muscata. notemuge*) ⚘ *GH* 307 (NUX MUSCATA, *nutmygge*); Tu 2.746 (NUTMEGGES, *nux muscata, nux myristica, moscocarydion, mescoryon*); *DL* 527 (NUTMEG AND MACIS, κάριον μυριστικὸν, μοσχοκάριον, *nux myristica, nux moschata*); *Ge* 1353 (NUTMEG TREE, κάρυον μυριστικὸν, *nux moschata, nux myristica*).
>
> C²S² (*Grad.*, *LS*, *Cl*, *TH*, *GH*, Tu, *DL*, *Ge*)

1542 take...1543 notte. Comparison with the source text makes it clear that the first half of the passage is missing, cf. Brodin 1950: 188 (quoting from MS L of the tradition): "þe vertu of þis fruyt is a man haue a wikked stomake take in the morwenyng an hol note *and* eet hur*e* and if he be lite he is þe betere *and* þ*at* schal hele hy*m*".

1550 orpyn. The Latin headword and the ME name suggest that the species must be orpine (*Sedum telephium* L.) but the lack of physical description (apparently skipped by the scribe from the source text, *AC*) means that identification is not absolutely positive but traditional only.

The species is described as an excellent vulnerary (**1551**). This is in keeping with the etymology of the plant name (ultimately from Lat *auripigmentum*, "orpiment", via OF *orpin*, in reference to the rusty colour of its stalk and leaves, which resembles somewhat that of a scab over a wound). The virtue is of course frequently found in the medical literature but missing, for instance, in Ge.

Literature: ORPINE (*Sedum telephium* L.): *MM* ii.186 (τηλεφώνιον); *NH* xxvii.137 (*telephion*); *SM* xii.140 (τηλέφιον); *RM* ii.266; *OEH* 147 (*herba aizon*); Alph. 34 (*crassula maior, faba silvestris*. $_{GA}$*orme*, $_{AN}$*alfuurt*); Sin.Bart. 17 (*crassula maior. orpin*), 23 (*halsewort. crassula major*); *AC* 173.22 (*crassula maior. orpin, oruale*) ⚜ Fu (ΤΗΛΕΦΙΟΝ, ἀείζωον ἄγριον, *telephium, illecebra, crassula maior, faba crassa*); DL 29 (ORPYNE, *liblong, liuelong, crassula maior, fabaria, faba crassa*); Ge 415 (ORPYNE, *liblong, liuelong*, τελέφιον, ἀείζωον ἄγριον, *telephium, semperuium syluestre, illecebra, crassula maior, fabaria*).

F^3 (DL) | C^1S^2 (*SM, RM,* Fu) | FS (Ge)

1553 origanum. This is a translation of the chapter *origanum* in *DVH*. Although the Latin name was applied *senso lato* to a number of labiates, including thyme (the synonym *brotherwort* is now generally used to mean *Thymus serpyllum* L., → **1631**), pennyroyal and dyttany, which were badly distinguished by Classical and medieval botanists (see André 1985: *s.v.*, and Literature), identification with wild marjoram (*Origanum vulgare* L.) is traditional and supported by textual and pharmacological evidence, as seen by its purported validity as an alexipharmic (**1555** = *DVH* 1287–1290), anticontusive (**1556** = *DVH* 1291), antitussive, antipruritic and cosmetic (**1557** = *DVH* 1297–1299), anticteric (**1559** = *DVH* 1300), antiuvulitic (**1560** = *DVH* 1301–1302), antiotalgic (**1561** = *DVH* 1306), antiaphthic (**1562** = *DVH* 1303), eupeptic (**1563** = *DVH* 1312–1313), anthelminthic and diuretic (**1564** = *DVH* 1318), antiodontalgic (**1566** = *DVH* 1319), tonic (**1567** = *DVH* 1320), diaphoretic (**1568** = *DVH* 1321–1322) and antipleurodynic (**1569** = *DVH* 1323–1324). Some of the medical qualities extolled in *DVH* are missing, probably due to a block of text in the Latin original that was skipped by the translator: anthydropic (*DVH* 1291–1292), cholagogue (*DVH* 1293–1294) antiemmenagoge (*DVH* 1295–1296). The recipe to make noxious beasts flee from one's bed (*DVH* 1307–1311) is also missing, but this may have been done on purpose as it asked for ingredients such as *rhos syriacus* which were not readily available (see the problems caused to other ME translators by that word in Frisk 1949: 222, note to 29a24). The same species will be treated again later in the text (→ **1634**).

Literature: WILD MARJORAM (*Origanum vulgare* L.): *HP* vi.2.3 (ὀρίγανος λευκή); *MM* iii.27 (ὀρίγανος ἡρακλεωτική); *NH* xx.175 (*origanum*); *SM* xii.91 (ὀρίγανος ἡ ἡρακλεωτική); *RM* ii.248; *Grad.* 372; *OEH* 124 (*herba origanum. organe*); *Dur.Glos.* 304 (*organum. organe*); *DVH* 1285–1324 (*origanum*); *LS* 300 (*fandenigi* [فتنغ *futanağ*], *origanum*); *EPN* ii (*origanum.warmelle*), iv (*pollegia. broðer-wyrt, hæl-wyrt, dweorges drostle | oreganum.ælepe*), v (*organe*), vi (*organum. organe | origanum. puliol real, wde-minte*); *Cl* 0.4 (*origanum, golona. origanie, piliole ryal*); *TH* 342 (*origanum, golena*); *DVH(NME)* 254r.24 (*pygyll*); *DVH(SME)* 28b.30 (*puliole haunt*); *Alph.* 130 (*origanum. golena, colena, chirchewrt*); *Sin.Bart.* 32 (*origanum ... pulegium majus, videlicet regale*); *AC* 211.4 (*organum. organe*) ⚜ *GH* 317 (ORIGANUM, *brotherworte*); *Fu* 208 (ΌΡΙΓΑΝΟΣ, *origanus*); *Tu* 2.474 (ORGAN, *origanum*); *DL* 169 (ORIGAN, *wild marierom*, ὀρίγανος, *origanum*); *Ge* 540 (WILDE MARIEROME, *bastarde marierome, groue marierome*, ὀρίγανος, ονίτις, *cunila, origanum, agriorganum*).

C^3S^3 (*SM, RM, Grad., DVH, LS, Cl, TH, GH, Fu, DL, Ge*)

1571 ostricium. The entry is a translation of *DVH* 907–927. Identification with soapwort (*Saponaria officinalis* L.) is sustained by textual and pharmacological evidence, as seen by its mentioning in the text as a hepatic and splenetic (**1572** = *DVH* 909–910), lithontriptic, emmenagogue and diuretic (**1573** = *DVH* 912–913), antitussive and antiasthmatic (→ **1575**), abortifacient (**1576** = *DVH* 915–916), leprostatic and antiherpetic (**1577** = *DVH* 917–921), and sternutatory (**1580** = *DVH* 922–925). Two references to the anticteric quality of the species at the beginning and end of the Latin chapter (*DVH* 910, 926–927) are missing from the ME account. The same species is described again later in the text (→ **2068**).

Literature: SOAPWORT (*Saponaria officinalis* L.): *HP* vi.4.3 (στρούθιον); *MM* ii.163 (στρούθιον); *NH* xxiv.96 (*struthion*); *SM* xii.131 (στρούθιον); *Grad.* 383 (*condisi*); *OEH* 146 (*herba strutius*); *Dur.Glos.* 304 (*ostricium. vude-rofe*); *DVH* 907–927 (*ostritium*); *LS* 352 (*condes* [كندس *kundus*], *condisi*); *TH* 424 (*saponaria, burit, herba fullonum, herba sancti Philippi*); *Pand.* 177 ($_{AR}$*condes, condisi, condos*, $_{GR}$*strutium*, $_{LA}$*condisi, obstricium*); *DVH(NME)* 254r.13 (*senykyll*); *DVH(SME)* 28a.20 (*bisshopeswort. structon, ostructon*); *Alph.* 158 (*saponaria, borax, boryth, herba fullorum. cowesope*); *Sin.Bart.* 37 (*saponaria. crowsope*); *AC* 156.15 (*saponaria. crowsope*) ⚜ *Fu* 299 (ΣΤΡΟΥΘΙΟΝ, *radicula, lanaria, condisi, herba fullonum, saponaria*); *DL* 242 (CRUCIASMA, *dwarfe gentian, sopewort, mocke gillofer, alisma, saponaria*); *Ge* 359 (SOPEWOORT, *brusewoort, saponaria, alisma, damasonium*).

CS (*DVH, Ge*) | C^3S^3 (*DL*) | C^4S^4 (*SM, Grad., LS, Fu*)

1575 helith þe jaundis. According to the edition of *DVH*, the passage in the Latin poem praises the merits of the species as a help to those who cannot breathe. The apparatus criticus yet records that some Latin textual families offer variants like ‹emoptoicis› (θ, κ) or ‹haemopthoicis› (κκ). The translator of

DVH(SME) must have used a MS from one of these families as his exemplar, for in the parallel passage the ME text states that the plant "helpiþ hem þat speten blode" (28a.29–30). Next to a mistranslation, it would not be impossible to argue that *Q* could have read *ICTERICIS instead of *DVH* 914 *orthopnoicis*.

1577 the scabbe. *DVH* 917–918 demonstrates that ‹scabbe› stands here for leprosy.

1581 oynowneis. An account of the medical virtues of the onion (*Allium cepa* L.) as given in *DVH* 1087–1126. The species had already been described in a previous entry that also derived ultimately from the same Latin source (→ **189**).

Identification with the onion is traditional, and sure on both lexical and pharmacological grounds: after the warning to choleric people and its recommendation to those of a phlegmatic temperament, the text praises the powers of the onion as a cosmetic (**1587** = *DVH* 1093–1094), laxative (**1587** = *DVH* 1098), against hound- and snake bite (**1589** = *DVH* 1099–1104), antiotalgic (**1592** = *DVH* 1105–1106), eloquent (**1594** = *DVH* 1107–1108), sternutatory (**1595** = *DVH* 1109–1110), emmenagogue and anticallus (**1596** = *DVH* 1111–1114), antiodontalgic and antiaphthic (**1598** = *DVH* 1115–1117), antidysenteric (**1601** = *DVH* 1119), antialopecic (**1602** = *DVH* 1120–1121), antihalitosic and orectic (**1603** = *DVH* 1122), antihemorrhoidal (**1604** = *DVH* 1123), ophthalmic (**1605** = *DVH* 1124–1125) and antiephelic (**1606** = *DVH* 1125–1126). Missing from the account is the reference to the soporific qualities of the species if chewed (*DVH* 1097).

> **Literature**: ONION (*Allium cepa* L.): HP vii.4.7 (κρόμνον), MM ii.151; NH xx.39–43 (*cepa*); SM xii.48 (κρόμμνον); RM ii.232 (κρόμυον); OEH 174 (*herba bulbus*); Dur.Glos. 301 (*cepa. henne leac*); *DVH* 1087–1126 (*cepa*); LS 344 (*basil* [بصل *baṣal*], *cæpe*); EPN ii (*cepa. ennelec*), iii (*ungio. yne-leac*), iv (*scalonia. ynneleac | cerefolium. enne-leac | unio. ynneleac*), vi (*cepe. oingnun. kue-lek*); Cl c.36 (*cepa*); TH 135 (*cepa domestica*); Pand. 78 (ARbasal, GRbulbus, LAcepe); DVH(NME) 245r.10 (*letus*); DVH(SME) 17a.9 (*oynones*); Alph. 36 (*cepa. eyngnon*); AC 177.26 (*cepa. onyoun*) ⚭ GH 107 (CEPE DOMESTICA, *onyon*); Fu 163 (KPOMMYON, *cepa*); Tu 1.267 (ONYONS, *unio, cepa, crommion*); DL 459 (ONIONS, κρόμμιον, *cepa*); Ge 134 (ONIONS, κρόμμιον, *cepa*).
>
> C⁴ (SM, RM, Tu, DL) | C⁴S (Fu) | C³S³ (TH, GH) | C⁴S⁴ (LS, Ge)

1582 Galyan saythe. → **189** for the ultimate origin of this passage.

1584 hote... 1585 degre. No information is given in the canonical version of *DVH* about the temperament of the onion, and moreover the complexion given here runs counter to most *auctoritates*, who assumed a dry nature for this species. While the possibility that this is an interpolation or else an addition of the scribe, who (mis)copied the temperament of the species in its customary place in entries derived from Macer's herbal (just before the list of virtues), cannot be discarded outright, the syntax of the sentence, which is verbless, is suggestive of a faulty exemplar.

1586 Plenius saith. This is a rendering of *NH* xx.43 through *DVH* 1092–1094: "Asclepiadis schola [dicit] ad colorem quoque validum profici hoc cibo, si ieiuni cotidie edant, firmitatem valetudinis custodiri, stomacho utile‹s› esse". Macer Floridus versified these ideas by stating that the author of these *dicta* was Asclepius, the god of Medicine himself, but in fact Pliny was referring to Asclepiades of Bithynia (see *NH* xxvi.12–21; Rawson 1982, Polito 1990). The same fragment is attributed to Galen in the other version of the entry (→ **191**).

1607 oynone gresse. MED: *s.v.* oitone gresse *n.* gives the name as a hapax and suggests identification with either oat grass (*Bromus hordeaceus* L./*B. sterilis* L.) or onion grass (*Arrhenatherum elatius* (L.) P.Beauv. ex J.Presl & C.Presl). The round form of the root and maritime habitat of the plant described in the entry, yet, do not match those gramineous species (the *bulbosum* variety of *Arrhenatherum*, which might qualify as a defendable candidate, is to be discarded as its bulbs look rather like small nodes, usually two or three, that are reminiscent of small onions threaded together). It seems safer to assume that the species meant here is the sea onion (*Drimia maritima* (L.) Stearn = *Scilla maritima* L.), which was historically an important medicinal plant. Comparison with the source text, *AC* supports this identification. There are also pharmacographic grounds for the emendation, as the powers of the species as emetic (**1608**), anthydropic (**1609**) and alexipharmic (**1610**) were already included in the Classical pharmacopea.

> **Literature**: SEA ONION (*Drimia maritima* (L.) Stearn): *HP* i.6–9 (σκίλλα); *MM* ii.171; *NH* xix.93 (*scilla*); *SM* xii.125; *RM* ii.260; *OEH* 43 (*herba bulbiscillica. glædene*); *Dur. Glos.* 300 (*bulbi scillici. gledene*); *LS* 294 (*haspel* [اِشْقِيل *išqīl*], *squilla*); *EPN* iii, iv (*scilla. glædene*), iv (*scilla et gladiola. glædene*); *CI* s.4 (*squilla. oynen of þe see*); *TH* 454 (*squilla*); *Pand.* 339 (ᴀʀ*haurifel, haulachach,* ɢʀ*sala,* ʟᴀ*squilla, cepe muris*); *Alph.* 173 (*scille*); *Sin.Bart.* 40 (*squilla. cepa marina*); *AC* p. 202.33 (*squilla. oynon*) ❊ *GH* 413 (SQUILLA, *cepa marina, squyll, see onyon, chyboll of the see, bulbe, scilla, albison, pantacron, cifanos*); *Fu* 300 (ΣΚΙΛΛΑ, *scilla, squilla*); *Tu* 2.560 (SEA UNYON, *squilla, skilla, squill unyon*); *DL* 463 (SEA VNION, *squilla, scilla,* σκίλλα); *Ge* 135 (SEA ONION, *squill,* σκίλλα, *scilla, cepa muris*).
>
> C^2 (*SM*, Tu, Ge) | C^2S^2 (*RM, TH, GH*, Fu) | C^2S^3 (DL) | C^3S^3 (*LS, CI*)

1613 osmunde. The Latin heading (→ **1462**), the ME name and the habitat indicate that the species treated here must be the royal fern (*Osmunda regalis*

L.). The same species was briefly mentioned earlier in the treatise (→ **663**), with reference to the consolidative powers that are mentioned in the usual literature. The garbled reference to salves (**1614**) on the other hand is missing from its source text (AC) but might be authorial: Ge states that the tender sprigs (i.e., the furled fronds) of this fern "are good to be put into balmes, oiles, and consolidatiues or healing plaisters, and into vnguents appropriate vnto wounds, punctures, and such like". On the other hand, there is always a possibility that ‹salvis› stands for *s a v i s "saves".

> **Literature**: ROYAL FERN (*Osmunda regalis* L.): *EPN* vi (*osmunda. osmunde. bon-wurt*); *Alph.* 132 (*osmunda, filex siluestris.* _{GA}*osmonde, feugerole.* _{AN}*euerfarn, moreclam*); *Sin. Bart.* 32 (*osmunda. everfern*); *AC* 211.1 (*osmund. osmund*) ⚕ *GH* 82 (FILEX DICTUS OS MUNDA, *filex masculus, heferue*); Fu 38 (ΆΦΑΚΗ, *aphace, syluestris uitia, Os mundi,* [*Wildwicken, S. Christoffelßkraut*]); *DL* 291 (OSMUNDE, *water ferne, St Christophers hearbe, filix aquatica, filicastrum, lunaria major*); Ge 970 (WATER FERNE, *Osmund the water man, Saint Christophers herbe, osmunda, filix palustris/aquatilis, filicastrum, lunaria maior*).

CS (Ge) | C¹S² (DL)

1616 oculus Christi. The Latin name is applied as a rule to some yellow-flowered plant, diversely identified as pot marigold (*Calendula officinalis* L.), hairy fleabane (*Inula oculus-christi* L.) or some *Chrysanthemum* L., but none of them applies here as the flower of the species must be blue. Stirling 1995–1998: *s.v.* oculus, drawing ultimately from a Latin synonyma, includes Michaelmas daisy (*Aster amellus* L.) which bears purple flowers. But the physical description and the woodcuts in Renaissance herbals for the species (see for example Fu and Ge) seems rather to picture some *Salvia* L. spp., traditionally identified as wild clary (*Salvia verbenaca* L.) or else meadow clary (*S. pratensis* L.). The description tallies as well as regards the seeds, for they are indeed round—more accurately, slightly egg-shaped. Brodin (1950: 283) recognized the wood forget-me-not (*Myosotis sylvatica* Hoffm.) in the description provided in the source text for this entry (AC), probably because the plant leaves are compared there to those of some *Symphytum* L. spp., cf. "þis herbe haȝt lewys lyk to conforie". Identification of the plant of the entry in *LH* with some *Salvia*, and particularly with *S. verbenaca*, is yet to be preferred on account of the medical powers traditionally allotted to this species, and would also explain the obscure ‹wilde worte› as a simple clerical error for *WILDE CLARY. On the other hand, the appearance of ‹scabwort› (rather than *stab-wort*, as read in MED: *s.v.* stab *n.*, drawing from *WG* and interpreted as an erroneous spelling for *stub-wort, i.e. wood-sorrel, *Oxalis acetosella* L.)

is perhaps to be explained as an instance of misuse of a synonyma: the name *scabwort* referred as a rule to another yellow-flowered species, elecampane (*Inula helenium* L., → **899**; note that, as stated above, L. *oculus Christi* was usually applied another member from the same genus).

Not surprisingly, *Salvia verbenaca*—just like any other Asteraceae—was praised medically as an excellent ophthalmic (**1618**; Renaissance apothecaries sometimes spelt *clary*, apparently from ML *sclarea*, as *clair-ye*, *clear-eye* through popular etymology; see OED: *s.v.*). The plant is additionally described as stomachal and eupeptic (**1620**), anticholeric and phlegmagogue (**1621**) and as a consequence deoppilant of the liver, brain and nostrils (**1623**).

Literature: WILD CLARY (*Salvia verbenaca* L.): *HP* viii.1.4 (ὅρμινον); *MM* iii.129 (ὅρμινον); *NH* xxii.159 (*horminum*); *SM* xii.152 (φόρβιον); *RM* ii.270 (φορμίον); *Cl* G.9 (*gallitricum, centrum galli*); *TH* 208 (*gallitricum, centrigalli*); *Pand.* 626 ($_{GR}$*sideritis, eraclia,* $_{LA}$*scariola agrestis, centrum galli, gerebotanum*); *DVH(SME)* 43a.4 (*sclarye*); *Alph.* 38, 71, 126 (*centrum galli, centrum grana, gallitricum, gallicresta, caride, nux moscata, oculus Christi, herba cancri*); *Sin.Bart.* 22, 32 (*gallitricum, galli crista, centrum galli, oculus Christi*); *AC* 210.13 (*oculus Christi*) ⚜ *GH* 193 (GALLITRICUM, *centrum galli, clarey*); Fu 193 (ʹOPMINON, *geminalis, gallitricum*); DL 181 (HORMINUM, *geminalis, wilde clarie, oculus Christi, double clarie*, ὅρμινον); Ge 627 (WILDE CLARIE, *oculus Christi,* ὅρμινον, *geminalis*).

CS (*Cl, TH,* DL) | C³S³ (Ge)

1625 paratory. The Latin headword and the first English synonym are traditionally applied to pellitory-of-the-wall (*Parietaria judaica* L.), and so does ⟨hemerworte⟩ by assuming that the scribe must have missed an *er*-brevigraph over **m** (see OED: *s.v.* hammerwort *n.*). On the other hand, ⟨lithwort⟩ is not fully clear. OE *liðwyrt* has been identified as a synonym for a number of species, above all danewort (*Sambucus ebulus* L., → **2385**) but including candidates as diverse as the wayfaring-tree (*Viburnum lantana* L.), rue (*Ruta graveolens* L., → **1947**), or madder (*Rubia tinctorum* L., → **1271**; see Bierbaumer 1975–1979: i.96, ii.79–80, iii.163 for details). But the evidence of *OEH* xxix = *HAP* 75, where *lyðwyrt*, translating La. *(h)ostriago*, is said to grow "abutan byrgenne & on beorgum & on wagum þæra husa" (*in monumentis aut parietibus*), may indicate the name could be used for a *Parietaria* already in Anglo-Saxon times (*contra* de Vriend 1984: 295, who takes it to mean the *Viburnum* on account of the accompanying illustration in the MS, even though this plant's habitat is in fact open woodland). The explanation probably lies in a confusion between *vitrago*, a synonym for *Parietaria* since Oribasius (see Stirling 1995–1998: *s.v.*), and *ostriago*. The possibility that it may also mean buck's-horn plantain (*Plantago coronopus* L.), tentatively suggested in

MED: s.v. lĭth-wort n., can be discarded as it surely rests on another scribal confusion, this time between *stellago* and *ostriago* (see André 1985: s.vv.). The entry follows AC.

The species is praised as stomachal (**1627**), anti-inflammatory of the kidneys and penis (**1628**), lithontriptic (**1629**), and antihemorrhoidal (**1630**). Indeed the species was used traditionally used by medieval and Renaissance physicians against problems of the genitourinary system.

> **Literature**: PELLITORY-OF-THE-WALL (*Parietaria judaica* L.): *HP* vii.7.2 (παρθένιον); *MM* iv.85 (ἐλξίνη); *NH* xxii.43 (*perdicium, parthenium, sideritis, herba urceolaris, astercum*); *SM* xi.874; *RM* ii.210; *OEH* 83 (*herba perdicalis. dolhrune*); *Dur.Glos.* 304 (*perdicalis. dolhrune*); *EPN* iv (*perdicalis. homor-wyrt*); *Cl* p.14 (*paritaria. paritorie*); *TH* 367 (*paritaria, vitreola, perdiciados*); *Pand.* 32 ($_{GR}$*alsmen, partenion, perdicali, perdicion, sideritis, eraclia querastri agreste, libatian, poliominon,* $_{AR}$*tugegraria,* $_{LA}$*paritaria*); *Alph.* 51 (*ebulus uel ebula* $_{GA}$*eble,* $_{AN}$*welleuort, licheuurt*), 134 (*paritaria, perniciades, uitreola, nitrago, herba muralis, paritarie*); *AC* p. 197.19 (*paritoria. parytorye, hethwort, hemerwort*) ⚘ Fu 106 (ΈΛΕΙΝΗ, περδίκιον, vrceolaris, pari(e)taria, muralium, muralis*); Tu 2.394 (PARIETORI, *helxine, pardition, parietariam*); DL 37 (PELLITORY OF THE WALL, ἐλξίνη, περδίκιον, *muralium perdicium, vrceolaris, pari(e)taria, muralis, perdicalis*); Ge 260 (PELLITORIE OF THE WALL, *pari(e)taria, muralis, helxine cissampelos, perdicium, vrceolaris, vitraria*).
>
> CS (*Cl*) | C³S³ (*TH*) | FH (*SM, RM,* Fu, DL, Ge)

1631 pulyoll monten. Identification with wild thyme (*Thymus serpyllum* L.; → **2314** about the garden counterpart), given in the entry as a synonym, is traditional but not really backed by any pharmacographic evidence. Although the text is a severely abridged version of *AC*, there is yet no reference to its vulnerary properties (**1633**) either in the Latin or in the ME versions. The English text only mentions its qualities as a purgative and restorative of the humoral balance (**1632**), while the Latin rendering (*Sl.*16r/16–17), which is longer than the version printed by Brodin, further mentions its assumed qualities as antiemetic and antacid, antitussive, emmenagogue and abortifacient.

A substantial part of the early English evidence, yet, suggests that *Thymus* must have become confused with some *Origanum* L. spp. (as a rule either wild marjoram, *O. vulgare* L., → **1553**, **1634**, or sweet marjoram, *O. marjorana* L. → **1265**), which is an akin labiate very much used in cookery (details in Bierbaumer 1975–1979: ii.90, iii.180). The virtues of these two *Origanum* included in the medical literature of the time, and particularly the vulnerary one, do not really match the ones recorded here either, but there is a third member of the same genus, dittany of Crete (*Origanum dictamnus* L., → **574**), which was universally commended as vulnerary and arrow expeller since Dioscorides's times. But supportive evidence is flimsy since there is no mention to arrows in the text, a feature that never fails to appear in the accounts of dittany.

Literature: WILD THYME (*Thymus serpyllum* L.): *HP* i.9.4 (ἕρπυλλος); *MM* iii.38; *NH* xx.245 (*serpyllum*); *SM* xi.877; *RM* ii.211; *OEH* 101 (*herba serpillus. organa*); *Dur. Glos.* 305 (*serpillus. organe, brade lec*); *DVH* 1325–1341 (*serpillum*); *LS* 289 (*nemen* [نمّام *nammān*], *serpillum*); *EPN* iii (*serpulum. crop-leac*), iv (*sarpullum. brade leac*), v (*serpillum, fille*), vii (*hoc sirpillum. petergrys*); *Cl* s.37 (*serpillum, erpillum*); *TH* 460 (*serpillum, erpetum*); *Pand.* 557 (_{AR}*numir, mestratir, miseri,* _{GR}*serpillum, herpillum,* _{LA}*serpillum*); *DVH(NME)* 252r.3 (*betone*); *Alph.* 120 (*montanum serpillum, timbra. brothwort*); *Sin.Bart.* 35 (*pulegium montanum. brotherwort*); *AC* p. 198.36 (*pvlogium montanum. puliole mountayn, hulwort, broþerwort*) ❦ *GH* 342 (POLIUM MONTANUM, *wylde tyme*); *Fu* 93 (ἙΡΠΥΛΛΟΣ, *serpyllum*); *Tu* 2.565 (WILD THYME, *serpillum*); *DL* 165 (WILD-TIME, *puliall montaine, pellamountaine, running time, serpillum, pulegium montantum*); *Ge* 455 (WILDE TIME, *puliall mountaine, pella mountaine, running time, creeping time, mother of time, ladies bedstrawe, serpillum, fulegium montanum*).
¶ DITTANY OF CRETE (*Origanum dictamnus* L.): → ditander [**574**].

CS (*Cl, TH*) | C³S³ (Fu, Tu, DL, Ge)

1634 pygele. The ME name *pig(e)le* usually referred to the greater stitchwort, *Stellaria holostea* L. (see PNME: *s.v.* pigula), but comparison with Latin pharmacopea indicates that this is in fact a translation of the chapter *origanum* in *DVH* 1285–1324 as given in *DVH(NME)*. In fact the stitchword does not seem to have been treated in Classical botanical literature (the Gk name apparently refers to some plantain, *Plantago bellardii* All. or *P. albicans* L., see André 1985: *s.v.* holosteon). Wild marjoram (*Origanum vulgare* L.) had been already treated above (→ **1553**, with discussion). The word *pulegium*, frequently used as a synonym for *origanum* in many medieval sources (see Literature), must have obviously misled the ME translator, but note the spelling ⟨pugile⟩ in *W*.31v/15, which probably maintains the original vocalism of Ω and which was erroneously emended in the other witnesses.

In comparison with the previous rendering of the species, this version includes the translation of *DVH* 1291–1296, containing the powers of the species as an anthydropic, cholagogue and emmenagoge (**1638**), and the recipe to make noxious beasts flee (**1647**). A copy mistake is behind the reference to an antipyrotic virtue (→ **1637**). On the other hand, several virtues are missing: antipruritic (*DVH* 1298), antiuvulitic (*DVH* 1302), antiotalgic (*DVH* 1306), anthelminthic and diuretic (*DVH* 1318), antiodontalgic (*DVH* 1319) and diaphoretic (*DVH* 1321–1322). Moreover, the last lines of this version include two virtues that are not found in the Latin text and may answer to an interpolation from some other chapter: against some pulmonary disease involving the effusion of a watery substance, probably bronchitis or edema, and as an ophthalmic (→ **1650, 1652**).

Literature: WILD MARJORAM (*Origanum vulgare* L.): → origanum [**1553**]. ¶ GREATER STITCHWORT (*Stellaria holostea* L.): *Grad.* 351 (*lingua auis*); *LS* 216 (*lisen hasafir* [لسان العصافير] *lisān al-'aṣāfīr*], *lingua auis*); *EPN* ii (*agrimonia. stic-wyrt*); *Cl* L.7 (*lingua auis. pigle*); *TH* 252 (*lingua avis*); *Pand.* 502 (ᴀʀ*lisenanalhasafir*, ɢʀ*lienula iafir*, ʟᴀ*lingua auis*); *Alph.* 103 (*lingua auis. pigula idem. sticheuurt*); *Sin.Bart.* 34 (*pigle. stichewort*); *AC* p. 197.42 (*pjgula maior. pygle, stichewort, bryddes tonge*) ⚶ *GH* 62 (LINGUA ANSERIS, *goosbyll, stychwort, bec d'oye*); *Fu* 48 (*ΑΓΡΩΣΤΙΣ, gramen*); *DL* 364 (STITCHWURT, κραταιόγονον, κραταίονον, κράταιος, *gramen leucanthemum*); *Ge* 42 (STITCHWOORT, ὁλόστεον, *tota ossea*).

C¹H¹ (*Grad., TH*) | C²H² (*LS*) | CS (DL) | C¹S¹ (*Cl*) | C⁴S⁴ (*GH*) | F¹H² (Fu)

1636 for²... 1637 brenynge. This virtue, recorded in all three copies derived from *RH*, is missing both in the Latin poem and in *B*. This is not a scribal addition but a copy mistake instead of the expected *BRISYNGE to translate *DVH* 1291 *conquassata*, cf. ⟨all brusynge⟩ in the other version of this chapter (**1556**). See another instance of the same error in → **2421**.

1644 hony and rose. *DVH* 1307 *cepis et rho syriaco*. While ⟨rose⟩ instead of *rho syriaco* (sumac, *Rhus coriaria* L.) is an evident *lectio facilior*, the translation of *cepa* as ⟨hony⟩ is unexpected and must answer to some copy error in either *Q* or *Ω* (perhaps standing metonymically for a misread *a p i s "bee"?).

1650 abatith þe. This virtue is not in the canonical edition of *DVH* so we cannot read the ME passage against it, but the sentence is obviously nonsensical as one should not reduce, but rather increase, the dryness to cure watery lungs. These two words should therefore have been expunctuated by the scribe, just like he did with the ⟨akynge⟩ that followed, as they are due to a homoioteleuton *y - v s i d ... v s y d in S_1 that the scribe managed to detect. That he chose to delete just the noun is revealing. He must have taken *DRYETH in his exemplar as the complement of ⟨abatith⟩, rather than as a verb (cf. *B*.254v/II ⟨dryse⟩, and similarly in *W* and *P*), hence the inclusion of the preposition ⟨of⟩ immediately after. Therefore the ending *-th* must have been used both as a noun and verbal morpheme in *Λ*: it is probable that the scribe of S_1 would have deleted the whole fragment if his exemplar had read *DRYIS.

1651 venym. There is no reference in the parallel passage of the Latin poem (*DVH* 1319) to poison, but rather to toothache.

1652 the juis. As in the previous note, this virtue is not found in the canonical version of *DVH*: the passage in the original Latin poem (1323–1324) explains how a mixture of the juice of the plant and gruel applied to the hips reduces the pain in the area.

1653 pulyoll. The entry is a translation of the chapter *pulegium* in *DVH* as rendered in *DVH(NME)*. As with *origanum* (→ **1553**), the Latin name was applied to a number of labiates (André 1985: *s.v.* pūleium), but in ME the name normally refers to either wild thyme (*Thymus serpyllum* L.) or pennyroyal (*Mentha pulegium* L.; see MED: *s.v.* pŭliol *n.*). The entry is taken to describe the latter species, not only because wild thyme appears to have been treated just a few lines before (→ **1631**) and was distinguished there through the addition of the adjective ‹monten›, but also because identification is reassured on textual and pharmacological grounds, cf. its qualities as abortifacient (**1654** = *DVH* 628), emmenagogue and mazolytic (**1655** = *DVH* 629–630), antiparalytic (**1657** = *DVH* 642–643), expectorant (**1658** = *DVH* 644–646), antacid and antiemetic (**1659** = *DVH* 647–648), anticoleric and alexipharmic (**1661** = *DVH* 649–650), tonic (**1663** = *DVH* 651–656), antigingivitic and antipodagric (**1665** = *DVH* 657–658), anti-inflammatory and antiephelic (**1666** = *DVH* 659–661), splenetic (**1668** = *DVH* 662), antipruritic and against endometritis (**1669** = *DVH* 664–665), antitussive and diuretic (**1670** = *DVH* 666–667). Missing from this account are the last ten lines from the poem (668–677), where the author described (again) the powers of the species as an anti-inflammatory and alexipharmic, and also as an aphrodisiac, galactogenous, pulmonic and hepatic, and as a remedy to dog bite. These same lines are missing as well in several of the Latin MSS consulted by Choulant for his edition (γ, η, λ, π), so this is surely a reflection of the entry as recorded in *Q*.

Literature: PENNYROYAL (*Mentha pulegium* L.): *HP* ix.16.1 (βλήχων); *MM* iii.31 (γλήχων); *NH* xx.152 (*Puleium*); *SM* xi.857; *RM* ii.205; *OEH* 94 (*herba pollegion. dweorgedwosle*); *Dur.Glos.* 304 (*pollegia. hyll vyrt, dveorge dveosle*); *DVH* 626–677 (*pullegium*); *LS* 300 (*fandenigi* [فتناغ *futanağ*], *origanum*); *EPN* ii (*pollegia. hyl-wyrt*), iv (*pollegia. broðer-wyrt, hæl-wyrt, dweorges drostle*), v (*pollegia, hyl-wyrt, dwyrge-dwysle*), vi (*pulegium. puliol, hul-wurt*); *CI* p.16 (*pulegium. piliole, hulwort*); *TH* 369 (*pulegium*); *DVH(NME)* 251r.10 (*puliole*); *Alph.* 76 (*gliconium. pulegium regale*), 148 (*polium*), 150 (*pulegium regale. gliconeum idem | pulegium ceruinum uel montanum, serpillum, herpillum,* ᴳᴬ*puliol,* ᴬᴺ*brotherwurt*); *Sin.Bart.* 22 (*glicon, gliconum, pullegium regale*); *AC* p. 198.14 (*pvlogium regale. puliole real, churche-wort*) ⚘ *Fu* 73 (ΓΛΗΧΩΝ, βλήχων, *pulegium*); *Tu* 2.532 (PENNY RYALL, *puddyng grasse, pulegium,* γληχων, βλήχων); *DL* 166 (PENNY ROYALL, *podding grasse,* γλήχων, *pulegium*); *Ge* 546 (PENNIE ROYALL, *pudding grasse, puliall royall, organie,* γλήχων, βλήχων, *pulegium*).

CS (*SM, RM*) | C³S³ (*DVH, LS, CI, TH, Fu, DL, Ge*)

1669 wormys of the body. There seems to be no references to intestinal worms in the corresponding Latin (half-)line, which reads *pruritus non patietur* (*DVH* 664). There seems to be no reference to any anthelminthic virtue in the pharmacological literature, so this is probably to be put down as an interpolation.

1672 pyany. The entry describes the medical qualities of peonies as described in *DVH* 1605–1640 and according to *DVH(NME)*. As indicated in the text, two species of *paeoniae*, male and female, were distinguished in Graeco-Roman and medieval pharmacopea. The female is universally acknowledged to be *Paeonia officinalis* L., while the male is usually identified as *P. mascula* (L.) Mill. (= *P. corallina* Retz.). Only the former was really known in medieval Western pharmacopea, as hinted by its modern binomen. (Macer Floridus avoided the issue and did not really provide with any separate virtue to the male counterpart in **1688–1689**.)

Identification with *Paeonia* L. spp., and particularly with *P. officinalis*, is traditional and sustained by textual and pharmacological criteria, cf. its value as a splenetic (**1673** = *DVH* 1607), emmenagogue and antidysenteric (**1674** = *DVH* 1608–1609), anticholecystic and anticteric (**1676** = *DVH* 1610–1613), lithontriptic (**1677** = *DVH* 1614), antiepileptic (**1678** = *DVH* 1617–1629), and as a postpartum tonic (**1687** = *DVH* 1638–1639). Some of the purposed qualities of the species are missing, viz. as a hepatic and nephretic (*DVH* 1607), antinephritic (*DVH* 1613), and antephialtic (*DVH* 1615–1616). A homoioteleuton in *RH* explains the missing virtues of the species as an antimetrorrhagic and antiacne (→ **1684**), but these were demonstrably recorded in Ω. The virtue against scotoma is also missing, the reading in *B* notwithstanding (→ **1675**). The last two virtues of the entry (antiparalytic and eloquent, **1690, 1692**) are not included in the canonical version of the Latin poem, and probably answer to an interpolation from another entry. Both were apparently already present in *Q*.

Literature: PEONY (*Paeonia officinalis* L.): *HP* ix.8.6 (γλυκυσίδη); *MM* iii.140; *NH* xxvii.84 ff. (*glycyside, paeonia, pentorobon*); *SM* xi.858; *RM* ii.205; *Grad.* 358 (*peonia*); *OEH* 66 (*herba peonia*); *DVH* 1605–1640 (*paeonia*); *LS* 61 (*foeonia* [فاوانيا] *fāwānyā*], *pœonia*); *EPN* iv (*peonia. peonia*); *CI* P.3 (*peonia*); *TH* 356 (*peonia*); *Pand.* 574 (_{AR}*pinufer, pionia,* _{GR}*penterebon, pentaboran, pernia, glikifide,* _{LA}*peonia*); *DVH(NME)* 254v.18 (*pyone*); *DVH(SME)* 31a.6 (*pyonye*); *Alph.* 145 (*pionia, glacida*); *Sin.Bart.* 23 (*glicida, pionia*); *AC* 212.9 (*piania. pyanye*) ❦ *GH* 328 (PEONIA, *pyony, penthoron, aglosotos, aliofotes*); *Fu* 75 (ΓΛΥΚΥΣΙΔΗ, παιονία, *pœonia, casta herba*); *Tu* 2.496 (PEONYE, *glyciside, pentoboron*); *DL* 244 (PEONIE, παιονία, *pœonia, dulcilida, idœus dactylus,* *aglaophotis, herba casta*); Ge 829 (PEIONIE, παιονία, *pæonia, dulcifida, rosa fatuina, herba casta, lunaris, idæus dactylus, aglaophotis*).

CS (*SM, RM,* Fu, Ge) | C¹S¹ (*LS*) | C²S² (*Grad., Cl, TH, DVH, GH*)

1675 abatith þe akynge of the blader. The Bodley version offers an extra virtue here: *B*.254v/20–21 ⟨abatis þe hede werke & þe werke of þe bledd*er*⟩. The reference to headache may then stand for *DVH* 1612 *scotosim*, since this disease (an alteration in the field of vision) is frequently paired with giddiness and migraines. Still, the reading in the other two MSS (*W*.34r/27–28 ⟨all þe hard werk⟩, *P*.276/18 ⟨þe harde ache⟩) indicate otherwise, as this perfectly translates *DVH* 1611 *duros ... dolores*. It seems rather that α was unclear here, and the scribe must have conjectured from the **h** and **d** that he read immediately before *WERK.

1677 Galean seiþ. The idea that the roots of peony are good against epilepsy, which Tu proved and confirmed in "two childer", is recorded in *SM* xi.859, 10–16 but there are a number of differences: in the Galenic version, the sick is an eight-month old infant (παιδίον ὀκτὼ μησί), rather than a boy, and he is bound to bear the root (τῆς ῥίζης) rather than a branch with leaves. The change in the patient's age is already present in *DVH* 1620 *annorum circa octo* and in *Grad.* "puerum octo annorum". The ME text is somewhat abridged, as Galen went on to explain that he took the root off the boy's neck again and the infant had an immediate seizure, which subsided as soon as the root was replaced. The whole episode was correctly translated in *DVH(SME)* 31a20–31 while, in contrast, *AC* 212.22–24 succinctly says "ȝef a chyld hawe þe fallyng ewyl. tak þe Rote of þis herbe and hang it abowtyn þe chyldis nekke and he schal be hol". The Northern MSS of *DVH(NME)* offer neither the story nor the Dioscoridean advice that follows (→ **1682**), although in the case of Bodley there is a textual clue (a mysterious *B*.254v/23–24 ⟨borne on hyate⟩ that seems to match ⟨to bere on hem⟩ in *P*.276/26–27 and ⟨to ber vpon ham⟩ in *S*₁ (**1683–1684**), apparently *BER(E) ON ÞAM) that suggests that the fragment may have been damaged in its exemplar. The omission in *W* is on the other hand clearly deliberate.

1682 Diascardias... 1683 saith. Pedanius Dioscorides of Anazarbus, military physician under Nero, herbalist and author of Περὶ ὕλης ἰατρικῆς (*De Materia Medica*) in five books. He described the physical features and the medical properties of a large number of *simples*, becoming the first pharmacological treatise to be widely read since Classical Antiquity and well studied during the Renaissance and beyond. The original Greek text was fully translated into Latin at least twice: first by Gargilius Martialis, which is now fragmentary, and later by the anonymous translator (Constantinus Africanus or some of his disciples? Riddle 1984: 102) of the *Dioscorides Langobardus*, an alphabetized version which has survived and is available in print (Hofmann/Auracher 1883, Stadler 1897a,b, 1899, 1901). These translations allowed Dioscorides to be known during the Middle Ages (in opposition to other sources, for example Theophrastus).

This fragment renders *DVH* 1628–1629 quite faithfully (although "young and old" for *cunctis ... caducis* is a somewhat free translation), but the passage is nowhere to be found in the appropriate entry of *MM*, where epilepsy is never mentioned. Beyond the expected policy of dropping names to impart more authority to this remedy, it is easy to suspect that Macer Floridus's mentioning of the Greek physician here answers to metrical reasons, as the syllabic structure of his name fits perfectly the gap in the hexameter. → **180** for another instance of the same.

1684 take... 1685 bed. This sentence does not record any virtue. In fact a homoioteleuton *DRYNKE ÞAM...DRYNKE ÞAM in γ explains that the virtues of the species explained in *DVH* 1631–1632 are missing both here and in *W*. Bodley (and, with variants, also *P*.276/28–277/2) reads as follows: *B*.254v/25–255r/1 ⟨drynke þame in wyne & it ste*m*mys þe flixe of þe mat*r*ice and also it dos a-way þe blacke cornys iff scho drynke þam⟩.

1694 papy. An account of the medical virtues of the poppies (common name for several *Papaver* L. spp.), according to the *DVH(NME)* translation of *DVH*. Other than in S_1, the entry is kept only in *B* (→ **1526** for another example). As customary at least since Dioscorides, a threefold division is made in the poem between a white, a black and a red species. The former two are probably varieties of the opium poppy (*Papaver somniferum* L.), *P. s.* L. var. *album* DC. and *P. s.* L. var. *nigrum* DC., but the red species described in *MM* remains unidentified. It stands to reason, however, that the medieval physician assumed that the species was the field poppy (*Papaver rhoeas* L.) which grows among cereal crops.

Identification is traditional and sustained by textual and pharmacological data, not only because of the references to the well-known value of its latex, opium, as a powerful soporific (recurrent in the text, starting in **1700** = *DVH* 1050–1051), but also for the medical value of seed as an antidiarrheic and antimetrorrhagic (**1704, 1712** = *DVH* 1057–1058, 1075), antitussive (**1706, 1712** = *DVH* 1059, 1075), antiherpetic (**1708** = *DVH* 1064), analgesic (**1715** = *DVH* 1077–1079) and antipodagric (**1717** = *DVH* 1083–1084). The antirheumatic and antiotalgic qualities are faultily recorded as well (→ **1713, 1716**), while its antitonsillitic powers appear in the Bodley version (→ **1708**). Missing from the translation is the passage where the species is used as a voice tonic (*DVH* 1065–1067).

Literature: POPPIES (*Papaver* L. spp.): *HP* ix.8.2 (μήκων); *MM* iv.63 (μήκων ῥοιάς), iv.64 (μήκων ἥμερος/κηπευτή); *NH* xix.168 (*papauer*); *SM* xii.72 (μήκων); *RM* ii.241; *Grad*. 346, 386 (*semen nigri papaueris*); *LS* 364 (*thaxthax* [خشخاش *ḥašḥāš*], *papauer*); *OEH* 54 (*herba metoria. hwit popig*); *Dur.Glos.* 304 (*metoria. hvit popig | papaver. popig*); *DVH* 1037–1086 (*papauer*); *EPN* ii, v (*papaver. popig*), iv (*astula regia. baso, popi | papaver. popig*) vi (*astula regia. popi | alimonis. wilde popi*), vii (*hec papaver. chesbolle*), viii (*papaver. a chespolle*), ix (*hoc papaver. a papy*); *Cl* P.4 (*papauer. popy*); *TH* 357 (*papaver*); *Pand*. 143 (ARcaxchax, chachili, caxax, caschafi, GRanimonie, miconium, LApapauer); *DVH(NME)* 249r.9 (*chesbole*); *DVH(SME)* 19b.24 (*popie*); *Alph*. 134 (*papauer album. whatpopy | papauer nigrum. blakpopy | papauer rubeum. redpopy*); *Sin.Bart*. 17 (*codium, papaver*); *AC* 212.25 (*papauard. wylde popy*) ❦ *GH* 329 (PAPAUER, *poppy*); Fu 194 (ΜΗΚΩΝ 'ΡΟΙΑΣ, *papauer rhœas/fluidum/erraticum/rubeum*), 195 (ΜΗΚΩΝ 'ΗΜΕΡΟΣ, *papauer satiuum*); Tu 2.486 (POPPY, *chesboule, papaver,* μηκων); DL 309 (POPPIE, μήκων, *papauer, oxytonon, prosopon, lethe, lethusa, onitron*), 310 (RED POPPIE, *cornerose,* μήκων ῥοιάς, *papauer erraticum/fluidum/rhœas/rubrum*); Ge 295 (GARDEN POPPIE, μήκων, *papauer*), 299 (CORNE ROSE, *wilde poppie,* μήκων ῥοιάς, *papauer erraticum/rubrum*).

F⁴ (*SM, RM,* Fu, Ge) | FS (*DVH, Cl, TH, GH*) | F¹S¹ (*Grad*. [plant]) | F⁴S⁴ (*Grad*. [seed], *LS,* DL)

1694 hote and drye. As seen from the previous note, this plant was almost universally considered to be cold in the fourth degree, and *DVH* is no exception: *vim gelidam siccamque* (1037). According to Choulant's apparatus, only MS π reads *calidam siccamque*. But of course the possibility that this is a mere mistranslation cannot be ruled out.

1696 tendryns. Cf *B*.249r/11 ⟨tend*er* hede⟩ and *DVH* 1042 *teneris ... capitellis*. Note moreover ⟨tendryn⟩ in **1709** and probably **2511**. The emendation was already suggested in MED: *s.v.* tendron *n*.

1708 sleyth the fire of helle. Bodley offers here *B*.249r/21–22 ⟨it helys þe temples⟩. Each of the two MSS has missed a portion of the complete translation, for the Latin text (*DVH* 1063–1064) reads:
> Eximie fauces dicunt curare tumentes,
> Quosque vocant sacros extinguere dicitur ignes.

The translation of *fauces ... tumentes*, likely to be a reference to tonsillitis, seems therefore quite inaccurate unless it derives from some variant in Ω.

1711 hony. A homoioteleuton somewhere in the transmission of S_1 explains the missing fragment *B*.249r/24–25 ⟨to it be als thike as hony⟩ that translates *DVH* 1074 *sit quasi mel*.

1712 stroiethe the womme. This has been emended after *B*.249v/1 ⟨wom⟩ and *DVH* 1075 *alvum*. The reference to kidneys later on the same sentence is also unexpected, as it translates *DVH* 1076 *vocalis venae bene rheumatismata siccat*, so ⟨reynes⟩ must then be a copy mistake for *REUME, cf. *B*.249v/1 ⟨rewme⟩. The word *rheuma* here is used etymologically (Gk ῥεῦμα "flow"), as morbid discharge of phlegm from the head.

1715 put sauery ther-to. There seems to be no references to savory in the Latin entry, and the parallel passage in Bodley reads *B*.249v/3 ⟨saltt þer-to don to þe erys it mak*is* men to herr*e* bett*er*⟩. Comparison with the original poem indicates that ⟨sauery⟩/⟨saltt⟩ must stand for *DVH* 1081 *croci redolentia fila* here. A second reference to savory later on the entry (**1717**, cf. also *B*.249v/4 ⟨sau*e*ray⟩) corresponds again with a recipe including saffron: *DVH* 1083 *crocoque*. Obviously the words in the MSS answer to *lectiones faciliores* but it is difficult to be sure about the authorial reading; perhaps Ω *SAFUR (→ **2104**)?

1716 to slepe. The reference to sleep must be a copy mistake, cf. *B*.249v/3 ⟨to herr*e*⟩. Ω must have innovated since the parallel passage in the Latin poem deals with pain in the ears: *DVH* 1082 *Auris curabis haec infundendo dolorem*.

1718 women papis. This stands for *DVH* 1085 *ano*. As in → **2420**, the reading in S_1 is opposed to *B*.249v/5 ⟨woma*n*s schape⟩. It is possible then to assume that the word used in Ω to refer to the rectum ended in *-APE or *-APIS. The candidate that best fulfills that condition seems to be *(ARS-)ROPE (surely a reference to the form of the intestines), a word used in the Wycliffite Bible and Chauliac's *Cyrurgie* (MED: *s.v.* ărs *n.*). A Northern *RAPE would elegantly explain the common presence of **a** before **p** in both S_1 and *B*. Another, less likely possibility is *CR(O)UPE (< OF *cr(o)upe*), and moreover this refers more exactly to the buttocks. *LURE (< ML *lūra*), used in the text (**1288**) but in an entry drawn from a different tradition, and *ÞARM (< OE *ðearm*) seem improbable on paleographical grounds, while *ARS(E) would have probably caused no problem to any copyist (other than to avoid a taboo word).

1720 pastyrnepe. The (mispelt) Latin heading and the ME name indicate that this entry describes the medical virtues of parsnip (*Pastinaca sativa* L.). The same species, or the akin *Daucus carota* L., had been described earlier in the herbal (→ **532**, with discussion); Fu and DL take *Pastinaca* to be the wild counterpart of *Daucus*, while Ge makes a distinction between both species drawing from the Classical evidence. The entry translates *DVH*, with some addition (see below).

Identification can be sustained both pharmacographically and textually, as the species is taken to be splenetic, hepatic and nephretic (**1722–1723**, again in **1731** = *DVH* 1267–1268), antiemetic (→ **1723**), alexipharmic (**1725**, again in **1728** = *DVH* 1274–1275, 1278–1279), anti-inflammatory and analgesic of the testicles (**1726–1727** = *DVH* 1271–1272), antitumoral (**1729** = *DVH* 1280–1281), anticancerous (**1731** = *DVH* 1282). The last two virtues, antidysenteric (**1732**, although this might be connected to an early passage in *DVH*, → **1723**) and aphrodisiac (**1734**), are not in the canonical edition of *DVH* but are frequently mentioned by the *auctoritates*.

Literature: PARSNIP (*Pastinaca sativa* L.): *MM* ii.113 (σίσαρον), iii.69 (ἐλαφοβόσκον); *NH* xix.90 (*siser*), xxii.79 (*elaphoboscon*); *SM* xi.873 (ἐλαφοβόσκος), xii.124 (σισάρου ἡ ῥίζα); *RM* ii.209, 259; *OEH* 82 (*herba pastinaca siluatica. feldmoru*); *Dur.Glos.* 304 (*pastinaca. mora | pastinaca siluatica. feld moru*); *DVH* 1264–1284 (*pastinaca*); *EPN* ii (*pastinaca. feldmora*), iii (*pastinaca. weal-more*), iv (*pastinace. wudu-cerfille*), v (*pastinaca. weal-mora*); *CI* B.5 (*baucia, pastinaca*); *TH* 63 (*baucia ... domestica, pastinaca, agriostasilon*); *DVH(NME)* 248r.2 (*pascuais*); *Alph.* 141 (*pastinaca agrestis. corioca, daucus*); *Sin.Bart.* 33 (*pastinaca. skirwhite*); *AC* p. 197.46 (*pastinaca domestica. pasnepe*) ⚘ *GH* 59 (BAUCIA, *skyrwyt*); Fu 263 (*ΣΤΑΦΥΛΙΝΟΣ, pastinaca*); Tu 2.573 (PERSNEPES, *skirwurtes, siser*); DL 432 (PARSENEP, *pastinaca, σίσαρον, σταφυλῖνος, branca leonina, baucia*); Ge 870 (PARSNEP, *mype, σταφυλῖνος, pastinaca, baucia, branca leonina, elaphoboscum*). ¶ WILD CARROT (*Daucus carota* L.): → dauke [**532**].

C^2H^1 (*Cl*) | C^2H^2 (*TH, GH*) | CS (Fu, DL, Ge) | C^2S^2 (*SM, RM*)

1723 gode...1724 myche. This mistranslates *DVH* 1269–1270, a passage where the plant is said to be beneficial to old asthmatics and dysenteric people (cf. **1732**).

1736 playnteyn. The Latin headword and the ME synonyms indicate that the entry describes the medical properties of some *Plantago* L. spp. When used without any modifier the plant name is traditionally identified with the waybread (*P. major* L.), while ⟨þe lesse playnteyn i-callid rubwort⟩ (**1763**) refers as a rule to ribwort (*P. lanceolata* L.; → **1938** for a more detailed rendering of that particular species). The entry, one of the longest of the treatise, is apparently a combination of several sources. The first half is a full—yet quite free—translation of the corresponding chapter in *DVH*, while **1774–1787** offer matter taken from a second source. From that line onwards some virtues are repeated a third time (for example the powers of the plant against dysentery). These two sources are untraced but probably derived from Macer's poem as well.

Identification with some species of *Plantago* is supported both textually and pharmacographically: the species is said to be antiseptic and vulnerary (**1737** =

DVH 204–205), antidysenteric (**1739, 1779, 1787** = *DVH* 206–209), hemostatic and antiacne (**1740** = *DVH* 210–211), antipyrotic (**1741** = *DVH* 212), antirabic and alexipharmic (**1742, 1781–1782** = *DVH* 213), anti-inflammatory (**1743, 1758, 1768–1769** = *DVH* 214, 251–253), anthydropic (**1744** = *DVH* 215), antiepileptic and antimanic (→ **1745**), antiaphthic (**1746, 1791, 1794** = *DVH* 217) and against fistulas (**1747**; → **858** for an explanation), antiotalgic and antiherpetic (→ **1748**), anthemoptyic (**1749** = *DVH* 221–222), antiphthisic (**1750** = *DVH* 223), ophthalmic (**1751** = *DVH* 225), antigingivitic and antiodontalgic (**1752** = *DVH* 226–228), antiemmenagogue (**1753–1755** = *DVH* 229–230), vesical and nephretic (**1756, 1774** = *DVH* 233, 260–264), antimalarial and febrifuge (**1761, 1770** = *DVH* 236–241), antiulcerous (**1765** = *DVH* 244–247), anthelminthic (**1767** = *DVH* 250), mazolitic (**1772** = *DVH* 256), and analgesic (rendered in the second source as antipodagric; **1773, 1782–1783, 1793** = *DVH* 258–259). The secondary sources further described the species as anticephalalgic (**1776**), vulnerary (**1778, 1784**), hemostatic (**1792**), and anticteric (**1796**).

> Literature: WAYBREAD (*Plantago major* L.): *HP* vii.8.3 (ἀρνόγλωσσον); *MM* ii.126; *NH* xxv.80 (*plantago*); *SM* xi.838; *RM* ii.196; *Grad.* 355 (*arnoglossa*); *OEH* 2 (*herba arniglosa. wegbræde*); *Dur.Glos.* 300 (*arnaglossa. vegbrade*); *DVH* 196–266 (*plantago, arnoglossa*); *LS* 223 (*lisen alhamel* [لسان الحمل *lisān al-ḥamal*], *lingua arietis, plantago, arnoglossa*); *EPN* iv (*arnaglosse. wegbrade* | *plantago. weg-brade*), v (*plantago. wegbræde*), vi (*arnoglossa. plauntein*), vii (*hic plantago. waybred*), viii (*hec plantago -nis. waybrede*), ix (*hoc plantago. weybrede*); *Cl* A.19 (*arnoglossa. playnteyn*); *TH* 379 (*plantago*); *Pand.* 57 (LA*plantago, quinqueneruia, lingua agni, lingua arietis,* GR*arnoglossa, heptapleuron,* AR*lisen alhamel*); *DVH(NME)* 250v.9 (*plantan*); *DVH(SME)* 4a.15 (*planteyn. arnoglossa*); *Alph.* 14 (*arnoglossa, lingua agni, lingua arietis, plantago maior.* GA*planteyne,* AN*weybrode*); *Sin.Bart.* 11 (*arnoglossa, plantago major*); *AC* p. 199.12 (*plantago maior. plantayn, weybrode*) ⚘ *GH* 344 (PLANTAGO, *quinque neruia, plantayne, weybrede, arnoglosse*); *Fu* 11 (ΆΡΝΟΓΛΩΣΣΟΝ, *plantago*); *Tu* 2.513 (PLANTAYN, *weybrede*); *DL* 64 (PLANTAINE, *waybrede,* ἀρνόγλωσσος, ἄρνειος, προβάτειος, πολύνευρος, ἑπτάπλευρος, *lingua agnina, plantago*); *Ge* 338 (LAND PLANTAINE, *weybred,* ἀρνόγλωσσος, *arnoglossa*).
>
> F^2S^2 (*SM, RM, Grad., LS, Cl, Fu, DL, Ge*) | F^3S^3 (*DVH*)

1741 oyle of eryn. A scribal conjecture to render *DVH* 212 *ovi ... lacrymo*, i.e. the white of an egg; the Latin expression must have posed problems to the ME translator (→ **12**).

1745 ham that ben lunatike. The canonical edition of the Latin poem does not mention lunacy but asthma in the expected passage, cf. *DVH* 216 *Sic iuvat asthmaticos, ferturque iuvare caducos.* Apparently the Latin exemplar must have read *LUNATICOS, a reading not recorded in Choulant's edition. Lunacy and epilepsy, which is mentioned next in the Latin sentence, seem in any case to have been akin concepts to most people in the Middle Ages. Lunatics were thought to be literally moonstruck by a horde of devils coming from the satellite, as seen from the following passages (both quoted in du Fresne 1938: *s.v.* lunaticus):

> Epilepsia fit e melancholico humore quoties exuberabit, ad cerebrum reversus fuerit. Haec passio caduca dicitur, eo quod cadens spasmos patiatur. Hoc etiam Lunaticos vulgus vocat, quod per Lunae cursum comitantur hoc insidiae daemonum. (Thierry de Chartres, *Vocabularium*)

> Deus ad hoc Lunam facit, ut tempora designet, et noctium tenebras temperet, non ut alicujus opus impediat, aut dementem faciat hominem, sicut stulti putant, qui a demonibus invasos a Luna pati arbitrantur. (*Vita St. Eulogii*, Ch. 15)

An assumed relationship between the phases of the moon, the humoral theory and epilepsy was also posited by some authors:

> Crescente luna omnes humiditates habent incremementum in corpore. Que igitur epilepsia crescit incremento lune, ex humida constat materia. Augmentum igitur lune cum habeat immutare corpus ad suam dispositionem. anget humiditates et fumos qui per nervos et venas dissoluti immutant: et expansi immutant alias humiditates donec ad cerebrum veniant et ipsum sua dispositione alterent et immutent. (*CM* 109v–110r)

1748 werkys of the eris. Emended after *DVH* 220 *dolor* [...] *auris*.

1799 persely. Both the Latin headword and the ME synonym refers to parsley, common name to refer to several *Petroselinum* Mill. spp., and especially *P. crispum* (Mill.) Fuss. Although many of the virtues given in the entry are common with those recorded in *AC*, the pedigree of the entry remains untraced.

Pharmacographically, the species is carminative (**1800**), emmenagogue (**1801, 1806**), anti-inflammatory and anthydropic (**1802**), hepatic, nephretic and anticholecystic (**1803**; the benefit for the kidneys is repeated in **1811**), antiulcerous (**1804**), abortifacient and mazolytic (**1806**), eupeptic (**1809**), antilumbalgic and splanchnic (**1810**), alexipharmic (**1812**), cardiac (**1814**, again in **1818**), lithontriptic (**1815**), antitussive and hematogenous (**1816**), antiphthisic and antimalarial (**1817**), stomachal (**1817**). Most of these virtues are in agreement with the usual medical literature of the period.

> **Literature**: PARSLEY (*Petroselinum crispum* (Mill.) Fuss): *MM* iii.66 (πετροσέλινον); *NH* xx.118 (*petroselinum*); *SM* xii.99; *RM* ii.251; *Grad.* 379 (*genus apii quod dicunt petroselinum*); *OEH* 129 (*herba petroselinum. petersilie*); *LS* 280 (*apium...petroselinum*); *EPN* ii (*petrosilion. stan-merce*), iv (*sigsonte. stan-merce*), v (*petrocilium. petersilium*), vi (*petrosillum. peresil. stoan-suke*), vii (*hoc petrocillum. percylle*), viii (*hoc petrocillum. persylle*), ix (*hoc petrocillum. persely*); *CI* P.6 (*petrosilinum. percil sed*); *TH* 359 (*petrosellinum*); *Pand.* 573 (*petroselinum, apium petre*); *DVH(SME)* 24b.3 (*persile. serpillum*); *Alph.* 169 (*petroselinum usuale, ortolanum uel domesticum.*

persile, quando simpliciter ponitur petrosillinum pro usuali intelligitur); AC p. 213.18 (*petrosilium. persely*) ❦ GH 331 (*petrocilium, percely, synomum*); Fu 253 (ΠΕΤΡΟΣΕΛΙΝΟΝ, *apium saxatile, petroselinum*); Tu 1.239 (PERSELY, *selinon*); DL 433 (*garden parsely*, σέλινον κηπαῖον, *apium hortense, petroselinum*); Ge 860 (*parsley*, σέλινον κηπαῖον, *petroselinum*).

C^2S^2 (*CI, TH, GH*) | C^2S^3 (Ge, DL) | C^3S^3 (*SM, RM, Grad., LS,* Fu)

1819 piretum domesticum. The original reading has not been emended into the expected *p i r e t r u m because the plant name is so spelt several times throughout the entry, cf. **1831, 1836**.

1820 pelletir. The ME name was applied as a rule to two separate plants (Hunt 1989: s.v. piretrum): pellitory of Spain (*Anacyclus pyrethrum* (L.) Lag.) and pellitory-of-the-wall (*Parietaria judaica* L.). Compilators sometimes mistook one for the other: *GH*, for instance, describes the medical properties of the former but uses a ME plant name that clearly refers to the latter (to be read *wallwort*, i.e. from OE *weall* rather than *wealh*, → **2385**). Although the entry provides no physical description and hence identification is largely traditional, the references to its powers against toothache and the excess of phlegm in the mouth, already present in *MM* and routinely repeated ever since, make it very plausible that the plant meant in the entry must be the *Anacyclus* (→ **1625** about the *Parietaria*). Comparison of the temperament of these two plants with those recorded in the usual medical literature also favours identification with *Anacyclus*, since *Parietaria* was generally regarded as a cold and humid species.

Pharmacographically, the species is said to be antiodontalgic (**1821**, again in **1832–1835**, including phlegmagogue and antiaphthic qualities), antiparalytic (**1822, 1839**), febrifuge (**1823, 1838**), anticephalalgic (**1826**), herpetofuge and alexipharmic (**1827**), diuretic (**1829**, and surely **1839**, where it is broadly described as a good nephretic), splenetic (**1830**), galactogenous (**1831**), and antiepileptic (**1836**). Most of these, and particularly the references to mouth diseases, poison and palsy, are to be found in the usual medical literature since Dioscorides. The entry in *LH* is a combination of the corresponding entries in *AC* and, from **1831** onwards, *DVH* (which obviously served as the basis for the former treatise and explains why so many virtues are repeated in roughly the same order).

Literature: PELLITORY OF SPAIN (*Anacyclus pyrethrum* (L.) Lag.): *MM* iii.73 (πύρεθρον); *NH* xxviii.151 (*pyrethrum*); *SM* xii.110; *RM* ii.255; *Grad.* 381 (*pyrethrum*); *DVH* 2086–2108 (*pyrethrum*); *LS* 356 (*macharcaraha* [عقرقرحا '*aqarqarḥā*'], *pyretrum*); *EPN* viii (*hoc cerbellum. pellatur*); *CI* P.1 (*piretrum. peleter*); *TH* 354 (*piretrum*);

Pand. 575 (_LA_*piretrum,* _GR_*dentanos,* _AR_*achiraraha, acharcharaha, harchancathara*); *DVH(SME)* 37a.10 (*peletre*); *Alph.* 145 (*piretrum. pelestre*); *Sin.Bart.* 34 (*piretrum*); *AC* 214.8 (*peretrum domesticum. pelethre*) ⚕ *GH* 326 (PIRETRUM, *walworte*); Fu 246 (ΠΥΡΕΘΡΟΝ, *saliuaris*); Tu 2.415 (LASERPITIUM, *pillitori of Spain*); DL 247 (BASTARD PELLITORIE, *bartram,* πύρεθρον, πύρινον, πύρωτον, πυρίτης, *saliuaris, pyrethrum*); Ge 618 (PELLITORIE OF SPAINE, *bertram,* πύρεθρον, *pyrethrum, saliuaris*).

C³S³ (Cl, TH, GH, Fu, DL) | C⁴S⁴ (Grad., DVH, LS)

1820 grene sause. Pellitory as an ingredient to cook green sauce is missing from the most famous gastronomic literature of the period (*Le Viandier, The Forme of Curye*, etc.), but it is referenced in a number of 15th-century ME cookery books, cf. the recipes "pur verde sawce" in Morris 1865: 27 and "sauce verte" in Austin 1888: 77, 110:

> Take persole, peletre an oyns, and grynde,
> Take whyte bred myude by kynde,
> Temper alle up with venegur or wyne,
> Force hit with powder of peper fyne.

> Take p*a*rcely, Mintes, Betany, Peleter, and grinde hem smale; And take faire brede, and stepe hit in vinegre, and drawe it thorgh a streyno*ur*, and cast thereto pouder of pep*er*, salt, and ser*u*e it forth.

> Take p*e*rcely, myntes, diteyne, peletre, a foil or .ij. of costmarye, a cloue of garleke. And take faire brede, and stepe it with vynegre and pip*er*, and salt; and grynde al this to-gedre, and tempre it vp wiþ wynegre, or wiþ eisel, and serue it forþe.

1841 prymerose. The ME name refers to primrose (*Primula vulgaris* Huds.). Earlier in the treatise, the species had been compared to oxlip, a very similar kind of *Primula* but offering a cluster of flowers dangling from the scape (→ **499** and below). Identification is traditional and very plausible, since the flowers of primrose were used in cookery as suggested in the opening line of the entry: kitchen use of primrose was so widespread at the time that it even gave name to a certain confection which included its flowers mixed with honey, almond milk and grated ginger (details in Austin 1888: 25). The entry follows *AC*.

Pharmacographic evidence also supports identification with some *Primula*. According to the entry, primrose is employed medically for diseases of the head, and particularly of the mouth (being anticephalalgic **1844**, anticatarrhal and deoppilant **1845**, eloquent **1846**, cosmetic of the teeth **1848**, and antidontalgic **1849**), as well as against disorders in the lower abdomen and reproductive organs (**1842, 1849**). The powers of primrose to help the head are mentioned in DL, where its value as a potherb is also remarked; the purgative virtue of the brain and against megrim is recorded in Ge.

The Latin headword is on the other hand unexpected. La. *ligustrum* seems to have referred to some shrub yielding dyes, generally identified with wild privet (*Ligustrum vulgare* L.) or else henna (*Lawsonia inermis* L.; André 1985: *s.v.*). Medieval scribes frequently confused that word with La. *levisticum*, i.e. lovage (*Levisticum officinale* W.D.J.Koch, → **1162**), which was frequently spelt ‹ligusticum› in manuscripts, and there is good textual evidence suggesting that 15th-century English scribes transmitted the idea that ‹ligusticum› (and, by extension, ‹ligustrum›) corresponded to some species of *Primula*, including not only primroses but also cowslips and oxlips (→ **499**, with discussion). Besides primroses, Latin *ligustrum* was widely misapplied at the time to refer to some vine, probably a *Lonicera* spp. (Daems 1993: 194, 361). Renaissance authors (and already *GH* as well, for *prymerose* is indexed to Chapter 350) thought that *Primula* spp. belonged to the same family as the great mullein (*Verbascum thapsus* L., → **1443**, hence the reference to "pettie mullein" in DL or Ge), perhaps because both offer a bunch of five-petalled yellow(ish) flowers stemming from a single scape.

Literature: PRIMROSE (*Primula vulgaris* Huds.): *NH* xvi.77 (*ligustrum*); *EPN* ii (*ligustrum. hunisuge*), iv (*ligustrum. hunisuce*), vi (*ligustrum. triffoil. hunisuccles*), vii (*hoc ligustrum. primerolle*), viii (*hoc ligustrum. a primerose* | *hoc ligustrum. a cowslowpe*), ix (*hoc ligustrum. a cowyslepe*); *DVH(NME)* 256v.16 (*primros*); *DVH(SME)* 26b.25 (*wodebynde. caprifolium, ligusticum*); *Sin.Bart.* 28 (*ligustrum, corrigiola*); *AC* 196.6 (*ligustrum. prymrose*) ⚜ Fu 326 (ΦΛΟΜΟΣ, *verbascum, tapsus barbatus, candela regis, candelaria, lanaria*); Tu 2.767 (COWESLIPPE, *herba paralysis, primula veris*); DL 85 (PETIE-MULLEIN, *prime-roses*, φλόμος, *verbasculum, primula veris*); Ge 635 (COWSLIPS, *pettie mullein, primula veris, verbasculum*, φλόμος)

CS (Fu, Ge) | CS³ (DL)

1851 pedelyon. According to the Latin heading and the ME phytonyms, this must be a description of the medical qualities of the black hellebore (*Helleborus niger* L.; → **1224, 2385** for other descriptions of the same species and its white counterpart). Indeed the virtue of the plant as antihematuric (**1854**) and as a rodenticide if mixed with gruel or wheatmeal (**1857**) are included in the account "Ellebo*u*rrus niger" in *AC* 185.2 that obviously served as basis for the entry in S_1—although the qualities were presented there in an inverted order. The reference to a scaly head and dead flesh are not found in *AC* but must surely be put in connection with the oft-repeated antiherpetic and leprostatic qualities of the species (**1235, 2397** in the other versions).

The physical description of the plant, on the other hand, does not correspond to that of a hellebore, for those species bear white to pinkish flowers. The use of ‹clofe-tonge› as a synonym and reference to the bitter taste suggest that the plant described by the ME writer must be the buttercup called *clufðung* and *clufwyrt* in OE that glossed Latin *sceleratus* in a couple of works (see BT: *s.v.* cluf-þung). The connection between these two species, which are physically so different, is surely explained by the strong purgative (or rather, toxic) powers of both. Ortoleva (2014: 283), drawing from a previous article by Gourevitch, has recently demonstrated that both the adjectives *elleborosus* and *apiosus* (*apius risus* was a Latin synonym for these buttercups, see the Literature quoted in **1076**) meant "maniac", apparently with the sense "intoxicated", already in the comic poet Callias, a contemporary of Socrates, and in Plautus.

OE *clufðung* is customarily identified as the celery-leaved buttercup (*Ranunculus sceleratus* L.), but the minute measure of its petals (2–5 mm) does not seem to fit the description of the source text, *AC* 185.4–7, where the plant is said to have "a brod flour more þa*n*ne a peny". Perhaps the species here is the hairy buttercup (*R. sardous* Crantz), which physically and chemically is very similar to the aforementioned but displays noticeably larger petals (7–10 mm). Akin species are described elsewhere in the herbal (→ **1180**, **1907**, with discussion). The unexpected reference in the source text to "an [*var.* he ys] horrible in syth", which refers to its black root and which Brodin left unexplained, may then be a reference to the infamous *risus sardonicus*, the spasm of the facial muscles that resembles a grotesque grin and which is caused by neurotoxines such as those found in these species (see André 1985: *s.v.* scelerāta; Ribichini 2000). The colour of the flower and the taste in any case precludes the possibility that the species treated in the Middle English text is a water dropwort, either *Oenanthe crocata* L. or *O. fistulosa* L., although these species were recently shortlisted as the likeliest candidate to be the authentic *herba sardoa* mentioned by Virgil (*Buc. VII*) and other Classical authors (see Appendino *et al.* 2009 and Ortoleva 2014, although he thinks that the possibility that the species is simply another name for hemlock, *Conium maculatum* L., should not be dismissed out of hand).

Literature: BLACK HELLEBORE (*Helleborus niger* L.): *HP* ix.10.2 (ἐλλέβορος μέλας); *MM* iv.162 (ἐλλέβορος μέλας); *NH* xxv.47 (*helleborus niger, veratrum nigrum*); *SM* xi.874 (ἐλλέβορος); *RM* ii.210; Grad. 371 (*elleborum nigrum*); *DVH* 1833–1858 (*helleborus niger*); *Cl* E.8 (*elleborus niger*); *DVH(SME)* 34a.10 (*blake ellebore*); *Alph.* 52 (*elleborus niger, radicula, poliorion. melampolion*); *Sin.Bart.* 18 (*elleborus niger*); *AC* 185.2 (*elebourrus niger. clowetungge, pedelyoun*) ⚭ *GH* 158 (ELLEBORUS NIGER, *pedelyon, lyons fote*); *Fu* 105 (HELLEBORUS NIGER); *Tu* 2.593 (VERATRUM *nigrum, helleborus melas, melampodion*); *DL* 253 (BLACKE HELLEBOR, ἐλλέβορος μέλας, *veratrum nigrum, helleborus niger, melampodium, prætiuum, polyrhizon, melanorhizon, luparia, pulsatilla*); *Ge* 824 (BLACKE ELLEBOR, *veratrum nigrum, melampodion,* ἐλλέβορος μέλας); → longwort [**1224**]. ¶ *HAIRY BUTTERCUP (*Ranunculus sardous* Crantz):

MM ii.175 (βατράχιον...ἐν Σαρδονίᾳ γεννώμενον); NH xxv.172 (ranunculus ... foliorum incisuris); SM xi.849; RM 200; OEH 9 (herba scelerata. clufþung); EPN iv (batrachium. clufþung), v (lappa. clate, clyf-wyrt); Cl A.8 (apium risus); TH 10 (appium risus); Alph. 11 (apium risus, herba scelerata, murtillana siue brutacea, brutaceoci, ferula); Sin.Bart. 11 (apium risus, herba scelerata) ❀ GH 10 (APIUM RISUS, crowfote, ache, borracium, corar, julien, statice, articoris, cloropis, raselmo, effistion, licopon, belliuageron, buccon, herba scelerata); Fu 57 (BATPAXION, batrachium, ranunculus, scelerata, pes corui, flammula, agreste apium, apiastrum); Tu 2.542 (CROWFOOT, kingeux, gollande [...] another kind which [...] groweth much in Sardinia, wild persely); DL 300 (CROWFOOTE, βατράχιον, herba scelerata, herba sardoa, apium syluestre, apium rusticum, apiastrum, apium risus, ranunculus illyricus); Ge 803 (CROWFOOTES, Illyrian crowfoot, wild smallage, σέλινον ἄγριον, γελωτοφυή, apium syluestre, herba sardoa, apium risus).

1859 pympirnell. The English name pimpernel has been historically applied to several species (OED: *s.v.*): *Sanguisorba officinalis* L. (great burnet), *Pimpinella saxifraga* L. (burnet saxifrage), and *Anagallis arvensis* L. (scarlet pimpernel). The description in the entry does not fit an umbellifer such as *Pimpinella*, while the reference to its growing low suggests that the species intended here is surely *Anagallis*. The Latin headword supports such identification too (Stirling 1995–1998: *s.v.* ippia).

As regards the ME synonyms, ‹wolshele› seems a variant of the more frequent *selfheal* that is used in many works of the period as a synonym of pimpernel (probably referring to *Sanguisorba*, which had vulnerary properties as suggested by its name, although *Anagallis* was said in *MM* to be good against wounds as well; Hunt 1989: *s.vv.* ippia maior, pimpernella, testiculus auris), while ‹kennyng-worte› probably refers to the ophthalmic qualities traditionally attached to *Anagallis* since Dioscorides (see Moreno Olalla 2007: 130). Finally, the MS reading ‹yworte› has been corrected on account of "weyewourth" in the probably source text (*AC*) and the "Supplement" to the table of English names in Ge, where "waywort" is given as a synonym of "pimpernell", and "weywort" as being the same as "ipia maior". *Wayworte* was chosen over the etymologically more conservative *weyworte* (cf. OE *weg*) because *a*-spellings are clearly hegemonic in the treatise for this word and its derivatives (108× : 7×).

Identification with *Anagallis* is supported pharmacographically as well: the plant is said to be alexipharmic (**1862**), anti-inflammatory (**1863**), vulnerary and ophthalmic (**1864**), and prophylactic (**1866**). The last virtue is missing from the usual Classical, medieval and Renaissance accounts, including *AC*, though this could be a distorted reference to the cosmetic powers of the plant, which were frequently commended in the medical literature of the period.

Literature: SCARLET PIMPERNEL (*Anagallis arvensis* L.): *HP* vii.7.1 (κιχόριον); *MM* ii.178 (ἀναγαλλίς); *NH* xxv.144 (*anagallis*); *SM* xi.829; *RM* ii.193; *OEH* 138 (*herba spreritis*), *Dur.Glos.* 304 (*pipinella. pipi neale*); *LS* 155 (*anagallis*); *EPN* vi (*pinpernele. pinpre. briddes-tunge*), vii (*hec pimpinella. primerolle* | *hec pimpernella. pimpernolle*), ix (*hic anagalidos. netylle-sede*); *TH* 389 (*pimpinella*); *Pand.* 42 (GR*anagallus, mioschays*, AR*xantala, ippia*, LA*auricula muris*); *DVH(SME)* 40b.16 (*pympernolle*); *Alph.* 196 (*ypia maior*, GA*pimpre*, AN*marie goldwert*); *Sin.Bart.* 25 (*ippia major, pimpernella cum flore rubeo*); *AC* 194.17 (*ipia maior. pympernol, selfhol, weyewourth, morcrop*) ✥ *GH* 355 (PIMPINELLA, *selfe heale, pympernell*); *Fu* 6 (ἈΝΑΓΑΛΛΙΣ, *anagallis*); *Tu* 1.232 (PIMPERNEL, *anagallis, corchorus*); *DL* 40 (*pimpernell,* ἀναγαλλίς, κοράλλιον, *corchorus, corallium*); *Ge* 493 (PIMPERNELL, ἀναγαλλίς, *corchorus, macia, phœnicion, corallion*).

CS (*SM, RM*, Fu, Tu, DL, Ge) | C²S² (*LS*)

1868 portulake. A description of the medical qualities of the purslane (*Portulaca oleracea* L.) drawn from *DVH(SME)* and translating *DVH* 748–764. The species had been already treated in the text (→ **976**, and *de facto* also in → **963**). In opposition to the other two renderings of the Latin text, this version offers a more faithful translation of the opening lines of the entry *portulaca* as given in the canonical edition and keeps the same arrangement: first the temperament, then its febrifuge quality if rubbed on the stomach or drunk, then against excessive heat if chewed or taken as a broth, and finally its antidysenteric value if drunk or eaten. Only the reference to the greenness of the leaves when used against fever is missing from this account (→ **963** about this).

Identification of the entry is positive on pharmacological and textual grounds, cf. its value as febrifuge (**1869** = *DVH* 752–754), antidysenteric (**1872** = *DVH* 756–757) and ophthalmic (**1875** = *DVH* 759), against sunstroke (**1875** = *DVH* 760) and hemoptysis (→ **1876**), as a mollifier of the intestines (**1876** = *DVH* 761), and for a hurt bladder (**1878** = *DVH* 762; → **982**). Some of these are missing from the other accounts of the species.

Literature: PURSLANE (*Portulaca oleracea* L.): *HP* vii.1.2–3 (ἀνδράχνη); *MM* ii.124; *NH* xiii.120 (*andrachle, porcillaca*), xxv.162 (*andrachne*); *SM* xi.830; *RM* ii.194; *OEH* 105 (*porclaca*); *DVH* 748–764 (*portulaca*); *LS* 339 (*bakle hancha* [بقلة الحمقا] *baqla al-ḥamqā'*], *herba stulta*); *Cl* P.15 (*portulaca. porslane*); *TH* 368 (*portulaca*); *Pand.* 330 (AR*hasdane*, GR*andrane*, LA*portulaca, herba stulta, piperella*); *DVH(NME)* 254r.6 (*hewe*); *DVH(SME)* 28a.1 (*purslane, fole-foot. adragmis*); *Alph.* 10 (*andrago, adraginis, portacla, portulaca. porceleyne*), 149 (*portulaca, portacla, andrago, andragnis, pes pulli. porsulaigne*); *Sin. Bart.* 34 (*pes pulli. purcelan*) ✥ *GH* 340 (PORTULACA, *porcelayne*); *Fu* 39 (ἈΝΔΡΑΧΝΗ, *portulaca*); *Tu* 2.526 (PORCELLAYN, *andrachne, portulaca*); *DL* 413 (PURCELAINE, ἀνδράχνη, *portulaca*); *Ge* 419 (PURSLANE, *porcelaine,* ἀνδράχνη, *portulaca*).

FH (*SM, Cl, TH*) | F²H³ (*DVH*) | F³H² (*RM, LS, GH*, Fu, Tu, DL, Ge)

1868 colde. Cf. *DVH* 751 *frig(id)oris*.

1876 also².. 1877 blode. This is an interpolation found in most Latin MSS (α, β, δ, κ, λ, μ, π, δδ, εε, ζζ, ηη, θθ, κκ): *DVH* 762b *Est haemoptoicis* [var. *haemophthisicis*] *haec saepe comesta salubris*. The line normally appears after, rather than before, the virtue against pain in the bladder (so for instance in the MHG translation: "vor der blasensuche und dem, der das blůt ressent"; Schnell/Crossgrove 2003: 356).

1881 polycary. Both the Latin heading and the ME plant name are usually taken to refer to some fleabane, be it *Pulicaria dysenterica* (L.) Bernh. or *P. vulgaris* Gaertn., but the physical description of the species provided in the text is very much against that notion. Both DL and Ge, and already *Pand.*, used *policaria* as a synonym of Gk. κονύζα, traditionally identified with three different *Inula* L. spp. Since the species in the text "growith in watry plac*is*", this would be the third kind, the British yellowhead (*I. britannica* L.), since according to *MM* iii.121, § 3, this plant grows on wetlands (φύεται δὲ ἐν ἐφύδροις τόποις). Still, and just like the fleabane, *Inula* are yellow-flowered Asteraceae and hence do not fit the description provided in the ME text.

Hunt 1989: *s.v.* policaria tentatively suggests a third candidate, fleawort (*Plantago indica* L.), a plant that will be treated in the next entry (→ **1888**). The physical description in the entry does fit that species quite well, particularly the reference to "coddis w*ith* sede", which must mean either the pyxidia that contain the seed, or else the whole round inflorescences. The small flowers that are "su*m*dell rede" would then refer to the petals of the corolla, which are of a light brown colour. The stalk and leaves of the fleawort are usually green, but they usually turn reddish, and particularly during the dry season. While the plant does not require a very watery environment, sandy areas near beaches is the preferred habitat. On the other hand, the comparison between the leaves of the plant with those of a fern is difficult to account for unless a mistranslation or copy mistake between *foenum* and *filex* is posited (cf. καὶ τὸ ὅλον δὲ βοτάνιον χορτῶδες, "the entire plant is grass-like" in *MM* iv.69, Gk. χόρτος "hay, grass"). But chances of that are of course slim, particularly since this fragment is missing in *NH*.

Moreover, neither the assumed medical virtues of neither the British yellowhead nor those of the fleawort match those in the entry, where the species is described as stomachal (**1885**), aphrodisiac (**1886**), and antimelancholic (**1887**). Only the last one, which is curiously missing from the source text (*AC*), is paralleled in the medical literature, as *Plantago indica* "purgeth downwardes adust and cholericke humours" (Ge, and similarly DL).

Literature: *British yellowhead* (*Inula britannica* L.): *HP* vi.2.6 (κονύζα); *MM* iii.121; *NH* xxi.58 (*conyza*); *SM* xii.35; *RM* ii.228; *Cl* p.7 (*policaria*); *TH* 360 (*policaria*); *Pand.* 577 (_{LA}*policaria*, _{GR}*coniza*, *conisia*, _{AR}*gafit*); *Alph.* 139 (*petila, policaria minor*), 149 (*policaria minor et maior*); *Sin.Bart.* 34 (*policaria*); *AC* p. 197.3 (*policaria. policarie*) ✣ *GH* 332 (POLICARIA, *policary*); Tu 1.283 (CONIZA, *conise*); DL 26 (CONYZA, *flebane*, κονύζα, *policaria, pulicaria*); Ge 390 (*fleabane mullet*, κονύζα, *cunilago, policaria, pulicaria*). ¶ Fleawort (*Plantago indica* L.): → psilium [**1888**].

C³S² (*GH, Cl*) | C³S³ (*SM, RM*, Tu, DL, Ge)

1888 psilium. Although the entry bears no Latin headword and the ME plant name needed emendation (the scribe seems to have been at a loss to decide whether the second letter in his exemplar was **s** longa, **l** or **h**), the synonym ⟨policarya⟩ makes it very plausible that this section of the herbal is devoted to fleawort (*Plantago indica* L.). A detailed physical description of the same species was probably given in the preceding entry (→ **1881**).

Although the textual pedigree of the entry has not been traced, comparison of the virtues provided here with the usual pharmacographic literature supports identification with the fleawort as well: as befits a cold and humid species, the plant is said to be refrigerant of sinews (**1890**), adipsic (**1891**), and anti-inflammatory of the tongue and feet (**1893**). Only the vulnerary powers of the species (**1896**) are missing from the usual medical accounts.

Literature: Fleawort (*Plantago indica* L.): *HP* vii.11.2 (κύνωψ); *MM* iv.69 (ψύλλιον); *NH* xxv.140 (*psyllion*); *SM* xii.158; *RM* ii.273; *Grad.* 363 (*psyllium*); *OEH* 169 (*herba psillios*); *LS* 220 (*bazarachatona* [بزر قطونا, *bizr quṭūnā*], *psilium*); *EPN* vi (*psillium. lusesed*); *Cl* p.11 (*psillum*); *TH* 364 (*psillium*); *Pand.* 342 (_{AR}*hazarachona, bestercaton*, _{GR}*piper silium*, _{LA}*psilium*); *Alph.* 147 (*persillium, herba policaris, herba pollicaris*), 198 (*zairaton, acaron, psillium*); *AC* 216.7 (*pillium, syil*) ✣ *GH* 336 (*psilium*); Fu 340 (ΨΥΛΛΙΟΝ, *pulicaris*); Tu 2.530 (PSILLIUM, *fleasede, fleawurt*); DL 72 (FLEAWVRT, *flebane*, ψύλλιον, *psyllium, herba pulicaris*); Ge 470 (FLEAWOORT, ψύλλιον, *pulicaria, herba pulicaris, psyllium*).

F²Æ (Tu, Ge) | F²H² (*Grad., LS, Cl, TH, GH*) | F²S² (*SM, RM*, Fu)

1899 polipody. Both the Latin heading and the ME name ⟨polipody⟩ were applied to at least two separate epiphytic ferns (→ **663**), but the synonym ⟨okeverne⟩ suggests that the species here must be the one traditionally identified as the oak-fern (*Gymnocarpium dryopteris* (L.) Newman). The entry follows *AC*, but the antidiarrheic virtue (**1901**) is given a fuller treatment here, rather than the succinct version in the source. (The author of *AC* must have made some mistake that was transmitted to *LH*: polypodies, both the "wall" and "oak" species, were pharmacographically taken to be laxative and purgative.) The species is moreover commended as anticholeric and antiphlegmatic (**1901**), a virtue attached to this fern since *MM*.

Since the *Gymnocarpium* was frequently treated together with a similar fern growing on walls, part of the references gathered in the *Literature* section may apply here, and viceversa. I include here only those references that either unmistakably mention trees or do not give "everfern" as ME synonym.

    Literature: OAK-FERN (*Gymnocarpium dryopteris* (L.) Newman): *MM* iv.187 (δρυοπτερίς); *NH* xxvii.72 (*dryopteris*); *SM* xi.865; *RM* ii.207; *Grad*. 368 (*polipodium*); *Dur.Glos.* 302 (*Fetillina arboratica. eofer fearn*); *LS* 248 (*bisberg* [بسفايغ *basfāyğ*], *polypodium*); *EPN* ii (*filix arboratica. eferfearn*), v (*polipedium. hremmes-fot*), vi (*pollipodium. poliol. reven-fot*), vi (*felix arboratica. pollipode. eververn*), viii (*hoc polipodicum. a pollypod*); *Cl* p.12 (*pollipodium. pollipody*); *TH* 365 (*polipodium*); *Pand.* 216 (GRdipteris, filicteron, saraxpteris, ARbisbeig, biste, LApolipodium, filicica, filix arbor, pliricon); *Alph.* 50 (*diapton, pollipodium. o[k]efarn*), 147 (*polipodium quercinum, filex quercina, felicula. okfarn*); *Sin.Bart.* 34 (*polipodium, filix quercina*); *AC* 213.12 (*pollipodie. polipodie*) ※ *GH* 338 (POLIPODIUM, *oke ferne*); *Fu* 223 (POLYPODIUM, *polypodium, filicula*); *Tu* 1.306 (DRYOPTERIS); *DL* 292 (POLYPODIE, *wall ferne, oke ferne*, πολυπόδιον, *filicula, polypodium*); *Ge* 972 (POLYPODIE, *wall ferne, polypodie of the oke*, πολυπόδιον, *polypodium, filicula, parua filix*); → ferne [**663**].

    S (Ge) | C²S² (DL) | C³S² (*Grad., Cl, TH*) | C³S³ (*LS, GH*)

1902 small y-choppid. Although MED: *s.v.* clippen *v.*² takes the original MS reading as a form for ME *clippen* "to cut off", a copy mistake instead of *y - c h o p p i d makes a better possibility, since an *o*-vocalism is difficult to explain here (the word derives from ON *klippa*).

1907 ram-ys-fote. The Latin plant name is missing in Daems 1993 and Stirling 1995–1998, while PNME gives *LH* as sole source, even though it is also recorded in *AC*. Since the species is said to be extremely similar to ‹crowe-fote›, the plant must belong to the extensive family of Ranunculaceae (→ **1180, 1851**). The headword must therefore be a translation of the ME name, which in turn is probably due to a scribal mistake for an original *RAU(I)NYS FOTE (cf. OE *hræfnes fōt*; note yet that *hræmnes* and *hræmmes* are known variants, see Bierbaumer 1975–1979: iii.143, and this would have evolved into *RAMMYS), which served to refer to several buttercups. The reference to a knob in the root and the fact that it grows on hard ground suggest that the species is probably the bulbous buttercup (*Ranunculus bulbosus* L.), which grows on dry pastures. If this identification is correct, then ‹crowe-fote› may well be meadow buttercup (*R. acris* L.), which is noticeably similar to *R. bulbosus* but grows in marshes, river banks and boggy areas.

The presence of ‹lode-worte› (apparently, *Potentilla reptans* L. if from OE *gelod-wyrt*) is a bit unexpected, but association of this plant name with some *Ranunculus* could go a long way in English, as it is found already in *Dur.Glos.* in case "leoth vyrt" there refers to the same species—which is unsure. Indeed there are some similarities between both species, for instance serrated leaves (although the shapes are different), and five-petalled yellow flowers. Usage of an illustrated herbal in Anglo-Saxon times might have been behind the confusion, which was then transmitted via synonyma.

The species is described as an antiarthritic in a very detailed recipe, spanning ten lines (**1911–1921**) which are not in the source text (*AC*) and hence likely to be an addition by Lelamour. The description in *LH* is also more detailed than the version provided in *AC*, as it includes the reference to the ‹knobe› and the different habitats that serve to tell apart the two *Ranunculus*.

Literature: BULBOUS BUTTERCUP (*Ranunculus bulbosus* L.): MM ii.175 (βατράχιον); NH xxv.172 (*ranunculus*); SM xi.849; RM ii.200; OEH 10 (*herba batracion. clufwyrt*); *Dur.Glos.* 300 (*batrocum. cluf vyrt, botration. cluf thunge, thung*), 301 (*chamedafne. leoth vyrt, hreafnes fot*); EPN iv (*batracion. cluf-wyrt*); Pand. 47 (*apium... raninum, apius risus, botrachion, natrachion*); AC p. 199.8 (*pes arietis. rammesfot, lodewort*) ✿ Fu 57 (BATPAXION, *batrachium, ranunculus ... tertia species, kleiner Hanenfüß*); Tu 2.542 (CROWFOOT, *kingeux, gollande, the third kind*); DL 303 (RAPE CROWFOOTE, *gold knop, yellow craw*, βατράχιον); Ge 803 (CROWFOOTES, *the sixt kinde, oinion rooted crowfoot, round rooted crowfoote*).

CS (*SM, RM*, Fu) | C⁴S⁴ (DL)

1923 radich. The Latin headword, ME synonym, and the physical description indicate that this entry must record the medical virtues of radish (*Raphanus sativus* L.) and particularly its edible taproot. The misreading of the final brevigraph of the original *RAP(H)ANUS in the headword was already present in the source text (*AC*).

The species is described as a good antiaphthic (**1925**), analgesic of the stomach (**1926**), and emollient of the spleen (**1927**). Radish had many uses in medieval and Renaissance pharmacopeia, among them indeed as a splenetic against several stomach diseases, particularly if caused by cold humours or dyspepsia. On the other hand, the power to heal sores in the mouth is apparently missing from the usual literature.

Literature: RADISH (*Raphanus sativus* L.): HP i.2.6 (ῥαφανίς); MM ii.112; NH xix.83 (*raphanus*); SM xii.111; RM ii.255; *Dur.Glos.* 304 (*raphanum. redic*); LS 297 (*fugel* [فجل *fuǧl*], *raphanus*); EPN ii (*raphanum, radix. rædic*), iv (*vermenaca. rædic*), v (*rafanum. rædic*), vi (*raffarium. raiz. redich*), vii (*hoc raparium. raddyk*); Cl R.2 (*rafanus. radich*); TH 401 (*raphanus*); Pand. (ARfinel, *fugel, haffagel*, GR*raffanus, scandix*, LA*radix*); Alph.

153 (*raphanum acre uel acutum. radich*); *Sin.Bart.* 36 (*raphanum. radiche*); *AC* p. 201.15 (*rappaner. radich*) ❊ *GH* 364 (RAFANUS, *rape rote*); *Fu* 255 (ΡΑΦΑΝΟΣ, ραφανίς, *raphanus, radix, radicula*); *Tu* 2.538 (RADICE, *radish*, ραφονις, ραφανος, *radix, radicula*); *DL* 428 (RADISH, *rabone*, ῥαφανὶς ἥμερος, *radicula satiua, raphanus minor*); *Ge* 182 (RADISH, ῥαφανὶς, *raphanus, satiua radicula*).

C²S² (*Cl*) | C³S² (*SM, RM,* Fu, Tu, DL, Ge) | C³S³ (*TH, GH*)

1930 ragworte. The ME name and the physical description, including the comparison with tansy (*Tanacetum vulgare* L., → **2283**), suggest that the species must be ragwort (*Jacobaea vulgaris* Gaertn.). The unpleasant smell mentioned in the entry is evident from such synonyms as "marefart", "stinking Davie", "stinking elshinder", or "stinking weed" (DEPN: 610; other known names include "stinking nanny" and "stinking Willie"). The ME synonym ⟨fly-fo⟩ (apparently a reference to the plant's virtue against flies that is not recorded in the entry), is a hapax according to MED: *s.v.* flī-fō *n*. The pedigree of the entry is unknown.

The only virtue of ragwort recorded in the entry is as an anti-inflammatory, as given in a long recipe (**1931**–**1936**). The plant was mainly praised as vulnerary and analgesic, but DL and Ge did recommend to make gargarisms of ragwort to heal inflammations of the throat. This is supported as well by the synonym "fellon-weed" (DEPN: *ibidem*).

Literature: RAGWORT (*Jacobaea vulgaris* Gaertn.): ❊ *Fu* 282 (SANCTI IACOBI FLOS); *DL* 49 (S. IAMES-WURT, *iacobea, herba S. Iacobi, Sancti Iacobi flos*); *Ge* 218 (SAINT IAMES HIS WOORT, *stagger woort, stauerwoort, Herba S. Iacobi, S. Iacobi flos, iacobea*).

CS (Fu) | C²S² (Ge) | C³S³ (DL)

1938 rybwort. The Latin headword and ME name suggest that the entry describes the medical powers of ribwort (*Plantago lanceolata* L.), which is reassured by the reference to waybread (*P. major* L.), traditionally regarded as its larger counterpart (→ **1736**, with discussion and additional literature). The entry offers the same matter as *AC* but in a severely abridged manner.

Pharmacographically, the species is described as anticancerous and vulnerary, which is in accordance with the usual literature, since all plantains were taken to be hemostatic.

Literature: RIBWORT (*Plantago lanceolata* L.): *OEH* 98 (*herba cynoglossa. ribbe*); *Dur.Glos.* 300 (*cynoglossa. ribbe*); *EPN* ii (*cinoglossa, plantago, lapatium. wegbræde*), iii (*cinoglosa. ribbe*), iv (*cynoglossa. ribbe* | *quinquenerbia. ribbe*), vi (*lanceolata. launceleie. ribbe*), viii (*hic costus. rybbe*); *Pand.* 57 (*plantago... habens folia stricta, lanceola*); 499 (LA*lingua canis,* GR*cinoglossa*); *DVH(SME)* 4b.31 (*planteyn þe lesse*); *Alph.* 152 (*quinqueneruia lanceola, lanceolata, plantago minor, centumneruia.* GA*launcele,* AN*ribbeuurt*); *Sin.Bart.* 36 (*quinquenervia, lanceolata plantago minor*); *AC* p. 200.1

(*plantago minor. rybwort, launcele*) ✥ GH 244 (LAUREOLA, *rybwort, messeron, laurell terrestre, mustilage, vsilien, alipiados*); Tu 2.513 (PLANTAYN, *weybrede, the less kind, way-bred, sharp plantayn, rybgrasse*); DL 64 (*ribwurt, the third kind of* PLANTAINE, *waybrede*, πεντάνευρος, *quinqueneruia, lanceolata, lanceola*); Ge 341 (RIBWOORT, πεντάνευρος, *quinqueneruia, lanceola, lanceolata*).

F²S² (Tu, DL, Ge)

1942 rodewort. The Latin headword applies to a number of heliotropic plants, and particularly to chicory (*Cichorium intybus* L.; see Literature, Stirling 1995–1998: *s.v.* solsequia) while, according to the vernacular synonyms provided in the entry, the information provided by PNME: *s.v.* solsequium and the opposition with ‹endyue› **1945**, the name seems to have referred to another Asteraceae, pot marigold (*Calendula officinalis* L.), in ME sources. Unfortunately the text includes neither a physical description nor a temperament that could help discriminate the exact species (the flowers of *Cichorium* are blue and the plant is taken to be cold, those of *Calendula* are yellow and, according to Renaissance authors, the plant is of a hot nature).

The species is described as alexipharmic (**1943**) and deoppilant of the liver (**1944**). The usual medical literature of the period, yet, does not mention such powers in connection with *Calendula* (there is just a brief reference to poison in Ge). Textually, the entry closely follows the appropriate chapter in *AC*. That chapter is in turn an abridgement of the section in *Cl*, which is surely the source for the ME entries (and for the one in *GH* as well), but the plant described there seems to have been either chicory or endive (*Cichorium endivia* L., frequently taken as garden version of *C. intybus*). Again, neither of the two virtues is attached to a *Cichorium* in Classical pharmacopeia, although diseases of the liver are mentioned in passing in *NH* xx.74, but *Cl* might have blended two separate entries from *Grad.*: this treatise refers to oppilation of the liver and the spleen in the section *endiuia* (one would assume, meaning endive), while biting of poisonous animals is referred to in the chapter that follows, *sponsa solis* (which would then be chicory, see Stirling 1995–1998: *s.v.*). All in all, the evidence suggests that, ME names notwithstanding, the entry in *LH* probably refers to some *Cichorium* L. spp., and particularly chicory (as the last line of the entry states the plant to be a different species from endive).

Literature: CHICORY (*Cichorium intybus* L.)/POT MARIGOLD (*Calendula officinalis* L.): *HP* i.10.7 (κιχόριον); *MM* ii.132 (σέρις); *NH* xx.73–76 (*intubus, ambubaia, cichorium, hedyopnis, seris*), xxi.28 (*caltha*); *SM* xii.119 (σέρις, πικρίς, κιχώριον); *Grad.* 353 (*endiuia | sponsa solis*); *OEH* 64 (*herba solago maior. helioscorpion*), 137 (*herba eliotropus. sigilhweorfa*); *Dur.Glos.* 300 (*calesta, calcesta. hvit cleaure*), 302 (*eliotropion. solago minor | eliotropia. sigelhverpha*); *LS* 143 (*dundebe* [هندبا *hindibā*], *endiuia*); EPN ii (*solsequium, heliotropium. solsece, sigel-hweorfe*), iv (*heliotropus. sigell-hweorfa* | *solsequia. golde*), v (*solsequium. solsæce*), vi (*eliotropium. solsegle. gloden*), vii (*hoc solsequium. sawsykylle*), ix (*solsequium. a rode*); Cl s.20 (*sponsa solis, eliotropia, intiba, cicorea, solsequium, dionysia. sonsecle*); TH 432 (*sponsa solis*); Pand. 159 ($_{LA}$*cicorea, sponsa solis, solisequia,* $_{AR}$*hundebe,* $_{GR}$*seris, intuba, gegucisi*); DVH(SME) 40b.27 (*rodewort. solsequium. eliotropia*); Alph. 53 (*elytropia, incuba, sponsa solis, mira solis, solsequium, cicoria. cicoree*), 88 (*kalendula, sponsa solis, incuba. golduurt, rodes*); Sin.Bart. 14 (*calendula, solsequium*), 19 (*elytropia, eloytropia, sponsa solis, solsequium*), 25 (*incuba, solsequium, cicorea, sponsa solis*), 26 (*kalendula*); AC p. 203.25 (*solseqium. roddys, marigoldys*) ✣ GH 392 (CICOREA, *sponsa solis, incuba, solsequium, elitropium, emachates, vertonon, chicory*); Fu 142 (CALTHA, *calthula, calendula*), 262 (ΣΕΡΙΣ, πικρίς, κιχώριον, *intubus, endiuia, scariola, ambubeia, cichoria*); Tu 2.403 (CYCORIE, *endive, seris, cichorium, intubus hortensis, garden succory*); DL 116 (MARIGOLDS, *ruds, calendula, caltha, calthula, chrysanthemon*), 404 (ENDIUE, *succory,* σέρις, πικρίς, κιχώριον, *cichorium, intubum syluestre, ambubeia, cichorea syluestris*); Ge 219 (GARDEN SUCCORIE, σέρις ἀγρία, πικρὶς, *intybum syluestre/agreste/erraticum, cichorium, cicorea, ambugia, ambubeia, rostrum porcinum, sponsa solis*), 222 (WILDE SUCCORIE, *hyos(c)iris, hedyopnis*), 599 (MARIGOLDES, *ruddes, calendula, chrysanthemum, caltha, gromphena Plinij*).

Cichorium: C^2 (Ge) | CS (Cl, Fu, DL) | C^2H^2 (GH)
Calendula: F^1H^1 (LS) | F^1H^2 (TH) | F^1S^1 (Grad.) | F^2S^2 (SM, RM, Fu, DL, Ge)

1947 rewe. The entry describes the medical qualities of the rue (*Ruta graveolens* L.) as provided in the DVH(NME) translation of DVH 267–331. Identification is traditional and supported by the textual and pharmacological evidence, cf. the value of the species as a stomachal, contraceptive, anaphrodisiac and emmenagogue (**1948** = DVH 269–270), antitussive (**1949** = DVH 271), carminative (**1950** = DVH 272–273), pulmonic and antipleuritic (**1950** = DVH 274–275), febrifuge (**1952** = DVH 276–278), antiarthritic (**1953** = DVH 276), anti-inflammatory to several parts of the body (**1954, 1968** = DVH 279), antihydropic (**1956** = DVH 283–285), anticephalalgic (**1957** = DVH 290–291), hemostatic (**1958** = DVH 292–293), antiotalgic (→ **1958**), wart-remover and antiherpetic (**1960** = DVH 296–299, → **1961**), alexipharmic (**1962** = DVH 304–313) and against diseases of the uterus and testicles (**1966** = DVH 314–317). A couple of virtues in the Latin text are missing: as an anthelminthic (DVH 282) and as an ophthalmic (DVH 285–288, yet → **2390**). Most importantly, the entry, just like the other witnesses from RH, does not offer a translation of the long recipe to make diapyganon that is included in the Bodley version (B.246v/2–7).

Literature: RUE (*Ruta graveolens* L.): HP i.3.1 (πήγανον); MM iii.45; NH xx.131 (*ruta*); SM xii.100; RM ii.251; Grad. 386; OEH 91 (*herba ruta. rude*); Dur.Glos. 305 (*ruta. rude* | *sarta montana. rude*); DVH 267–331 (*ruta*); LS 290 (*sadeb* [سداب *sidāb*], *ruta*); EPN ii, iv, v (*ruta. rude*), vi (*ruta. rue*), ix (*hec ruta. rew*); *Cl* R.7 (*ruta. rew*); *TH* 407 (*ruta*); *Pand.* 597 (₍GR,LA₎*ruta*, ₍AR₎*radeb, aselep*); *DVH(NME)* 246r.11 (*rewe*); *DVH(SME)* 5a.15 (*rue*); *Alph.* 158 (*ruta domestica*); *Sin.Bart.* 37 (*ruta agrestis, stafisagria secundum quosdam*); *AC* p. 200.28 (*rvta domestica. ruwe*) ❧ *GH* 363 (RUTA, *rue, piganium*); Fu 235 (ΠΗΓΑΝΟΝ ΚΗΠΕΥΤΟΝ, *ruta hortensis*); Tu 2.552 (RUE, *herbe grace, ruta, pyganon*); DL 186 (RUE, *herbe grace,* πήγανον κήπευτον/ἄγριον, *ruta, eriphion*); Ge 1070 (RUE, *herbe grace, ruta hortensis/syluestris,* πήγανον).

C²S² (*TH, GH*) | C³S³ (*SM, RM, Grad., DVH, LS, Cl,* Fu, Tu, DL, Ge)

1953 þe archangeles. A *lectio facilior* in AS_1, cf. *W*.29r/6 ⟨arthatikes⟩ and *P*.266/17 ⟨gowte artetike⟩. The scribe chose a word with religious overtones for his emendations (→ next note and also **149, 188, 784**, and perhaps **282, 708** for other examples). Note that this virtue should have appeared before the one dealing with fever, which may be due to a transposition of lines in *Q*. The word ⟨curnelid⟩, therefore, must mean "crooked, bent at an angle" and is probably the same as *corneled* in MED, where this sense is not recorded.

1955 cromyn. This translates *DVH* 283 *caricis* "dried figs". Pepys reads together with S_1 and offers *P*.266/19-20 ⟨cro*m*mes⟩, while Bodley reads *B*.246r/16 ⟨Gru*m*mok⟩. The word is missing in *W*, since the anthydropic virtue is not recorded in that MS. The reconstructed original reading is unclear, but the presence of final **k** in *B* makes it likely that the ME translator borrowed the Latin word as *CARIK*IS*, which was wrongly expanded. As for the reading "crumbs" in the *RH* branch, it looks like a *lectio facilior.* Note in any case that the same Latin word will be correctly rendered as ⟨figis⟩ later in the entry (→ **1963**).

1958 put...hede-ake. *DVH* 294–295 offers a recipe against earache. The mistranslation derives from *Ω*, as all witnesses offer the same reading.

1959 of rose. An imperfect rendering of *DVH* 296 *roseoque oleo.* Both Wellcome and Pepys read together with S_1 here, which suggests that the expected word *o y l (e) was already missing in *RH*. Bodley read ⟨enoros⟩, which is perhaps a chaotic rendering, almost an anagram, of *ROSYNE.

1961 for¹...stynkande. The fragment translates *DVH* 300–303, which describe the powers of the plant against *achoras*, defined as *ulcera ... capitis humore fluentia pingui* (*DVH* 301), and *ozinas*, which according to the text are stinking ulcers in the nose (*DVH* 303). All MSS render the Latin text faultily.

1962 the kynge Perys. Mithridates VI Eupator Dionysus, king of Pontus (120–63 B.C.) and the fiercest enemy of Rome at the time. Obsessed with being poisoned while eating, he used to drink the blood of geese that had been fed every day with little quantities of poison and contrived several antidotes that made him proof to it, most famously his namesake, the complex mithridate, that involved 54 ingredients (see *NH* xxix.24). When his son Pharnaces led a revolt against him, he tried to commit suicide by ingesting some poison but naturally it failed and a Gallic bodyguard had to run him through with a sword. The name of the king is not mentioned in *B* or *P* but must be authorial as he is referred to by name in *DVH* 305; the spelling in Branch γ suggests a confusion **p** *pro* **þ**.

1963 ij vnces of figis. At first sight, just a reading mistake *u n c i b u s instead of *nucibus* in Ω, cf. *DVH* 307 *magnis nucibus binis caricisque duabus*, but note *P*.266/28–267/1 ‹ij ounces of figges and note kernelis›.

1964 that²... 1965 day. Probably a mistranslation of *DVH* 309–310 *quascunque ... insidias*, as if from *d i e s, but the fragment is only found in S_1.

1965 wessyll bitt. *W*.29r/17 reads together with Sloane, while *B*.246r/24 offers ‹wolfe byttynge› and *P*.267/3–4 ‹adderys bytyng›. The Latin text is of little use to decide which version—if any—best maintains the reading in Ω, for it mentions both weasels (*DVH* 311 *mustelae*) and snakes (*DVH* 313 *serpentibus atris*). But the version in Pepys, next to the other readings (all of which begin with **w-**) could lend some support to *wormis in the original translation; cf. a very similar case in → **1356–1357**.

1969 rosse. The entry describes the medical properties of the roses (*Rosa* L. spp.), according to the *DVH(NME)* translation of *DVH* 776–807. The frequent reference in the ME text to the red colour of its petals suggests that *R. gallica* L., *Rosa* × *damascena* Mill. or a similar variety was in the mind of the scribe, rather than any white species or hybrid. Identification is traditional and sustained by textual and pharmacographic evidence as well: the species is antiherpetic and antacid (**1970** = *DVH* 781–782), antimetrorrhagic and antidiarrheic (**1971** = *DVH* 783), antiaphthic (**1973** = *DVH* 784–786), febrifuge (**1973** = *DVH* 787–788), deoppilant (**1975** = *DVH* 791–792), anticephalalgic (**1977** = *DVH* 793), antipyrotic and antiodontalgic (**1977** = *DVH* 796–797), and ophthalmic (against chalazia in particular: **1979** = *DVH* 798). Missing from the account are the powers of the species as antiseptic (*DVH* 794–795), antipruritic (*DVH* 799) and against hysteropathies (*DVH* 800).

> **Literature**: Roses (*Rosa* L. spp.): *HP* i.13.2 (ῥόδον); *MM* i.99; *NH* xxi.121 (*rosa*); *SM* xii.114; *RM* ii.256; *Grad.* 344; *OEH* 170 (*herba cynosbatus*); Dur.Glos. 305 (*rosa. rose*); *DVH* 776–807 (*rosa*); *LS* 108 (*nard* [ܘܪܕ], *rosa*); *EPN* ii, v (*rosa. rose*), iv (*rosa. rosa*), vii (*hec rosa. rose*), ix (*hec rosa. a rose*); *Cl* r.1 (*rosa*); *TH* 400 (*rosa*); *Pand.* 322

416   Explanatory Notes

($_{AR}$hard, $_{GR}$rodon, $_{LA}$rosa); DVH(NME) 248v.11 (ros); DVH(SME) 10a.26 (rose); Alph. 154 (rosa, rodon); Sin.Bart. 36 (rosa); AC p. 200.39 (rosa rubea. reed rose) ⚘ GH 362 (ROSA, rose); Fu 254 ('POΔON, rosa); Tu 2.545 (ROSE, rosa, rodon); DL 469 (ROSE, rosa, ῥόδον); Ge 1077 (ROSES, rosa, ῥόδον).

Æ (SM, RM, Fu, Ge) | FS (DL) | F¹S¹ (DVH, LS) | F¹S² (Grad., Cl, TH, GH, Tu)

1980 Palydius techith. Rutilius Taurus Aemilianus Palladius was the Latin author of the 15-volume *De Re Rustica* (Rodgers 1975; a verse ME translation in Lodge 1873–1879). A popular medieval *auctoritas* on natural sciences and virtually the sole one on husbandry, Frisk 1949: 329 oddly took "Pallidius" appearing in the parallel passage of *DVH(SME)* to mean Palladius Iatrosophista, an obscure Greek medical scholiast of Hippocrates who lived sometime between the 3rd and the 9th centuries (Choulant 1956: 131–132). The recipe to make oil of roses is recorded in the book devoted to the month of May: "[i]n olei libras singulas rosae purgatae singulas uncias mittis et septem diebus in sole suspendis et luna" (vi.15).

The ME version, drawing directly from *DVH* 802–807, includes some details, like using a glass jar, that are not found in Palladius's original text but were added by Macer Floridus (*DVH* 805 *vitreo* […] *vase*), obviates that the petals must be plucked from the flowers (*DVH* 803–804 *foliorum* […] *floris* […] *purgatorum*), and offers some oddities of its own as well. For example, the quantities of the two ingredients are reversed, which makes little sense since you cannot possibly combine a pound of rose petals and an ounce of oil and still expect to obtain a liquid. The Latin poem, just like his source, of course states that one should put an ounce of rose petals into a pound of oil: (*DVH* 804–805 *uncia ... iungatur olivi in libra*); cf. also "[i]n every pounde of oil an unce of rose / ypurged putte, and hange it dayes seven / in sonne and moone" in the ME translation of Palladius's work (Lodge 1873–1879: i.156) and "of þat þat is red of þe rose flour an vnce and […] a pounde of oile de oliue" in *DVH(SME)* (Frisk 1949: 93). The mistranslation must have existed already in Ω, which may have offered something like *VNCE OF OIL OLYUE & A POUNDE OF ROSE (cf. *W*.25v/11–12 ⟨an unce of oil olif & a pond of rose⟩); the scribes of the other copies must have noticed the incoherence and emended their exemplars' reading as best they could, cf. *B*.248v/19 ⟨an vnce of oill olyue & an vnce of þe ros⟩, *P*.280/19 ⟨leuys of roses and oyle of olyue⟩.

The phrase ⟨sum-whate of roysyng⟩ also deserves comment. MED: *s.v.* rōsĭn(e *n.* takes ⟨roysyng⟩ to be a mere writing variant of "rosin" (i.e. colophony, the solid residue of the distillation of oil of turpentine). That spelling is odd: it would be a hapax in ME, and forms ending in -*ng* will not (re)appear until well into the sixteenth century—and then very sparsely: OED: *s.v.* rosin *n*. could only quote a single instance, dated *ca*. 1550. Moreover, there is no reference to this product in the Latin text and in fact it would be a bit odd to find rosin, which is solid, in a recipe for a medical oil. The phrase seems to translate the first hemistich of *DVH* 803 *quod rubeum* [var. *rubrum*] *fuerit foliorum sumito floris*, meaning that the petals of the rose used for the recipe must be the red ones, as seen by the quotation from *DVH(SME)* above. The readings in other MSS of the tradition suggest that the archetype was either garbled or misunderstood by the several scribes, who either innovated or dropped the fragment altogether (as did the scribe of *P*). Wellcome, for example, reads *W*.25v/11 ‹a nunce of þe rosyn› while Bodley offers the *lectio facilior B*.248v/18 ‹þe somet [*MS* fomet] of the ros›. The usage of ‹rosyn› in the Wellcome version together with the parallel reading of S_1 suggests that the exemplar must have offered a bisyllabic word containing a final nasal and that it was not a weak plural morpheme (cf. OE *rōsan*), since they were virtually unknown in that dialect and the scribe of *W* would surely had turned it into *r o s i s without a second thought (Mossé 1968: § 55). Bodley's ‹somet› is obviously connected with ‹sum-whate› in S_1 and hence cannot be a scribal emendation but must represent an authorial reading. The Latin line is syntactically clumsy and the author of Ω seems to have interpreted *sumito* "take [2nd sg. fut. imp. of *sūmo*]" as if some declined form of La. *summitās* "summit, the highest part"—even though the word had already been translated as ‹thou shalt take›. All in all, Ω probably read *ÞE SUMMITE OF ÞE ROYSYNG, meaning "the topmost of the rosy (part of the leaves)", and where the adjective *ROYSYN(G) traslated either *rubeum* or *rubrum*. If this is correct, then the appearance of ‹roysyng› in S_1 would antedate the other known instance of the word (Henryson's *Testament of Cresseid* 464 "ȝour roising reid to rotting sall retour"). Usage of the word by the makar could be used as evidence to posit an origin around the Anglo-Scottish Borders for the *DVH(NME)* tradition (which is concurrent with the spelling ‹oy› to indicate *ō*).

1985 rose-mary. Although it neither bears a Latin headword nor contains a physical description, the ME name indicates that the entry is devoted to the well-known herb rosemary (*Rosmarinus officinalis* L.). The section is a translation of a Latin text variously called the *Anonymous Prose Treatise on Rosemary*, the *Virtues of Rosemary*, the *Twenty-six Virtues of Rosemary*, the *Virtues and Marvels of Rosemary*, etc. (see Keiser 1998: 3644 and Keiser 2008, particularly Appendix B, where the entry from *LH* is also edited in full). The treatise was copied over more than 30 MSS and reproduced in handwritten and printed form until 1637 (Keiser 2008: 198–199), but there is no modern critical edition, so for comparative purposes the version included in London, British Library, Sloane 3545, ff. 4r–5v as edited in Keiser 2008: 203–204 will be used instead. According to the information provided in the same source, the translation in *LH* is closest to Cambridge, Trinity College, MS O.1.13, ff. 148v–150r, Exeter, Cathedral Library, MS 3521, pp. 410–412, and Oxford, Corpus Christi College, MS 226, f. 25r–v.

Concerning the contents of the entry, it pays particular attention to husbandry matters (herpetofuge and pest controller, **2009, 2029, 2036**; food preservative, **2011**; fertilizer, **2020**) that are very briefly touched upon in other sections of the herbal. Pharmacographically, rosemary is described generally as a panacea (**1987**) and specifically as antialopecic and cosmetic (**1990, 2041**), exhilarant (**1993**), anticaries (**1996**), calefacient of the head (**1998**), corroborant of the feet (**2000**), antephialtic (**2002**), anti-inflammatory (**2003, 2014**), rejuvenatory and reinvigorant (**2005**), anticancerous (**2007**), antidiaphoretic and antitussive (**2018**), orectic (**2022**), antidysenteric (**2025**), antimanic (→ **2026**), antiarthritic (**2030**), refrigerant of the stomach and adipsic (**2032**), antiphthisic (→ **2038, 2043**), and prophylactic (**2045**). Some virtues appear in a different position than the Latin version, and one of them (to help breathing) is missing in the English account.

> **Literature**: ROSEMARY (*Rosmarinus officinalis* L.): *MM* iii.75 (λιβανωτίς); *NH* xix.187 (*libanotis, rosmarinus*); *SM* xii.60; *RM* ii.235; *OEH* 81 (*herba rosmarinum. boðen*); Dur. Glos. 305 (*rosmarinum. sun deav, bothen, feld medere*); *LS* 317 (*xaieralmerien* [شجر المريم *šağar al-Maryam*], *rosmarinus*); *EPN* iv (*rosmarinum. feld-mædere | rosmarinus. sun-deaw*); *Cl* R.8 (*rosmarinus. ros maryne*); *TH* 696 (*ros marinus*); Pand. 380 (_AR_*laieralmarien, alkelilgebel* [الأكليل الجبل\ *al-iklīl ğabal*], _GR_*libanotida*, _LA_*rosmarinus, corona montana*); Alph. 49 (*dendrolibanum, libanotidos, libantus, ros marini. rosemaryn*), 55 (*ros marinus. ros maryn*); Sin.Bart. 28 (*libanotides, ros marinus*); AC p. 201.32 (*ros marinus. rosmarine, feld madere*) ❧ *GH* 370 (ROSMARINUS, *rosemary, anthos, libramondos, dendrolibanos, liantis, ycterycon, luim*); Fu 180 (ΛΙΒΑΝΩΤΙΣ, *rosmarinus, coronaria*); Tu 2.423 (ROSMARY, *libanotis stephenomatike, rosmarinus*); DL 188 (ROSEMARY, λιβανωτὶς στεφανωματικὴ, *rosmarinum coronarium, rosmarinus*); Ge 1108 (ROSEMARIE, λιβανωτὶς στεφανωματικὴ, *rosmarinus coronaria*).
>
> CS (*Cl*, *GH*, Fu) | C²S² (DL, Ge) | C²S³ (*LS*) | C³S³ (Tu)

1998 the colnes þat is y-take on the hevede. This stands for *catemsatus*, glossed in the Latin text as *infrigidatus*. The word was not emended in the edition but looks like a botched attempt at reproducing *CATARRATUS or *CATARRIZATUS (a word used in some Medical treatises of the 16th century), i.e. having a runny nose. Mucus was thought to generate in the forehead usually due to excessive cold ("coryza est extra naturam humiditas, descendens a prora capitis per nares, quæ semper frigore, uel calore augmentatur, sed multo magis ex frigore"; Costantinus Africanus, *De morborum cognitione*, ii.14), and hence the ME equivalent is accurate.

2026 oute of his witt. The cross-reference to the powers of rosemary against madness, which would make number 18 in the list, is missing in Keiser 2008: 204, but the ME text mirrors item 20 in the Latin original:
> Item si quis amens aut stultus effectus fuerit ex aliqua infirmitate pregravante flores et folia eius bullias in aqua et in ea paciens balneatur et liberabitur.

Judging from this passage, the reference to the head in the English version when rendering *balneatur* must have been a scribal addition.

2038 ete þe levis. A scribal conjecture due to a faulty exemplar, or else a *lectio facilior*, instead of the correct *e t i k (cf. La. *ethicus*, i.e. *hecticus* "suffering from consumptive fever", in Sloane 3545).

2046 savory. An account of the medical qualities of savory (either the annual *Satureja hortensis* L., frequently referred to as "summer savory" and the perennial *S. montana* L., or "winter savory"; as described by the *DVH(NME)* translation of *DVH* 843–869. Identification with *Satureja* is traditional and supported both by textual and pharmacological data: the species is diuretic and emmenagogue (**2047** = *DVH* 845), abortifacient and purgative (**2047, 2054** = *DVH* 845–846, 858–859), expectorant (**2049** = *DVH* 847–849), carminative (**2050** = *DVH* 850–851), antilethargic (→ **2052** = *DVH* 852–857), antiemetic (**2055** = *DVH* 860–861), and aphrodisiac (**2056** = *DVH* 862–865). The text in *DVH* is complete, other than the opening of the chapter, where the Greek and Latin names of the species are given, and the closing lines, where the Latin name is put in etymological connection with *satyrus* on account of its aphrodisiac powers (see André 1985: 227) and the possibility of substituting thyme in case savory is missing (both labiates were easily confused by early botanist; see Andrews 1958, part of the Literature apparatus, and below, → **2314**).

> **Literature**: SAVORIES (*Satureja* L. spp.): *HP* i.3.1 (θύμβρα); *MM* iii.37; *NH* xix.165 (*thymbra, satureia*); *RM* ii.216; *DVH* 843–869 (*satureia*); *LS* 303 (*sahater* [صعتر *ṣa'atar*], *thymbra*); *EPN* vi (*satureia. satureie. timbre*), viii (*hec scurera. saveray*), ix (*hec samina. a saveryn*); *Cl* s.38 (*saturegia*); *TH* 461 (*saturegia*); *Pand.* 602 (_AR_*sahanc, sahater,* _GR_*tymbra,* _LA_*saturegia*); *DVH(NME)* 247r.15 (*saueray*); *DVH(SME)* 11b.18 (*sauerey. saturia. tymbra*); *Alph.* 158 (*satureia, saturegia, timbra, timbria. sauerey*), 167 (*serpillus, satureia, saturegia | serpillum, herpillum, timbra, pulegium ceruinum uel montanum. brotherwort*), 186 (*tymbra, timbria, serpillum. brotherwrt*); *Sin.Bart.* 37 (*satureia, tymbra. saverey*); *AC* p. 203.10 (*saturea. saueroye*) ⸿ *GH* 420 (SATUREIA, *sauerey*); *Fu* 113 (ΘΥΜΒΡΑ, *thymbra, cunila, satureia*); *Tu* 2.557 (SAVERYE, *satureia,*

420   Explanatory Notes

cunila, thymbra); DL 163 (COMMON GARDEN SAUORIE, *cunila, satureia, saturegia*); Ge 460 (SAUORIE, θύμβρα, *satureia*).

CS (*DVH, Cl, TH*) | C³S³ (*RM, LS, GH, Fu, DL, Ge*)

2052 hede akynge. This appears to be a mistranslation of *DVH* 855–857, where the person afflicted with lethargy is advised to wash his head with a mixture of savory and vinegar. The reference to that disease as *pigri … morbi* must have misled the translator.

2054 distroieþ that childe and sleyth hit. All other versions of *DVH(NME)* have a shorter reading (cf. for instance B.247r/23 ‹slays þe barne›). *(Di)stroy* is used in S_1 as a dialectal translation of *SLE in reference to pustules, boils and the like, cf. ‹distroy þe cankyr› **46**, ‹stroyeth scabbis› **420**. The scribe must have recognized only too late that the passage was not dealing with an illness and had to add the coda to make the sense clear. Alternatively, *distroy* may have conveyed a sense of "purposeful abortion" to the reader that was certainly unintended by the Latin text or the ME translator.

2055 yf… 2056 lechery. This translates *DVH* 862 *hocque modo mire Venerem solet illa movere*. S_1 stands out against the other witnesses in addressing the reader directly, cf. on the other hand the more neutral approach of B.247r/25 ‹& þat maner iffe it be largly dronkyne it mevys lychory› (and similarly *W* and *P*). S_2.105v/18 provides a very succinct version that is completely opposed in meaning to the other witnesses: ‹and on þe same wyes it abat*is* lychery›. It is possible that Ω read *MEVIS (cf. *B*) rather than *m o v i s, and the vocalism confused the scribe of S_2, who conjectured wrongly—even though the aphrodisiac qualities of savery are stressed in the next sentence.

2058 sawyn. An account of the properties of the shrub savin (*Juniperus sabina* L.), according to the rendering in *DVH(NME)* of lines 492–506 in *DVH*. Identification is traditional and reassured by textual and pharmacological evidence, cf. its value as a vulnerary and antiseptic (**2059** = *DVH* 494–495), emmenagogue and abortifacient (**2060** = *DVH* 497–499), and antidinic (**2064** = *DVH* 502–504). The cosmetic powers of the species (→ **2062**) were faultily rendered in this translation, while its value as an antianthracic (*DVH* 496) went missing.

Literature: SAVIN (*Juniperus sabina* L.): *MM* i.76 (βράθυ); *NH* xxiv.102 (*herba sabina, brathy*); *SM* xi.853; *RM* ii.201; *Grad.* 367 (*sauina*); *OEH* 82 (*herba sabina. safinæ*); *DVH* 492–506 (*bratheos, sabina*); *LS* 245 (*abel* [أبهل *abhal*], *savina*); *EPN* v (*sabina. savine*); *Cl* s.27 (*sauina, saveyn*); *TH* 441 (*savina*); *Pand.* 3 (₍ₐᵣ*abel*, ₍ɢᵣ*brachi*, ₍ₗₐ*sauina*); *DVH(NME)* 247v.19 (*sayin*); *DVH(SME)* 8a.3 (*saueyne*); *Alph.* 158 (*sauinia, bracteos. saueyne*); *Sin. Bart.* 13 (*brateos, bracteos. savina*); *AC* p. 203.5 (*sauina. sauyne*) ❧ *GH* 400 (SAUINA, *sauyne, blancheos, vilopapilion, papicion, cathacieron, herbe sabyne*); Fu 54 (ΒΡΑΘΥΣ, βάρυθρον, sabina); Tu 2.553 (SAVIN, sabina, brathys); DL 552 (SAUINE, βράθυς, sabina, sauimera); Ge 1192 (SAUIN, βράθυ(ς), sabina, sauimera).

C¹S¹ (*Grad.*) | C²S² (*Cl*) | C³S³ (*SM, RM, DVH, LS, TH, GH,* Fu, Tu, DL, Ge)

2062 slakiþ the hede-ake. This must correspond to *DVH* 500–501, but these lines describe the value of the species as a cosmetic if mixed with *cerotum*, i.e. a salve of wax and some animal or vegetal grease, and applied to the face. While the possibility of an interpolation in *Q* can never be discarded out of hand, it is likelier that the ME translator was misled by the usage of the word *nitentem* "shining", which he may have not known and associated with ME *nit*. The reference to headache must have came naturally to him after he read *DVH* 501 *Omnibus et morbis prodest de frigore factis*.

2063 an autor of medicyne. *DVH* 506 *Oribasius auctor*. Oribasius (ca. 320–403), personal physician to Julian the Apostate, composed several works, most importantly the Ἰατρικαὶ Συναγωγαί or *Collectiones medicae*, a huge collection of medical excerpts (seventy or seventy-two books, now in a very fragmented state, see Raeder 1928–1933) that is our sole textual source for many medical writers.

Comparison of the ME text with its original Latin source (*DVH* 505–506) indicates that the translation was erroneous: Macer Floridus stated that savin in double dose will do in a recipe that asks for cinnamon whenever the spice is wanted. Oribasius's quoted text must be therefore *CMR* xv.1.2.23: ἔνιοι δὲ καὶ ἀντὶ κινναμώμου διπλάσιον αὐτὸ βάλλουσιν "some people double the quantity of this instead of cinnamon." In fact, the same suggestion was already mentioned by Pliny and Galen in their own accounts of the plant (see Literature).

2065 washe the ovyr-hede. The original reading ‹ovyn hede› makes no sense and unfortunately the Latin text (*DVH* 503 *si lotum sit caput inde*) is of little use here as the presence of ‹ovyn› remains unexplained. The proposed emendation, which syntactically is not completely satisfactory, is based on MED: *s.v.* ŏver-hēd *adv.*, meaning "above, overhead", thus taking ‹the› as a personal pronoun rather than an article, while the verb would convey the idea of sprinkling the water over one's head.

2068 savygill. This is a translation of the chapter *Ostrutium* in *DVH* 907–927 as it was recorded in the *DVH(NME)* textual tradition (→ **1571**, with discussion, for another translation of the same text). This version records the two references to the species as an anticteric (**2069, 2079** = *DVH* 910, 926) that are missing from the previous account but misses its diuretic and antiasthmatic powers (*DVH* 913–914).

The Latin plant name is usually identified as the soapwort (*Saponaria officinalis* L.). The spelling in S_1, rather than stemming directly from *s a n i c l e (cf. *B*.254r/13 ⟨senykyll⟩ and *W*.37v/5 ⟨senigle⟩) must have kept the v from the archetype (cf. OF *savon* "soap") and hence has not been emended. Assuming an original *SAUENEL in Ω (cf. Norman French *savenelle*, *savonelle* in FEW: *s.v.* *saipôn- *n.* to refer to this species) or *SAUENER (according to PNME, *savener* and *savuner* are found in synonyma contained in London, Sloane 282 and Exeter, Cathedral Library 3519, respectively) that was then deformed via scribal conjectures and *lectiones faciliores* would explain why the word *sanicle* (which refers to a number of species with perceptible vulnerary qualities and above all to *Sanicula europaea* L.) appears here, even though the two species are hardly confusable and there is not even a reference to wounds in the entry.

Literature: SOAPWORT (*Saponaria officinalis* L.): → ostricium [**1571**].

2075 well akynge. The original passage dealt with skin diseases, as indicated by the mention of leprosy and the parallel readings *B*.254r/19 ⟨vncommys⟩, *W*.37v/12 ⟨werk of oncomes⟩, suggesting Ω *WELK OF VNKOMYS that apparently translates *DVH* 920 *pustula*. The change l *pro* k in the first word is of course very frequent (as is the *lectio facilior* ⟨werk⟩ in *W*), while the presence in his exemplar of *v, *k, and *n which was obviously read as *r (again, an ubiquitous copy mistake), naturally suggested *w e r k to the scribe of AS_1, who rendered the Northern word into his idiolect as ⟨akynge⟩ as a matter of course. The coda ⟨where-to he is layde⟩ that is missing in *B* is similarly authorial, as it translates *DVH* 921 *superaddideris*.

2078 helith…2079 eyne. The references to children and to a mysterious "jaundice in the eyes" are not in the Latin poem, which states that a mixture of soapwort juice and woman's milk is good against jaundice if snorted. The mention of the eyes is probably due to a mistranslation of *DVH nare trahant*, or else to a variant *OCULI in Ω. Note nevertheless that *B* does not include the coda, which is only recorded in γ. The Bodley version, moreover, reads ⟨men⟩ instead of ⟨childrene⟩, but the appearance of these words is a bit puzzling. It may be that the English translator associated woman's milk and children and added the word of his own accord.

2080 sagge. The ME names indicates that the entry describes the medical properties of sage (*Salvia officinalis* L.). *LH* follows most pharmacological treatises since the Middle Ages in making a distinction between the cultivated species, the one described here, and the wild counterpart, called ‹ambros› and ‹eupatorye› in the text (about the virtues of which, → 133). The entry renders the appropriate chapter in *DVH*, but lines **2091–2095** belong to a different, untraced tradition, where the benefits of the species for diseases of the liver and against bleeding wounds are repeated together with febrifuge powers that are unknown in the usual literature.

Pharmacographically, sage is taken to be hepatic (**2082** = *DVH* 871), abortifacient and emmenagogue (**2083** = *DVH* 872), alexipharmic (**2084** = *DVH* 873), hemostatic (**2085** = *DVH* 874–875), antitussive and mucolytic, antiphthisic and antipleurodynic (→ **2087**), antipruritic of the genitals (**2089** = *DVH* 878–879). The species is also praised as a cosmetic, since it can be used to dye the hair black (**2091** = *DVH* 880–881).

> Literature: SAGE (*Salvia officinalis* L.): HP vi.1.4 (ἐλελίσφακον); MM iii.33; NH xxii.146 (*salvia, eleliphacum*); SM xi.873; RM ii.209; OEH 103 (*herba salfia*); Dur.Glos. 305 (*salvia. saluie*); DVH 870–906 (*saluia, elelisphacus*); LS 154 (*aelisfacos, saluia*); EPN ii (*salvia. fen-fearn*), v (*salvia. salvige*), vi (*salvia. sauge. fenvern*), vii (*hec saliva. salwe*), ix (*hec salgea. sawge*); CI s.34 (*saluia, sawge*); TH 447 (*salvia*); Pand. 234 (_{GR}*eliffagus, lilifagus*, _{AR}*geliffagos, alsamuet, tussilago, sache*, _{LA}*saluia*); DVH(NME) 247v.8 (*saygge*); DVH(SME) 12b.1 (*sauge. saluia. liliphagus*); Alph. 161 (*saluia. sauge*); Sin.Bart. 28 (*lilifagus. salvia agrestis*); AC p. 202.40 (*salgia. sauge*) ❧ GH 406 (SALUIA, *sawge, eupatory, lilifagus*); Fu (ΈΛΕΛΙΣΦΑΚΟΝ, *saluia romana, syderatio*); Tu 2.556 (SAGE, *salvia, elilisphacos*); DL 179 (SAGE, ἐλελίσφακος, *saluia, corsaluium*); Ge 622 (SAGE, ἐλελίσφακος, *saluia*).
>
> CS (SM, RM, Fu, Tu) | C¹S² (CI, TH, GH) | C²S² (LS) | C³S³ (DL, Ge)

2087 brekithe the tisyke. The parallel line in the Latin poem (*DVH*) does not contain a reference to phthisis: it simply reads *Compescit veterem tussim laterisque dolorem*. The variants *ventrem* and *venerem* recorded in Choulant's apparatus are naturally of no consequence here. Rather, it seems as if the ME translator were unsure of the reading *tussim* in his exemplar (perhaps because the line was blotted or defective) and to be on the safe side added a equivalent for *TISIM. As seen from the Latin text, the reference of sage having powers to "open the voice" (apparently, acting as a mucolytic) must be also a scribal addition suggested by the presence of cough in the same line.

2097 safe. While the heading *iris* was used to refer to the blue-flowered orris (treated earlier in the herbal, → **724**, as was the akin species ‹gladoyne› → **835**), La. *ireos*—a fanciful construction, it seems, after *ammi* : *ammeos*— was applied to its white variant, the Florentine iris (*Iris* × *germanica* L. var. *florentina* (L.) Dykes). The physical description supports that identification although, contrary to the information provided in the text, the plant does not grow in water but on dry slopes. The ME name must be a *lectio facilior* for *FANE (< OE *fana*) via an intermediate *s a u e , cf. ‹sane› **733**. The entry belongs to the *AC* tradition.

Identification with some *Iris* is borne out pharmacographically as well. The plant is described in the entry as analgesic (→ **2098**), antitussive (**2099**), expectorant (**2100**), alexipharmic and antispasmodic (**2101**), abortifacient (**2102**). Most of them, and particularly the powers of the species against mucus and the cramp are well recognized in the usual medical literature of the period. The value to help sore sinews is infrequent but referenced in *Pand.* ("valet *con*tra duricie*m* neruoru*m*"); Mattheus Sylvaticus, its author, claims to have drawn the information from "Pavl." (used in this work to refer to Paulus of Aegina), but the virtue is not recorded in *RM*.

> **Literature**: FLORENTINE IRIS (*Iris* × *germanica* L. var. *florentina* (L.) Dykes): *Cl* 1.4 (*iris*); *TH* 234 (*iris*); *Pand.* 691 (*yreos*); *Alph.* 54 (*elpha, elpheon. fone*), 68 (*folium elphion. fane*), 196 (*yreos*); *Sin.Bart.* 25 (*yri*), 28 (*lilium celeste, cujus radix dicitur yreos*); *AC* 193.9 (*ireos. fane*) ⚜ *GH* 215 (IRIS, *ireos, gladiolus, sifolifus, iris afrike, craticon, matricilon*); *Fu* 118 (*ΊΡΙΣ, iris*); *Tu* 2.404 (FLOUR DELYCE, *iris, irios*); *DL* 138 (FLOURE DE LUCE, *iris, ἴρις, iris florentina, ireos*); *Ge* 47 (FLOWER-DE-LUCE OF FLORENCE, *ἴερις, ὀυρανία, θαυμαστὶς, iris*). → flour delice [**724**].
>
> C²S² (*Cl*, *TH*, *GH*, *Ge*) | C²S³ (*Fu*) | C³S³ (*DL*)

2104 safur. The Latin headword indicates that the entry describes the medical powers of saffron, the dried stigmas of *Crocus sativus* L. The ME spellings ‹safur› and ‹safar› (**97**) are peculiar, for as a rule they mean "sapphire". Since they are recorded in *LH* only (see MED: *s.v.* saf(f)rŏun *n.*), a *lectio facilior* can be easily posited here.

The text follows the same tradition as *AC*, although the account in *LH* is somewhat more accurate: the last virtue is missing in the latter tradition, which reads "þis he*r*be grow*ith* in gardy*n*ggi*s*" (177.1) instead. This is probably a reference to the *ortensis* species mentioned in some sources (for instance *Cl* and *TH*).

The species is described as anticteric (**2105**), stomachal and antiemetic (**2106**), soporific (**2107**) and ophthalmic (**2108**). All of them are regularly found in the medical literature of the period.

> **Literature**: SAFFRON (*Crocus sativus* L.): *MM* i.26 (κρόκος); *NH* xxi.31 (*crocus*); *SM* xii.48; *RM* ii.232; *Grad.* 353; *LS* 173 (*zahafaran* [زعفران *zaʻfarān*], *crocus*); *EPN* vii (*hic crocus. safurroun*), viii (*hic crocus. sapherone*), ix (*hic crocus. safryn*); *Cl* c.21 (*crocus. safron*); *TH* 108 (*crocus*); *Pand.* 364 (ₐᵣ*iamfaran*, ₉ᵣ,ₗₐ*crocus*); *DVH(SME)* 41b.29 (*safron*); *Alph.* 46 (*croci. saffron*); *AC* 176.24 (*crocus. safron*) ⚜ *GH* 103 (CROCUS,

saffron); Fu 166 (ΚΡΟΚΟΣ, crocus); Tu 1.289 (SAFFRON, krokos, crocus); DL 155 (SAFFRON, κρόκος, crocus, castor, cynomorphos, herculis sanguis); Ge 123 (SAFFRON, κροκός, crocus).

C¹S¹ (Grad., Cl) | C²S¹ (SM, RM, Pand., Fu, Tu, DL, Ge) | C²S² (LS)

2111 sowtheryne-wode. The Latin headword and the ME name indicate that the entry describes the medical properties of southernwood (*Artemisia abrotanum* L.). Textually, the entry is a combination of two traditions: *AC* (up to ⟨a-yene⟩ **2119** but missing the minute physical description offered there), then *DVH*.

Identification with southernwood is well established both textually and pharmacographically. The species is described as lithontriptic and antiparalytic (**2113**), alexipharmic (**2115**), maturative (**2116**), trichogenous (**2118**), antineuropathic and thoracic (**2120** = *DVH* 33–34), antipruritic (→ **2120**), nephretic and hysteric (**2121** = *DVH* 36), diuretic, expectorant and antiemmenagogue (**2122** = *DVH* 37–39), herpetofuge (**2124** = *DVH* 40–41), febrifuge (**2124** = *DVH* 41–43), anthelminthic (**2127** = *DVH* 44), ophthalmic (→ **2129**), thorn-remover (**2130** = *DVH* 48–49), aphrodisiac (**2131** = *DVH* 50–51). The entry moreover adds a final virtue against sleep-talking (**2133**) that is missing in the original Latin.

Literature: SOUTHERNWOOD (*Artemisia abrotanum* L.): *HP* i.9.4 (ἀβρότονον); *MM* iii.24 (ἀβρότονον); *NH* xxi.60 (*habrotonum*); *SM* xi.798 (ἀβρότονον); *RM* ii.186; Grad. 363 (*abrotanum*); *OEH* 135 (*herba abrotanus. supernewuda*); Dur.Glos. 299 (*abrotanum. sutherne vude*); *DVH* 31–52 (*abrotanum*); *LS* 307 (*catsum* [قيصوم *qayṣūm*], *abrotanum*); *EPN* ii (*abrotonum. superne-wude*), iv (*abrotanum. sœprene-wuda*), v (*aprotanum. suðerne-wudu*), vi (*abrotanum. averoine. supe-wurt*), vii (*hoc albatorium. sothernwode*); *Cl* A.31 (*abrotanum. sowpernwod*); *Pand.* 4 (GR,LA*abrotanum*, AR*hesum*); *DVH(NME)* 244v.8 (*auerone*); *DVH(SME)* 1b.4 (*sowthernwode*); *Alph.* 1 (*abrotanum, linerinum. southerneuuode*); *Sin.Bart.* 9 (*abrotanum. southrenwode*), 12 (*averoyn. southrenwode*); *AC* 163.7 (*abrotanum. sothernwode*) ⚶ Fu 2 ('ABPOTONON, *abrotonum*); Tu 1.219 (SOTHERNWOOD, *abrotonon, abrotonum*); DL 1 (SOTHRENWOOD, ἀβρότονον, *abrotonum*); Ge 947 (SOTHERNWOOD, ἀβρότονον, *abrotonum*).

C²S¹ (Grad., Cl) | C³S³ (SM, RM, DVH, LS, Fu, Tu, DL, Ge)

2117 woll oylle. This is not a reference to lanolin ("the cholesterin-fatty matter extracted from sheep's wool, used as a basis for ointments", OED: *s.v.* lanolin), since the parallel passage in the immediate source reads "olde olye" (*AC* 163.17; Brodin 1950: 127 records no variant for this reading in his apparatus criticus) and so do the Latin version of *Agnus Castus* (*Sl.*2v/7) and *Cl*, the ultimate source for the entry, both of which duly read ⟨vetusto oleo⟩. ⟨Woll⟩ then must be taken as a *lectio facilior* for *WOLD "old". Breaking of initial OE *(e)ā-* into *wǭ*- via intermediate ME *ǭ*- is found in several dialects, "predominantly in the more western parts of the South" (Jordan 1974: § 283).

2120 ichinge and clawynge. The corresponding Latin passage actually refers to breathlessness and coughing: *sic quoque dysnoicis* [var. *dismaticis*] *prodest tussimque repellit* (*DVH* 35). Although the meaning of La. *dy(p)noicus* might have been unknown to the scribe, *tussis* was correctly translated many times in the text so at least the word *c o (u) 3 (e)* would have been expected. Any explanation for such a free rendering into ME cannot be therefore but a mere hypothesis. Perhaps an original *PRODEST TUSSIMQUE (for the abbreviation p̄d3 of *prodest*, see Cappelli 1990: 266) was badly copied in the exemplar and/or misread by the translator as *p r u r i t u m q u e*, which naturally elicited ‹clawynge›, then *dypnoicis* was regarded as a synonym—although the collocation ‹icching and clawynge› had already appeared in **1558** to translate *DVH* 1298 *pruritus*.

2129 the empatyk. This stands for *DVH* 46–47 *oculorum* [...] *dolori* [...] *vel fervori*. The meaning of the ME word is unclear; it seems to be a blending of *epatik* (i.e. a disease of the liver) and *empetik* (theoretically meaning *impetigo*, see MED: *s.v.* impetīgo *n.*, but used in the text to translate *haemoptoicis*, → **151**). As with the previous note, it is very difficult to ascertain the reason(s) behind the scribal choice of this word, but a *lectio facilior* for an exemplary reading *EGILL PACE (→ **378**) may be not far off the mark.

2137 serfoyle. The Latin headword and the ME synonym refer to wild chervil (*Anthriscus sylvestris* (L.) Hoffm.; → **1061, 1105** for two other (and closely related) accounts of the medical qualities of that species). The physical description, on the other hand, points to the vine woodbine (*Lonicera periclymenum* L.; → **2484**). The confusion undoubtedly arose because of the similarity between *chevirfoil(e)* (< La. *caprifolium*), which designated the woodbine, and *CERFOYL(E) (< La. *chaerephyllum*); the scribe himself must have suspected the mistake as it was probably he who added the last line of the entry (he also committed a dittography in **2143–2146**). Although the text ultimately derives from *DVH*, the direct source of the entry is untraced.

Pharmacographically, most virtues are attached to chervil: the species is described as antiaphthic (**2140**), anticolic (**2142**), antidinic (**2143**), and antilumbalgic (**2144**), and they are included in the usual medical literature. The assumed powers of the species as calefacient of sinews and limbs (**2147**), on the other hand, are not found in the usual literature related to that plant.

Literature: WILD CHERVIL (*Anthriscus sylvestris* (L.) Hoffm.): → kerwell [**1061**].
¶ WOODBINE (*Lonicera periclymenum* L.): → wodebynd [**2484**].

2151 stonecrop. The Latin headword, ME synonym, physical description and habitat refer to some stonecrop (*Sedum* L. spp.), traditionally identifed with common stonecrop (*S. acre* L.). Although modern scholarship—at least since Sprengel 1829–1830: II.615—has associated stonecrops with Dioscorides's third kind of ἀείζωον (diversely known as ἀνδράχνη ἀγρία, τηλέφιον, ἀείζωον τὸ μικρόν, πετροφυές, ἀείζωον ἄγριον, and *illecebra* in Latin), the supposed anaphrodisiac qualities of the species (cf. **2154**) speak against that identification. The Dioscoridean species was thought to possess a fiery hot temperament (as already pointed by the sentence δύναμιν δὲ ἔχει θερμαντικήν, "[i]t has properties that warm", and made clear as well by such synonyms as "wild prick-madam", "wallpepper" or "country pepper" recorded in Renaissance herbals), and this as a rule would have caused the opposite effect.

Comparison of the entries and woodcuts in Fu (*Sedum minus mas/klein haußwurtz mennle*), Tu (*Sedum minus*) and Ge (*Sedum minus hæmatoides*), on the other hand, makes very likely that some *Sedum* L. sp. was identified at the time with the *second*, or minor, kind of Dioscoridean ἀείζωον, a plant that modern scholars regularly identify with houseleek (*Sempervivum tectorum* L. → **709, 1031**; so Aufmesser 2000: 165, Beck 2005: 286, although Sprengel 1829–1830: ibid. had already suggested *Sedum rupestre* L.), a flowering succulent just like a *Sedum* but having a cold temperament, which would be in keeping with the pharmacographic power mentioned in the ME text. Fu, moreover, used *crassula minor* as a synonym of the *minor* species, while DL and Ge used it to refer to a subspecies of the same plant. Be it a *Sedum* or a *Sempervivum*, it must be noted that neither were recommended to quench sexual desire in the usual medical literature—in fact, both MM iv.88 and NH xxv.160 mention στέργηθρον, i.e. "love-charm", as a synonym for the latter species, but aphrodisiac qualities are missing in the medieval and Renaissance herbals (although the Greek name was mentioned in DL and Ge to refer to ἀείζωον μέγα).

The source for this entry has not been traced.

Literature: COMMON STONECROP (*Sedum acre* L.): MM iv.90 (ἀνδράχνη ἀγρία); NH xxv.162 (*andrachne agria*); OEH 139 (*herba aizos minor*); EPN viii (*hec vermicularis. ston-croppe*); Alph. 34 (*crassula minor* [...] ₐₙ*tecesorite*), 190 (*vermicularis minor*); Sin.Bart. 17 (*crassula minor, vermicularis. stancroppe*); AC 173.28 (*crassula minor. stonore, stoncrop*) ❀ Fu 10 (ʼΑΕΙΖΩΟΝ, [...] *sedum minus*, τριθαλὲς, *vermicularis, crassula minor*); Tu 2.563 (HOUSLEKE, *sedum, sempervivum, aeizoon* [...] *the second kind, stone crop, sedum minus*); DL 79 (HOVSELEEKE, *the third kind of sengreene, wild prickmadame, great stonecrop, wormegrasse, crassula minor, vermicularis*); Ge 413

(LITTLE HOUSLEEKE, *great stonecrop, wilde prickmadam, wormegrasse, crassula minor, vermicularis*); → jubarbe [**1031**].

F (Ge) | F³S³ (Fu) | C⁴S⁴ (DL)

2156 sparowe-tonge. The Latin headword and the ME synonyms suggest that the entry deals with knotgrass (*Polygonum aviculare* L.; note that the entry ‹knotwort› does not refer to this species but probably refers to butcher's broom, *Ruscus aculeatus* L. → **1098**). The entry probably belongs to the *AC* textual tradition, although the reference to its growing in gardens and orchards is missing there, as is the mysterious synonym ‹stryle› (perhaps a scribal blunder). The position of the temperament also varies in each tradition.

Pharmacographically, the species is said to be lithontriptic (**2159**). While a stone-breaking virtue is not found in the medical literature other than in *AC*, knotgrass was used in many diseases of the lower abdomen, including excretory, genito-urinary and gynaecological ones (constipation, dysentery, dysury and strangury, menorrhagia, gonorrhea, etc.). The temperament does not fit the description either: medical authorities since Galen agreed in assuming a cold and dry temperament for this species.

Literature: KNOTGRASS (*Polygonum aviculare* L.): *MM* iv.4 (πολύγονον ἄρρεν); *NH* xxvii.113 (*polygonum, sanguinaria*); *SM* xii.104 (πολύγονον); *RM* ii.253; *OEH* 19 (*herba proserpinaca. unfortredde*); *Dur.Glos.* 299 (*appolligonius. unfortreden vyrt*), 304 (*proserpinata. unfortredden*); *EPN* iv (*pilogonum, sanguinaria. unfortredde*); *TH* 382 (*polligonia*); *Pand.* 325 (ₐᵣ*harsiarbay* [الرّعي عص *'aṣa ar-ra'ī*], *persoidami*, ₢ᵣ*proserpinata, poligonia, porcinatia, sanguinaria, multigonia*, ₗₐ*centumnodia, corrigiola minor, lingua passerina, geniculata*); *Alph.* 38 (*centinodium, populus, popluus. swynegrece, cattesgres*), 104 (*lingua passeris, poligonia, proserpinata, centinodium. swynesgarce*), 147 (*poligonia, proserpinata, corrigiola, lingua passerina, lingua passeris, genicula, centumnodia, centinodia, pupulus, uua major. swynesgres*); *Sin.Bart.* 15 (*centinodium, corrigiola*), 34 (*poligonia, lingua passerina.* [...] *geniculata, proserpina*); *AC* 177.3 (*centenodium. centenodye, sparwystungge, swynys grees*) ❧ *GH* 348 (LINGUA PASSERINA, *polygonia, proserpina, corrigiole, centynode, swynes grasse, knotrasse, sparow tongue*); *Fu* 234 (ΠΟΛΥΓΟΝΟΝ ΆΡΡΕΝ, *proserpinaca, seminalis, sanguinalis, corrigiola, centumnodia*); *Tu* 2.517 (KNOT GRASS, *swinesgrass*, πολυγονον αρρεν, *polygonum mas, sanguinalis*); *DL* 68 (KNOTGRASSE, πολύγονον ἄρρεν, καλλίγονον, πολύκαρπον, *seminalis, centumnodia, corrigiola, sanguinaria, sanguinalis, proserpinaca*); *Ge* 451 (KNOT GRASSE, *swines grasse, birdes toong*, πολύγονον ἄρρεν, *seminalis, sanguinalis, centumnodia, corrigiola, proserpinaca*).

F²S (*SM, RM,* Fu, Tu, Ge) | F²S³ (DL)

2161 skyrwhite. The ME name (< OF *esch(i)ervie*) generally refers to an umbellifer, the parsnip (either *Pastinaca sativa* L. or *Sium sisarum* L.), but the Latin heading suggests that the species intended here is a Brassicacea, the rocket (*Eruca vesicaria* (L.) Cav.). Comparison of the ME entry with *DVH* 1016–1036 suggests that this is actually a rendering of the latter plant. Assimilation of the skirret and rocket is not privative to *LH* but seems to have been used in other traditions, cf. *Sin.Bart.* 20: "Eruca, tam semen quam herba, an. skirwhit" (further references in MED: *s.v.* skĭrwhĭt(e *n.*, § b).

The text derives from *DVH* and hence the medical qualities of the species were already treated in *LH* under the entry *costmaryn* (→ **313**), but the opening lines of this version include a few virtues not found in the Latin poem (antaphthic, **2162**; lithontriptic and antimelancholic, **2163**), which were apparently taken from *AC*.

   Literature: ROCKET (*Eruca sativa* Mill.): → costmaryn [**313**].

2161 no3te drye. A mistranslation of the original poem, which actually states that the rocket is hot to a moderate degree, and also dry but less so: *DVH* 1016–1017 *Erucam calidam dicunt mediocriter esse, / Siccam non adeo*. A copy mistake for *(ɪ)NO3E translating *mediocriter* in the original is hence quite plausible, unless the translator somehow mistook *siccam non* as a syntactic unit.

2171 hardith wonderly the wytt. This stands for *DVH* 1028 *Indurare ferunt hanc contra verbera sensum*, where La. *sensus* "capacity for feeling, sense" was misunderstood as "mind, reason". Since it is doubtful that the translator did not know the meaning of *contra verbera* "against lashes", which could have helped the translator to arrive at the correct sense of the word, either the exemplar missed the phrase or was faulty here, or else the scribe was unaware of that particular meaning of *sensus*. The ME sentence is closer to the Latin original, but still clumsy, in the other version of the entry (→ **320**).

2175 spereworte. The Latin headword (for the emendation, → **1180**) and the ME synonyms make it obvious that the intended species must be some spearwort (*Ranunculus* L. spp.), but the detailed physical description fits no European ranunculi. On the one hand, those bearing white petals (including the section *Leucoranunculus* Boiss.) cannot be properly called spearworts, since their leaves are not lanceolate and/or else their white flowers do not grow in ‹smale stalkys›, i.e., panicles. (The form of the leaves is not mentioned in the description but becomes evident from the ME synonyms, and cf. also "þis herbe ha3t scharpe lewys as a spere", in the source text, *AC* 185.28). On the other hand, the Latin and English plant names, most features of the physical description (including the form of the leaves) and the species's habitat strongly point to the greater spearwort (*R. lingua* L.), but then this species bears bright yellow flowers. One could assume a copy or translation mistake here; still, the same colour is mentioned in all copies of *AC* collated by Brodin for his edition, and so does the parallel Latin text, which reads ⟨flore*m* albu*m* h*abet*⟩ (*Sl*.9v/2).

Pharmacographically, the species is described in the text as febrifugue (→ **2178**) and maturative (**2179**). Both of them, particularly the second one, are included in medical literature of the period in connection with the great spearwort (as seen from the Renaissance woodcuts, Ge in particular). All things considered, then, it seems that the traditional identification of this plant name with *R. lingua* L. can be sustained, the reference to white flowers notwithstanding.

Literature: GREATER SPEARWORT (*Ranunculus lingua* L.): → lasse sper-wort [**1180**].

CS (*SM*, *RM*, Fu) | C⁴S⁴ (*Cl*, *Sin.Bart.*, *GH*, DL, Ge)

2178 he shal be hole. The sentence is unclear as it never mentions the disease that the species will help cure. Comparison with the source text shows that there is a missing part: "ʒef a ma*n* hawe þe feue*re*s & hys pouuse be anoy*n*ted þ*er-with* he schal be*n* hol" (*AC* 186.2–4). A febrifuge quality ("co*n*tra q*u*artana") for this species is similarly recorded in *Cl*.

2181 strawbery. The Latin headword and the ME name are traditionally taken to refer to wild strawberry (*Fragaria vesca* L.). Textually, the entry follows the same tradition as *AC*, but misses misses the final sentence about the habitat of the plant ("þis he*r*be grow*ith i*n wodys & in dyrk placys" 186.21–22).

The species is medically described as ophthalmic (**2182**), vulnerary (**2183**) and splenetic (**2184**). Strawberries will not appear regularly in pharmacographic treatises until the late Middle Ages. Before that date (and still in Fu), the virtues of *Fragaria* were assimilated to those of some *Rubus* L. spp., either blackberry (*R. fruticosus* L., *R. ulmifolius* L.) or raspberry (*R. idaeus* L.). These plants were praised *inter alia* as vulnerary (antiaphthic in particular), and ophthalmic. As for the benefits of strawberries on the spleen, they are recorded in just a few sources, including *TH* and *GH*.

Literature: WILD STRAWBERRY (*Fragaria vesca* L.): *HP* i.5.3 (βάτος); *MM* iv.37; *NH* xxiv.117 (*rubus*); *SM* xi.848; *RM* ii.200; *OEH* 38 (*herba fraga. streaberge*); Dur.Glos. 302 (*fraga. stravberian, mersc mealeve*); *LS* 124 (*bvleich* [علّيق *'ullayq*], *rubus*); *EPN* ii (*fraga. strea-berige*), iii (*fraga. streowberge*), iv (*fraga. straw-berige*), v (*fraga. streaw-berian wisan*), vi (*fraga. fraser. streberi-lef*), vii (*hoc stragum. strabery*), viii (*hic fragus. a strebere-wise* | *hoc fragum. a strebere*); *Cl* R.9 (*rubus*); *TH* 185 (*fragula, fragia*); *Pand.* 645 (ₐᴿ*sulach, suleich,* ɢᴿ*batus,* ʟᴀ*rubus*); *Alph.* 63 (*fragaria, stauberie*); *Sin.Bart.* 22 (*fragaria, fraser. straubery*); *AC* 186.16 (*fragra. streberye. fresere*) ✥ *GH*

175 (FRAGRARIA, *strawberyes*); Fu 327 (FRAGARIA); Tu 2.384 (STRAUBERRIES, *fragaria*); DL 59 (STRAWBERIES, *fragaria, fragula, fraga*); Ge 844 (STRAWBERRIES, *fraga*).

FS (*SM, RM, Cl*) | F¹H¹ (Fu, Ge) | F¹S¹ (*LS*)

2186 swynes-fenyll. The Latin and ME names have been traditionally identified as hog's fennel (*Peucedanum officinale* L.). The distorted syntax of the first sentence suggests that ⟨o*þer* wormesede⟩ was added on second thoughts, or else the scribe realized that he had missed that piece of information just after he had written the temperament. The entry seems to belong to the same tradition as *AC*, since it offers the same synonyms and the anthelminthic virtue (→ **2187**), but it is too short to be completely sure, all the more so since the scribe dropped the physical description provided in the probable source.

Literature: HOG'S FENNEL (*Peucedanum officinale* L.): *HP* ix.14.1 (πευκέδανον); *MM* iii.78; *NH* xxv.117 (*peucedanum*); *SM* xii.99; *RM* ii.251; *OEH* 96 (*herba peucedana. cammoc*); *Dur.Glos.* 304 (*peucedanum. cammoc*); *LS* 276 (*harbatum* [يَرْبَطُور *yarbaṭūr*], *peucedanum*); *EPN* iv (*peucidanum. cammoce*); *Cl* p.5 (*paucedanum. howndis fenel*); *TH* 358 (*peucedanum*); *Pand.* 349 (ₐᵣ*herbaturum, herbaturis,* ₉ᵣ*peucedanum,* ₗₐ*cauda porcina*); *Alph.* 140 (*peusedanum, cauda porcina, fenicularis, feniculus porcinus, feniculus agrestis, masmaratrum, cauda pecorina*); *Sin.Bart.* 21 (*feniculus porcinus, peucedanum*), 33 (*peucedona, feniculus porcinus | peucedona. cammoc secundum quosdam*); *AC* 188.15 (*ferniculus porcus. swynys fenkel, wyrmsed*) ⅋ *GH* 330 (PENCEDANUM, *dogfenell, mydde consolde, swynefenel*); Fu 227 (ΠΕΥΚΕΔΑΝΟΣ, *peucedanus, fœniculum porcinum, pinastellum*); Tu 2.495 (PEUCEDANUM, πευκεδανος, *har strang*); DL 212 (HORESTRANGE, *sulphurwoort, horestronge, sow fenell,* πευκέδανον, ἄγαθον δαίμον, *peucedanum, pinastellum, stataria, fœniculum porcinum*); Ge 896 (HORESTRANGE, *sulphurwoort, horestrong, sow fennell, hogs fennel, brimstone woort,* πευκέδανον, *peucedanos, pinastellum, fœniculum porcinum, stataria*).

CS (*Cl, TH, GH*) | C²S³ (*SM, Fu, DL, Ge*) | C³S³ (*RM, LS*)

2189 sowe-þistill. The ME name is applied to several compositae belonging to the genus *Sonchus* L. Identification with the common sowthistle, *S. oleraceus* L., is traditional. The word ⟨labi*um*⟩ in the Latin heading is an evident *lectio facilior* for *l a b r u m "bath". The names δίψακος and *dipsacus* that are sometimes quoted as an equivalent seem to have referred to common teasel (*Dipsacus fullonum* L.) in part of the literature, but the physical description provided in the entry, including the reference to its latex, the English synonym provided and the mention of Saint Mary's seed support identification with a *Sonchus*. The entry derives from *AC* but is much abridged.

Pharmacographically, the species is febrifuge (**2191**), and alexipharmic (**2192**). Dioscorides and many medical writers since (even one as late as DL; see the dry remarks of Ge against that notion) mentioned that the maggots found in the head of the plant can be used against quartan fever if they were put in a leather bag and hung from the neck or the arm, so it seems likely that the virtues allotted to the species in the entry stem from here.

Literature: COMMON SOWTHISTLE (*Sonchus oleraceus* L.): *HP* iv.7.1 (δίψακος); *MM* iii.11; *NH* xxv.171 (*labrum Venerium*), xxvii.71 (*dipsacus*); *SM* xi.864; *RM* ii.207; *Grad*. 374 (*virga pastoris*); *OEH* III (*herba carduus siluaticus. wudupistel*); *Dur.Glos*. 304 (*carduus silvaticus. vude thistel*); *LS* 341 (*basialrahagi* [عص الرّعي 'aṣa ar-ra'ī], *virga pastoris*); *Cl* v.3 (*virga pastoris*); *TH* 506 (*virga pastoris*); *Pand*. 214 (GR*dipseus, dipsecus,* AR*presenda, dipsacos haresana, harsiarbai, albsacos,* LA*virga pastoris, cardo fullonis*); *Alph*. 27 (*cameleonta alba, cardus coagulatus, ixion. southistel*), 89 (*labrum Ueneris, cardo idem. sough thistil*); *Sin.Bart*. 27 (*labrum Veneris, wokethistel*); *AC* 198.6 (*labrum. sowesthystyl*) ⚘ *GH* 497 (CARDUS BENEDICTUS, *sowthystle, holy thystle*); *Fu* 82 (*ΔΙΨΑΚΟΣ, labrum ueneris, carduus ueneris, virga pastoris, cardo fullonum*); *Tu* 1.305 (WYLDE TASEL, *dipsacos, labrum veneris, virga pastoris*); *DL* 375 (TEASELL, *fullers teasell, carde teasell, Uenus bath, bason,* δίψακος, *labrum Veneris, chæmaleon crocodilion, onocardion, cneoron, meleta, cinara rustica, moraria, carduus Veneris, Veneris lauacrum, sciaria, virga pastoris, carduus fullonum*); *Ge* 1005 (TEASELS, *carde teasell, Venus bason,* δίψακος, *labrum Veneris, carduus Veneris, lauer lauacrum, virga pastoris, carduus fullonum*).

F³H³ (*LS*) | FS (*Cl*) | F³S³ (*Grad., TH*) | S² (*SM, RM,* Fu, Tu, DL, Ge)

2195 standilgose. The Latin heading and the ME names ‹scandilgose› and ‹skandylwelkys› suggest that the entry describes the medical virtues of some orchid, but the exact species is very difficult to ascertain as there is no physical description. The use of ‹ʒekesterris›, which normally refers to *Arum maculatum* L. (→ **1018** for a number of virtues traditionally attached to *Arum* and → **970** for another instance of misapplication of a synonym of that species), must probably be read as evidence that the species displays speckled leaves. The fact that the plant described in *GH* is good against "spottes that abyde after sores" also suggests the presence of those speckles, in keeping with the doctrine of signatures (Prior 1863: xiv). Crossreferencing this information with the woodcuts in Fu and Ge makes it extremely likely that it is the same plant called "orchis mas angustifolia/gesprengt Knabenkraut mennle" and "cynosorchis morio mas", apparently early purple orchid (*Orchis mascula* (L.) L.)—though the inflorescences in Fuchs's woodcut are actually wrong (see Künkele 1987: 229–230 for details). The entry stems from *AC*, but as usual obviates a great part of the description.

Emendation of the MS readings is based on the evidence of "stondenegousse" in *Alph*., "standelwelkes" in *AC*, "standelwort", "standergrasse" in DL, and the equation "standelwelks is satyrion" in the "Supplement" to English names of Ge. These ME names have probable SW origins (Moreno Olalla 2007: 130–131).

Pharmacographically, the species is described as being carminative (**2197**), vulnerary (**2198**), and ophthalmic (**2199**). Orchids were mainly praised as powerful aphrodisiacs, but the virtue of the species against flatulence is found in *Grad.*, and the ophthalmic qualities are mentioned in *TH* and *GH*. The vulnerary virtue, on the other hand, is found neither in the source text nor in the usual literature, hence it looks like an independent addition in *LH*.

Literature: *EARLY PURPLE ORCHID (*Orchis mascula* (L.) L.): MM iii.128 (σατύριον); NH xxvi.97 (*satyrion*); SM xii.118; RM ii.257; Grad. 379 (*satyrion*); OEH 16 (*herba satyrion. hreafnes leac*); Dur.Glos. 305 (*satyrion. hrefnes lec*); LS 91 (*chasi alkeb* [خصي الكلب *ḥuṣī al-kalb*], *testiculus canis, cinos arcos*); EPN ii (*satirion. suðerige*); Cl s.19 (*satirion. ȝekestrus*); TH 431 (*satirion*); Pand. 154 (ᴀʀ*chasialchel*, ɢʀ*orchis, afrodisia, priapismon,* ʟᴀ*testiculus vulpis, satirion, leporina*); Alph. 140 (*pes uituli, interficiens patrem. stondenegousse*), 158 (*satirion. stondenegousse*); Sin.Bart. 37 (*satyrion, priapismus, herba leporina*); AC p. 202,7 (*saturion maior. ȝekes, standelwelkes*) ⚘ GH 391 (SATYRION, *gangelon, hares ballockes, priapismus, guyos, eucarion, sarapias, orcis, testiculi leporis, neme, baram*); Fu 209 (ʹΟΡΧΙΣ, κυνὸς ὄρχις, *testiculus canis*); Tu 2.586 (ADDERS GRASSE, *cynosorchis, fox stone, hare stone, dogstone*); DL 156 (STANDELWORT, *standergrasse, the first kind… orchis, ragwort, priest pintell, ballock grasse, adders grasse, bastard satyrion*, ὄρχις, κυνὸς ὄρχις, *testiculus canis, satyrion*); Ge 158 (FOOLES STONES, *cuckoo orchis, cynosorchis morio, orchis mas, satyrion, orchis delphinia*).

CH (*SM, RM*, Fu, DL, Ge) | C¹H¹ (*LS*) | C³H³ (*Cl*) | C³S³ (*Grad., TH, GH*)

2201 saxfrage. The Latin headword, ME name and physical description make it clear that the entry deals with the medical virtues of burnet saxifrage (*Pimpinella saxifraga* L.). The chapter derives from *AC* but misses much information provided there, including the temperament—which, in opposition to all consulted *auctoritates*, is thought to be "colde & drye" (p. 203.36).

As suggested by its Latin name and confirmed by the medieval and Renaissance pharmacopea, the species is described as a lithontriptic for both the urinary bladder and the kidneys (**2203**).

Literature: BURNET SAXIFRAGE (*Pimpinella saxifraga* L.): HP vii.7.1 (καυκαλίς); MM ii.139; NH xxi.89 (*caucalis*); SM xii.15; RM ii.222; OEH 99 (*herba saxifragiam. sundcorn*); Dur.Glos. 305 (*saxifrigia. sund corn*); EPN ii (*saxifraga. sund-corn*), vi (*saxifragium. saxifrage. wai-wurt*); Cl s.28 (*saxifragia. saxifrage*); TH 442 (*saxifraga*); DVH(SME) 42a.15 (*saxifrage*); Alph. 163 (*saxifragia.* ɢᴀ,ᴀɴ*saxifrage*); AC p. 203.31 (*saxifrage. saxfrage, stone-breke*) ⚘ GH 401 (SAXIFRAGIA, *amaucus, aprogio, aspiron, saxyfrage*); Fu 231 (PIMPINELLA MAIOR); Tu 2.731 (DUCH PIMPINELL, *saxifrage*); DL 204 (SAXIFRAGE, *saxifragia, petra findula, bibinella*); Ge 887 (BURNET SAXIFRAGE, *saxifragia, petrafindula, bipinella, bipenula*).

CS (*SM, RM*) | C²S² (Fu) | C³S³ (*Cl, TH, GH*, DL, Ge)

2206 scabyeus. The Latin headword and ME name traditionally refer to field scabious (*Knautia arvensis* (L.) Coult.). Textually, the entry combines virtues apparently drawn from *AC* (against scab and for hair growth) with other borrowed from one or more untraced source(s). The description of the species in *AC* cannot be *Knautia arvensis* since, in opposition to the statement of the scribe, the leaves of that species are slit. Brodin (1950: 246) suggests some *Scabiosa* L. spp., but these species usually display lobed leaves as well. While its leaves are not slit, the species meant in the text cannot be elecampane (*Inula helenium* L.), as suggested in *Alph.* as the flowers of this plant are bright yellow. According to the description, the plant in *AC* (and perhaps also *LH*) must be devil's-bit scabious (*Succisa pratensis* Moench; → **1306**).

Pharmacographically, the species is, as expected, recommended against skin diseases (scabs **2209**; apostemes **2210**; swellings **2213**; sores **2211**); other than this, the entry praises it as trichogenous (**2209**), expectorant (**2211**), alexipharmic (**2212**), hepatic (**2215**) and stomachal (**2215**). The powers to clean the breast and as an antitussive are mentioned in several sources in connection with *scabiosa*, but the rest seems not to be found in any treatise of the period. On the other hand, *morsus diaboli* is recommended for the same diseases as *scabiosa*, and also against poison. The temperament provided in the text is the exact opposite to the one mentioned in the literature for both species.

Literature: *DEVIL'S-BIT SCABIOUS (*Succisa pratensis* Moench): ⚕ Fu 271 (SUCCISA); Tu 2.748 (DEVILS BITE, *morsus diaboli, succisa*); DL 77 (DEUILS-BIT, *morsus diaboli, succisa*); Ge 587 (DIUELS BIT, *morsus diaboli*); → morre y-bitt [**1306**]. ¶ *FIELD SCABIOUS (*Knautia arvensis* (L.) Coult.): *Cl* s.32 (*scabiosa*); *TH* 448 (*scabiosa*); *Pand.* 613 ($_{LA}$*scabiosa*, $_{GR}$*stibes, stibeos*); *Alph.* 53 (*elena campana, enula, ortolana et campana differunt, ortolana maior, elena campana minor, scabiosa maior. horshelne*), 163 (*scabiosa maior, elna campana, enula campana.* $_{GA}$*scabiouse,* $_{AN}$*scabwrt, brodewed, horsneferte*); *Sin.Bart.* 38 (*scabiosa maior*); *AC* p. 203.37 (*scabiosa maior. scabyose*) ⚕ *GH* 407 (SCABIOSA, *scabious, galiynary*); Fu 272 (SCABIOSA); DL 76 (SCABIOUS, *scabiosa, χώρα*); Ge 582 (SCABIOUS).

CS (Fu, DL) | C^{2}S^2 (*Cl, TH, GH,* Ge)

2217 spurge. The ME name refers to some species with purgative qualities, traditionally identified with caper spurge, *Euphorbia lathyris* L. (→ **2332** for an akin species). The Latin headword (a *lectio facilior*, cf. La. *ēlectuārium* 'electuary'), on the other hand, means the juice of the squirting cucumber (*Ecballium elaterium* (L.) A.Rich., cf. *Alph.*, *Sin.Bart.*). *Cl*, and consequently *TH* and *GH*, distinguished between *lacterides* (caper spurge), *electerides* (squirting cucumber) and *electerium* (the fruit and juice extracted from the latter):

Aliud est lacterides, sunt enim cataputie, aliud electerides, quia cucumer agrestis. Alio nomine dicitur siccidum, aliud eletherium. Electerium est fructus cucumeris agrestis (*TH*).

And there is dyfference betwene electerides ad electerium, for electerides is the sedes of cathapucia spurge, but electeriumis the iuce of wylde cowcomers (*GH*).

The fact that the author of *Cl* had to comment on it makes clear that confusion between these three terms was frequent during the Middle Ages and beyond: Fu still used ἐλατήριον as a synonym of σίκυς ἄγριος, although he was aware that "sic autem propriè uocatur succus eius". In the case of *LH*, identification with squirting cucumber is the best possibility, if only because the text states that the seed of ‹spurge› is ‹nought so myghty as the þat is callid catapusia› (**2223–2224**), catapuce being a regular synonym for *Euphorbia lathyris*, as seen from the quotations above.

An akin species, *Daphne laureola* L., was treated in → **1149** offering virtually a twin entry, which suggests that the same source was used in both cases.

Literature: SQUIRTING CUCUMBER (*Ecballium elaterium* (L.) A.Rich.): *MM* iv.150 (σίκυς ἄγριος); *NH* xx.3 (*cucumis silvestris*); *SM* xii.122; *RM* ii.259; *Dur.Glos.* 301 (*cucumeris. hservhete, verhvete*); *Cl* E.7 (*elacterium*); *TH* 166 (*electerium*); *Pand.* 535 (*mezaharan, mezereon, elacterium*); *Alph.* 53–54 (*elacterium, succus cucurbite agrestis*); *Sin.Bart.* 18 (*elactarium, sucus cucumeris asinini*) ⚕ *GH* 156 (ELECTERIUM, *iuse of wylde cowcomers called asinines*); Fu 267 (ΣΙΚΥΣ ἈΓΡΙΟΣ, ἐλατήριον, *cucumer anguinus/syluestris/erraticus/asininus*); Tu 1.292 (WYLDE CUCUMBER, *cucumis sylvestris, cucumis anguinus, sicis agrios, cucumer asininus, lepying cucumbre*); DL 269 (WILDE SPIRTING CUCUMBER, σίκυς ἄγριος, *cucumis agrestis/syluestris/errraticus/anguinus/asininus*); Ge 765 (WILDE CUCUMBERS, σίκυς ἄγριος, *agrestis/errraticus/asininus cucumis*); → lawreoll [**1149**].

C^2 (Ge) | CS (Fu) | C^2S^2 (DL) | C^4S^4 (*Cl, TH, GH*)

2226 stafisagre. The Latin headword and ME name (both of them misspelt in the MS) and the reference to ‹wilde vyne› indicate that the entry must describe the medical virtues of stavesacre (*Delphinium staphisagria* L., cf. Gk. σταφὶς ἀγρία "wild raisin"). The confusion between **f** and long **s** in the MS can be traced back to the source text (*AC*) and may have been helped by the similarity with La. *saxifraga* (→ **2201**).

Pharmacographically, the species is said to be emetic of humours (**2229**) and antipruritic (**2233**). The first virtue is found everywhere in the usual literature, where it is commended particularly as an excellent drug to to purge the head (cf. the synonyms in the Literature, including Ar. ḥabb ar-rās, lit. "grain of the head"), while the second is mentioned in many medical sources together with the well-known antiphtheiriac powers of the plant, highlighted by the synonym *herba pedicularis*—and Gk φθειροκτόνον and φθείριον, cf. φθείρ "louse".

Literature: STAVESACRE (*Delphinium staphisagria* L.): *MM* iv.152 (σταφὶς ἀγρία); *NH* xxiii.17 (*astaphis agria, staphis agria*); *SM* xi.842 (ἀσταφίς); *RM* ii.197; *Grad.* 371 (*staphisagria*); *OEH* 181 (*herba stauisagria*); *LS* 267 (*alberas* [حبّ الرّاس ḥabb ar-rās], *staphysagria, granum capitis*); *Cl* s.8 (*staphisagra, caput purgium*); *TH* 457 (*staphisagria*); *Pand.* 302 (_{AR}*haberas, nunbafas,* _{GR}*pediculicida,* _{LA}*stafisagria, pedicularia, granum capitis, passula montana, rosa regis*); *Alph.* 81 (*herba pedicularis, stafisagria*), 164 (*sataffisagria* [...] *staffisagria, campurrigium*); *Sin.Bart.* 14 (*caputpurgium, stafisagria*), 37 (*ruta agrestis, stafisagria*), 41 (*staphis agria, herba pedicularis*); *AC* 156.1 (*scafisagia. scafisage*) ❦ *GH* 416 (STAPHISAGRIA, *pyllulary, lyke grasse*); *Fu* 301 (ΣΤΑΦΙΣ ΆΓΡΙΑ, *pedicularis, pituitaria, staphisagria*); *Tu* 2.583 (STAVIS AKER, *staphis agria*); *DL* 268 (STAPHIS-AKER, σταφὶς ἀγρία, φθειροκτόνον, φθείριον, *herba pedicularis, pituitaria, staphis agria*); *Ge* 398 (STAUES AKER, *lowsewoort, lowse powder,* σταφὶς ἀγρία, *herba pedicularis, peduncularia, vua taminia, pituitaria, passula montana, staphisagria*).

C³S³ (*Grad., LS, Cl, TH, GH*) | C⁴S⁴ (*Fu, DL, Ge*)

2236 synkefoly. The Latin headword, ME synonym and the reference to the creeping habits of the species strongly suggest that the entry describes the properties of the cinquefoil (*Potentilla reptans* L.), even though the temperament does not match. The chapter combines information from at least two sources (which explains why some virtues are repeated); one of them may have been *AC* (although the wording is different), while the other remains untraced.

The species is above all described as an excellent remedy for diseases of the digestive system, from the mouth to the intestines (teeth, **2257**, **2259**; mouth, tongue and throat, **2240**; tongue again, **2248**). Other than this, it is also presented as antilumbalgic (**2239**), anticephalalgic (**2240**), analgesic (**2242**, **2245**), anti-inflammatory (**2246**), anthemoptyic (**2243**), lithontriptic (**2244**), antiepistactic (**2249**), alexipharmic (**2252**), antipyrotic (**2253**). All of them are routinely recorded in the medical literature of the period, bar the powers to break kidney stones.

Literature: CINQUEFOIL (*Potentilla reptans* L.): *HP* ix.13.5 (πεντάφυλλον); *MM* iv.42 (πεντέφυλλον); *NH* xxv.109 (*quinquefolium*); *SM* xii.96 (πεντάφυλλον); *RM* ii.250 (πεντάφυλλος); *OEH* 3 (*herba pentafilon. fifleafe*); *Dur.Glos.* 304 (*pentaphilon. refnes fot | quinque folia. fif leaf*); *EPN* ii (*quinquefolium, pentufillon. fif-leafe*), iii (*quinquevolium. fiif-leafe*), iv (*quinquefila. hræfnes fot | pentaphyllon. fif-leafe*), v (*quinquefolium. fif-leafe*), vi (*quinquefolium. quintfoil. fiflef*), vii (*hoc pentifolium. filife*); *TH* 381 (*pentaphilon*); *Pand.* 584 (_{LA}*quinquefolium,* _{GR}*pentafilon*); *Alph.* 27 (*camolee, quinquefolium, pentaphilon. fifuuedgresse*), 152 (*quinquefolium, pentafilon. fiueleuedgras*); *Sin.Bart.* 36 (*quinquefolium, pentafilon*); *AC* p. 200.6 (*qvinquefolium. fyfleued gras*) ❦ *GH* 347 (PENTHAFILON, *synkefoyle, v-leued grasse*); *Fu* 238

(*ΠΕΝΤΑΦΥΛΛΟΝ*, *quinquefolium*); Tu 2.537 (CINKFOLY, *five-fingred grasse*, *quinquefolium*, πέντε φύλλον); DL 57 (CINQUEFOYLE, *fiue finger grasse*, πεντάφυλλον, *pentaphyllum*, *quinquefolium*); Ge 835 (CINKEFOILE, *fiue finger grasse*, *fiue leafed grasse*, *sinkfield*, πεντάφυλλον, *quinquefolium*, *pentaphyllon*).

S³ (*RM*, DL, Ge) | C¹S³ (*SM*, Fu)

2241 Galean sayth. The sentence seems to be a scribal addition to impart more authority to it, for it seems to be recorded nowhere in the Galenic corpus. There a passage in the fifth book of *De compositione medicamentorum secundum locos* (Περὶ συνθέσεως φαρμάκων τῶν κατὰ τόπους) that may have served as source in case that the ‹sore akyng› refers in fact to toothache, but the ingredients and preparation are different, so that the relationship between both texts is dubious: Πρὸς ὀδόντων βρῶσιν καὶ πόνους. Πενταφύλλου ῥίζας σὺν οἴνῳ ἑψήσας δίδου διακλύζεσθαι μετὰ τὸ δεῖπνον, ἀφέψου δὲ εἰς τὸ τρίτον μέρος (Kühn 1821–1833: xiii.879; "Against decay and pain of the teeth. Make the sickman have the roots of cinquefoil, rinsed and boiled in wine, with his supper. Boil until it is reduced to a third part.").

2262 souredok. The Latin headword applies to a number of bitter species (traditionally, *Rumex* L. spp. and *Oxalis* L. spp.), most of the times *R. acetosa* L., *R. acetosella* L., or *O. acetosella* L. Although there is no physical description that may help decide which of these is the actual species, the ME synonym is usually identified with common sorrel, *R. acetosa* L. (see for instance OED: *s.v.* sour dock, DEPN: *s.vv.* dock, sour; and docken or docking, sour). The entry translates the appropriate chapter in *DVH*, which in fact seems to deal with some *Sempervivum* L. sp. (→ **1031**, with discussion), cf. its opening line: *dicimus acidulam, quam Graecus dicit aizon* (i.e. ἀείζῳον). Since the poem talks later about the *minor* counterpart of the plant (→ **2273**), this would be the tree *major* species, i.e. houseleek (*Aeonium arboreum* Webb & Berthel. = *Sempervivum arboreum* L.).

Medically, the plant is mainly described as a good ophthalmic (**2266** = *DVH* 719, **2271** = *DVH* 733, and → **2273**), but it is also said to be a good antiemetic and anticaustic (**2264** = *DVH* 715, 718), antiulcerous and antipodagric (→ **2266** = *DVH* 720–723), anticephalalgic (**2267** = *DVH* 725–726), antidysenteric (**2269** = *DVH* 727–728), anthelminthic (**2270** = *DVH* 731), alexipharmic (**2270** = *DVH* 732, and again on **2272** = *DVH* 735–736), acoustic (→ **2273**). Missing from the account is the antiemmenagogue virtue (*DVH* 729–730). All of them are included in the chapter ἀείζῳον μέγα in *MM* and all the usual medical literature dealing with *Sempervivum*.

Literature: COMMON SORREL (*Rumex acetosa* L.): *HP* vii.1.2 (λάπαθον); *MM* ii.114; *NH* xx.231 (*lapathum*); *SM* xii.56; *RM* ii.234; *OEH* 34 (*herba lapatium. wududocce*); *Dur. Glos.* 303 (*lapatium. vude docce*), 304 (*oxilapatium. eorth vealle, scearpe docce*); *DVH* 711–747 (*acidula, aizon*); *LS* 111 (*humadh* [حُمَّاض *ḥummāḍ*], *acetosa*); *EPN* ii (*oxylapation. anes cynnes clate*), iv (*lappacium. docce*); *CI* L.8 (*lapacium*); *TH* 254 (*lapatium*); *Pand.* 362 ($_{AR}$*humad*, $_{GR}$*oxilapatium*, $_{LA}$*acetosa*), 382 ($_{LA}$*lapatium, pratella*, $_{GR}$*lapaton hemason, acetosa, origma, lapagos*); *DVH(NME)* 253v.14 (*sowredoke*); *DVH(SME)* 27a.20 (*sorell, souredok. assidula. aizon*); *Alph.* 2 (*acedula, ribes, herba acetosa. sourdocke*); *Sin.Bart.* 33 (*oxilapacium, acedula. soure-dock*); *AC* 200.18 (*lapasium. rede dokke*) ❧ *GH* 51 (ACETOSUM, *huma, oxilapatium, sorell*); *Fu* 174 (ΛΑΠΑΘΟΝ, *quartum genus rumicis*, ὀξαλὶς, *acetosa*); *Tu* 2.549 (DOCKES, *rumex*, [...] *oxilapathon*); *DL* 401 (*the fourth kinde of* DOCKS, ὀξαλὶς, *acetosa, sorrell*); *Ge* 318 (SORRELL, ὀξαλὶς, ἀναξυρὲς, ὀξυλάπαθον, *acetosa*). ¶ TREE HOUSELEEK (*Aeonium arboreum* Webb & Berthel.): *MM* iv.88 (ἀείζωον μέγα); *NH* xxv.160–161 (*sedum magnum*); *SM* xi.815; *DVH(SME)* 27a.20 (*sorell, souredok*) ❧ *Fu* 10 (ΆΕΙΖΩΟΝ, *sedum, semperuiuum, Iouis barba*); *Tu* 2.563 (HOUSLEKE, *sempervivum*, [...] *sedum magnum, aeizoon mega, singren, aygrene*); *DL* 79 (HOUSELEEKE, *sengreene*, ἀείζωον, *sedum, semperuiuum, vitalis*); *Ge* 411 (HOUSLEEKE, *sengreene, aygreene, Iupiters eie, bullocks eie, Iupiters beard, Iouis barba*). → jubarbe [**1031**].

ÆS³ (*DL*) | C³S³ (*CI*) | FS (*GH*, *Ge*) | F¹S¹ (*LS*) | F²S² (*Fu*) | F³S³ (*DVH*)

2266 crepynge goutys. Comparison with the Latin poem indicates that the power of the plant served to cure not the mysterious "creeping gout" but rather the apparition of creeping ulcers (probably meaning herpes), cf. *DVH* 720 *Ulcera, quae serpunt, cohibet combustaque curat.*

2273 eryn. The ME text lacks the final part, but the exemplar must have dealt with deafness and otalgia, as seen from the parallel passage in *DVH* 737–738: *Auribus expressus si succus funditur eius /Adiuvat auditum mire pellitque dolorem.*

2273 anoynte the eyne-lyddis. According to the parallel Latin line (*DVH* 744–747), this virtue does really not belong to acidula, but to its *minor* counterpart, which is identified as the houseleek, a species described at least three times in the treatise (→ **709**, → **1031**, with discussion, and → **2151**).

2277 Seynt Mary seall. Lack of physical description makes identification difficult. Traditionally, the Latin and ME names were taken to mean Solomon's seal (*Polygonatum multiflorum* (L.) All.; so PNME: *s.v.* sigillum Sancte Marie, Brodin 1950: 244, etc.), but in Renaissance herbals the Latin headword was applied to some sort of wild vine, identified with black bryony (*Dioscorea communis* (L.) Caddick & Wilkin = *Tamus communis* L.). The physical description in *GH* mixes both species (*contra* OED: *s.v.* lady's seal *n.*, § 1), cf. "bereth reed sedes on a rowe", which points to the *Dioscorea* while "hathe a whyte knotty rote" refers to the *Polygonatum* (cf. the synonyms "white woort", "white roote" in DL and Ge); naturally, the same applies to *TH*. The references to the straight stalk and the rough leaves of the plant indicate that bryony is also meant in *Alph.* and *Sin.Bart.*, cf. *Pand.* "hastas h*abet* longas & lignosas & asp*eras*" in the description of "ampelos agria"/"vitis siluestris". As for *AC*, the comparison of the leaves of this species with those of "playntayn" (some *Plantago* L. spp.) and the small size of the stalk suggest that the *Polygonatum* was intended, as this species grows to about 100cm while the *Dioscorea* is a vine that will climb several metres.

The entry is among the few to describe husbandry uses for this species; in this case, to cure oxen (**2280**; other instances in → **656**, → **970**, → **1985**). Pharmacographically, the species is described as anaphrodisiac (**2278**) and antisciatic (since ⟨tisayne⟩ is likely to be a *lectio facilior*, as in → **595**, → **900**, and **1336**; cf. the parallel readings in → **338** as well), but these are indifferent for identification purposes as they are found in the literature of the period in connection with neither candidate. The reference to ⟨piment⟩ (**2279**, "an aromatic ointment, perfume", MED: *s.v.* pĩment *n.*, § b), on the other hand, is crucial to this argument: the inflorescences of wild vines, called *oenanthe* (Gk. οἰνάνθη, lit. "wine flower"), were the main ingredient to create οἰνανθίνος "unguent of wild vine inflorescence" (*MM* i.46, also mentioned in *NH* xii.132 and xxxiii.8), a perfume used by the kings of Parthia (Groom 1992: 164). Hence the text in *LH* seems to refer to a wild vine, such as the black bryony.

> **Literature**: BLACK BRYONY (*Dioscorea communis* (L.) Caddick & Wilkin): *MM* v.2 (ἄμπελος ἀγρία); *NH* xxiii.19 (*labrusca*); *SM* xi.826; *RM* ii.193; *LS* 35 (*harin* [ڕ karm], *vitis ... sylvestris*); *TH* 480 (*sigillum sancte Marie*); *Pand.* 299 (ᴀʀ*haarim, harin,* ɢʀ*ampeleos ... agria,* ʟᴀ*vitis ... siluestris*); *Alph.* 169 (*sigillum Sancte Marie*); *Sin.Bart.* 39 (*sigillum beatæ Mariæ*) ⚭ *GH* 437 (SIGILLUM SANCTE MARIE, *sigillum Salomonis, Salomons seale, our ladyes seale*); *Tu* 2.601 (BLACK BRIONYE); *DL* 278 (WILDE VINE, *brionie, our Ladies seale,* ἄμπελος ἀγρία, *vitis silvestris, tamus, salicastrum, sigillum beatæ Mariæ*); *Ge* 721 (BLACKE BRYONIE, *wilde vine*). ¶ SOLOMON'S SEAL (*Polygonatum multiflorum* (L.) All.): *MM* iv.6 (πολυγόνατον); *NH* xxvii.113 (*polygonum, sanguinaria*); *SM* xii.106; *RM* ii.253; *AC* p. 202.21 (*sigillum Sancte Marie. Seynt Marie seal*) ⚭ *Fu* 222 (ΠΟΛΥΓΟΝΑΤΟΝ, *sigilum Salomonis*); *Tu* 2.517 (POLYGONATUM, *scala caeli, sigillum Salomonis, whyte wurt*); *DL* 71 (WHITE ROOTE, *Salomons seale, scala cæli, white-wurt,* πολύγονατον, *sigillum Salomonis*); *Ge* 755 (SALOMONS SEALE, *Scala cæli, white woort, white roote,* πολυγόνατον, *sigilum Salomonis, scala cæli*).

CS (DL) | C¹S¹ (*LS*) | C³S³ (Ge)

2283 tansy. Identification of the Latin headword and the ME name with tansy (*Tanacetum vulgare* L.) is traditional. Textually, the pedigree of the entry is untraced. Pharmacographically, the plant is said to be anthelminthic (**2283**), febrifuge (**2284**), anti-inflammatory of the feet (**2285**), lithontriptic (**2287**) and alexipharmic (**2289**). Other than this, the plant is also praised as a condiment for meat (**2289**). The powers of the species to kill tapeworms is well recognized in the literature and the properties against the ague are found in a few sources (*TH* and DL), but the rest are not generally included in the appropriate entries for this species. Even so, the anti-inflammatory virtue might be read as a reference to gout, while the assumed stone-breaking powers could be connected to dysury; both diseases are indeed routinely found in the medieval and Renaissance herbals. Concerning the culinary value of the plant, Ge states that newly-sprung tansy leaves were cooked with eggs into cakes called *tansies*, "which be pleasant in taste" (see also OED: *s.v.* tansy *n.* § 3.a.

Literature: TANSY (*Tanacetum vulgare* L.): Dur.Glos. 305 (*tanacetum, tanaceta. helde*); *EPN* iv (*artemesia. tagantes, helde | tenedisse. helde*), v (*tanicétum. helde*), vi (*tanecetum. taneseie. helde*); *TH* 31 (*arthemisia media*); *Pand.* 37 (*ambrosia, athanasia*); *DVH(SME)* 41a.5 (*tansey*); *Alph.* 16 (*atanasia, athasia. tansie, bemp*), 181 (*tanacetum, athanasia*); *Sin.Bart.* 12 (*athanasia. tanacetum*) ⚘ Fu 13 (ΆΡΤΕΜΙΣΙΑ, *tertia species artemisia monoclonos, tanacetum, tagetes*); Tu 2.489 (FEVERFEW, *parthenium, amaracus* [...] *tansey*); DL 14 (TANSIE, *tanacetum, athanasia, artemisia vnicaulis, artemisia tragante, tragetes*, ἀρτεμίσια μονόκλωνος); Ge 524 (TANSIE, *tanacetum, athanasia*).

$$C^2S^2 \text{ (Fu)} \mid C^2S^3 \text{ (DL, Ge)} \mid C^3S^3 \text{ (TH)}$$

2291 tutesayne. The ME names suggest that the entry describes the medical properties of tutsan (*Hypericum androsaemum* L.), but the Latin headword and the reference to chastity suggest that the species intended must be the chaste tree (*Vitex agnus-castus* L.). Both of them produce black berries. The fact that *Vitex* did not grow in Britain at the time naturally points to the first candidate, but the medical powers allotted to the species in the entry are actually associated with that Mediterranean tree (see below). Substitution of one for the other was common in English apothecaries, as indicated in Tu: "in England they abuse shamefully tutsam [*sic*] for agno". Textually, the section follows *AC*.

Pharmacographically, the species is said to be anaphrodisiac (**2293**, and again in **2295**), deoppilant (**2294**), anthydropic (→ **2295**), antilethargic (**2299**), hemostatic of the anal zone (**2302**), hepatic and splenetic (**2303**), and anticephalalgic (**2305**). All of them are found in the usual literature in connection with *Vitex*, *Hypericum* being praised as purgative, vulnerary and hemostatic (cf. the ME name, apparently from OF *toute sain* "all healthy", yet see OED: *s.v.* tutsan).

Literature: CHASTE TREE (*Vitex agnus-castus* L.): *HP* iii.12.1 (ἄγνος); *MM* i.103; *NH* xiii.14, xxiv.59 (*vitex, agnos*); *SM* xi.807; *RM* ii.187; *Grad.* 378 (*agnus castus*); *LS* 299 (*famanchest* [فنجنكشت *fanǧankišt*], *agnus castus, arbor Abrahæ*); *Cl* A.6 (*agnus castus*); *TH* 6 (*agnus castus*); *Pand.* 35 (_{AR}*amarichest, pentafilem,* _{GR}*aligos, ligos,* _{LA}*agnus castus, salix marina, alexandrina, arbor abae*); *Alph.* 3, 235 (*zucchozaria, agnus castus, salices marini*); *Sin.Bart.* 9 (*agnus castus. bischopeswort*); *AC* 157.15 (*agnus castus. totsane, parkleuys*) ❦ *GH* 6 (AGNUS CASTUS, *tutson*); Tu 2.600 (VITEX, *agnos, ligos, vitex agnus castus*); DL 496 (AGNUS CASTUS, *hemp tree, chaste tree,* ἄγ(υ)νος, λύγος, *vitex, vitex, salix marina, salix amerina, piper agreste, agnus castus*); Ge 1201 (CHASTE TREE, *hempe tree,* ἄγ(υ)νος, λύγος, *vitex, salix marina, salix amerina, piper agreste, agnus castus*). ¶ TUTSAN (*Hypericum androsaemum* L.): *MM* iii.156 (ἀνδρόσαιμον); *NH* xxvii.26 (*androsaemon, ascyron*); *SM* xi.829; *RM* ii.194 ❦ Fu 25 (*ΑΝΔΡΟΣΑΙΜΟΝ, androsæmon*); Tu 1.234 (TUTSAN, *androsemom, agnus castus*); DL 47 (TUTSAN, *parke leaves,* ἀνδρόσαιμον, *agnus castus*); Ge 434 (TUTSAN, *parke leaues,* ἀνδρόσαιμον, *dionysias, herba siciliana*).

C²S² (*Pand.*) | C³S³ (*SM, RM, Grad., LS, TH, GH,* Tu, DL, Ge) | C⁴S⁴ (*Cl*)

2293 the porrys. MED: *s.v.* paunch(e *n.* takes the original MS reading ⟨pomys⟩ to be a scribal misreading of *p o u n s "belly" (< OF *pauns*), but comparison with the Latin text rather suggests that the exemplary word was actually *PORRYS "pores", cf. *Sl*.1r/10–11 ⟨*secundum* dias & plac*es* d*icitu*r ad ap*er*iend*um* poros & sp*iritu*s euap*or*and*um*⟩. The same reading ⟨pomys⟩ seems to refer to "pulse" elsewhere in the treatise (→ **1438**).

2295 Places saith. The quotation does indeed originate in the chapter devoted to the chaste tree in *Cl* and reads:

> Alia [*sc.* vis] inaniendo spiritus et consumendo sperma [...]. In succo agnicasti semen feniculi .ʒ.iij. et esule .ϴ.iij. decoquatur mane detur cum vino calido leucophlegmatico colatura.

Similarly, the Latin version of *AC*, where the actual meaning of leucophlegmacy is glossed, offers:

> dic*it* & idem auctor quod eius decocc*io* valet *contra* leu[c]oflegma*m* frigida*m* i. frigida*m* ydropis[i]m si c*um* seme*n* feni*c*uli & modica esula decoquatur.

In keeping with the usual ideas of the humoral theory, four different types of dropsy were distinguished, to wit *leucophlegmancy* (phlegm); *hyposarca*, also called *anasarca* (black bile); *ascites* (blood); and *tympanites* (yellow bile):

> [Q]uattuor species [*sc.* hydropisi] esse dicunt: assignant eas secundum quattuor causas humorales, et secundum eas quattuor nomina attribuuntur vt illi speciei que est ex flegmate attribuant nomen leucoflegmancia a leucos quod est album. et flegma, quasi album flegma. Illa que est ex [MS est] melancholia denominatur yposarca, ab ypos quod est sub, quasi sub cute, creos autem caro est, vel anasarca quasi iuxta carnem. Que est ex sanguine vocatur archis vel archites, archis enim vter est; sonat enim venter ad modum vtris semipleni. Que est ex colera vocatur tympanites a tympano eo quam venter percussus resonat ad modum tympani

(*CM*: f. ccxlviij, bis).

2307 totheworte. The Latin headword and ME names are traditionally identified with shepherd's purse (*Capsella bursa-pastoris* (L.) Medik.). In a number of sources (*OEH, LS, EPN,* Fu) Classical θλάσπι was identified with some pepperwort (*Lepidium campestre* (L.) R.Br./*L. ruderale* L., to judge from the woodcuts in *Fu*), but the properties of this species (purgative, hematogogue, emmenagogue) are wholly different from those assumed for the *Capsella*. The name ⟨totheworte⟩ is recorded in the "Supplement" to English names in Ge and probably connected to ⟨toywoort⟩ in the same source (where it is said to be used "in the North part of England") if this is due to the printer's confusion between þ and y in Gerard's handwritten autograph (see OED s.v. †toywort for another explanation). The textual pedigree of the entry remains untraced.

As expected from the ME synonyms ⟨stanche⟩ and ⟨sanguynary⟩, the species is universally praised as antidysenteric/hemostatic (**2310**) and vulnerary (**2312**).

> **Literature:** SHEPHERD'S PURSE (*Capsella bursa-pastoris* (L.) Medik.): *MM* ii.156 (θλάσπι); *NH* xxvii.139 (*thlaspi*); *SM* xi.886; *RM* ii.216; *OEH* 150 (*herba thyaspis*); *LS* 349 (*nartucium tectorum*); *EPN* iv (*pissli. reosan* | *thiaspis. lambes cerse*); *TH* 77 (*bursa pastoris*); *Alph.* 34 (*capsellula, herba sanguinaria, bursa pastoris. pursewurt*); *AC* 172.5 (*bursa pastoris. scheperdys purs, tothwort*) ❀ *GH* 72 (BURSA PASTORIS, *cassewed, shepherdes purs, sanguynarye*); Fu 114 (ΘΛΑΣΠΙ, θλασπίδιον, σίνηπι ἄγριον, *capsella, scandulaceum, nasturtium tectorum, sinapi rusticum, bursa pastoris*), 232 (PASTORIA BURSA, *pera pastoris*); Tu 2.733 (BURSA PASTORIS, *shepeherdes pouche*); DL 57 (SHEPHEARDS PURSE/*scrip/pouch, casseweed, pastoria bursa, pera/bursa pastoris*); Ge 214 (SHEPHEARDES PURSE/*scirp* [sic]*/pouch, poore mans parmacetie, toywoort, pickepurse, caseweede, pastoris bursa, pera pastoris*).
>
> CF (Tu) |CS (Ge) | C³S³ (DL) | C⁴S⁴ (*LS,* Fu)

2314 tyme. The ME name generally refers to garden thyme (*Thymus vulgaris* L.; → **1631** about the wild counterpart), while the Latin headword could refer either to the flower of that species (cf. "flos eius [*sc.* thymi] inde dicitur epithimum, quasi supra thimum" in *TH*, and similarly in *Sin.Bart.*; ⟨athemon⟩ in *Pand.* is probably connected as well, cf. Gk ἄνθεμον "flower"), or else to that type of dodder that grows on thyme (*Cuscuta epithymum* L.). Ge, on the authority of Pietro Andrea Mattioli and Pierre Pena (a helper of Matthias de L'Obel, with whom he published *Stirpium Adversaria Nova* in 1571; Legré 1899), seems to have used the name *epithymum* to refer to the fourth type of thyme (called *Epithymum Græcorum/Laced time* in the corresponding woodcut), which some scholars thought more prone to suffer parasitical infestation from *Cuscuta*. The English botanist, moreover, paraphrased Galen to state that "epithymum [...] is of more effectuall operation in physicke then time, [...] more mightily clensing, heating, drying, and opening then *cuscuta*" (cf. ἐπίθυμον τῆς θύμου δυνάμεώς ἐστιν ἰσχυρότερον, τὰ πάντα ξηραινούσης τε καὶ θερμαινούσης κατὰ τὴν τρίτην ἀπόστασιν, Kühn 1821–1833: xi.875). This surely explains the lack of an entry for *thymus* but the inclusion of one for *epithymum* in the textually related *Cl*, *TH* and *GH*. The pedigree of the entry is unknown.

Regardless of whether the entry describes the medical powers of thyme or thyme dodder, emendation of the temperament that is missing in the manuscript is supported by most *auctoritates* since Galen (only *Pand.* and *Sin. Bart.* differ, as *epithymum* is said there to be hot and dry in the second degree, which makes little sense after the Galenic dictum).

Pharmacographically, the species is said to be lithontriptic (**2315**), diuretic (**2316**), emmenagogue and abortifacient (**2317**), expectorant (**2319**), carminative (**2320**), anticephalalgic and antilethargic (**2321**). All of them are routinely included in the accounts for *Thymus* and *Cuscuta*. As mentioned in the last sentence, savory and thyme could be used interchangeably in recipes, as both were assumed to have similar medical qualities and indeed the virtues are roughly the same for both plants (→ **2046**).

> **Literature**: GARDEN THYME (*Thymus vulgaris* L.): *MM* iii.36 (θύμος); *NH* xxi.56 (*thymus*); *SM* xi.887; *RM* ii.216; *Grad.* 368; *LS* 271 (*hasce* [حاشا *ḥāšā*], *thymus*); *EPN* iii (*timus. hæp*); *Alph.* 186 (*timus*); *Sin.Bart.* 42 (*thimus* [...] *cujus flos dicitur epithimum*); *AC* p. 198.36 (*pvlogium montanum. puliole mountayn, hulwort, broþerwort*) ৠ *Fu* 319 (ΘΥΜΟΣ, *thymus, serpyllum romanum*); *Tu* 2.565 (WILD THYME, *garden serpillum*), 2.590 (THYME, *thymus*); *DL* 163 (TIME, θύμος); *Ge* 458 (GARDEN TIME). ¶ THYME DODDER (*Cuscuta epithymum* L.): *MM* iv.177 (ἐπίθυμον); *NH* xxvi.55 (*epithymum*); *SM* xi.875; *RM* ii.210; *Grad.* 368; *LS* 246 (*epithymum*); *EPN* vi (*epitime. epithimum. fordboh*), viii (*hec epitimeum. tyme*); *Cl* E.3 (*epithimum*); *TH* 159 (*epithimum*); *Pand.* 67 (ᴀʀ*athemon*, ɢʀ*epithimon*, ʟᴀ*epithimum*); *Alph.* 57 (*epithinum* | *epithimum*, ɢᴀ*epytyme*); *Sin.Bart.* 19 (*epithumi*) ৠ *GH* 149 (*epithimium*); *Tu* 1.265 (DODER, *casitas, cassutha, cuscuta, podragra lini, epithimum Mesues*); *DL* 288 (DODER, *cuscuta*, κασσύθα, *epithymum*); *Ge* 462 (DODDER, *cuscuta, cassutha*, ἐπίθυμον).
>
> C³S³ (*SM, RM, Grad., LS, Cl, TH, GH,* Fu, Tu, DL, Ge)

2314 þe þyrde. Emendation is based on the Literature sources, which universally agree in attaching this temperament to thyme.

2324 turmentile. Although the Latin headword generally refers to tansy (*Tanacetum vulgare* L., → **2283**), the ME synonym and the physical description (in particular, the reference to its rhizomatous root) indicate that the species must be in fact the common tormentil (*Potentilla erecta* (L.) Raeusch.). The confusion is probably connected with the names *tanacetum agreste/album* used in *Alph.*$_{181}$ and *Sin.Bart.*$_{41}$ to refer to "gosegres(se)", i.e. silverweed (*Potentilla anserina* L.), which is very similar to tormentil but lacks its noticeable rhizome. The source for the entry remains untraced.

Medically, the species is described as alexipharmic (**2327**), ophthalmic (**2328**), and antidysenteric (**2330**). The powers of *Potentilla* against poison were well known (cf. the Latin synonyms *antipharmacum*, *vicetoxicon* in PNME; the entry "vicetoxicon" in *GH*$_{468}$ may refer to another plant since "poudre of tormentyll" is to be mixed with it in order to make a good antidote), and its powers against dysentery are also recorded in the usual literature. The reference to eye diseases is referenced in *TH* and *GH*, although the recipe is completely different and makes no mention to children: "contra maculam oculi succus eius vino albo oculo instillatus mire valet"/"for the webbe in the eye, medle the iuce with whyte wyne, and droppe therin".

Literature: COMMON TORMENTIL (*Potentilla erecta* (L.) Raeusch.): OEH 118 (*herba eptafilon. seofonleafe*); *Dur.Glos.* 302 (*eptafilon. gelod vyrt, vii.folia*); EPN iv (*heptaphyllon. gelod-wyrt*), vi (*turmentine. nutehede*), viii (*hec tormentilla. tormentyne*); TH 498 (*torbentilla*); *Pand.* 98 ($_{LA}$*bistorta, consolida rubea,* $_{GR}$*cataphilon, tormentilla, porentilla,* $_{AR}$*buseke*); *Alph.* 187 (*termentilla. tormentille*) ⚕ GH 453 (TORMERTILLA, *fistularia, tormentyll, taglafayre*); Fu 98 ('ΕΠΤΑΦΥΛΛΟΝ, *septifolium, tormentilla, bistorta*); Tu 2.763 (TORMENTILL, *tormentilla, heptaphyllon*); DL 59 (TORMENTILL, *setfoyle, tormentilla,* ἑπτάφυλλον, *septifolium*); Ge 840 (SETFOILE, *tormentill, tormentilla,* ἑπτάφυλλον, *septifolium*).

S³ (DL) | CS³ (Fu, Ge) | F³S³ (*Pand.*)

2332 tvtymallys. The name τιθύμαλλος/*tithymallus* was applied since Antiquity to seven separate species of strong purgative qualities. The uncharacteristically detailed physical description provided in the entry suggests that the plant intended must be sun spurge (*Euphorbia helioscopia* L., identified with the fourth type of spurge in *MM, SM,* Fu, Tu or DL) since this species—in opposition to other spurges, as seen from Renaissance woodcuts—displays most of their leaves at the top of the stem (→ **2334**).

Pharmacographically, the species is described as antipruritic (→ **2339**), which was one of the main uses of spurges together with their purgative qualities. Textually, the pedigree of the entry remains untraced.

Literature: SUN SPURGE (*Euphorbia helioscopia* L.): HP ix.11.7 (τιθύμαλλος); MM iv.164; NH xxvi.62 (*tithymallus, herba lactaria, lactuca caprina*); SM xii.141; RM ii.266; *Grad.* 387 (*thitymallus*); OEH 110 (*herba tytymallus calatites. lacterida*); *Dur. Glos.* 305 (*temolus, titemallos. singrene*); LS 350 (*xauset* [عشى *yatū'*], *lacticinium,* *tithymallus*); *EPN* iv (*titemallos. singrene* | *tytymalosca. lib-corn*), vii (*hic tintimalius. spowrge*); *Cl* T.2 (*titimallus. titimal*); *TH* 490 (*titimallus*); *Pand.* 664 (~LA~*titimallus,* ~AR~*xencua*); *Alph.* 9 (*anabulla maior, spurga, mezereon, rapiens uitam, faciens uiduas, leo terre.* ~GA,AN~*spurge*), 185 (*titimallus, uericaria.* ~GA~*ueroyne,* ~AN~*wertewert*); *Sin. Bart.* 11 (*anabulla. spurge*), 42 (*titimallus*); *AC* 167.26 (*anabulla. sporge*) ✥ *GH* 446 (TYNTYMALLUS, *tyntymall, anabule*); *Fu* 313 (*TIΘYMAΛOΣ, lactaria herba, lactuca caprina/marina, esula, quartus genus heliosopius, solsequus*); *Tu* 2.588 (TITHYMALES, *spourges, the fourth* [kind], *helioscopius, wartwurt, sun(-following) spourge*); *DL* 258 (TITHYMALE, *spourge, the fourth kind ... sunne spourge, wartwurt,* τιθυμάλος ἡλιοσκοπιος, *tithymalus solsequius, lactaria solsequia*); *Ge* 401 (SPURGE, *seconde kynde...sunne spurge, time tithymale, helioscopius, solsequium*).

C³S³ (*TH, GH*) | C⁴S⁴ (Fu, DL, Ge)

2334 compas. The sense "in shape" given in MED: *s.v.* cŏmpăs *adv.*, § c, quoting this passage as sole instance, is probably unnecessary since the regular sense "in a circle" (§ a) makes sense: the flowers of sun spurge are borne on an umbel of five rays and bracts similar in shape to leaves but of a more yellow tinge (which explains the synonym "umbrella milkweed").

2337 flayne. An uncertain word. The general sense of the passage indicates that this is a verb probably meaning "to mix with a liquid into a mushy substance". It could therefore be related to the OE feminine *flyne* "batter", but the different vocalism makes this unclear.

2341 woderofe. The Latin headword refers as a rule to some asphodel (*Asphodelus* L. spp. → **91**; Stirling 1995–1998: *s.v.* hastula) and dubiously to peony (*Paeonia officinalis* L.; Fischer 1929: 277) or St. John's wort (*Hypericum perforatum* L.; PNME: *s.v.* hastula regia), but the ME name is applied to sweet woodruff (*Galium odoratum* (L.) Scop. = *Asperula odorata* L.). This is reinforced by the reference to the sweet taste of the plant, reminiscent of vanilla, which is due to the presence of coumarin ($C_9H_6O_2$) and which explains its use as a flavouring agent in Germany (where it is called *Waldmeister*). As seen from the Literature section, association of *hastula regia* and sweet woodruff is not peculiar to *LH* but can be traced back to Anglo-Saxon times and probably lies in an early confusion between OE *wudurife*, which indicates woodruff, and *wudurofe*, which referred to the *Asphodelus* (de Vriend 1984: 300–301, with an etymological explanation; see also Bierbaumer 1975–1979: i.146, ii.132–133, iii.267–268 regarding the links with μολοχή ἀγρία and *ostricium*). As seen from the synonyms provided in the Literature section (clearly *Pand.*, in all likelihood also *TH*), in the treatises composed outside England the Latin word probably refers to the asphodel. The source for the entry is unknown.

Identification with *Galium* is not sustained pharmacographically: the species is said to be antiherpetic (**2342**), stomachal (**2343**), hemostatic (**2344**), antirheumatic (**2345**), antipodagric (**2346**), antiaphthic (**2347**), antidysenteric (**2348**), anti-inflammatory of the throat (**2349**), but only the powers of against mouth diseases are recorded in a small part of the medical literature (*TH* and *GH*, which probably refer to some *Asphodelus* as indicated above).

> **Literature**: SWEET WOODRUFF (*Galium odoratum* (L.) Scop.): *OEH* 33 (*herba astularegia. wudurofe*), 53 (*herba malochinagria. wudurofe*); *Dur.Glos.* 300 (*apodillis. vude roue, bara popig | astula regia. vude roue, bare popig*), 303 (*malachin agria. vude rofe*), 304 (*ostricium. vude rofe*); *EPN* ii (*astula regia. wuderofe*), iv (*astula regia. baso, popig*), vi (*hastula regia. muget de bois. wuderove | astula regia. popi*), viii (*hec hastula. wodruffe*), ix (*hec artimatia. wodrofe*); *TH* 44 (*astula regia*); *Pand.* 17 (*affodillus, albutium, lappa, astula regia*); *Alph.* 16 (*asta regia. muget, woderowe*); *Sin.Bart.* 12, 23 (*astula regia. woderove*) 24 (*herba muscata*); *AC* 191.23 (*hastilogia. woderowe*) ❀ *GH* 41 (ASTULA REGIA, *woodroue*); *Tu* 2.738 (WOOD ROSE, *wood rowell, cordialis, asperula, spergula odorata*); *DL* 388 (WOODROW, *woodrowell, asperula, cordialis, herba stellaris, spergula odorata, iua muscata*); *Ge* 965 (WOODROOFFE, *woodrowe, woodrowell, asperula/aspergula odorata, cordialis, stellaria*). ¶ ASPHODEL (*Asphodelus* L. sp.): → affodill [**91**].

CS (DL, Ge)

2350 wermode. The entry describes the medical properties of wormwood (*Arthemisia absinthium* L.) as described in *DVH* 52–114 and translated in the *DVH(NME)* tradition. Identification is traditional and supported by textual and pharmacological evidence, although a substantial number of lines from the canonical edition of the Latin poem are missing (*DVH* 95–114), apparently due to an atelous exemplar, and the translation is noticeably less close to the original text than the rest of the entries from this family. Both texts agree in assuming that the species is stomachal (see next note), anthelminthic (**2357** = *DVH* 57–58), carminative, diuretic and emmenagogue (**2358** = *DVH* 58–60), anticteric (**2366** = *DVH* 73), and splenetic (→ **2367**), alexipharmic (**2368** = *DVH* 76–78, although the references to toadstools and hemlock are missing), ophthalmic and anticontusive (**2368** = *DVH* 79), anticatarrhal (→ **2370**), anti-inflammatory of the tonsils (**2373** = *DVH* 83–84), soporific (**2375** = *DVH* 91–82) and dyer (**2378** = *DVH* 93–94). The virtue of the species as an abortifacient (**2362**) looks like a very broad rendering of *DVH* 61–64 (which reprises the value of the plant as an emmenagogue), as seen from the common mention of wool in the recipe.

Apart from the missing lines at the end of the entry, the following qualities are not recorded in S_1: as an insect repellent (*DVH* 71–72; it seems dubious that *culices* "gnats, mosquitoes" corresponds to ‹nit*is*› **2373**, unless it is a copy mistake for *MIT*IS*), vulnerary (*DVH* 84), antiemetic (*DVH* 87–88) and against inguinal hernia (*DVH* 89–90). Conversely, the ME text offers a few virtues that are not in Choulant's edition and which may be due to interpolations in *Q*: cholagogue and phlegmagogue (**2358**), cardiac and hepatic (→ **2362**), and antiphtheiriac (**2373**). The English translation, moreover, greatly expands *DVH* 55–56 by providing not only the recipe, but also a detailed explanation on the ellaboration and the exact posology of the stomachal potion.

> **Literature**: WORMWOOD (*Arthemisia absinthium* L.): *HP* i.12.1 (ἀψίνθιον); *MM* iii.23; *NH* xxvii.45 (*absinthium*); *SM* xi.844; *RM* ii.199; *Grad.* 344; *OEH* 102 (*herba absinthius. wermod*); *Dur.Glos.* 299 (*absinthium. vermod*); *DVH* 52–114 (*absinthium*); *LS* 14 (*afsinthium* [أفسنتين *afsantyum*], *absinthium*); *EPN* iv (*absynthium. weremod*), v (*absíntium. wermod*), vi (*absinthium. aloigne. wermod*), vii (*hoc absinthium. wormode*), viii (*hoc absinthium. wormwod*); *CI* A.19 (*absinthium. warmot*); *TH* 22 (*absinthium*); *Pand.* 5 ($_{LA}$*absinthium,* $_{GR}$*absinthion,* $_{AR}$*saricom*); *DVH(NME)* 244v.19 (*wormode*); *DVH(SME)* 1b.33 (*wermode*); *Alph.* 1 (*absinthium, herba fortis*); *Sin.Bart.* 9 (*absintheum. wermode*); *AC* 160.6 (*absinthium. wyrmmod*) ⚘ *GH* 22 (ABSINTHIUM, *saxicon, wormwood*); *Fu* 1 (*ΑΨΙΝΘΙΟΝ, absinthium*); *Tu* 1.217 (*pontyke* WORMWODE, *absinthium, apsinthion);* DL 5 (WORMEWOOD, ἀψίνθιον, βαθύπικρον, βαρύπικρον, *absynthium*); Ge 936 (WORMEWOOD, ἀψίνθιον, *absinthium*).
>
> C^{1}S^1 (*LS*) | C^{1}S^2 (*DVH, CI*) | C^{1}S^3 (*SM, RM,* Fu, Tu, DL) | C^{2}S^2 (*TH, GH*) | C^{2}S^3 (Ge)

2350 stroyeth. Cf. *DVH* 53 *corroborat*, i.e. the exact opposite to the MS reading. Each MS from the tradition offers a different word here, which is an indication that *Ω* was either unclear here or else used a dialectal word that most scribes ignored. Only Wellcome offers the expected ‹strenthis›, while B.244v/20 ‹strehenys› looks like a botched attempt to reproduce verbatim an exemplary reading that may have been *STRE*N*THNYS, with a confusion **e** *pro* **t**, via an intermediate **c** *pro* **t**. Just like ‹stroyeth›, *P.*273/27 ‹streyneþ› seems a scribal conjecture.

2357 the wombe². This corresponds to *DVH* 58 *alvum*. Wellcome reads together with S_1, while the other witnesses offer B.244v/26 ‹vaynes› and *P.*274/5 ‹bodi›. The spelling of the Bodley scribe, who usually had no trouble with the word *WAME, suggests that *Ω* may have read *VAME here. The reading in Pepys is, just like → **2350**, a scribal conjecture.

2362 cerementayne spyknard and aloyne. While sermountain and spikenard are mentioned in *DVH* 65 and ‹aloyne› is a synonym for wormwood, the sense of this long sentence is different in the Latin and the English text. While the ME translation extols the potion as a cardiac and a hepatic, according to the original poem such drink will actually cleanse *noxia ... fastidia* (*DVH* 66), i.e. noxious squeamishness or nausea. The reference to the liver may stand for *DVH* 74 *curat epar*, although the place is somewhat unexpected unless some transposition of lines in *Q* is assumed.

2367 the mydryd. There seems to be no references to the diaphragm in the Latin chapter. The position of the virtue within the entry suggests that this corresponds to *DVH* 75, a passage praising the medical qualities of the plant as a splenetic. It is possible therefore that ⟨mydryd⟩ is in fact a copy mistake instead of Ω *MILTE. The same reading appears in *W* and *P*, which would indicate that the change was already complete in *RH*.

2370 þrow. The original reading has been emended since the two other MSS of the tradition that offer the passage (*W*.33r/4–5 and *P*.274/20–21) assume that ⟨the evill of the hede⟩ functions as complement of ⟨stoppid⟩ when translating *DVH* 81 *Decoctaeque vapor obstrusas liberat aures*. The "disease in the head" must therefore be a catarrh, that is, a copious discharge of humours from the brain that oppilates the ears. It is possible nevertheless that the Latin sentence was wrongly interpreted by the ME translator and that ⟨evill of the hede⟩ simply stands for *vapor*.

2379 wolde. The ME name refers to weld (*Reseda luteola* L.), which was better known in the Middle Ages as a source of yellow dye than as a medicinal plant (which goes to explain the sparse collection of references in the Literature section) although, according to Dioscorides, the species could be used as an emetic. In fact, the text is an abridged rendering of the chapter *asarum* (asarabacca, *Asarum europaeum* L.) in *DVH* 1532–1568 as translated in the *DVH(NME)* tradition. Identification is therefore based on textual and pharmacological criteria only, but it is very clear: cf. the medicinal value of the plant as a diuretic and emmenagogue (**2380** = *DVH* 1535), hysteric (**2381** = *DVH* 1538), anticteric and emetic, being softer than hellebore for the task (**2382** = *DVH* 1539–1542; → **2385** for the identification of ⟨walworte⟩). Missing from the ME account is a block of references to the species being a good hepatic, anthydropic and antisciatic (*DVH* 1536–1537). Most importantly, none of MSS holding a version of the entry keeps the long explanation on the posology according to age, disease, place and season which make up two-thirds of the Latin entry (*DVH* 1543–1568).

Other than the fact that both species were considered emetic, there seems to be no obvious reason why weld and asarabacca should be confused. There is yet a gloss "vulgago, anglice uod" in London, British Library, Sloane 282, 206v–210r, a Latin-ME synonyma apparently drawn from *DVH* (inc. "Hic tractat Macer de virtutibus diversarum herbarum"; quoted in PNME: *s.v.* asarab) which may be related to this equation.

Literature: ASARABACCA (*Asarum europaeum* L.): MM i.10 (ἄσαρον); NH xxi.29–30 (*baccar*); SM xi.840; RM ii.197; Grad. 369 (*asarum*); DVH 1532–1568; LS 244 (*asaron* [أسارون] *asārūn*], *asarum, nardum agreste*); CI A.32 (*assarum*); TH 46 (*asara, bachira*); Pand. 14 (_{AR}*aerma, aerba*, _{GR}*assarum,* _{LA}*bachara, nardus agrestis*); DVH(NME) 254v.13 (*wald*); DVH(SME) 30a.9 (*softe, moleyn*); Alph. 15 (*Asarabacca, uuluago, gariofilata agrestis*), 16 (*asarus*), 19 (*baccara*), 106 (*matricaria aquatica*), 192 (*uulgago*); Sin. Bart. 11 (*asara baccara, gariofilus agrestis*), 30 (*milvago*) ✽ GH 43 (ASARA, *asarium, brathea, vulgago, asarabaca*); Fu 3 (*ΑΣΑΡΟΝ, asarum*); Tu 1.244 (FOLLFOTE, *asarabacca, asarum, asaron*); DL 230 (ASARABACCA, *folefoot, haselwurt,* ἄσαρον, *asarum, nardus rustica, perpensa, vulgago*); Ge 688 (ASTRABACCA, *folefoote, hasell woort,* ἄσαρον, αἷμα ἄρεως, *asarum, nardus rustica, perpensa, vulgago*). ¶ WELD (*Reseda luteola* L.): HP ix.9.2 (σησαμοειδὴς τὸ μέγα); MM iv.149; NH xxii.133 (*sesamoides*); SM xii.120; RM ii.258 ✽ DL 49 (DIERS-WEED, *herba lutea, flos tinctorius*); Ge 398 (DIERS WEED, *welde, lutea*).

CS (Tu, Ge) | C³S³ (DVH, LS, CI, TH, GH, Fu, DL)

2385 walworte. The ME name is a synonym of danewort, *Sambucus ebulus* L., (and in, some late ME textual traditions such as *AC*, it can also refer to the elder, *Sambucus nigra* L.; some Renaissance authors followed *MM* and treated both as separate kinds of the same species, cf. Tu$_{2.554}$), but the reference to a "white" and a "black" plant makes clear that the entry is in fact a combination of the chapters in *DVH* devoted to the black and white hellebores (*Helleborus niger* L. and *Veratrum album* L., respectively) as translated in the *DVH(NME)* textual tradition. These species had been previously treated in the ME text (→ **1224**, with discussion, and **1851**, where the plant described was actually a buttercup). Here too the common use of the *Sambucus* and the *Veratrum/Hellebore* as a very powerful purgative is probably behind the confusion of species. Note that the equation *helleborus = walworte* was also made in the previous entry (**2383**).

In comparison to the previous translation of the chapters on *hellebori* in *DVH*, this version is fuller, as it contains not only the same abortifacient, apophlegmatic, ophthalmic, rodenticide and muscicide virtues of the white species and the acoustic, leprostatic and antiodontalgic powers of the black species, but also translates the long fragment that was missing there, cf. its value as an emetic (**2394** = *DVH* 1786–1787), antimanic (**2395, 2407** = *DVH* 1789–1790, 1836–1837), anthydropic (**2396, 2413** = *DVH* 1791, 1838–1839), antimelancholic and antiepileptic (**2396** = *DVH* 1789–1790), leprostatic (**2397, 2416** = *DVH* 1792, 1852–1853), carminative (**2398** = *DVH* 1793), antipodagric and febrifuge (**2408** = *DVH* 1837–1838), antiparalytic (**2409** = *DVH* 1839), chola- and phlegmagogue (**2411** = *DVH* 1841), ophthalmic (**2411** = *DVH* 1842), emmenagogue, abortifacient and acoustic (**2414–2415** = *DVH* 1849–1851), antiodontalgic (**2417** = *DVH* 1854–1855). The discussion on the correct posology of the *Veratrum* (*DVH* 1798–1832) is maintained here, but severely abridged and stripped of the references to the works of *auctoritates* (**2398–2401** = *DVH* 1797–1832). The short final remark on the posology of the black hellebore is given in full (**2417** = *DVH* 1856–1858). Only a few of the many medical virtues of these species were left out from the account: as an antidinic (*DVH* 1788), antitetanic (*DVH* 1792), spasmolytic (*DVH* 1793), antisciatic (*DVH* 1794), antarthritic (*DVH* 1840) and antipernius (*DVH* 1843–1846). On the other hand, the ME text contains a recipe that is not in the canonical version of *DVH* (→ **2401**).

> **Literature**: BLACK & WHITE HELLEBORES (*Helleborus niger* L., *Veratrum album* L.):→ longwort [**1224**], → pedelyon [**1851**]. ¶ DANEWORT (*Sambucus ebulus* L.): MM iv.173.2 (χαμαιάκτη); NH xxiv.51 (*chamaeacte*); SM xi.820; RM ii.190; OEH xxix (*herba ostriago. liðwyrt*), xciii (*herba ebulus. wealwyrt*), cxxvii (*herba erifion. lyþwyrt*); Dur. Glos. 302 (*ebule, eobulum. veal vyrt, ellenvyrt | erifeon. lith vyrt*), 304 (*ostriago. lith vyrt*); LS 274 (*kameacti, sambucus*); EPN ii (*ebulum. wal-wyrt*), iv (*eripheon. lið-wyrt | ebolum. ellen-wyrt | ostriago. liþ-wyrt*), vi (*ebulum. eble. wal-wurt | ostragium. herbyve. liþe-wurt*), viii (*hic ebolus. wal-wortte*), ix (*hec ebula. a walle-wurte*); Cl 300 (*ebulus. walwort*); TH 171 (*ebulus*); Pand. 374 (₍ₐᵣ₎*kameactis, iacta*, ₍GR₎*meation*, ₍LA₎*ebulus*); AC 185.23 (*ebullus minor. lesse walwourt*) ⚜ GH 162 (EBULUS, *walworde, cameatus*); Fu 20 (᾿ΑΚΤΗ ... χαμαιάκτη, *humilis sambucus, ebulus*); Tu 1.307 (WALWURT, *danewurt, chameacte, ebulus*); DL 274 (WALWORT, *danewort, bloodwort,* χαμαιάκτη, *ebulus*); Ge 1237 (DANEWOORT, *wall-wort, dwarfe elder,* χαμαιάκτη, *ebulus*). ¶ ELDER (*Sambucus nigra* L.): HP i.5.4 (ἀκτή); MM iv.173; NH xxiv.51 (*sambucus*); SM xi.820 (ἀκτή μεγάλη); RM ii.190; Grad. 361; OEH 148 (*herba samsuchon. ellen*); Dur.Glos. 305 (*samsuchon. ellen, cinges-vyrt*); LS 274 (*iaphacti* [ايفاقي] *rafagā'*], *sambucus*); EPN iii (*sambucus. ellen*), iv (*actis, sambucus. ellen*), vi (*sambucus. suev, ellarne*); Cl s.5 (*sambucus. elarun*); TH 453 (*sanbucus*); Alph. 161 (*sambucus. ellen*); Sin.Bart. 37 (*sambucus, hellarne*); AC p. 153.1 (*ebulus. walwort*) ⚜ GH 412 (SAMBUCUS, *eldre*); Fu 20 (᾿ΑΚΤΗ, *sambucus*); Tu 2.554 (ELDER TREE, *walworte, daynwurt, elder, bourtre, sambucus, acte*); DL 273 (ELDER, *bourtree,* ἀκτή, *sambucus*); Ge 1233 (ELDER TREE, ἀκτή, *sambucus*).

2390 with juis of celydonum and rew. This renders *DVH* 1782 *confecturis quae lumina purgat* in a very free way. Celandine was of course renowned as a powerful ophthalmic (→ **322**), but the reference to rue is somewhat unexpected, if only because the benefits of this species to the eyes were never mentioned in the ME translation (→ **1947**). The ophthalmic value of the plant is recorded in *DVH* 285–288, and can already be found in *MM* iii.45, § 3 (ἔστι δὲ καὶ ὀξυωπὲς ἐσθιόμενον ὠμὸν καὶ ταριχευτὸν καὶ τὰς ἐν ὀφθαλμοῖς περιωδυνίας σὺν ἀλφίτοις καταπλασθὲν πραΰνει, "[e]aten either raw or preserved, it sharpens the vision, it assuages severe eye pains when applied as a plaster with barley groats") or *LS* 290 ("quando fit emplastrum ex ea cum sauich super oculum sedat dolorem eius"), but the excerpt that made rue so commendable to cure ailments in the eyes is probably *NH* xx.134:

> Pythagoras [...] oculis noxiam putavit, falsum, quoniam sculptores et pictores hoc cibo utuntur oculorum causa cum pane vel nasturtio, caprae quoque silvestres propter visum, ut aiunt. multi suco eius cum melle Attico inuncti discusserunt caligines vel cum lacte mulieris puerum enixae vel puro suco angulis oculorum tactis.

2393 wekyd humeris. The correct translation of *DVH* 1786–1787 *varios ... humores* is only found in *B*.255v/9 ‹dyuers homaurs›. The Wellcome version conveys the same idea as S_1, cf. *W*.36v/28–37r/1 ‹ill humours›. Ω might have read *DYWERCE HUMO(U)RS, perhaps curtailed to something similar to *WERCE in *RH* (unfortunately the word is missing in *P*, probably because the exemplary reading made no sense to the scribe of π), which must have been conjectured into *WEKYD in γ.

2395 at... 2397 lepir. The syntax of the passage is odd and it must have been like that already in *RH*, for S_1 reads together with *W*.37r/2–4 and *P*.283/22–24. On the other hand, *B* presents the information in a much neater way by continuing the previous sentence rather than beginning a new one and offering a different arrangement for the diseases: *B*.255v/10–11 ‹helpis þame þat ere wode & to þe falland euyll & to þe ydrope & clencis þe lepir›. Comparison with *DVH* 1789–1792 indicates that Bodley is closest to the original poem:

> Insanis, melancholicis valet atque caducis,
> Saepeque curatur sumpto lymphaticus isto.
> Hydropicis in principio mire medicatur,
> Emundat lepram.

But while the order of the diseases is correct in *B*, this version does not keep all the information provided by the original, as it is obvious that the references of melancholy and early stages of dropsy must have been also in Ω. The mention to the "lymphatic" (i.e. one suffering from an excess of watery substances, which was believed to cause frenzy) seems to have been skipped in the original translation, perhaps because *insanis* already conveyed a similar idea.

2398 Ypocras and Plenyus comaundith. The sentence is an extremely abridged version of the last lines of the chapter on white hellebore (*DVH* 1807–1832), which explain the correct posology of the species in a detailed way. The Hippocratic quotation (*DVH* 1814–1815) paraphrases either *Aphorisms* iv.14 or iv.15: ἐπὴν πίῃ τις ἐλλέβορον, πρὸς μὲν τὰς κινήσιας τῶν σωμάτων μᾶλλον ἄγειν, πρὸς δὲ τοὺς ὕπνους καὶ μὴ κινήσιας, ἧσσον ("when one takes a draught of hellebore one should be made to move more about, and indulge less in sleep and repose"); ἐπὴν βούλῃ μᾶλλον ἄγειν τὸν ἐλλέβορον, κίνει τὸ σῶμα· ἐπὴν δὲ παῦσαι, ὕπνον ποίει, καὶ μὴ κίνει ("when you wish the hellebore to act more, move the body, and when to stop, let the patient get sleep and rest"; translated in Adams 1849: ii.725). The reference to Pliny (*DVH* 1825–1828; repeated at *DVH* 1856–1858) derives from *NH* xxv.58: "Themison binas, non amplius, drachmas datavit; sequentes et quaternas dedere claro Herophili praeconio, qui helleborum fortissimi ducis similitudini aequabat". The same posology is recommended in the description of black hellebore (→ **2417**), even though the original weights are different in each case.

2401 the levis sodyn in watir. This recipe is neither in the canonical version of *DVH* nor in any medieval tradition that I know of. While all three MSS from the *RH* branch read alike (other than the usual minor dialectal changes), Bodley mentions nothing about a bath but after the ingredients it offers ⟨& done to both þe naturs of þe erbe⟩ instead, which looks like a *lectio facilior* due to a corrupt passage in α, since the authorial word to translate Latin *species in this textual tradition was not *NATURS but *MANER(I)S, as seen from **322, 335, 905, 1355, 1685, 2385** and **2431**. (The only noted exception is ⟨kyndis⟩ in **561**, but this is a scribal change in the ΛS_1 branch, as demonstrated by *BWP* ⟨man*er*s⟩.) As seen from the readings in *W* and *P*—which, just like *B*, offer ⟨don⟩ instead of ⟨i-put⟩ (turning *DO into *put* is a regular feature of S_1, see for instance **11, 16, 167, 200, 352, 1379**, etc.)—Ω must have read *DON IN BATH, which the scribe of the α*B* branch must have mistaken as *bāth.

2406 also mekyll. Although S_1 reads together with $W.37r/11$ ⟨als mikil⟩ here, all medieval *auctoritates* agreed that the effects of eating black hellebore, a laxative, were less dangerous than those derived from the ingestion of the white counterpart, an emetic. Macer Floridus of course was no exception and *DVH* 1833–1834 stated that *Elleborum nigrum non est adeo violentum, / Nec formidandum quantum quod diximus album*. The other two MSS do offer the expected reading, cf. *B*.255v/17 ⟨not so miche⟩, *P*.284/7 ⟨nouȝt so myche⟩, hence the error must have originated in γ.

2409 all...2410 humeris. This corresponds to *DVH* 1840 *Et varios bibitum morbos levat articulorum*. The fragment is missing in *B* but—other than ⟨all⟩, which seems authorial to translate *varios*—is recorded also in *W* and *P*, which suggests that the passage was already in Ω, perhaps in some corrupt form.

2411 blacke colour. A translation mistake, already present in Ω since it is common to all MSS, of *DVH* 1841 *choleras varias*, i.e. both yellow and black bile—unless *Q* read *NIGRAS.

2417 Plenius... 2418 biddith. This sentence translates *DVH* 1856–1858 and derives ultimately from *NH* xxv.54: "datur ad leniter molliendam alvum plurimum drachma una". Note that in → **2398** the same posology was suggested for white hellebore even though Pliny recommended half the dosage, *Veratrum album* being stronger and more dangerous than *Helleborus niger*.

2420 wylwe. Notwithstanding the headword, which would seem to refer to the willow, comparison with *DVH* shows that this is an account of the medicinal properties of the marshmallow (*Althaea officinalis* L.) as rendered in the *DVH(NME)* textual tradition (→ **849** for another, less informative description of the same species that provides different virtues, and → **1290** for the wild species). Ω must have read *WYMAWE, the Anglo-Norman spelling parallel to Francien *guimauve*. This is still kept, albeit faultily, in *W*.39v/17 ⟨wyniwe⟩. A change **ll** pro **w** is probably behind *B*.250r/5 ⟨wymalle⟩, which should be construed as a clue that α was copied in an Anglicana hand or else derived from an exemplar in that script. The form in S_1 would be a mere *lectio facilior*. Alternatively, Ω could have read *WYMALWE, whence the reading in *B* through simplification of **lw** into **ll**, a change which may have been strictly graphical (if the exemplar was misread by the scribe as *lll) or dialectal (it is surely not amiss to mention here that *mall* is a Northern word for "mallow", see EDD: *s.v.* maul *n.*⁷). S_1 would again be explained as a *lectio facilior*, while for *W* we must assume dropping of **l**.

A careful reading of the ME entry and the original poem strongly suggests that many lines of the Latin chapter in *Q*, mostly in its first half, must have been corrupt or else substantially edited, for several of the medical powers of the plant are mistraslated or rendered in a distorted way. Even so, identification with the marshmallow seems secure on textual and pharmacographic grounds, as the species is deemed to be antiseptic (see next note), relaxant (→ **2424**), anti-inflammatory (**2424** = *DVH* 379), antidysenteric (**2426** = *DVH* 382–383), mazolytic (→ **2426**), anticholecystic (**2427** = *DVH* 386), antiacne (**2429** = *DVH* 387–388), and antipyrotic (**2430** = *DVH* 393–394). Missing from the account are the purported values of the plant as antiscrofulous, analgesic and anticontusive for the rectum (yet → **2420**), anthemoptyic and lithontriptic (*DVH* 385), and vulnerary (*DVH* 390–391). The value of the plant as an emollient and against animal bites (*DVH* 392, 394) was kept in α, cf. *B*.250r/13–14 ⟨it &

hony to-ged*er* swag*is* & neschys þe hardnes & þe leyues sodyne in oill helys brymmynge & euyll bytt*is*›, but went missing in γ—although the word ‹to-ged*er*›, which is an obvious remnant of the authorial text, was added after ‹oil› in *W*.39v/27.

Literature: MARSHMALLOW (*Althaea officinialis* L.): → holyhok [**849**]. ¶ WILLOWS (*Salix* L. spp.): → wythi [**2511**].

2420 the rote sodyn wiþ wyn. According to *DVH* 371, the vulnerary powers of the species were in the flowers, rather than in its root. There is yet a reference to the roots only two lines above, where they are compared to the mistletoe, and this must have confused the translator.

The idea of boiling the root in wine is not found in the canonical version of *DVH*. The corresponding passage (*DVH* 372–374) deals with the powers of the plant against scrofula and pain in the rectum, but there are some clues that allow to assume that the ME fragment does correspond (albeit just partially) to those Latin lines. There are references to wine and the crushing of the ingredient (cf. *DVH* 372 *cum vino tritum*), and the word ‹akynge› may stand for *DVH* 373 *dolentem*. Concerning ‹womanys pappe› (and *W*.39v/18 ‹woman*is* pappe›), which opposes *B*.250r/6 ‹woma*n*s shape› and stands for *DVH* 374 *anumque*, → **1718**. Finally, the appearance of ‹brenynge› can be explained as a copy mistake for Ω *BRISYNGE to translate *DVH* 374 *conquassatis* (→ **1636** for another instance of the same).

2423 anoynte ham. Dialectal choices aside, both *W* and S_1 offer here the same sentence, which stands for *DVH* 375–377 but is syntactically odd: one would expect the singular noun ‹mawe› to appear before, rather than after, the plural pronoun ‹ham› that obviously refers to it. As stated in the previous note, this part of the entry must have been corrupt in *Q* or somehow unclear to the scribes. Bodley provides a solution that does not maintain faithfully the original reading, since it includes dislodging *BRISYNGE from its original place, but at least makes sense and moreover keeps the word *SMERE (translated as ‹gresse› in this copy and which stands for *DVH* 375 *adipique*), which was interpreted as a verb in γ: *B*.250r/7–8 ‹þe rott stampit & sothen is gud for brymmynge and it mengid w*ith* gresse helys all bolnynge of þe matr*ice*›.

The word ‹mawe› later in the line is a bit unexpected insofar as it translates *DVH* 377 *matricis*, for in this textual tradition the word *SCHAPE was used for the purpose (see **20, 1324, 1954, 1966, 1972, 2060, 2073**). The parallel readings in the other MSS (‹matrice› in Bodley as already mentioned, and *W*.39v/21 ‹mat*er*›) indicate that Ω must have offered the synonym *MATR*I*S here, which in S_1 is normally rendered as ‹matrice› (see **800, 1669**).

2424 makiþ syneous harde. The Latin text (*DVH* 378) states the exact opposite: *nervos sic ipsa relaxat*. The mistranslation goes back to Ω.

2426 longe… 2427 holdyn. This translates *DVH* 384 *tardas*, which belongs to the line where the properties to expel the placenta are described. Either the translator blended this with *DVH* 383, which is in fact an expansion on the antidysenteric qualities of the plant, or else the missing words were not copied in either *Q* or Ω. The second possibility in particular would explain why the whole passage was dropped in the Bodley version: perhaps α was already nonsensical.

2431 verveyn. This is a translation of the plant *verbena* (*DVH* 1859–1902) as given in the *DVH(NME)* textual tradition. The chapter mentions two species, diversely referred to in pre-Linnaean botanical literature as *mas* or *recta*, and *foemina* or *supina*. Ge translated these names as *vpright* and *creeping veruaine*, respectively. Such distinction was mainly based on the absence or presence of basal leaves. The male or upright species, judging from the Renaissance woodcuts provided by Fu and Ge, must be the hedge mustard (*Sisymbrium officinale* (L.) Scop.), while the female or creeping species is the vervain (*Verbena officinalis* L.).

Identification of the species is traditional and assured on textual and pharmacological grounds, as seen by its perceived value as an anticteric (**2432** = *DVH* 1862), vulnerary, and particularly antiaphthic (**2434** = *DVH* 1865–1866), prognostic (**2439** = *DVH* 1881–1883), anticephalalgic (**2442** = *DVH* 1884–1886), splanchnic (**2444** = *DVH* 1888–1890), lithontriptic and febrifuge (**2448** = *DVH* 1895, 1900). The plant was particularly renowned as an alexipharmic and exhilarant since Classical times, hence the several references to these virtues in the entry (**2433, 2436** = *DVH* 1863–1865, 1871; and **2437, 2446** = *DVH* 1878–1880, 1899, respectively). The second mention to the species as a consolidative, in particular to cure slit veins (**2449**), is not in the Latin poem and looks like an addition by the translator. Missing from the translation are the references to the species as anticaries (*DVH* 1867–1868), antimalarial (*DVH* 1872–1877), and antiphthisic (*DVH* 1890) and antiparotiditic (*DVH* 1891).

Literature: Vervain/hedge mustard (*Verbena officinalis* L./*Sisymbrium officinale* (L.) Scop.): *MM* iv.60 (ἱερὰ βοτάνη); *NH* xxv.105 (*hiera botane, aristereon, verbenaca*); *SM* xii.98 (περιστερεών); *RM* ii.251; *OEH* 4 (*herba uermenaca. æscþrotu*); *Dur.Glos.* 305 (*vervena. berbena*); *DVH* 1859–1902 (*verbena, ierobotanum, peristereon*); *EPN* ii (*gerobonana, verbena, sagmen. biscop-wyrtil*), vi (*vervena. verveine. iren-harde*), vii (*hec vervena. warwayn*), viii (*hec verveta. a verveyn*), ix (*hec vervene. vermyne*); *TH* 75 (*berbena*); *Pand.* 282 (_GR_*gerebotanium, ierobotanum, peristereon*, _AR_*albea*, _LA_*herbena, sacra herba*); *DVH(NME)* 256r.2 (*veruayne*); *DVH(SME)* 34b.5 (*verveyne. ierobatanum,* *peristerion*); *Alph.* 43 (*columbaria, peristereon, uerbena. fleguurt*), 74 (*gerabotonum, peristerion, uerbena.* ᴳᴬ*ueruayne,* ᴬᴺ*flegheuurt*), 190 (*ierobotonon, bona herba ueneris idem.* ᴳᴬ*uerueyne,* ᴬᴺ*fleghewrt*) ⚜ GH 473 (UERBENA, *sacra herba, centrum galli, gallinatica*); Fu 225 (ΠΕΡΙΣΤΕΡΕΩΝ, ἱερὰ βοτάνη, *verbenaca, verbena, columbaris, columbina, herba sagminalis*); Tu 2.595 (VERVINE, *peristereon, hierobatone, verbena, verbenaca*); DL 88 (VERVAINE, περιστερεών ὀρθίος, *verbenaca columbina recta, columbaris, herba sanguinalis, crista gallinacea, exupera, feria, ferraria, trixago, verbena recta*); Ge 580 (VERUAINE, περιστερεών, *verbena, verbenaca, herculania, ferraria, exupera, matricalis, hierabotane, sacra herba, sagmina*).

s (SM, RM, GH, Fu, DL, Ge)

2437 pepill that fastith. The original translation in Ω was demonstrably misunderstood and altered in all the extant MSS of the tradition. See Moreno 2017: 684–685 for further details.

2439 aske howe he faryth. While the passage maintains the same idea as the original Latin lines (*DVH* 1881–1883), the story has been substantially redacted (and dramatically enhanced, note for instance the usage of ‹trewly› and ‹withoute doute›) in *ΛS*₁, cf. *B*.256r/9–10 ‹if he say wall [*W*39r/09 ‹wele›] he shall varys & if he say euyll [*W*39r/10 ‹il›] he sal dye›.

2442 Plenius comaundiþ. This translates *DVH* 1887–1890, which ultimately derives from *NH* xxvi.37: "verbenaca vero omnibus visceribus medetur, lateribus, pulmonibus, iocineribus, thoraci". The position of ‹gisser› (= La. *iocineribus*) has been altered in relation to Pliny's original text due to metrical reasons in Macer Floridus's poem:

> Plinius affirmat hanc omnibus esse salubrem
> Visceribus, lateris morbis, iecorisque querelis,
> Pectoris et viciis [...].

2446 all folke shall loue the. As with a previous note on prognostics, this passage was rephrased in either *Λ* or *S*₁, cf. *B*.256r/14 ‹it shall make 30*ur* frenschype›, *W*.39r/25 ‹ʒif þ*u* will haue lofredene›. The reference to ‹loue› in *S*₁ may be an indication that Wellcome maintains the authorial reading, which may have been Ω *LOFREDEN (< OE *luf-rǣden*). Other than that, the virtue (*DVH* 1899, drawing from an idea already found in *MM*) is misplaced within the entry, as this should appear after, rather than before the lithontriptic qualities of the plant (*DVH* 1892–1895).

2453 watyr-cars. Since there is no physical description of the species, identification of the Latin headword and the ME name with watercress (*Nasturtium officinale* R.Br. = *Rorippa nasturtium-aquaticum* (L.) Hayek) is traditional. Textually, the pedigree of the entry remains untraced.

From a medical viewpoint, the species is described as antihemorrhoidal (**2454**), antiulcerous (**2458**), anti-inflammatory (**2460**), antiasthmatic (**2463**), and lithontriptic (**2467**). The stone-breaking powers are found in a few sources since Galen, but the rest is unknown in the usual medical literature.

Literature: WATERCRESS (*Nasturtium officinale* R.Br.): *MM* ii.128 (σισύμβριον); *NH* xx.247 (*sisymbrium silvestre*); *SM* xii.124; *RM* ii.259; *Grad.* 384 (*nasturcium*); *OEH* 21 (*herba nasturcium. cærse*); *Dur.Glos.* 304 (*nasturcium. vilde cerse*); *EPN* ii (*nasturtium. tun-kerse*), iii (*nasturcium. leac-cersan, tun-c.*), iv (*nasturtium. tun-cærse*), vi (*nasturtium. kersuns, cressens*), vii (*hoc nausticium. water-kyrs*); *Cl* N.1 (*nasturcium. carces*); *TH* 327 (*nasturcium*); *Pand.* 352 (₄ᵣ*herochalchay, saxabram*, ₆ᵣ*camelea, senition, hirigontis*, ₗₐ*senatio, apium aque, nasturcium aquaticum*); *Alph.* 122 (*narstucium aquaticum*), 165 (*senacio, narstucium aquaticum idem.* ₆ₐ*crissouns ewages*, ₐₙ*watercresses*); *Sin.Bart.* 17 (*cresso. nasturcium aquaticum*), 31 (*nasturcium aquaticum* [...] *cresso ovis, senacio ovis*); , *AC* 209.12 (*nascorium aquaticum. water cresse*) ⚜ *GH* 303 (NASTURCIUM [...] *water cresses*); *Fu* 275 (ΣΙΣΥΜΒΡΙΟΝ, *cardamine, nasturtium aquaticum*); *Tu* 2.575 (*sisimbrium, the second kind, cardamine, water cresses*); *DL* 448 (WATER CRESSES/*kars, nasturtium aquaticum*); *Ge* 199 (WATER/*browne* CRESSES, *sium, sysymbrium aquaticum*).

CS (Ge) | C¹S³ (Fu) | C²S² (Tu, DL) | C³S³ (SM, RM) | C⁴S⁴ (Grad., Cl, TH, GH)

2469 wodesoure. The Latin and ME names, together with the physical description, make it clear that the plant treated must be wood sorrel (*Oxalis acetosella* L.). Textually, the entry is a composite: the first virtue (up to the end of **2474**) belongs to the *AC* tradition, but from that line onwards the source is unknown.

The plant is praised pharmacographically as the main component in remedies for diseases that involve skin hypertrophy: exfoliant (**2474**), anticallus (**2475**), and antipernius (**2481**). Such powers are not found in the usual literature. Note as well that the temperament stated in the chapter is also at odds with the one suggested in the Renaissance herbals.

Literature: WOOD SORREL (*Oxalis acetosella* L.): *NH* xxvii.112 (*oxys*); *Dur.Glos.* 299 (*acitulium. geaces sure*), 300 (*calciculium. geacessure*), 305 (*trifolium siluaticum. eaces sure*); *EPN* ii (*trifolium. geaces-sure, pri-lefe*), iii (*accitulium. iaces-sure*), iv (*calcilum. iaces sure*); *TH* 54 (*alleluia, pane de cuccho*); *Alph.* 5 (*alleluia, panis cuculi, trifolium siluestre. wodesoure*); *Sin.Bart.* 10 (*alleluia. wodesour*), 33 (*panis cuculi, alleluia*); *AC* 163.30 (*alleluya. wodesowr, stopwourt*) ⚜ *GH* 50 (ALLELUYA, *wood sorell, cukowes meate*); *Tu* 2.482 (OXYS, *alleluya, wodsore, wod sour, sorell*); *Fu* 212 (ΟΞΥΣ, *trifolium acetosum, alleluya, panis cuculi*); *DL* 361 (WOOD SORRELL, *sorrell de boys, cuckowes meat, sower trifoile, stubwoort, woodsower,* ὀξύς, *aleluya, trifolium acetosum, panis cuculi, alimonia*); *Ge* 1030 (WOOD SORRELL, *stubwoort, woode sower, sower trefoile, sorrell du bois, trifolium acetosum, alleluya, panis cuculi*).

FS (Fu, DL, Ge)

2470 stokwort oþer sorell de boys oþer cokkowe-brede. The first synonym probably answers to a scribal mistake instead of *s t o b w o r t, as seen from "stopwourt" in *AC* and the headwords in MED (*s.v.* stub-wort) and OED (*s.vv.* stubwort, stobwort), but it has yet been left uncorrected since *stok* also means "stump" (*s.v.* stok *n.*¹) and hence could be regarded as a valid synonym. OED also recorded the variant *stabwort* (*s.v.* stab *n.*¹, § 5: "a wound produced by stabbing"), quoting John Parkinson's 1640 *Theatrum Botanicum* and Robert Lovell's 1665 Παμβοτανολογία as authorities, but this is surely connected with stab *n.*² ("stump"), which is a variant of northern *stob* (< ON *stabbi*, the *o*-grade of the same Germanic root whence also OE *stubb*). The explanation provided there ("believed to be so called with reference to its supposed healing properties") is therefore to be discarded—even though the plant appears in several sources as a vulnerary (particularly antiaphthic). As regards ‹cokkowe-brede›, a transcription mistake in *WG* has meant the inclusion of the ghost word *cŏkkŏu hed* in MED (s.v. cokkŏu, cŏkkŏu n., § 3).

2484 wodebynd. The Latin headword and the ME names are traditionally associated with both woodbine (*Lonicera periclymenum* L.) and perfoliate honeysuckle (*L. caprifolium* L.). Lack of a physical description makes species identification impossible, but one could argue that the plant must be the former since the latter is a Mediterranean species while the other is pan-European (cf. Gerard's remark that "[t]he double Honisuckle [i.e., *L. caprifolium*] groweth now in my garden, and many others likewise in great plenty, although not long since, [it was] very rare and hard to be found, except in the garden of some diligent herbarist"). The species had been confused with wild chervil (*Anthriscus sylvestris* (L.) Hoffm.) earlier in the treatise (→ **2137**). The entry belongs to the same tradition as *AC* up to **2486**, then another, unknown textual family is followed.

Pharmacographically, the plant is described as anticancerous and maturative (**2485**), antiodontalgic and antiulcerous (**2486**), alexipharmic (against bees and wasps; **2487**), and hematogogue (**2488**). None of these are found in the usual medical literature of the period.

Literature: WOODBINE (*Lonicera periclymenum* L.): *HP* ix.8.5 (κλύμενον); *MM* iv.14 (περικλύμενον); *NH* xxv.70 (*clymenon*), xxvii.120 (*periclymenon*); *SM* xii.98; *RM* ii.251; *Dur.Glos.* 301 (*caprifolium. vudebinde*); *EPN* ii (*viticella. wiðwinde* | *hedera nigra. wudebinde*), iv (*viticella. weodu-binde*), vi (*mater silva. chevefoil. wudebinde*); *TH* 316 (*matrisilva, periclimeno*); *Pand.* 135 (LA*caprifolium, mater siluarum,* AR*grimath, periclimenon,* GR*periclemon, liceos, exacanton*), 522 (LA*matrissilua, caprifolium,* GR*splemon, splenon, splenaria, linealis, periclimenos*); *DVH(SME)* 26b.25 (*wodebynde. caprifolium, ligusticum*); *Alph.* 29 (*caprifolium, oculus lucii, perichenon, mater* *siluana, uolubilis maior. wodebynde, honisocles*); *Sin.Bart*. 17 (*corrigiola maior, caprifolium. wodebinde*), 43 (*volubilis, caprifolium, mater silvarum, oculus licii*); *AC* 177.7 (*caprifolium. wodebynde*) ❧ *GH* 140 (CAPRIFOLIUM, *daprificus, matrisilua, orialum, woodbynde*); Fu 249 (*ΠΕΡΙΚΛΥΜΕΝΟΝ, volucrum maius, syluæ mater, caprifolium, matersylua, lilium inter spinas*); Tu 2.493 (WODBYNDE, *periclymenon, matrisylva, honysuckle*); DL 282 (WOODBINE, *honisuckle, caprifolie,* περικλύμενον, αἰγίνη, κάρπαθον, σπλήνιον, ἐπαιτίτις, κλεματίτις, καλυκάνθεμον, *volucrum maius, periclymenum, syluæ mater, caprifolium, mater sylua, lilium inter spinas*); Ge 743 (WOODBINDE, *honisuckle, caprifoly,* περικλύμενον, *volucrum maius, syluamater, caprifolium, matrisylus, lilium inter spinas*).

CS (*SM, RM, TH,* Fu, Ge) | C³S³ (DL)

2490 wolfe-ys þistill. According to the words used to refer to the plant, the entry must describe a thistle or thistle-like plant of dubious identification, but apparently not the carline thistle (*Carlina acaulis* L.; *contra* DEPN: 498 and OED: *s.v.* wolf *n.*, § 11.f), since that plant bears yellow flowers. A distinction between white and black chameleons (Gk. χαμαιλέων λευκός/μέλας, La. *chamaeleon candidus/niger*) was customary in Classical pharmacography since Theophrastus. The white one is traditionally identified with the pine thistle (*Carlina gummifera* (L.) Less. = *Atractylis gummifera* L.), while the black counterpart is thought to be the black chameleon (*Cardopatium corymbosum* (L.) Pers.; André 1985: *s.v.* chamaeleōn). Judging from the available evidence in the Literature section—*contra* Bierbaumer 1975–1979: i.148, ii.135, iii.268–269, who only accepts wild teasel (*Dipsacus fullonum* L. = *Dipsacus sylvestris* Huds., *Dipsacus silvester* A.Kern.) as candidate for both; the same is valid for PNME: *s.v.* cameleon—the same opposition seems to have been maintained in OE, so that *wulfes camb* must equate *chamaeleon niger*, if only because the *candidus/albus* version was referred to either by employing a different name (*wulfes tæsl*) or else by adding an adjective to the general name (*se brāda wulfes camb*). This idea is reinforced also by the sentence "[a]lba d*icitu*r cameleon alba, nigra d*icitu*r cameleon" in *Pand.*, the synonyms in *GH*, and by the woodcuts of the chapter *Chamæleon thistle* in Ge, which seem to depict *Cardopatium corymbosum* (L.) Pers. (called *Chamæleon niger/The blacke chamæleon thistle*) and *Picnomon acarna* (L.) Cass. (called *Chamæleon niger Salmaticensis/The Spanish blacke chamæleon*). The problem with this identification is that the flower of the species is blue, rather than red.

Brodin suggested Scotch thistle (*Onopordum acanthium* L.) for the plant described in *AC*, which served as source text for the entry in *LH*, but identification with that species is not firmly sustained. The description in that treatise is certainly fuller than the one offered here, as it states that the plant bears "quyte lewys grete & brode" and grows "by weyes", but these remarks could also apply to the *Carlina* (assuming that the purple colour of its inflorescences is called ‹rede›, as was the rule in ME, see MED: s.v. rēd *a*., § 1a), and indeed to a large number of species from the Carduoideae subfamily (*Cirsium heterophyllum* (L.) Hill, *Cynara cardunculus* L., or *Carduus tenuiflorus* Curtis, to mention a few). While this carries but little weight by itself, the fact that *Onopordum* was as a rule called ἀκάνθιον/ *acanthium* in the medico-botanical literature (see Fu$_{54}$, DL$_{378}$, Ge$_{987}$) is against such identification as well.

The entry is also problematic from a pharmacographic point of view, since it provides no proper medical use for this species but describes it rather as an amulet to be used as a prophylactic measure. There is no reference to such magical powers in the entries dealing with the two chameleons, but in the Dioscoridean section dealing with thistles and other species having thorns (*MM* iii.8–22), only the plant called ἄκανθα λευκή (iii.12), identified as either *Picnomon acarna* (L.) Cass. = *Cnicus acarna* L. or *Cirsium ferox* (L.) DC. = *Cnicus ferox* L., is used with a similar talismanic powers as it "automatically chases away wild beast when hung upon a person" (περίαπτον ἐξ αὐτοῦ θηρία διώκει). Interestingly, either *Picnomon* or *Cirsium* is probably depicted as one of the woodcuts under the chapter "Chamæleon thistle" in Ge.

Literature: *BLACK CHAMELEON (*Cardopatium corymbosum* (L.) Pers.): *HP* ix.12.1 (χαμαιλέων μέλας); *MM* iii.9; *NH* xxii.47 (*chamaeleon niger, ixia*); *SM* xii.154; *RM* ii.271; *OEH* 26 (*herba chameæleæ. wulfes camb*); *Dur.Glos.* 300 (*cameleon, camedris. vulues-comb*), 301 (*camerion. mete thistel*); *LS* 265 (*kameleon melanos, cameleonta nigra*); *EPN* ii (*cameleon, wulfes camb*), iv (*camellia. wulfes-camb*); *Pand.* 125 ($_{AR}$*cameleombante, suchaa,* $_{GR}$*cameleonta alba, spina iudaica, scoltea, acantahani, acantis egyptiaca, spina arabica,* $_{LA}$*cardus albus*); *Sin.Bart.* 14 (*cameleon, carduus benedictus, senecion*); *Alph.* 27 (*cameleonta nigra, cardus assinius, cardus uarius, labrum ueneris*), 113 (*melus*); *AC* 179.3 (*camalion. wolwysthystyl*) ⚭ *GH* 121 (CAMELEONTA, *wolues thystle, black cameleonte, coccodyllus, dyspata, anacardion, semerit, astradace locer, amelita, labrum veneris*); *Fu* 338 (ΧΑΜΑΙΛΕΩΝ ΜΕΛΑΣ, *carduus niger, vernilagium*); *DL* 372 (THISTLE CHAMELEON, χαμαιλέων μέλας, *pancarpon, viophonon, cynomazon, cynoxylon, ocymoides, cnidos coccos, carduus niger, veruilago, vstilago*); *Ge* 997 (CHAMÆLEON THISTLE, χαμαιλέων μέλας, *carduus niger, vernilago, crocodilion*). ¶ *PINE THISTLE (*Carlina gummifera* (L.) Less.): *HP* ix.12.1 (χαμαιλέων λευκός); *MM* iii.8; *NH* xxii.45 (*chamaeleon candidus*); *SM* xii.154; *RM* ii.271; *OEH* 156 (*herba camelleon alba. wulfes tæsl*); *Dur.Glos.* 300 (*camemileon alba, camemelon. sebrade, vulues teals*), *LS* 264 (*kemeleon leuce, cameleonta alba, accia*); *EPN* iv (*camemelon alba. se brada wulfes camb*); *TH* 127 (*camelleunta alba, camelleon*); *Pand.* 125 ($_{AR}$*cameleombante, suchaa,* $_{GR}$*cameleonta alba, spina iudaica, scoltea, acantahani, acantis egyptiaca, spina arabica,* $_{LA}$*cardus albus*); *Alph.* 27

(*cameleonta alba, cardus coagulatus, ixion. southistel*) ⚘ Fu 337 (*ΧΑΜΑΙΛΕΩΝ ΛΕΥΚΟΣ, carduus suarius/uarius, cardopatium*), DL 372 (THISTLE CHAMELEON, χαμαιλέων λευκός, *carduus syluaticus/varinus/irinus/lacteus, erisisceptrum, ixia*); Ge 995 (WHITE CARLINE THISTLE, *car(o)lina, cardopatium, leucanthes*).

C²S³ (*SM*, Fu, DL, Ge) | C³S³ (*RM, LS*)

2495 wylde hempe. The Latin headword, either a scribal innovation from an original *c a n (n) a b i n a (cf. similar names such as *fabaria, persicaria*, or *policaria*) or else some sort of contraction from κάνναβις ἀγρία/*cannabis agrya (so Brodin 1950: 217), and the ME names (→ **2496** on the last one) are traditionally refer to hemp agrimony (*Eupatorium cannabinum* L.). The brief physical description and the habitat of the species support such identification as well. The entry derives from *AC*.

Pharmacographically, the plant is described as febrifuge (**2497**), which is recorded in DL and Ge but missing elsewhere.

Literature: HEMP AGRIMONY (*Eupatorium cannabinum* L.): *MM* iii.149 (κάνναβις ἀγρία); *NH* xx.259 (*cannabis*); *OEH* 116 (*herba cannaue silfatica*); *Dur.Glos*. 302 (*canafel siluatica. camepithis henep*); *LS* 207 (*scehedenegi* [شهداج *šahdānīǧ*], *canabis*); *EPN* iv (*canafel sylvatica. hænep*); *TH* 126 (*canapa ... silvatica, agrion canabin)*; *Pand*. 619 (ₐᵣ*sechedenichi*, ₉ᵣ*canabis*, ₗₐ*canapis*); *Alph*. 30 (*canabaria*); *AC* 177.13 (*canabarya. wylde hemp, holyrop, doumnetele*) ⚘ *GH* 120 (CANAPIS ... *wylde hempe, agryon canabyn*); Fu 100 (EUPATORIUM ADULTERINUM, *herba S. Kunigundi*); Tu 2.740 (EUPATORIUM, *water hemp*); DL 44 (BASTARD AGRIMONIE, *eupatorium aquaticum/ adulterinum*); Ge 574 (WATER HEMPE, *bastard/water agrimonie, hepatorium cannabinum, eupatorium adulterium, cannabina*).

C²H² (*TH*) | CS (DL) | C²S² (*GH*, Fu, Ge)

2501 wylde tansy. The ME synonyms and the comparison of the leaves with those of tansy (*Tanacetum vulgare* L.; → **2283**) suggest that the species here must be silverweed (*Potentilla anserina* L.). The Latin headword, on the other hand, is traditionally ascribed either to the greater knapweed (*Centaurea scabiosa* L.; PNME: *s.v.*) or to the similar-looking devil's-bit scabious (*Succisa pratensis* Moench; Stirling 1995–1998: *s.v.* iacea). The two species are quite different from each other, so the confusion is probably pharmacographic or (more likely) lexical, but the link between both words is unclear. In any case the mistake seems not to be due to the scribe of *LH* but was transmitted from the likely source text, *AC*—even though the virtues are different in each treatise.

Pharmacographically, the species is described as preservative (→ **2503**) and detergent (**2504**).

Literature: SILVERWEED (*Potentilla anserina* L.): *Alph.* 83 (*iacea alba, scabiosa. scabwort*), 125 (*nimpha aquatica*); *Sin.Bart.* 24 (*jacia alba, scabiosa*); *AC* 194.9 (*iasia alba. gosgres, wyldtanse*) ✿ Fu 236 (POTENTILLA, *agrimonia syluestris, tanacetum syluestre*); Tu 2.728 (WILD TANSEY, *anserina, tanacetum sylvestre, potentilla*); DL 60 (SILVER-WEED, *wild-tansie, wild-agrimonie, potentilla, argentina, agrimonia syluestris, tanacetum syluestre*); Ge 841 (WILDE TANSIE, *siluerweede, argentina, potentilla, agrimonia syluestris, anserina, tanacetum syluestre*).

S³ (DL) | C¹S³ (Fu, Ge)

2503 chafe. According to MED: *s.v.*, the main intransitive senses of ME *chaufen* are "to rot, disintegrate" (§ 2b) and "to grow or be excited, fervent, passionate, or provoked" (§ 4d). Both of them fit the general idea of the sentence quite well, but the clause ⟨will kepe the⟩ must probably be read as evidence that the first sense was in fact intended here. The suggestion that the plant is also beneficial to have clean limbs supports that sense as well. Note moreover that the meaning "?suffer illness", given in MED: *s.v.* thāven *v.*, § e and which quotes this passage as sole source, is a ghost due to a mistranscription "thafe" in *WG*.

2506 white pepir. Although the Latin headword generally refers to white charlock (*Raphanus raphanistrum* L.), the form of the leaves and the colour of the seed suggest that the species described here is rather white mustard (*Sinapis alba* L.). As seen from the Literature section and PNME: *s.v.* rapistrum, in botanical treatises the ME name seems to have been applied not to the ripe seeds of black pepper (*Piper nigrum* L.) but to a number of Brassicaceae having a pungent taste (some mustard, rocket and, above all, charlock). Textually, the entry seems to belong to the *AC* tradition, although the version of the chapter edited in Brodin 1950: 201 (drawn from MS *L*) misses the medical virtues and only mentions the culinary uses. The Latin version (*Sl.*17r/32–37) does mention its vulnerary powers.

Pharmacographically, the species is antiseptic and vulnerary (**2508**), and regenerative of skin on old wounds (**2509**).

Literature: WHITE MUSTARD (*Sinapis alba* L.): *EPN* viii (*hec eruta. whytte pepyre*); *DVH(SME)* 19a.3 (*white peper, white senuey. eruca*); *AC* p. 201.22 (*rapistrum domesticum. whitpepur*) ✿ Tu 2.571 (MUSTARDE, *napi, sinepi, sinapis ... white mustarde*); DL 443 (SENUY, *mustard... the first kind,* σίνηπι κηπαῖον, *sinapi(s) hortense, eruca, white senuy*); Ge 189 (MUSTARD, νάπι, *sinapi ... white mustard*). → mostarde [**1327**]. ¶ WHITE CHARLOCK (*Raphanus raphanistrum* L.): *Alph.* 14 (*armoceren, rapistrum*), 153 (*rapistrum, armoceren, kenekel, carlokes*); *Sin.Bart.* 20 (*eruca, sinapis albus. cherloc*), 36 (*rapistrum. kerloc*) ✿ GH 375 (RAPIASTRUM, *wylde rape*); Tu 2.538 (RADICE, *radish, wild kole, wild radice*); DL 445 (RAPISTRUM, *charlocke, sinapi syluestre*); Ge 179 (WILDE

TURNEP, *charlock, kedlock, carlock, wild mustard, rapistrum, rapum syluestre, sinapi syluestre*).

C³S³ (DL) | C⁴S⁴ (Tu, Ge) | FS (*GH*)

2511 wythi. The Latin headword, the ME name and the temperament of the species indicate that the entry describes the medical properties of willows (*Salix* L. spp.). The name "withy" (OE *wīðig*, related to OE *wiððe* "cord, band, throng") is currently applied to the flexible willow stems used in thatching, basket-weaving, and in husbandry (for instance to make wattle fences), but it was historically used to refer to the osier willow (*S. viminalis* L.), as this was the preferred species to obtain wicker. It is therefore quite likely that this is the actual species meant by the author, but definitive evidence is lacking. The textual pedigree of the entry is similarly unknown, the plant being missing in the main two sources for *LH*, i.e. *DVH* and *AC*.

Pharmacographically, the plant is described as hemostatic (**2512**), antiemmenagogue (**2513**), anesthetic (**2514**), antiverrucous and anaphrodisiac (**2516**). All of them are recorded in the usual medical literature (DL being particularly close).

Literature: WILLOWS (*Salix* L. spp.): *HP* iii.1.3 (ἰτέα); *MM* i.104; *NH* xxiv.56 (*salix*); *SM* xi.891; *RM* ii.218; *Grad*. 358; *LS* 136 (*bvlef* [خلاف] *ḥilāf*], *salix*); *EPN* ii (*salix. wiþig*), iii (*salix. welig*), v (*salix. wiðig*); *TH* 452 (*salix*); *Pand*. 196 (ₐᵣ*culef*, ᴳᴿ*ytee*, ʟᴀ*salix*); *Alph*. 87 (*isacotidis, isacotidix, salix. salgh*), 160 (*salix, icea*) ⚜ *GH* 411 (SALIX, *wylowe tree*); Fu 125 (ΊΤΕΑ, *salix*); Tu 2.555 (WILLOW, *sallow tree, saugh, salix, itia*); DL 535 (WITHY, *willow,* ἰτέα, *salix*); Ge 1202 (WILLOWE TREE, *sallow, withie,* ἰτέα, *salix*).

S (*SM, RM,* Fu) | F¹S¹ (*LS*) | F¹S³ (*TH*) | F²S¹ (*Grad.*) | F²S² (*GH*, DL, Ge)

2511 tendryns. The MS reading ⟨tendyrst⟩ could have stood with a sense "take the tenderest [part] of willow", but it is quite weak as well, since the exact part of the tree that is to be used (leaves, shoots, catkins, bark?) is never mentioned. Moreover, the scribe of *LH* experienced demonstrable problems with the exemplary reading *TENDRYN (OF *tendron*; → **1696**), which he must have obviously confused with *t e n d e r (OF *tendre* < La. *tener*).

2518 vyolett. The entry translates the appropriate *Violae* in *DVH* but, as seen below, includes a number of departures from the canonical version, some of which suggest a faulty exemplar. Comparison of the entry with the usual medical authorities indicates that as a whole this is ultimately based on the Dioscoridean chapter ἴον, traditionally identified as the sweet or English violet (*Viola odorata* L.), which displays purple petals and with which it agrees in temperament and virtues, rather than with λευκόϊον (identified as gilliflower,

Matthiola incana (L.) R.Br. in Beck 2005: 236, but probably covering also the yellow wallflower, *Erysimum* × *cheiri* (L.) Crantz = *Cheiranthus cheiri* L.; Sprengel 1829–1830: ii.550–551, Berendes 1902: 345), which provided little more than the Latin headword and the idea that the petals of the species come in three colours. The (con)fusion between both entries is already detectable in *NH*, which was Macer Floridus's probably direct source, but is found neither in *LS* nor (as expected) in Renaissance treatises.

Pharmacographically, the plant is described as antipyrotic (**2519** = *DVH* 1349), cephalgic (→ **2520**), antiepileptic (**2521** = *DVH* 1353–1354), ophthalmic (**2523** = *DVH* 1355–1356), (**2524** = *DVH* 1357–1359), antitussive (**2525** = *DVH* 1374), refrigerant (→ **2526**), and eloquent (**2533** = *DVH* 1382–1389). Missing from this account are its antitonsillitic powers (*DVH* 1352) and the collection of virtues included between *DVH* 1360–1373, which perhaps went unrecorded due to a faulty Latin exemplar. On the other hand, a passage describing the consolidative and antitussive powers of the species (**2529–2532**) is not in Choulant's canonical edition, while the hemostatic qualities (**2528** = *DVH* 1390–1394) were shifted from the original final position in Macer Floridus's poem.

Literature: SWEET VIOLET (*Viola odorata* L.): *HP* vi.6.7 (ἴον); *MM* iv.121; *NH* xxi.130 (*viola*); *SM* xi.889; *RM* ii.235; *Grad.* 344; *OEH* 165 (*herba viola. banwyrt*); *Dur.Glos.* 305 (*viola. cleafre, ban-wyrt*); *DVH* 1342–1394 (*violae*); *LS* 141 (*seneffigi* [بنفسج *banafsağ*], *violy*); *EPN* ii (*viola. hofe*), iv (*viola. simering-wyrt*), v (*viola. clæfre*), vi (*viola. violé. appel-leaf*), vii (*hec viola. wyolet*), viii (*hec viola. vyolytte*), ix (*hec violeta. a violet*); *CI* v.1 (*viola. violet*); *TH* 504 (*violla*); *Pand.* 259 (ₐᵣ*feneflig, fenefigi*, ɢʀ*leucis*, ʟₐ*viola*); *DVH(NME)* 249v.5 (*vyolett*); *DVH(SME)* 6a.1 (*violet*); *Alph.* 191 (*viola*); *Sin.Bart.* 43 (*viola*) ❀ *GH* 459 (VIOLA, *vyolette*); *Fu* 116 ('ΙΟΝ ΠΟΡΦΥΡΟΥΝ, *viola muraria/purpurea*); *Tu* 2.597 (VIOLET, *viola, ion, viola nigra, viola purpurea*); *DL* 105 (MARCH/garden/sweete VIOLET, ἴον πορφυροῦν, *viola nigra, viola purpurea, vaccinium, violaria, mater violarum*); *Ge* 698 (VIOLET, ἴον, *nigra viola, herba violaria, mater violarum*). ¶ GILLIFLOWER (*Matthiola incana* (L.) R.Br.)/WALLFLOWER (*Erysimum* × *cheiri* (L.) Crantz): *MM* iii.123 (λευκόϊον); *LS* 210 (*keiri* [خيري *ḫīrī*]) ❀ *Fu* 173 (ΛΕΥΚΟΙΟΝ Dioscoridis, *viola alba, cheiri, keirim*); *Tu* 2.597 (WALLGELOVER, *stock gelovers, viola alba, leucoion*); *DL* 107 (WALL-FLOURE, *yellow gillofer, harts-ease*, λευκόϊον, *leucoium luteum, viola lutea, keyri*), 108 (STOCKE-GILLOFER, *garnsie violet, white/stocke/castle gillofer*, λευκόϊον, *viola alba*); *Ge* 370 (WALL FLOWER/*gilloflower, yellow stocke/winter gilloflower*, λευκόϊον, *viola lutea, leucoium luteum, keyri*), 372 (STOCKE/*castle* GILLOFLOWER, *garnsey violet*, λευκόϊον, *viola alba*).

FH (*SM, RM, Ge*) | F¹H¹ (*DVH, LS*) | F¹H² (*Grad., CI, TH, GH, Fu, DL*)

2520 gode for þe hede. The sentence is actually an over-simplification of *DVH* 1350–1351, where the plant is praised as acrepalous (*crapula discutitur*) and anticatarrhal *(capitis gravedo)*, since the symptoms of both conditions are felt in the head. On the other hand, the possibility that the translator did not know the Latin words *crapula* and *gravedo* and simply made an inference after the references to *capitis* and *caput*, should perhaps not be discarded.

2526 all hote evillys. Comparison with the original poem indicates that this corresponds to *DVH* 1375–1379, but the expected virtues (antitinnitus, antiotalgic and anticephalalgic) are missing. The oil was used against ear buzzing (*DVH* 1375), while the reference to body heat is recorded in *DVH* 1379. Assuming a homoioteleuton from an English exemplar is a convenient solution, but textual support for this is lacking and it is likely that the scribe would have realized the mistake, the sentence in *LH* being flawless—which is exceptional in cases of eye-skipping. As for the Latin passage, it is very simple both syntactically and lexically, so it would have posed no problem to any competent translator, while assuming a homoioteleuton here would be difficult to defend on textual grounds. It is still possible that the intervening three lines were botched or missing in the poem, leaving thus something along the lines of **ex violis oleum sicut de flore rosarum* [...] *leniter infrigidans corpusque sopore resolvens*. The fragment, while ungrammatical, would yet be understandable enough to allow an easy rendering into ME.

2538 wylde sanagrene. The Latin headword suggests that this entry describes the medical virtues of darnel (*Lolium temulentum* L.), a species already treated in the herbal (→ **1078**, with discussion and where this section was actually interpolated). Still, the medical virtues recorded there suggest that the entry deals in fact with black cumin (*Nigella sativa* L.), a plant that was usually confused in medieval and Renaissance sources with corn cockle (*Agrostemma githago* L.), which in turn was a weed that, just like *Lolium*, is usually found in wheat and rye fields. The English synonym is apparently a hapax, and its etymology is unclear. The spelling *sanagrene* given by MED: s.v. sānāgrẹne *n.* is used here although *s a u a g r e n e would be also possible, cf. ⟨wyldsauagre⟩ in *AC*. The source of the entry remains untraced.

Identification with *Nigella* seems positive also on pharmacographic grounds: the plant is said to be emmenagogue (**2539**), galactogenous and resolvent (**2540**), and carminative (**2542**); all of these virtues are routinely mentioned in medical texts of the period. On the other hand, the antihalitosic quality of the species (**2543**) is not recorded in the usual literature. In fact ⟨breth⟩ is likely to be a copy mistake for *b r e d : black cumin was used as a condiment in bakery, as routinely repeated in the literature since *MM*, cf. τὸ σπέρμα μέλαν, δριμύ, εὐῶδες, καταπασσόμενον εἰς ἄρτους, "[the seed] is black, sharp, and fragrant and they sprinkle it on breads", or *NH* xx.184 "semen gratissime panes etiam condiat"; cf. also ⟨greynes amendith brede⟩ in **1080**.

Literature: BLACK CUMIN (*Nigella sativa* L.): *MM* iii.79 (μελάνθιον); *NH* xx.182 (*git, melanthium, melaspermon*); *SM* xii.69; *RM* 240; *Grad.* 375 (*nigella*); *LS* 318 (*xamim* [شونيز *šūnīz*], *nigella*); *EPN* ix (*hoc lollium/hoc git. kokylle*); *CI* N.4 (*nigella*); *TH* 336 (*nigella*); *Pand.* 139 (ARcaruum, stanix, GRmelanchium, git, LAnigella); *DVH(SME)* 43a.17 (*git*); *Alph.* 2, 75 (*acrimulatum, agrimulatum, melancium, gyth, cyminum ethiopicum, nigella*), 77 (*giter*), 215 (*gimpreti, melanthium, nigella*), 222 (*mellalia, nigella*); *Sin.Bart.* 16, 22 (*gith, ciminum Ethiopicum, nigella*), 30 (*melancium, nigella*); *AC* 200.4 (*lolium. cokkyl, popy, wyldsauagre*) ⚘ *GH* 312 (NIGELLA, *cokyll*); Fu 191 (*ΜΕΛΑΝΘΙΟΝ, papauer nigrum, nigella, gith*); Tu 2.390 (NIGELLA ROMANA, *git, melathion, melaspermon*); DL 198 (GIT, *nigella*, μελάνθιον, *melanthium, papauer nigrum*); Ge 924 (GITH, *nigella, bishops woort, Saint Katharines flower*, μελάνθιον, *melanthium, salusandria, papauer nigrum*). ¶ DARNEL (*Lolium temulentum* L.): → kokkyll [**1078**].

C³S³ (*SM, RM, Grad., LS, Cl, TH, Pand., GH,* Fu, DL, Ge)

2546–2547 Macer the philozofur. The ⟨boke in Latyn⟩ that John Lelamour is claimed to have translated is *De Viribus Herbarum,* an extremely popular Latin poem in (frequently clumsy) hexameters composed by someone who was called "Macer Floridus" in a number of early MSS. That name, borrowed from the Augustan poet Aemilius Macer who apparently wrote a now lost treatise on herbs variously called *De herbis* or *Alexipharmaca,* is generally identified now as the pseudonym of Odo Magdunensis/Odo de Meung-sur-Loire, a French physician living during the late 11th or early 12th century (Moreno Olalla 2007: 120). See the discussion on Macer Floridus and the validity of the various claims of the *explicit* in the Sources section of the Introduction.

Glossary

abate *v.* mitigate pain; lessen an inflammation; eliminate poison
abhominacion *n.* nausea
a-bide *v.* remain
abortyve *n.* stillbirth, foetus
aboue *adv.* above; (*in relation to evacuation*) upwards, i.e. throwing up
a-boue *prep.* above
a-boue-saide *a.* above-mentioned
aboue-saide *prep.* above-mentioned
ab(o)ute *prep.* about; around
a-brode *adv.* wide, open, over a broad surface
acces(se *n.* fit, sudden attack of an illness ¶ **þe a.** sudden and violent attack of fever ¶ **a. of flourys** unexpected discharge of catamenia
ake* *v.* ache, suffer pain
ache *n.*[1] ache, pain
(h)ache *n.*[2] smallage, wild celery (*Apium graveolens* L., → **1**)
akyng(e *n.* aching, feeling of continuous pain
a-corde *a.* in agreement
acorde *v.* agree, be in accordance
adde* *v.* increase
addyr → **(n)addyr**
addyrworte *n.* dragons (*Dracunculus vulgaris* Schott, → **38**)
adeleth *n.* face
a-down(e *adv.* downwards; down
afferme* *v.* affirm
affodill *n.* summer asphodel (*Asphodelus aestivus* Brot., → **91**)
aforsaid(e *a.* aforesaid, already mentioned
after *adv.* afterwards
after *conj.* after

after *prep.* after, subsequent to; according to; like
a-gayne → **aye(y)n(e**
age *n.* age
agry- → **egry-**
aye(y)n(e *adv.* against; near; again, once more
a-yene *prep.* against (*both physically and figuratively*)
air → **eire**
aysel(le *n.* vinegar
ale *n.* ale
alym(e *n.* alum
alixsandir *n.* horse parsley (*Smyrnium olusatrum* L., → **85**)
all *adv.* all; completely
al(l *a.* all
al(l)moste *adv.* almost
almond* *n.* almond, fruit of the *Prunus dulcis* (Mill.) D.A.Webb
aloyne *n.* wormwood (*Artemisia absinthium* L.)
a-longe *adv.* along
alonge *prep.* along
a(l)s *conj.* as
also *adv.* also, equally; as (*in comparisons*)
ambros(e *n.* ?wood germander, ?agrimony (*Teucrium scorodonia* L., *Agrimonia eupatoria* L., → **133**)
amen *int.* amen (*used as a concluding formula*)
amende *v.* cure or improve an illness; emend, correct a mistake
ameos *n.* ammi, bishopsweed (*Ammi majus* L., → **124**)
amonge *prep.* among
a(n *a. (indef. art.)* a

an → **on**
ana *adv.* in the same amount
ancle* *n.* ankle
and *conj.* and; if
angrely *adv.* fiercely, painfully
any → **eny**
annete *n.* dill (*Anethum graveolens* L., → **105**)
annys *n.* dill (*Anethum graveolens* L., → **15**)
anoynte *v.* anoint, rub over with oil or unguent
anoyntynge *n.* anointing
anon(e *adv.* anon
a-noþer *a.* another
an-oþer *pron.* another
antracas *n.* carbuncle, malignant boil (→ **301**)
a-peire* *v.* impair, worsen
apon → **vpon**
appet(id)e *n.* appetite, craving for food; bodily desire, inclination
appill *n.* fruit, and particularly the one of the *Malus domestica* Borkh.
ar → **be**, **ere**
arbuste *n.* mistletoe (*Viscum album* L., → **1462**)
archangeles *n.* arthritis (→ **1953**)
aryse* *v.* arise, come above the horizon; appear (a boil)
Armany *n.* Armenia
arme *n.* arm
arme-hole *n.* armpit
aron *n.* cleavers (*Galium aparine* L., → **970**)
arsmeche *n.* water-pepper/willow-weed (*P. hydropiper* (L.) Delarbre/ *Persicaria maculosa* Gray, → **517**)
as → **a(l)s**
aske *v.* require; ask
aske* *n.* ash
astrologie *n.* birthwort (*Aristolochia* L. spp., → **67**)
aswage *v.* mitigate pain
at *prep.* at
atter-cop* *n.* spider
attribut* *n.* genital organs
a-two *adv.* in two parts
auto(u)r *n.* author, medical authority
avance *n.* wood avens (*Geum urbanum* L., → **30**)
avoyde* *v.* clear, cleanse
away(e *adv.* away
ax(c)es → **acces(se**

bak(ke *n.* back
bay* *n.* berry
bal(l)ok* *n.* testicle
ballok-stone* *n.* testicle
balme *n.* balsam-tree (*Commiphora gileadensis* (L.) C.Chr., → **267**)
bank* *n.* bank, ridge near a water current
barly *n.* barley
barow* *n.* barrow, castrated boar
basilicon *n.* basil (*Ocimum* L. spp., → **283**)
basyn *n.* basin
bat *n.* blow (→ **318**)
bate* *v.* reduce
bathe *n.* bath
baþe *v.* bathe
be *v.* be
be* *n.* bee
beate* *n.* onion (*Allium cepa* L., → **189**)
be-cause *adv.* (+ **of**) because
bed(d *n.* bed
begyn *v.* begin
begyn(n)yng(e *n.* beginning
bellyre, -y *n.* narrow-leaved water-parsnip (*Berula erecta* (Huds.) Coville, → **240**)
bene *n.* bean, seed of many Leguminosae; used as a measure
bene-hyve *n.* beehive

Lelamour Herbal 469

be-nym* *v.* take away
berde *n.* beard
ber(e *v.* bear, carry upon someone; display certain characteristic ¶ **b. child(e** be pregnant
bere *n.* barley
bery* *n.* berry
best(e, better → **gode**
beste *n.* beast
betayn(ne, betony *n.* betony (*Stachys betonica* (L.) Trevis., → **150**)
bete *n.* beet (*Beta* L. spp.)
bete *v.* beat, pound, triturate; flog
betynge *n.* beating
be-twene *prep.* between
by *prep.* by
bidde* *v.* command, prescribe
bide *v.* remain
byfor *adv.* before
bile* *n.* boil, swelling; callus; festering sore
bynde *v.* bind; oppilate; constipate
byndynge *a.* accumulation of mucus
by-nethe *adv.* downwards; (*in relation to evacuation*) downwards, i.e. passing stool
byrd(e *n.* bird; chick
birdis-neste *n.* wild carrot (*Daucus carota* L., → **532**)
bit(e *v.* bite
bityng(e *n.* biting; bite, an instance of biting
bit(te *n.* bite
bittyr *a.* bitter
bittirnes *n.* bitterness
by-twyx *prep.* between, within
bla(c)k(e *a.* black
blacknes(se *n.* blackness, dirt
blad(d)er *n.* urinary bladder; gall-bladder; blister, pustule
blankett *n.* white lead, ceruse
blawe* *v.* blow, produce a current of air;

be driven by the wind
blede *v.* bleed
bledyng(e *n.* bleeding
bleyn* *n.* blain, swelling
bler, -ther *n.* bleariness
blered *a.* having watery eyes
blew(e *a.* blue
blynde-nettill *n.* dead nettle (*Lamium* L. spp.)
blyþe *a.* merry
blode *n.* blood
blody *a.* bleeding, bloody
blossum *n.* blossom
blot* *n.* spot, stain, blemish
boc(c)he *n.* bubo, swelling, tumor
boke *n.* book
body *n.* body
boyl(le *v.* boil, cook in a liquid; inflame, make fervent
bol(o)wyng(e, boln- *n.* swelling, tumour
bolwing *a.* swelling, suffering from inflammation
bond* *n.* nerve, ligament
bon(e *n.* bone
bon-worte *n.* daisy (*Bellis perennis* L., → **522**)
borage *n.* alkanet (*Anchusa officinalis* L., → **214**)
bord *n.* board, piece of timber
bore* *n.* boar, uncastrated male swine
bornete* *n.* burnet (*Sanguisorba* L. spp., → **230**)
borþen *n.* that which is carried in the womb, foetus ¶ **laste/second b.** secundines, placenta
boþe *a.* both; second
boþe *pron.* both
bothe *prep.* both
boþ(e *conj.* both
bowel(l)is *n.* intestines, entrails
box *n.* box
bray(e *v.* crush

brayne *n.* brain
branne *n.* bran
brasse *n.* brass
bra(u)nche *n.* branch
breke *v.* break, shatter; snap; dissolve an obstruction; make to flow (by dissolving an obstruction)
brede *n.* bread
bren, -a- *v.* burn, consume by fire; be in combustion
bren(n)yng *a.* burning, having great heat
bren(n)yng(e, bryn- *n.* burning, sensation of heat
brest* *v.* burst, suffer from hernia
brest(e *n.* breast
breth(e *n.* breath
brew* *n.* brow
bright *a.* bright, shining
brymstone *n.* sulphur
brynge *v.* bring
bryony *n.* bryony (*Bryonia cretica* subsp. *dioica* (Jacq.) Tutin, → **1006**)
brysewort *n.* daisy (*Bellis perennis* L., → **522**)
broke* *n.* brook
broke-vilmyd *a.* ruptured
brokleuys *n.* brooklime (*Veronica beccabunga* L., → **245**)
brode *a.* wide
broyse *v.* hit; crush in a mortar
brome *n.* common broom (*Cytisus scoparius* (L.) Link, → **251**)
brothe *n.* broth
broþer-worte *n.* wild marjoram (*Origanum vulgare* L., → **1553**)
browne bugill *n.* bugle (*Ajuga reptans* L., → **223**)
brusid → **broyse**
brusinge *n.* contusion, fracture
bugill *n.* borage (*Borago officinalis* L., → **205**)
bustous *a.* rough, coarse in texture

but(e *conj.* but; except
but(t)yr *n.* butter ¶ **may(e b.** unsalted, purified butter

kake *n.* cake, a flat mass
kayre *n.* rowan tree (*Sorbus aucuparia* L., → **656**)
calamynte *n.* calamint (*Calamintha* Mill. spp., → **383**)
kalketrap *n.* ?Celtic spikenard, ?caltrops (*Valeriana celtica* L., *Centaurea calcitrapa* L., → **1049**)
call* *v.* call, give a name
camamyll *n.* camomile (*Anthemis* L. spp.)
kammok *n.* restharrow (*Ononis spinosa* subsp. *procurrens* (Wallr.) Briq., → **1054**)
canker* *v.* to become cancerous
cankyr(e, -cre *n.* ulcerous wound; cancer, tumour (→ **36**)
canell *n.* cinnamon (bark of the *Cinnamomum verum* J.Presl)
capon* *n.* capon, castrated cock
cardiake *n.* garlic mustard (*Alliaria petiolata* (M.Bieb.) Cavara & Grande, → **466**)
cardiacle *n.* disease of the heart, perhaps some kind of violent palpitation
cars(se, cra- *n.* garden cress (*Lepidium sativum* L., → **300**)
carw(e)y *n.* caraway (*Carum carvi* L., → **407**)
caste *v.* cast, toss; get rid of an ailment ¶ **c. oute** vomit, throw up
castynge *n.* vomiting
catapusia *n.* caper spurge (purgative seed of *Euphorbia lathyris* L.)
catte *n.* cat
catt-mynte *n.* calamint (*Clinopodium nepeta* (L.) Kuntze, → **1504**)
caule, -ou- *n.* cabbage, common name for several *Brassica* L. spp., particularly

B. *oleracea* L., → **422**); pottage of garden greens in which cabbage is a principal ingredient
cause *n.* cause, reason
cause* *v.* cause, produce, bring about
kele *v.* cool, make cold; become cold
celedony(e *n.* celandines (*Chelidonium majus* L./*Ranunculus ficaria* L., → **322**)
ken(n)yng(e *n.* some disease of the eye, perhaps a cataract
kene *a.* pungent or sharp to the taste
kennyng-worte *n.* scarlet pimpernel (*Anagallis arvensis* L., → **1859**)
centory(e *n.* centauries (*Centaurea centaurium* L./*Centaurium erythraea* Rafn, → **335**)
kepe *v.* keep
cerelonge *n.* hart's tongue fern (*Asplenium scolopendrium* L., → **923**)
cerementayne *n.* sermountain (*Laserpitium siler* L.)
kerwell *n.* wild chervil (*Anthriscus sylvestris* (L.) Hoffm., → **1061, 1105, 2137**)
keuerchiff *n.* headcloth
chafe *v.* ?rot (→ **2503**)
chafynge *n.* ?bad animal smell caused by sweat or fear (→ **638**)
chambur *n.* chamber, room
chauuede *n.* cudweed/cottonrose (*Filago germanica* (L.) Huds./*F. pyramidata* L., → **884**)
cheke* *n.* cheek
cheppe *n.* chap, side of the jaw
cheruell → **kerwell**
chese *v.* choose
chessboll *n.* poppy (*Papaver* L. spp., → **1694**)
cheuyrfoyl(le *n.* woodbine (*Lonicera periclymenum* L., → **2484**)
chewe *v.* chew

child(e *n.* child; foetus; stillborn, abortion
chyne *n.* chin
choppe *v.* chop, cut into small pieces
kill* *v.* kill
cilsper *n.* garlic mustard (*Alliaria petiolata* (M.Bieb.) Cavara & Grande, → **466**)
kynde *n.* nature, type, class; genital organs; sperm; temperament
kyndely *adv.* naturally, by its own natural disposition
kynge *n.* king
kyrnyng *n.* rumbling sensation in the stomach (→ **108**)
kyt(t *v.* cut
clawyng(e, clo- *n.* scratching; itching
clene *a.* clean
clene *adv.* clean
clene *v.* clean
clense *v.* cleanse, free from filth or noxious matter; eliminate
clenser *n.* cleansing substance
clepe* *v.* call, have a name
clere *a.* clear; free from sediments
clere* *v.* clear, mundify, free from obstruction or obscurity
cleue *v.* stick, adhere
clyuer *n.* cleavers (*Galium aparine* L.; → **970**)
clofe-tonge *n.* black hellebore (*Helleborus niger* L., → **1851**)
close *v.* close, stop up the flow of sth.; heal up by bringing separated parts together
cloþ(e *n.* cloth
cluster *n.* cluster
knawleche *n.* knowledge
knyt(te *v.* sold a broken bone, conjoin closely and firmly
knytter *n.* a medicine causing broken bones to sold
knob(be *n.* knot, hump

knot* *n.* knot, a protuberance in the tissue of a plant; a hard lump in a body
knotwort *n.* ?butcher's broom (*Ruscus aculeatus* L., → **1098**)
knowe *v.* have knowledge; distinguish
cokkyll *n.* corn cockle, black cumin, darnel (*Agrostemma githago* L., *Nigella sativa* L., *Lolium temulentum* L., → **1078, 2538**)
cokkowe-brede *n.* wood sorrel (*Oxalis acetosella* L., → **2469**)
codd* *n.* pod, husk
cold(e *a.* cold
cold(e *n.* coldness; catarrh, inflammation of the mucose membrane of the respiratory organs.
coldnes *n.* coldness
cole* *n.* coal, piece of carbon glowing without flame
cole* *v.* cool off
colik *n.* colic, griping pains in the intestines (→ **1168**)
colnes *n.* cool sensation
colombyne *n.* wall germander (*Teucrium chamaedrys* L., → **344**)
colour *n.* colour, hue; appearance
colour* *v.* have a certain complexion
col(ou)r(e *n.* bile, gall ¶ **brannyd c.** adust choler
coltisfote *n.* coltsfoot (*Tussilago farfara* L., → **963**)
coluer* *n.* dove, pigeon
coluyrfote *n.* long stalked cranesbill (*Geranium columbinum* L., → **511**)
comford *n.* strengthening
comfort(e, -d *v.* comfort; strengthen
comyn, -ovn *a.* common, normal, usual
comynly *adv.* usually
com(m)a(u)nde* *v.* command, prescribe
com(me *v.* come, reach a place; happen, occur; appear
com(m)yn *n.* cumin (*Cuminum cyminum* L., → **477**)
compas *adv.* in a circle, around (→ **2334**)
confery(e *n.* comfrey (*Symphytum officinale* L., → **490**)
consayve *v.* conceive, become pregnant
conseyvyng(e *n.* conception
consume* *v.* reduce
contayne *v.* hold, restrain
coryandyr *n.* coriander (*Coriandrum sativum* L., → **355**)
corne *n.*¹ corn, seed
corne *n.*² horny induration of the cuticle of the toes or feet
corner* *n.* corner
cost[if]nys *n.* constipation
costmaryn *n.* rocket (*Eruca sativa* Mill., → **313**)
cotidian(e *a.* quotidian, a type of fever recurring every day
co(u)gh(e *n.* cough
coule → **caule**
cow → **co(u)gh(e**
cowe *n.* cow
cow(e)slop(p)e *n.* some cowslip; oxlip (*Primula elatior* (L.) Hill, → **499**)
crampe *n.* cramp, spasm
crede* *n.* Creed
crepe* *v.* crawl
crepynge *a.* crawling ¶ **c. goute** *app.* herpes (→ **2266**)
croke* *v.* twist, bend
crokid *a.* curved
crom* *n.* crumb
crop(pe *n.* top of a plant
crosse *n.* cross, two perpendicular lines; such lines used as a symbol of Christianity
croswort *n.* ?Northern bedstraw/common marsh-straw (*Galium boreale* L./*G. palustre* L., → **472**)
crowefote *n.* meadow buttercup
crowesope *n.* soapwort

cubit* *n.* cubit, a measure of length
cvlrage *n.* water-pepper/willow-weed (*P. hydropiper* (L.) Delarbre/*Persicaria maculosa* Gray, → **517**)
curnelid *a.* crooked, bent at an angle
customable *adv.* habitually

day(e *n.* day
daysye *n.* daisy (*Bellis perennis* L., → **522**)
dare* *v.* (+ *neg.*) need not
dauke *n.* wild carrot (*Daucus carota* L., → **532**)
decoccioun *n.* medicinal preparation made by boiling
dede *a.* dead
defaute *n.* lack
defe *a.* deaf
defend* *v.* forbid
defye *v.* digest
degre(e *n.* degree
dele *v.* have sexual intercourse
delyuer *v.* release, liberate; deliver, give birth; expel harmful matter from the body; evacuate
delle *n.* ?leprosy (→ **1529**)
dent de lyon(ne *n.* dandelion (*Taraxacum* F.H.Wigg. spp., → **556**)
dente *n.* dint, wound or mark left by a blow
departe *v.* expel
depe* *adv.* low
derknes, dy- *n.* dimness of vision
deth(e *v.* death
dew → **du**
dewe *n.* dew
diche verne *n.* royal fern (*Osmunda regalis* L.)
diche* *n.* ditch
dye *v.* die
digestio(u)n *n.* digestion
dilicious, de- *a.* having a pleasant taste; voluptuous, given to sensous pleasures
dyll *n.* dill (*Anethum graveolens* L., → **105**)
dym *a.* devoid of clear vision
dyrkyn *v.* become blurred
dispose *v.* make ready
disses *n.* pain, suffering
dissolue *v.* dissolve, disintegrate
distroy(e *v.* distroy, render useless; kill, eliminate, do away with sth.
distroyenge *n.* impairment
ditander *n.* pepperwort (*Lepidium latifolium* L., → **574**)
diuee *n.* coltsfoot (*Tussilago farfara* L., → **963**)
dyuerse *a.* several; different
dokk *n.* dock (*Rumex* L. spp., → **561**)
doctor* *n.* physician, medical authority
dodyr *n.* dodder (*Cuscuta epilinum* Weihe, → **745**)
dogfynell *n.* stinking camomile (*Anthemis cotula* L., → **856**)
donge *n.* manure
do(ne *v.* do, perform; put, place; add (a new ingredient); be useful
donnetyl *n.* hemp agrimony (*Eupatorium cannabinum* L., → **2495**)
dor *n.* door
dosell *n.* syringe
do(u)nwarde *adv.* downwards (i.e. passing stool); downwards
doust *n.* dust
doute *n.* doubt, suspicion
doute *v.* mistrust, fear
doutous *a.* dangerous, terrifying
dowechs *n.* deadly nightshade (*Atropa bella-donna* L., → **579**)
downe *adv.* down
doworte *n.* deadly nightshade (*Atropa bella-donna* L.)
dragans(ia *n.* dragons (*Dracunculus*

vulgaris Schott, → **38, 539**)
dram *n.* dram, a weight equal to three scruples (*ca.* 3.9g)
draw(e *v.* draw, pull after one, drag; remove ¶ **d. togeder** mix
dred(e *v.* dread
dreme* *n.* dream
drest* *n.* dregs, lees
dry(e *v.* dry, desiccate; shrink or wipe away by desiccation
dry(e *a.* dry
dryeth *n.* dryness, dry condition
drynk(e *v.* drink ¶ **d. in** imbibe, absorb
drynke *n.* drink, beverage; an instance of drinking
dryve *v.* drive, move from one place to another
dronknes(se *n.* intoxication, drunkenness
drope *v.* drop, let a liquid fall in small portions; trickle, fall in globules
drop(e)sy(e *n.* dropsy
dropwort *n.* dropwort (*Filipendula vulgaris* Moench, → **673**)
drowe* *v.* dry up
du *a.* due, proper
dwale *n.* deadly nightshade (*Atropa belladonna* L.)

earthnote *n.* sow-bread (*Cyclamen hederifolium* Aiton, → **458**)
egge *n.* egg
egge-shill *n.* eggshell
eghe *n.* edge, tingling in the teeth
egill pace *n.* aegilops, fistula in the inner angle of the eye (→ **378**)
egrymo(y)n(e, a- *n.* agrimony (*Agrimonia eupatoria* L., → **56**)
ey* *n.* egg
eye *n.* eye
eye-brer *n.* eyelid
eye-lid* *n.* eyelid
eyre *n.* air

eysell → **aisell**
eiþer *conj.* either
elebyr(e *n.* hellebore (*Helleborus niger* L., *Veratrum album* L., → **1224**)
elefancia(sys *n.* a very virulent form of leprosy (→ **392**)
elena campana *n.* elecampane (*Inula elenium* L., → **587**)
elisaunder → **alixsandir**
ellryne *n.* elder (*Sambucus nigra* L.)
els(e else, otherwise
em(e)rodis *n.* haemorrhoids
empetik *n.* impetigo
ench(e)yson *n.* attack of illness
enchafe *v.* make warm
enclyse *n.* enema
encrese* *v.* increase; grow
ende *n.* end
endintd *a.* indented, having a serrated figure
endyue *n.* bristly ox-tongue (*Helminthotheca echioides* (L.) Holub, → **606**)
engender* *v.* produce, generate
engendir *n.* foetus
Englishe *a.* English
eny *a.* any
enplaster *n.* plaster
entra(il)le(s *n.* viscera, inner organs
epatica *n.* disease of the liver
(h)erbe *n.* herb
(h)erbe-benet *n.* hemlock (*Conium maculatum* L. → **641**)
erbe Christofyr male *n.* ?spiny starwort (*Pallenis spinosa* (L.) Cass., → **622**)
herbe yue *n.* buck-horn's plantain (*Plantago coronopus* L., → **1018**)
erbe Johann *n.* St. John's wort (*Hypericum perforatum* L., → **646**)
erbe moyntayne *n.* ?garden angelica (*Angelica archangelica* L., → **656**)
herba Plenius *n.* ?garden angelica

(*Angelica archangelica* L., → **1045**)
erbe Robert *n.* herb Robert (*Geranium robertianum* L., → **636**)
erbe Waltir *n.* ?sweet woodruff (*Galium odoratum* (L.) Scop., → **630**)
(h)ere *n.* ear
ere, ar *conj.* before
eryn → **ey**
erly *adv.* early, in the first part of the morning
erþen *a.* earthen
ese* *v.* alleviate, mitigate
esyle, estampit → **aisell, stamp(e**
esily *adv.* easily
(h)ete *v.* eat
etynge *n.* act of eating
euche *pron.* each
eufrase *n.* eyebright (*Euphrasia* L. spp., → **616**)
eupatorye *n.* wood sage (*Teucrium scorodonia* L.)
eve(n *n.* evening
even *a.* same, equal, uniform
euer *adv.* always, constantly ¶ **e. as whenever**
euere-verre[n]e *n.* common polypody (*Polypodium vulgare* L., → **670**)
euery *a.* every
euery *pron.* every one
evil(l *a.* harmful; evil; unpleasant, disagreeable
evill *adv.* badly, poorly
evill *n.* disease, malady ¶ **fallyng(e e.** epilepsy ¶ **montayne e.** an unknown disease of cattle
evyn *adv.* straight, directly

face *n.* face
fail(le *n.* failure
fair(e *a.* good; beautiful to behold; clean; clean, pure
fair(e *adv.* beautifully; properly; carefully

fall *v.* be taken ill; happen
fallyng(e *a.* falling
fare *v.* fare, get on, do (well or badly)
faste *a.* firmly set
faste *adv.* firmly; quick
faste *v.*¹ fix firmly, make fast
faste *v.*² fast, abstain from food; follow a diet on some food
fastyng(e *a.* fasting, abstaining from food
fat(te *a.* fat
faute* *n.* imperfection, defect
febill *a.* feeble, weak
febilnes *n.* weakness, lack of strength
February *n.* February
feche *v.* fetch ¶ **f. away** remove
fedyrfewe → **fethir-foy**
fele *adv.* much
fele *v.* feel
fel(l)on *n.* suppurative abscess, boil, carbuncle
fem(m)al(l)e *a.* female
fenel(l *n.* fennel (*Foeniculum vulgare* Mill., → **694**)
fenygrek, -crek *n.* fenugreek (*Trigonella foenum-graecum* L., → **750**)
ferne → **verne**
feste *n.* feast, banquet
fester *n.* fistula, festering wound
festeryng(e *n.* festering, rankling of a wound
festrynge *a.* festering, that festers
feþer *n.* feather
fethir-foy *n.* feverfew (*Tanacetum parthenium* (L.) Sch.Bip., → **713**)
feuer *n.* fever ¶ **hote f. causus** ¶ **colde f. ague**
fig* *n.* fig, fruit of the *Ficus carica* L.
filipendula *n.* dropwort (*Filipendula vulgaris* Moench, → **673**)
fill *v.* fill
fille *v.* defecate
filth(e *n.* filth, dirt; filthy body matter

(tartar, mucus, pus, etc.)
fynde *v.* find
fynger* *n.* finger
fir(e *n.* fire ¶ **f. of helle** herpes ¶ **wilde f.** some skin disease, probably erysipelas
first *pron.* first one
first(e *a.* first
first(e *adv.* first ¶ **f. and laste** the first and last action in a day
fistula *n.* fistula, pipe-like ulcer with a narrow orifice
flayne *v.* ?mix with a liquid into a mushy substance (→ **2337**)
fla(u)nke *n.* side of the abdomen
flax *n.* flax (*Linum usitatissimum* L., → **741**)
fle* *n.* flea
fle(e *v.* flee, run away
fl(e)y* *n.* fly
fleshe *n.* flesh, muscular part of an animal body; meat
fle(w)matik(e *a.* suffering from an excess of phlegm
flewme *n.* phlegm
fly-fo *n.* ragwort (*Jacobaea vulgaris* Gaertn., → **1930**)
flour delis(e *n.* German flag (*Iris* × *germanica* L., → **724**)
flour(e *n.*^{1} flower, reproductive organ of angiosperms
flour(e *n.*^{2} flour, finely-powdered ground seeds
flour(e *n.*^{3} menstrual discharge, catamenia
flux *n.* pathological flowing of a body fluid ¶ **blody f.** dysentery
fnese *v.* sneeze
folke *n.* people
foldyng *a.* folding
fole-fote *n.* coltsfoot (*Tussilago farfara* L., → **963**)
fome *n.* foam
fomyte → **vomyte**

for *conj.* for
for *prep.* for; from; against
forbede *v.* forbid, prohibit
forhede *n.* forehead
for-saide *a.* mentioned previously
forse *n.*^{1} gorse, furze (*Ulex europaeus* L.)
forse *n.*^{2} effect
forthe *adv.* continuously
fote *n.* foot
foule *a.* purulent, corrupt
foule *adv.* in a manner offensive to the smell
fo(u)ndement *n.* anus, lower extremity of the rectum
foure *a.* four
fourthe *a.* fourth
fox *n.* fox
fox-gloue *n.* foxglove (*Digitalis purpurea* L.)
franke-encens(e *n.* frankincense, the aromatic gum resin from several *Boswellia* Roxb. spp.
frantikle*, fre- *n.* freckle
frekylnes *n.* freckle
frenesy *n.* frenzy (→ **411**)
frentekill *a.* delirious
fresh(e *a.* recent; pure, not salted or smoked; retaining its original qualities
freting, v- *a.* ulcerous, corrosive ¶ **f. evill** some cutaneous disease, probably herpes
fret(te *v.* gnaw, corrode; rub
fry(e *v.* fry, cook in a pan with a little oil
fro(m *prep.* against; from
frote *v.* rub
frotinge *n.* friction
fru(y)te *n.* fruit
fu de inferne *n.* a corroding skin disease (→ **1375**)
full *a.* full
full *n.* houseleek (*Sempervivum tectorum* L., → **709**)

fullich *adv.* completely, entirely
fvmyter *n.* fumewort (*Corydalis solida* (L.) Clairv., → **681**)

gader *v.* gather; bring together as a mass
gaderinge* *n.* accumulation of morbid matter
galynga *n.* English galingale (*Cyperus longus* L.)
gall *n.* gall, bile
galon *n.* gallon
gardyne, -thyn *n.* orchard
garland *n.* garland, wreath
garlek(e *n.* garlic (*Allium sativum* L., → **759**)
garofull, -ill *n.* clove-scented basil; wood avens (*Geum urbanum* L., → **844**)
garse *v.* scarify, make incision in order to drain off venom or let blood
gasar *n.* ?butchers broom (*Ruscus aculeatus* L., → **1098**)
gencyan *n.* gentian (*Gentiana amarella* (L.) Börner, → **804**)
gender* *v.* produce
gentill *a.* noble, excellent
germandir *n.* rattles (*Rhinanthus* L. spp., → **812**)
geser, gi- *n.* liver; gizzard of birds (→ **258**)
gettyng *n.* conception
gib* *n.* chilblain
glad(de *a.* cheerful, merry
glade(y)n(e *n.* gladdon (*Iris pseudacorus* L., → **835**)
glasse *adv.* glass
gletous *a.* viscous
glet(te *n.* viscous matter, mucus; congestion of phlegm
gnawynge *a.* corrosive
go *v.* go, travel; expand; (*in comparisons*) be similar ¶ **g. away, his way** leave; fall away; wither ¶ **g. to-geder** heal up
God *n.* God
gode *a.* beneficial; correct; of excellent quality; agreeable to taste; abundant
godely *a.* excellent; noble, intelligent
godhishond *n.* black bryony (*Dioscorea communis* (L.) Caddick & Wilkin, → **2277**)
gom(me* *n.* toothgum, the fleshy integument of the jaws
gose gresse *n.* silverweed (*Potentilla anserina* L., → **2501**)
gose *n.* goose
goste *n.* ghost
gote* *n.* goat
gounde *n.* morbid matter in the eye
goute *n.* gout
gracious *a.* merciful, that dispenses grace
grape* *n.* grape, fruit of the *Vitis vinifera* L.
graunt* *n.* favour, boon
graunt* *v.* bestow, confer
greyn* *n.* grain, seed
grene *a.* green; not yet ripe
gres(se *n.*¹ grass
gres(se *n.*² grease, animal fat
gret(te *a.* physically large; plentiful; excessive
gretly *adv.* greatly
greue *v.* cause injury; have a bad influence
greuous *a.* severe, causing hurt or pain
grevance *n.* ailment, disease
grewe *n.* the Greek language
grewell *n.* porridge
grynde *v.* grind
grynding(e *n.* cramps, sharp pains
gryniswelly → **growndswelow**
grip* *n.* drain, trench
grom(m)ill *n.* gromwell (*Lithospermum officinale* L., → **784**)
growe *v.* grow; produce, cause to grow
growyng *a.* growing

gro(w)nd(e *n.* ground; soil
growndswelow *n.* common groundsel (*Senecio vulgaris* L., → **794, 824**)
gutte* *n.* drop of liquid

hayme *n.* membrane (→ **1357**)
hayreff *n.* cleavers (*Galium aparine* L., → **970**)
halfe *a.* half
halfe *adv.* half
halfe *n.* half
halfyndell *n.* half
hall *n.* hall, public room
hanse* *v.* enhance
hard(e *a.* hard; constipated
harde *adv.* very, extremely
harde *v.* harden, make hard; render callous and difficult to remove; sharpen, make penetrating
hardnes *v.* rigidity; morbid hardening
hare-fote *n.* wood avens (*Geum urbanum* L., → **30**)
harme *n.* harm
hart-worte *n.* bugle (*Ajuga reptans* L., → **223**)
hastely *adv.* quickly, in a short time
hasty* *a.* quick
haue *v.* own, possess; ingest (*a medicine*); enjoy or suffer (*good or bad health*); obtain (*a name*)
hauyng(e *a.* having
he *pron.* he
hed(e *n.* head, upper division of the body; poppy capsule
hede-ake, -ache *n.* headache; vertigo
heyhofe *n.* ground ivy (*Glechoma hederacea* L., → **893**)
hele *v.* heal
hele* *n.* heel
heler(e *n.* something that heals, medicament
helynge *n.* healing

helle *n.* hell
helow *n.* purslane (*Portulaca oleracea* L., → **976**)
helpe *n.* help
helpe *v.* help, be useful
hem[er]worte *n.* pellitory-of-the-wall (*Parietaria judaica* L., → **1625**)
hemloke *n.* hemlock (*Conium maculatum* L., → **872**)
hempe *n.* hemp (*Cannabis sativa* L.)
hen *n.* hen
henbane henbane (*Hyoscyamus* L. spp., → **905**)
herbe → **(h)erbe**
herdis purse *n.* shepherd's purse (*Capsella bursa-pastoris* L., → **2307**)
her(e *n.* hair
here-of *adv.* from this
hery *a.* growing in sandy places
heryn → **(h)ere**
herynge *n.* sense of hearing
hersgall *n.* feverfew (*Tanacetum parthenium* (L.) Sch.Bip., → **713**)
hert → **hard(e**
hert *n.* hart
hert(e *n.* heart
hertishorne *n.* buck-horn's plantain (*Plantago coronopus* L., → **1018**)
hertis-tonge *n.* hart's tongue fern (*Asplenium scolopendrium* L., → **923**)
hertwort *n.* bugle (*Ajuga reptans* L., → **919**)
hervyste *n.* autumn
hete → **(h)ete**
hete *n.* heat; body temperature
hete *v.* heat
heve *v.* raise, lift
hevede → **hed(e**
hevy *a.* heavy, possessing great weight; deep, profound
hyde *n.* hide, skin
hilwort *n.* wild thyme (*Thymus serpyllum*

L., → **1631**)
hyndale *n.* ?wood sage (*Teucrium scorodonia* L., → **133**)
hinder *a.* rear
hyng, hirt(e → **hong(e, hurt(e**
hokk* *n.* common mallow (*Malva sylvestris* L., → **1290**)
hoyle* *n.* husk
hol(ee *a.* healthy, whole; cured
hold(e *v.* hold
hole *n.* hole
holy fire *n.* some corroding skin disease, prob. herpes (→ **877**)
holy-hok *n.* marshmallow (*Althaea officinialis* L., → **849**)
holy rope *n.* hemp agrimony (*Eupatorium cannabinum* L., → **2495**)
holsom(e *a.* wholesome
hond(e *n.* hand
hondful *n.* handful
hong(e *v.* hang, suspend; be suspended; cling, adhere
hongynge *a.* dangling
hony *n.* honey
hony-sokyll *n.* melilot (*Melilotus* Mill. spp./*Trifolium* L. spp./*Medicago* L. spp., → **1448**)
hore *n.* filth, dirt
horehound(e *n.* white horehound (*Marrubium vulgare* L., → **935**)
horeworte *n.* cudweed/cottonrose (*Filago germanica* (L.) Huds./*F. pyramidata* L., → **884**)
hory *a.* dirty, foul
horne *n.* horn; awn, glume of the Gramineae
hors(e)mynte *n.* water-mint (*Mentha aquatica* L., → **863**)
horse-þistill *n.* bristly ox-tongue (*Helminthotheca echioides* (L.) Holub, → **606**)
horshele *n.* elecampane (*Inula elenium*

L., → **587, 899**)
horsho(ue *n.* purslane (*Portulaca oleracea* L., → **963, 976**)
horting *n.* injury, damage
hosyng *n.* ?pain (→ **1002–1004**)
hosnes(se *n.* hoarseness
host *n.* cough
hote *a.* hot, that has been heated; radiating heat
houndbery *n.* black nightshade (*Solanum nigrum* L., → **1519**)
hounde *n.* dog
houndfynell *n.* stinking camomile (*Anthemis cotula* L., → **856**)
houndystonge *n.* hound's-tongue (*Cynoglossum officinale* L., → **930**)
house *n.* house
houseleke *n.* houseleek (*Sempervivum tectorum* L., → **1031**)
howe *adv.* how
howndbene *n.* white horehound (*Marrubium vulgare* L., → **935**)
humo(u)r *n.* moisture; humour, one of the four chief fluids of the body
hurlyng *n.* rumbling sensation
hurt(e *v.* hurt

y(ch)chyng(e *n.* itching; itch
yarowe *n.* yarrow (*Achillea millefolium* L., → **1376**)
yate *n.* path
ydell *a.* foolish, delirious
ydrop *n.* dropsy
ye *pron.* ye
ȝekesterris *n.* ?early purple orchid (*Orchis mascula* (L.) L., → **2195**)
yel(l)ow(e *a.* yellow
yer *n.* year
yerde *n.* penis, virile member
yett *adv.* nonetheless
yeue *v.* give ¶ **y. oute** cause to discharge
yf *conj.* if

yf(f- → **yeue**
yl *a.* diseased
ilke *a.* same
ylike, -che *a.* similar
y-like *adv.* similarly, alike
in *adv.* inside; in
in *prep.* in
ynde *a.* indigo
Ynglis *n.* English language
inhanse* *v.* promote
inne *adv.* inside
inne *prep.* in
inner *a.* inner
ynnyrer *a.* inner
y-nowe *adv.* enough
in-to *prep.* into (*used to indicate directions and transformations*); until
in-warde *a.* inner, internal
yonge *a.* young
yongliche *a.* youthful, having a juvenile appearance
yongthe *n.* youth
yo(u)xe *n.* hiccup
yoxinge *n.* hiccupping
ypocandria *n.* abdomen, the soft part of the body between the ribs and the navel, particularly as a seat of body humours
ire-mole* *n.* rust spot
yryn *n.* iron
yrne *a.* made of iron
isope *n.* hyssop (*Hyssopus officinalis* L., → **986**)
(h)it *pron.* it
ive *n.* buck-horns plantain (*Plantago coronopus* L., → **1018**)
ivy *n.* ivy (*Hedera helix* L., → **1006**)

jaundys(e *n.* jaundice
jaw* *n.* jaw
joynt* *n.* joint
jornaye *n.* journey
ju(i)s(e *n.* juice
jubarbe *n.* houseleek (*Sempervivum tectorum* L., → **709, 1031**)
jule *n.* July
june *n.* June

labour *n.* painful work, toil
lack* *v.* lack
lady *n.* Lady, the Virgin Mary
lay *v.* place, lay
la(i)ste *adv.* last
land *n.* soil, ground
langage *n.* language
large *a.* abundant, copious; wide
largely *adv.* copiously, abundantly
lask* *v.* purge
lass(e *adv.* less
lasse *a.* smaller; lesser
lasse centorye *n.* common centaury (*Centaurium erythraea* Rafn., → **335**)
lasse sper-wort *n.* lesser spearwort (*Ranunculus flammula* L., → **1180**)
laste *a.* last
laste *v.* remain, continue
Latyn *n.* Latin
lat(te → **let(te**
launcell *n.* ribwort (*Plantago lanceolata* L., → **1938**); greater spearwort (*Ranunculus lingua* L., → **2175**)
lauandyr *n.* English lavender (*Lavandula angustifolia* Mill., → **1172**)
lavandyr coton *n.* sea wormwood (*Artemisia maritima* L., → **1175**)
law(e, lo- *a.* tepid
lawreoll *n.* spurge laurel (*Daphne laureola* L., → **1149**)
laxatife *a.* laxative, that causes diarrhoea; loose in the bowels, suffering from diarrhoea
laxatife *n.* laxative medicine
lax(e *a.* loose, unconstipated
leke *n.* leek (*Allium porrum* L., → **1112**)

leche* *n.* physician
lechery(e *n.* lechery, sexual lust
lecour(e, ly- *n.* liquid
lectuary* *n.* a medinal conserve or paste
leder *n.* a medicine that draws broken bones together
lefe *n.* leaf; petal
leg* *n.* leg
leynthe *n.* length
lemys → **lym**
lendys *n.* loins
lenthe *v.* lengthen, prolong
lepir(e *n.* leprosy
lese *v.* lose
lesior *n.* deadly nightshade (*Atropa bella-donna* L., → **579**)
less- → **lass-**
let(te, la- *v.* let, allow
lett *v.* hinder, impede; put an end to an illness
lettynge *n.* bloodletting, phlebotomy
letuse *n.* lettuce (*Lactuca sativa* L., → **1207**)
leþer, li- *a.* harmful, dangerous; wicked
leu(e)r(e, leuke- → **lyuer(e, luke-**
leuyr *n.* yellow flag (*Iris pseudoacorus* L.)
levirwort *n.* liverwort (*Marchantia polymorpha* L., → **1241**)
ly *v.* lie down, be prostrate
like *a.* similar
like *adv.* equally ¶ **l. moche** in the same quantity
like *prep.* like
lycorys *n.* licorise (rhyzome of *Glycyrrhiza glabra* L., → **1248**)
lyfe *n.* life
lyfe *v.* live
lyfte *a.* left
light *a.* cheeful, merry
light *v.* alight, settle on a horizontal surface

liȝtly *adv.* carefully, gently; easily, without difficulty
lyl(l)y *n.* white lily (*Lilium candidum* L., → **1136**)
lym *n.* limb
lymbryk* *n.* helminth, intestinal worm (prob. the threadworm, *Enterobius vermicularis* Linnaeus, 1758)
lynclope *n.* piece of linen
lyne *n.* flax (*Linum usitatissimum* L., → **741**)
lynyn *a.* linen, made of flax
lynsede *n.* linseed, seed of *Linum usitatissimum* L.
lyon* *n.* lion
liste *v.* please
litarge *n.* lethargy, morbid drowsiness (→ **1352**)
lite *adv.* little, not much
litell *a.* little, having a small size; scarce
literge, -y *n.* litharge, protoxide of lead (PbO).
lithwort *n.* pellitory-of-the-wall (*Parietaria judaica* L., → **1625**)
lyuer(e *n.* liver
lokk* *v.* join firmly; shut
loke *v.* take care, observe, make sure
lod* *v.* stick together
lode-worte *n.* bulbous buttercup (*Ranunculus bulbosus* L., → **1907**)
long *n.* lung
longe *a.* long
longe *adv.* for a long time
longe de beffe *n.* alkanet (*Anchusa arvensis* (L.) M.Bieb, → **1183**)
longwort *n.* hellebore (*Helleborus niger* L., *Veratrum album* L., → **1224**)
lord *n.* lord
lorrey *n.* laurel (*Laurus nobilis* L.)
lose *v.* lose
loue *v.* love, feel affection
louse* *n.* louse

louse* *v.* loose, release; dissolve
lovache *n.* lovage (*Levisticum officinale* W.D.J.Koch, → **1162**)
lowe *a.* set in the lower side; lowered, adulterated with water
lowe, la- *adv.* in a low position, little above the ground
luke *a.* lukewarm
luke-warme *a.* lukewarm
lvnary *n.* Italian starwort (*Aster amellus* L., → **1253**)
lunatike *a.* insane
lupyn(e *n.* lupin (*Lupinus albus* L., → **1192**)
luste *n.* desire

make *v.* make, produce; cause ¶ m. **vryn(e** urinate; cause to urinate ¶ m. **neshe** cure costipation ¶ m. **rome** clear up the breast
madyr *n.* madder (*Rubia tinctorum* L., → **1271**)
magiron *n.* sweet marjoram (*Origanum majorana* L., → **1265**)
may *v.* may, be able to; have the power of
mayden *n.* young woman
maidenhere *n.* maidenhair spleenwort (*Asplenium trichomanes* L., → **1301**)
may(e *n.* May
maister *n.* master, teacher; medical authority
maistrey *n.* efficacy
maythe *n.* stinking camomile (*Anthemis cotula* L., → **856**)
mal de fla(u)nke *n.* pain in the side
malady *n.* disease, illness
male *a.* male
malencoly *n.* black bile; excess of black bile, melancholy
maloue *n.* common mallow (*Malva sylvestris* L., → **1290**)
malt *n.* malt, grain prepared for brewing

mandrag(ge *n.* mandrake (*Mandragora* L. spp., → **1416**)
maner(e *n.* manner, method of action; species, kind, sort
many *a.* abundant in number; diverse
man(ne *n.* human being; male human being
marche *n.* some celery (*Apium* L. spp.)
marice *n.* uterus, womb
marygoldye *n.* chicory (*Cichorium intybus* L., → **1942**)
mastik *n.* mastic, gum resin from *Pistacia lentiscus* L.
mater *n.*[1] womb
mater *n.*[2] body fluid
matrice *n.* uterus, womb
maufete *n.* a sudden turn for the worse in an illness
mawe *n.* liver; uterus, womb
maworte *n.* ?bloody cranesbill (*Geranium sanguineum* L., → **1286**)
mekyll *adv.* much
mede* *n.* meadow
medemynt *n.* water-mint (*Mentha aquatica* L., → **863**)
medewort *n.* common balm (*Melissa officinalis* L., → **1355**)
med(i)cyne *n.* the science of healing; medicament
medill *n.* middle
medill *v.* mix, combine ingredients
melilote *n.* melilot (*Melilotus* Mill. spp./*Trifolium* L. spp./*Medicago* L. spp., → **1448**)
mel(le *n.* meal, flour
mell(e *v.* mix
membre *n.* member; virile member
memorye *n.* memory
men *pron.* one
meng(e mix
menysoun *n.* dysentery
menstrue *n.* menses, catamenia

merke *n.* mark, sign
mercury *n.* allgood (*Chenopodium bonus-henricus* L., → **1312**)
mery *a.* merry
mesell *a.* afflicted with leprosy, leper
mete *n.* solid food (*as opposed to* **drynke**); the fleshy pith of a stalk of cabbage; meal
meting *n.* nightmare
meve*, **mo-** *v.* move; stir
myche *a.* large; much
myche, **mo-** *adv.* in great quantity; frequently
mydday *n.* midday
mydryd *n.* diaphragm
mighty *a.* potent, efficacious
mygrane *n.* migraine, strong headache
myys *n.* crumb
milk(e *n.* milk; sap, latex
milken *v.* extract the juice
mill *n.* mill
myl(le)foly *n.* yarrow (*Achillea millefolium* L., → **1376**)
mylt(e *n.* spleen
mynde *n.* memory
mynte *n.* mint (*Mentha* L. spp., → **1318**)
myr(re *n.* myrrh, gum resin exuded from *Commiphora myrrha* (Nees) Engl.
myschefe *n.* misfortune, calamity
myssay* *v.* say something amiss or erroneous
mistilte *n.* mistletoe (*Viscum album* L., → **1462**)
myte* *n.* mite, a parasitic arthropod that burrows into skin and causes scabies (*Sarcoptes scabiei* Linnaeus 1758)
mo *a.* more
modir *n.* mother; uterus
mogwort *n.* mugwort (*Artemisia vulgaris* L., → **1385**)
moyle *n.* chilblain, mole
moist(e *a.* moist

molayne *n.* great mullein (*Verbascum thapsus* L., → **1443**)
mone *n.* moon
mon(e)th *n.* month
montayne *n.* mountain
morall n white horehound (*Marrubium vulgare* L., → **935**)
mor(e *a.* larger in size; greater in degree or extent
more *n.*¹ root
more *n.*² moor, wasteland
more *adv.* more
more centory *n.* some knapweed (*Centaurea centaurium* L./*C. nigra* L., → **646**)
more centuary *n.* St. John's wort (*Hypericum perforatum* L., → **646**);
more morel *a.* deadly nightshade (*Atropa bella-donna* L., → **579**)
morell *n.* black nightshade (*Solanum nigrum* L., → **1371**)
morfue *n.* morphew, a skin disease (→ **102**)
mornyng *n.* morning, beginning of the day
morow(e *n.* morning, beginning of the day; the day after the present
morre y-bitt *n* autumnal hawkbit (*Scorzoneroides autumnalis* (L.) Moench, → **1306**)
morter *n.* mortar, vessel used to pound ingredients with a pestle
mostarde *n.* black mustard (*Brassica nigra* (L.) K.Koch, → **1327**)
moste *v.* must, have to
moste *a.* main, principal
moth* *n.* clothing moth (*Tineola bisselliella* (Hummel, 1823)), a well-known pest of fabrics
mount syon *n.* ?lesser water-parsnip/marsh speedwell (*Berula erecta* (Huds.) Coville/*Veronica scutellata*

L., → **784**)
mouse* *n.* mouse
m(o)ust(e *n.* must, grape juice
mo(u)th *n.* mouth
mowsere *n.* mouse-ear hawkweed (*Pilosella officinarum* Vaill., → **1468**)
multiply* *v.* enlarge, make bigger; augment the quantity of sth.

nakyd *a.* naked
(n)addyr *n.* snake, serpent, adder
nayl* *n.* fingernail
name *n.* name
namely *adv.* especially, in particular
narthe *n.* congestion in the breast, asthma (→ **840**)
nase- → **nose-**
nature *n.* nature, temperament; feature; physical condition
navill *n.* navel
ne *conj.* no; nor
nec(ke *n.* neck
n(e)y *adv.* almost; almost
nepe *n.* lesser calamint (*Clinopodium nepeta* (L.) Kuntze, → **1526**)
nepte ryall *n.* lesser calamint (*Clinopodium nepeta* (L.) Kuntze, → **1504**)
nerue* *n.* nerve
nese *v.* sneeze
nese-þrell*, **nestryll*** *n.* nostril
nesh(e *a.* soft in texture, not dense; loose; flexible ¶ **be n.** suffer from diarrhoea ¶ **n. egg** soft-boiled egg
neshe* *v.* soften; loosen the bowels
nesse *n.* nose
nettyll *n.* nettle (*Urtica* L. spp., → **1477**)
neuer *adv.* never
new(e *a.* recent; not yet used
newe* *v.* renew, make new again
new(e)fratik *n.* nephritis
newfratik *a.* suffering from nephritis

nyght *n.* night (as opposed to **day(e**); night used as a time measure
nyght-shade *n.* black nightshade (*Solanum nigrum* L., → **1519**)
nys → **be**
nyt* *n.* nit, egg of a louse
no *a.* no, none
no *adv.* not
nobill *a.* good, efficacious; agreeable to the taste
noy *v.* harm
noyse *n.* noise
non(e *a.* none
none *pron.* no one
norys(he *n.* wet nurse
norish* *v.* nourish; supply with the necessary to promote growth or formation; strengthen
nose-holle* *n.* nostril
nos(s)e *n.* nose
nos(se)t(h)ril(l, na- *n.* nostril
not(e *adv.* not
notemyge *n.* nutmeg, seed of *Myristica fragrans* Houtt. (→ **1539**)
not(te *n.* nut
noþing(e *pron.* nothing
noþinge *adv.* not at all
nothir *conj.* neither
no(u)ght(e *adv.* not

o *a.* one, a single
oke *n.* oak
oke-verne *n.* oak-fern (*Gymnocarpium dryopteris* (L.) Newman, → **1899**)
oculus Christi *n.* ?wild clary (*Salvia verbenaca* L., → **1616**)
od(o)ur(e *n.* odour; aroma
of *prep.* of; from; for
oft(e *adv.* often
of(te)-tyme(s *adv.* often
oftyn *adv.* often
oyl(le *n.* oil; albumen ¶ **paynter o.**

linseed oil
oynement, oynt- *n.* ointment
oynone gresse *n.* sea onion (*Drimia maritima* (L.) Stearn, → **1607**)
oyno(w)n *n.* onion (*Allium cepa* L., → **1581**)
oiþer → **oþer(e** *conj.*
olde *a.* that has lived long (*opp.* yonge) ¶ that has existed for a long time (*opp.* new(e)
olifant *n.* elephant
olyfe, -ue *n.* olive, fruit of the *Olea europaea* L.
on, an *prep.* on
on(e *a.* one
on(e *pron.* (the first) one; one
one *adv.* by itself
ony → **eny**
onys *adv.* once
only *adv.* only
opon → **vpon**
op(p)yn *v.* give access to what was locked; discover what was closed; clear an obturation
or, er *adv.* before
or *conj.* or
origanum *n.* wild marjoram (*Origanum vulgare* L., → **1553**)
orpyn *n.* orpine (*Sedum telephium* L., → **1550**)
osm(o)unde *n.* royal fern (*Osmunda regalis* L., → **667, 1613**)
ostricium *n.* soapwort (*Saponaria officinalis* L., → **1571**)
oþer → **od(o)ur(e**
oþer *pron.* other
oþer(e *a.* other, different; second
oþer(e *conj.* or
oþer-w(e)ys(se *adv.* differently; otherwise
otyn *a.* made of oat
ouercome* *v.* overcome, cure an illness
oute *adv.* out

ovyn *n.* oven
ovir *prep.* over
ovir-all *adv.* especially
ovyr-hede *adv.* above, over the head (→ **2065**)
ovir-myche *a.* excessive
ox *n.* ox
oxetonge *n.* alkanet (*Anchusa arvensis* (L.) M.Bieb, → **1183**)

payne *n.* pain
paynter *n.* painter
pal(le)sy *n.* palsy
pan(e *n.* pan
papy *n.* poppy (*Papaver* L. spp., → **1694**)
pappe *n.* woman's breast
papwort *n.* allgood (*Chenopodium bonus-henricus* L., → **1312**)
paralityk(e *n.* palsy; a person afflicted with palsy
paratory *n.* pellitory-of-the-wall (*Parietaria judaica* L., → **1625**)
park-levis *n.* chaste tree (*Vitex agnus-castus* L., → **2291**)
part(e *n.* part
party *n.* part, fraction; zone, area
passe *v.* pass
passyng *adv.* exceedingly, very
passyon *n.* disorder, disease
paste *n.* pasty, dough
pas(tyr)nepe *n.* parsnip (*Pastinaca sativa* L., → **1720**)
pedelyon *n.* black hellebore (*Helleborus niger* L., → **1851**)
pelletir *n.* pellitory of Spain (*Anacyclus pyrethrum* (L.) Lag., → **1820**)
pen *n.* feather
peny *n.* penny
peny-wight *n.* pennywight, one third of a dram
pepill *n.* people
pepir *n.* pepper, seed of *Piper nigrum* L.

percil(y *n.* parsley (*Petroselinum crispum* (Mill.) Fuss, → **1799**)
pere* *v.* damage, deteriorate, impair
perill *n.* danger, risk
perle *n.* pearl
pers *v.* perforate, pierce
pese *n.* pea, seed of *Pisum sativum* L.
pest(i)lens(e *n.* (bubonic) plague
pety morell *n.* black nightshade (*Solanum nigrum* L., → **1519**)
philozofur *n.* philosopher, scholar, wise man
pyany *n.* peony (*Paeonia* L. spp., → **1672**)
pichon* *n.* dove, pigeon
pigil(le *n.* wild marjoram (*Origanum vulgare* L., → **1634**)
piletir of Spayne *n.* hellebore (*Helleborus niger* L., *Veratrum album* L., → **1224**)
pyment *n.* an aromatic ointment
pympirnell *n.* scarlet pimpernel (*Anagallis arvensis* L., → **1859**)
pyntill *n.* virile member, penis
pipe *n.* fistula (→ **857**)
pisse *v.* urinate
pithe *n.* medulla, the central column of spongy cellular tissue in the stems and branches of dicotyledonous plants; inward part of an organ
place *n.* place
playne *a.* smooth, free from unevenness
pla(y)nteyn(e *n.* waybread (*Plantago major* L., → **1736**)
pla(i)ster *n.* plaster
plaster* *v.* apply or cover with plaster
plaster-wyse *adv.* in the manner of a plaster
plente *n.* abundance
plowe *n.* plough, make furrows
podyng *n.* pudding, a kind of sausage
poyson *n.* poison
polycary(a *n.* fleawort (*Plantago indica* L., → **1881**, **1888**)

polypody *n.* oak-fern (*Gymnocarpium dryopteris* (L.) Newman, → **665**, **1899**)
pol(l)ucyon *n.* involuntary seminal emission
pomigarnet *n.* pomegranate, fruit of *Punica granatum* L.
pon(d)e *n.* pound, crush
porke *n.* pork, flesh of swine
porcion *n.* portion
pore *n.* leek (*Allium porrum* L.)
porre* *n.* pore, orifice of the sweat-glands (→ **2293**)
portulake *n.* purslane (*Portulaca oleracea* L., → **976**, **1868**)
pose *n.* catarrh, cold in the head
postem(e *n.* morbid swelling, gathering of noxious humours
potage, -che *n.* thick soup, stew
potager(e *n.* podagra, gout in the foot
potell *n.* pottle, half a gallon
pot(t *n.* pot, round vessel
pouder *n.* powder
pounce *n.* pulse
pounde *n.* pound, a weight equal to twelve ounces (*ca.* 373 g)
po(u)n(d)e *v.* crush, grind
poure *v.* pour, scum liquids so that the heaviest matter remains in the bottom of the vessel
pray* *v.* pray, beseech
precious *a.* valuable, excellent
preu- → **priu-**
preue *v.* prove
prikk *v.* cause a pricking sensation
prykk* *n.* thorn, spine
prym(e)rose *n.* primrose (*Primula vulgaris* Huds., → **1841**)
principale *n.* main, principal
priue *a.* sexual
priuete *n.* genitals
profit* *v.* be helpful

profitable *a.* beneficial, useful
pulyoll *n.* pennyroyal (*Mentha pulegium* L., → **1653**)
pulyoll monten *n.* wild thyme (*Thymus serpyllum* L., → **1631**)
purgacion *n.* purgative medicine, emetic
purge *v.* purge, cleanse through emetics
purpill *a.* purple
purpur(e *a.* purple, reddish
put(te *v.* put

quake* *v.* tremble
quakyng(e *n.* trembling spasm
quantite *n.* quantity
quarte *n.* quart, a liquid measure
quarteyn *a.* quartan
quarten *n.* quartan fever
quell *v.* kill; alleviate
quench- → **quynch-**
quyk *n.* quick, ungual bed
quy(c)k *a.* raw, not covered by the epidermis; fiery, readily inflammable
quik-syluer *n.* quicksilver, mercury
quynacy → **squynacy(e**
quynche *v.* quench, extinguish sth. by cooling it
quynfoyly *n.* cinquefoil (*Potentilla reptans* L., → **2236**)
quyt(t)er(e *n.* pus, suppurating matter

radich *n.* radish (*Raphanus sativus* L., → **1923**)
raggid *a.* pinnated
ragworte ragwort (*Jacobaea vulgaris* Gaertn., → **1930**)
rayne rain
ram(m)ys-fote *n.* bulbous buttercup (*Ranunculus bulbosus* L., → **1907**)
rat* *n.* rat
rawe *a.* raw, uncooked
rede *a.* red

rede dokk *n.* some undescribed *Rumex* spp., perhaps wood dock (*R. sanguineus* L.)
rede mader *n.* (*prob. a mistake*) sarrasine (*Aristolochia longa* L., → **67**)
rede nettill *n.* red deadnettle (*Lamium purpureum* L., → **1477**)
reder *n.* reader
r(e)yn* *n.* kidney; zone of the loins under which the kidneys are located
relesse *n.* relief, deliverance from pain
relesse *v.* relieve, alleviate
releue* *v.* alleviate, mitigate
relowse* *v.* relieve
remedy *n.* remedy, cure
ren(e *v.* flow freely; discharge; suppurate; deoppilate by draining out the dangerous humour ¶ **r. oute** let liquids flow freely; cleanse the body by the flowing off of dangerous humours
renewe *v.* renew, restore to the previous conditions
ren(n)yng(e *a.* flowing
rennyng *n.* flow
res(c)eyue *v.* ingest, take into the body
reseyte *n.* medical prescription
rest *v.* lie undisturbed, macerate
restore *v.* restore, bring to a healthy state
restreyn* *v.* staunch, stop the flow of a body liquid
reve* *v.* remove, take away
rew(e *n.* rue (*Ruta graveolens* L., → **1947**)
rewme *n.* catarrh in the head; morbid defluxion of humours; rheumatism, inflammation of the joints
rib* *n.* rib
rybwort *n.* ribwort (*Plantago lanceolata* L., → **1938**)
ryk(k)yll(s *n.* frankincense
rige *n.* back, spine
right *a.* right (as opposed to **lyfte**)
right *adv.* very, completely

rynde *n.* bark
ripe *a.* ripe, mature
rip(p)e *v.* ripen, become mature; come to a head
rise* *v.* rise ¶ **r. vp** spring up; be on one's feet
rysynge *n.* eruption on the skin
roche *n.* rock
rodewort *n.* chicory (*Cichorium intybus* L., → **1942**)
roysyng *a.* made of roses
romayne *a.* Latin language
rome *a.* clear from congestion
ronde *a.* round
ronde astrologi *n.* smearwort (*Aristolochia rotunda* L., → **67**)
rose-mary(e *n.* rosemary (*Rosmarinus officinalis* L., → **1985**)
rosyn *n.* rosin, distillate of turpentine
rosyne *n.* raisin
ros(s)e *n.* rose (*Rosa* L. spp., → **1969**)
roste *v.* roast
rote *n.* root
rottynge *n.* putrefaction
rounde *a.* round
rowme* *v.* clear from congestion
rub- → **rib-**
rub(be *v.* rub, smear
rwe → **rew(e**

sache, safe → **(h)ache** *n.*², **saue**
saf(f)ron *n.* saffron, dried stigmas from *Crocus sativus* L. (→ **2104**)
sag(g)e → **sa(ug)ge**
say *v.* say
salt(te *n.* salt
salue *n.* healing ointment, salve
sam(e *pron.* same
same *a.* same
sanke dragon *n.* resin of the dragon tree (*Dracaena draco* L.)
sanguynary *n.* shepherd's purse (*Capsella bursa-pastoris* L., → **2307**)
sangwyne *a.* blood-red
saucere *n.* saucer
saue *n.* Florentine iris (*Iris × germanica* L. var. *florentina* (L.) Dykes, → **2097**)
saue *v.* save
sauer(a)y *n.* savory (*Satureja* L. spp., → **2046**)
sauery *a.* tasty; pleasant in breath
sa(ug)ge *n.* sage (*Salvia officinalis* L., → **2080**)
sauo(u)r(e *n.* odour; taste; scent; smell
sause *n.* sauce
saute *n.* heat, sexual arousal
sav(e)yn(e *n.* savin (*Juniperus sabina* L., → **2058**)
savygill *n.* soapwort (*Saponaria officinalis* L., → **2068**)
saxfrage *n.* burnet saxifrage (*Pimpinella saxifraga* L., → **2201**)
scabbe *n.* eczema, scabies (→ **413**)
scabbid *a.* scabby, mangy
scabyous *n.* devil's-bit scabious (*Succisa pratensis* Moench, → **2206**)
scabwort *n.* ?wild clary (*Salvia verbenaca* L., → **1616**)
skal(le *n.* a scabby skin disease
scall*, **sha-** *v.* scald, burn with a hot liquid
scamony *n.* root of scamony (*Convolvulus scammonia* L.)
skap(e → **shap(pe**
skem* *v.* skim, remove impurities from a liquid
schale* *n.* scale, crust on the skin
skyn(ne *n.* skin
skyrwhite *n.* parsnip (*Pastinaca sativa* L.); rocket (*Eruca sativa* Mill., → **2161**)
scle- → **sle-**
sclepy *a.* sleepy, lethargic
scolemaister *n.* schoolmaster
skolle *n.* skull

scome of syluer litharge obtained from silver
scome *v.* skim impurities
scroffe *n.* ?scurf, dandruff (→ **1353**)
scropion* *n.* scorpion
se *v.* perceive with the eyes; have the faculty of sight
seke *a.* ill, diseased
seke *n.* sick person
sek(e)man* *n.* sick person
sekenes(se *n.* sickness
seconde *pron.* second
sec(o)und(e *n.* afterbirth, placenta
sec(o)und(e *a.* second
sed(e *n.* seed
see *n.* sea
seynt Mary seall *n.* black bryony (*Dioscorea communis* (L.) Caddick & Wilkin, → **2277**)
seynte Mary sede *n.* common sowthistle (*Sonchus oleraceus* L., → **2189**)
seme *v.* seem
sercle *n.* circle
serfoyle → **kerwell**
serpent* *n.* serpent
serpentary *n.* dragons (*Dracunculus vulgaris* Schott, → **38**)
ses(s)e *v.* cease pain; soothe, appease; heal from fluxes by cutting down the flow
set(t *v.* set, put; cause to be
seþ(e *v.* boil, cook in a liquid
shall *v.* shall (aux. to indicate necessity or future fulfilment)
shape* *v.* form in a certain way
shap(pe, sk- *n.* shape, form; female genitals
sharpe* *v.* make keen, render more acute
sharpe *a.* rough; sharp (*prob. a mistake,* → **920**); pricky, spiny
shaue *v.* scrape
she *pron.* she
shelowe *a.* ?emaciated (→ **508**)

shepe *n.* sheep
shere *v.* shear, cut
shyne* *v.* shine
shorte *a.* having small physical extent; brief, lasting but little time
shortly *adv.* recently, not long ago
shred(e *v.* shred, cut into thin slices
shrink* *v.* wither
sykynge *n.* difficult breathing, fit of asthma
syde *n.* side
siʒt(e *n.* sight
silfe-hele *n.* bugle (*Ajuga reptans* L., → **223, 919**)
siluer *n.* silver ¶ **s. fome** litharge obtained from silver
synkefoly *n.* cinquefoil (*Potentilla reptans* L., → **2236**)
synew* *n.* sinew, tendon; nerve
synge *n.* sign of the zodiac
singe *v.* sing
sit *v.* sit
slak* *v.* relieve, mitigate
sle *v.* kill; supress poison; resolve an abscess, cure a skin disease; rot
slepe *n.* sleep, repose
slepe *v.* sleep
slyt *v.* divide
smalache *n.* smallage (*Apium graveolens* L.)
smal(le *a.* small
smal(le *adv.* into small pieces
smell *n.* smell; aroma, pleasant odour
smell *v.* smell, inhale, sniff
smere* *v.* apply a medical preparation
smere-worte *n.* allgood (*Chenopodium bonus-henricus* L., → **1312**)
smert *n.* waterpepper (*Persicaria hydropiper* (L.) Delarbre)
smyll → **smell**
smyte *v.* attack, affect suddenly ¶ **s. þrowe** cut through

smoke *n.* smoke
smoke *v.* emit smoke
snake *n.* snake
so *adv.* so
sodeyn *a.* sudden
sode(y)nly *adv.* suddenly, without warning
softe *a.* soft
softely *adv.* softly, gently
sole *n.* sole of foot
solibyll *a.* loose, free from constipation
somdel(le *adv.* somewhat
som(e *a.* some
somer *n.* summer
somertyme *n.* summertime
som-tyme *adv.* sometime, now and then
sone *adv.* soon, within a short time
son(ne *n.* sun
sop* *n.*[1] piece of bread dipped in a liquid
sop* *n.*[2] draught, small amount of drink
soper *n.* supper
sore *n.* pain; wound, sore, ulcer
sore *a.* grievous; suffering from pain
sore *adv.* severely
sorell de boys *n.* wood sorrel (*Oxalis acetosella* L., → **2469**)
soþe *n.* truth
soþly *adv.* assuredly, certainly
soude* *v.* heal a fracture, knit
soupe *v.* sip, drink in small mouthfuls
soure *a.* sour
souredok(ke *n.* common sorrel (*Rumex acetosa* L., → **2262**)
souerayn(e *a.* outstanding, very efficient or potent, excellent
sowble* *v.* mollify
sowe-þistill *n.* common sowthistle (*Sonchus oleraceus* L., → **2189**)
sowtheryne-wode *n.* southernwood (*Artemisia abrotanum* L., → **2111**)
space *n.* space, lapse between two points in time

sparowe-tonge *n.* knotgrass (*Polygonum aviculare* L., → **2156**)
spasom *n.* spasm ¶ **cold(e s.** shiver
speke *v.* speak
spece, -i- *n.* species, type
speche *n.* faculty of speech
spere *n.* spear
spereworte *n.* greater spearwort (*Ranunculus lingua* L., → **2175**)
sper-hede *n.* greater spearwort (*Ranunculus lingua* L., → **2175**)
spet* *n.* spit out
spettill *n.* saliva
spewyng(e *n.* spitting
spice* *n.* spice
spikynter* *n.* splinter
spyknard *n.* spikenard (*Nardostachys jatamansi* (D.Don) DC.)
spill* *v.* ruin, spoil
spirit(e *n.* vital principle; ghost
spit(t *v.* spit
splene *n.* spleen
spone *n.* spoon
sponefull *n.* spoonful
sporge *n.* squirting cucumber (*Ecballium elaterium* (L.) A.Rich., → **2217**)
spot* *n.* spot
spotill *n.* saliva
spo(u)rge *v.* cleanse
sprakle* *v.* speckle, mark with speckles
sprynge *v.* sprinkle
spume of siluer *n.* litharge obtained from silver
spv- → **spew-, spo-**
(s)quynacy(e *n.* quinsy, tonsillitis
stafe *n.* staff, stick, rod
stafisagre *n.* stavesacre (*Delphinium staphisagria* L., → **2226**)
stalke *n.* stalk
stale *a.* stale, clear from lees and impurities
stamp(e *v.* pound, bray in a mortar

stanche *n.* shepherd's purse (*Capsella bursa-pastoris* L., → **2307**)
standilgose *n.* ?early purple orchid (*Orchis mascula* (L.) L., → **2195**)
standylwelkys *m* ?early purple orchid (*Orchis mascula* (L.) L., → **2195**)
stang *n.* animal bite; sting
stannmarche *n.* horse parsley (*Smyrnium olusatrum* L., → **85**)
sta(u)nche *v.* stop the flow of a flux; cease flowing
stek* *v.* stick, lock, prevent from delivery
stede *n.* place
stench *n.* offensive odour
stiken *v.* fasten with a nail
stiche *n.* stich, sharp pain in the side
stife → **styve**
still *v.* distil
stynk* *v.* emit an offensive odour
stynke *n.* offensive odour
stynkyn(ge *a.* foul smelling
styng(e *n.* sting, the sharp-pointed organ in certain insects; stinging, bite of an insect
styng(g)yng(e *n.* stinging, bite of an insect
stir* *v.* move, set in motion; stimulate
styve *v.* boil slowly; take a hot bath
stok(e *n.* stem or trunk of a plant
stokwort *n.* wood sorrel (*Oxalis acetosella* L., → **2469**)
stofe *v.* stuff, fill the inside of an animal
stoyne* *v.* stun, stupefy, cause to be numb
stomak(e *n.* stomach
ston(e *n.* stone; calculus, kidney stone
stond(e *v.* stand up; stop the flow; remain undisturbed
stonecrop *n.* common stonecrop (*Sedum acre* L., → **2151**)
stonge* *v.* sting
stony *a.* growing in rocky places
stoppe *v.* stop; oppilate, obstruct; cover tightly, seal
stop(p)yng(e *n.* oppilation, obstruction
strayn* *v.* strain, filter
straitnes *v.* constriction of the breast, asthma
strawbery *n.* wild strawberry (*Fragaria vesca* L., → **2181**)
streynth(e *n.* strength, physical vigour; intensity; healing power
streite *a.* constricted, tight
strenth *v.* strengthen
stri(c)chell, -e- *n.* uvula; some disease of the uvula, ?staphyledema (→ **449**)
stryle *n.* knotgrass (*Polygonum aviculare* L., → **2156**)
stroke *n.* blow, slash
str(o)y *v.* destroy; neutralize; strengthen (*a copy mistake,* → **2350**)
strong(e *a.* strong, vigorous; intense; having great healing powers
stronge *adv.* intensely; abundantly
strongly *adv.* intensely; strongly
strow(e *v.* scatter
subiugacioun *n.* suffumigation, the process of causing fumes to penetrate a part of the body
suche *a.* such
suche *pron.* such
suffyr *v.* suffer, resist pain; tolerate
sum *pron.* someone; a small quantity, a bit
sum-whate *pron.* somewhat, a small quantity
superfluyte *n.* overabundance, excessive quantity
sursanour* *n.* superficially healed wound
suspecion *n.* suspicion
swage *v.* relieve pain; reduce swelling
swalowe *n.* swallow (*Hirundo rustica* Linnaeus, 1758)
swarme *n.* swarm, colony of bees
swell *v.* swell, increase

swel(l)yng(e *n.* swelling, tumour; inflammation
swellyng(e *a.* swelling
swellow *v.* swallow
swete *a.* sweet, having the taste of sugar or honey; having a pleasant aroma
swete *v.* sweat
sweting *n.* sweating
swyne* *n.* swine (*Sus scrofa* ssp. *domestica* Linnaeus, 1758)
swynes-carsse *n.* knotgrass (*Polygonum aviculare* L., → **2156**)
swynes-fenyll *n.* hog's fennel (*Peucedanum officinale* L., → **2186**)
swython *n.* common groundsel (*Senecio vulgaris* L., → **824**)

t(o)uche *n.* touch
take *v.* take, seize; ingest, swallow; receive; remove; attack suddenly
tayl* *n.* tail
talent *n.* sexual appetite
talo(we *n.* suet, animal fat
tame *a.* cultivated
tans(e)y *n.* tansy (*Tanacetum vulgare* L., → **2283**)
taperwort *n.* great mullein (*Verbascum thapsus* L., → **1443**)
taste *n.* taste, savour
tawarde *prep.* towards
teche* *v.* teach
tell* *v.* tell, narrate
temper *n.* mood, mental state
temper *v.* soften ⁋ **t. togeder** mix in equal proportions
temple* *n.* temple of the head
tendir *a.* tender, yielding easily to pressure
tendryn *n.* tendril, tendron, sprout (→ **1696**)
tenture *n.* medicated roll
tercian *a.* tertian

tercian *n.* tertian fever
tesyll *n.* teasel, some *Dipsacus* L. sp.
teter* *n.* tetter, some skin disease causing a burning sensation, probably ringworm (→ **953**)
tyas- → **tysa-**
tike* *n.* tick (*Ixodes ricinus* Linnaeus, 1758)
tyde *n.* time of day
tyle *n.* tile, slab of burnt clay
till *conj.* till, until
till *prep.* to; over
tyme *n.*^{1} time; each of the several instances of a recurring action
tyme *n.*^{2} garden thyme (*Thymus vulgaris* L., → **2314**)
tynd* *n.* antler
tysain(e *n.*^{1} ptisan, medical decoction
tysayn(e *n.*^{2} sciatica
tysik(e *n.* phthisis
tit* *n.* nipple; prolapsed varicose vein
to *n.* toe
to *adv.*^{1} too
to *adv.*^{2} to a place
to *prep.* to; to (*before infinitives*); into; against (*when referring to illnesses*); similar to
to → **two(o**
tobbe *n.* tub, open wooden vessel
to-for *adv.* earlier, previously
to-for *prep.* before
to-gad(e)rys *adv.* together
to-geder *adv.* together
tole *n.* tool, instrument
ton *n.* large cask
tong(e *n.* tongue; language
top(pe *n.* top, highest part
tornynge *n.* translation
toþe *n.* tooth
toþe-ake, -ache *n.* toothache
totheworte *n.* shepherd's purse (*Capsella bursa-pastoris* (L.) Medik., → **2307**)

toun *v.* store in a vessel
toune-carse *n.* garden cress (*Lepidium sativum* L.)
to(u)rne *v.* turn; translate
travaill *n.* toil, hard physical labour; labour, pains of childbirth
tre *n.* tree
tremlyng *a.* trembling, shaking
trewly *adv.* confidently
trodel* *n.* pellet of animal dung
trowe *v.* believe, trust
turmentil(le *n.* common tormentil (*Potentilla erecta* (L.) Raeusch., → **2324**)
tutesayne *n.* chaste tree (*Vitex agnus-castus* L., → **2291**)
tvtymallys *n.* sun spurge (*Euphorbia helioscopia* L., → **2332**)
two(o *a.* two

þan *adv.* then, immediately afterwards
thar → **thurfe***
that *pron.* that one
that *dem. a.* that
that *conj.* that; so that
þe *dem. a. (def. art.)* the
þe *adv.* the... the... (*in comparisons*)
þey *conj.* though
þei *pron.* they
þen *conj.* than (*with comparatives*)
ther *adv.* in that place; in that moment; in that case, then; on the other hand
þer(e *adv.* where
þere-by *adv.* thereby
ther-fro *adv.* from that place
þer(e)-of(fe *adv.* from that place; for that reason
þer(e)-to *adv.* thereto, to that place
þer(e)-vp(p)on(e *adv.* thereupon
þer(e)-with *adv.* therewith, with that
þer(e-for *adv.* therefore, for that reason
þer-in(ne *adv.* in that place; with that

þer-on *adv.* thereon, on that place
þer-ovir *adv.* above that
þerst → **þorst**
þik(k *a.* dense; fleshy
þick *adv.* densely
þiesse *n.* thigh
thyn(e *a.* thin
þinge *n.* thing
þird(e *a.* third
þirde *pron.* third
þis *pron.* this one
this *dem. a.* this
þorn* *n.* thorn
thorsday *n.* Thursday
þorst *n.* thirst
þ(o)u *pron.* thou
þre *a.* three
þrede *n.* thread; stigma of saffron
þre-levid-grasse *n.* melilot (*Melilotus* Mill. spp./*Trifolium* L. spp./*Medicago* L. spp., → **1448**)
þryse *adv.* three times
þrote *n.* throat
þrow(e *prep.* through; from one end to the other; by means of; because of
þrowe *adv.* fully, completely
thurfe* *v.* need

v-levys *n.* cinquefoil (*Potentilla reptans* L.)
vnbynde* *v.* make loose, release; deoppilate
vnce *n.* ounce, a weight equal to eight drams (*ca.* 31.1 g)
vnkynde *a.* unnatural, injurious to health
vncome* *n.* boil
vndir *prep.* under
vndirlay* *v.* lay underneath
vndir-pitt *v.* apply as a suppository
vndirstond *v.* understand
vndirstonder *n.* one who understand, i.e. a learned person

vnneth *adv.* with difficulty; never
vnremeve *v.* leave undisturbed
vnto *prep.* until; (*in the collocation* **like vnto**) similar, resembling to
vnworthy *a.* unworthy, of no value
vpon, a-, o- *prep.* upon
vp(pe *adv.* up
vppyn *a* open
vpwarde *adv.* upwards; (*in relation to evacuation*) upwards, i.e. throwing up
ureste *n.* wrist
vryn(e *n.* urine
vse *v.* use, employ
vtmost *a.* outmost, most external

valey* *n.* valley
veccy* *n.* blister
veyne *n.* vein
venym(e *a.* poisonous
venym(e *n.* poison
venymous, -ys *a.* venomous
verne, f- *n.* fern, species from phylum Pteridophytae
vertyne *n.* vertigo
vertu(e *n.* strength; healing power
vertu(u)s *a.* full of medicinal powers; wholesome, beneficial
verv(e)yn(e *n.* vervain/hedge mustard (*Verbena officinalis* L./*Sisymbrium officinale* (L.) Scop., → **2431**)
vessell, f- *n.* vessel, vase
vigill *n.* vigil, day before a holy day
vyne → **wyne** *n.*²
vyneger, ve- *n.* vinegar
violent *a.* violent, excessively intense
vyolet(t *n.* sweet violet (*Viola odorata* L., → **2518**)
virgyn *a.* virgin
vl-, vr- → **wl-, fr-**
voide* *v.* cure
vo(y)mit(te, f- *n.* vomit
vo(i)se *n.* voice

way(e *n.* way
waybred(e *n.* waybread (*Plantago major* L., → **1736**)
wayworte *n.* scarlet pimpernel (*Anagallis arvensis* L., → **1859**)
walkyne *n.* sky, firmament
wall* *n.* wall
walworte *n.* hellebore (*Helleborus niger* L./*Veratrum album* L., → **2385**)
wane* *v.* wane
wanyng *n.* waning, last quarter of the moon
warance *n.* madder (*Rubia tinctorum* L., → **1271**)
warke *v.* be in pain
ware *a.* aware
wariche, -she *v.* recover from illness
warme *a.* warm
wash, we- *v.* wash
wasp* *n.* wasp (*Vespula vulgaris* Linnaeus, 1758)
waste* *v.* consume completely
wat(e)ry *a.* suffused with water, damp; growing in damp places
water *n.* water
water-mynte *n.* water-mint (*Mentha aquatica* L., → **863**)
watyr-cars *n.* watercress (*Nasturtium officinale* R.Br., → **2453**)
wawing *a.* moving, loose
wax *n.* wax ¶ **virgyn w.** purest and finest quality bees-wax
we *pron.* we
webb(e *n.* film in the eye
wek(k)yd, -þ *a.* harmful, bad for the health; poisonous; malignant, evil
wedder* *n.* castrated ram
wey-hor *n.* cudweed/cottonrose (*Filago germanica* (L.) Huds./*F. pyramidata* L., → **884**)
wel(l *adv.* well

wen* *n.* maculation in the skin
werk* *n.* pain
wery *a.* weary, tired
wermod(e, wo- *n.* wormwood (*Artemisia absinthium* L., → **2350**)
wert* *n.* wart
wesill, wy- *n.* weasel (*Mustela nivalis* Linnaeus, 1766)
wete *a.* wet, humid
wete *v.* know
wet(te *v.* soak; moisten
wex* *v.* increase, swell; turn, evolve, become
wexing *n.* growth
whate *a.* whatever
w(h)elk* *n.* pimple
when *pron.* when
wher *pron.* where
where-to *conj.* whereto
wher-in *conj.* wherein
wher-of *conj.* whence
whete *n.* wheat, seed of *Triticum aestivum* L.
whiche *pron.* which
while *n.* portion of time
while *conj.* while, during the time that; (+ þat) whereas
white *a.* white
white *n* albumen, the white part of an egg
white mynte *n.* horsemint (*Mentha longifolia* (L.) L., → **1454**)
white pepir *n.* white mustard (*Sinapis alba* L., → **2506**)
white-horyd *a.* greyish white
whityn more *n.* silverweed (*Potentilla anserina* L., → **2501**)
whityngtre *n.* guelder rose/wayfaring tree (*Viburnum opulus* L./*V. lantana* L.)
who *pron.* who ¶ w. þat anyone who
who-so *pron.* anyone who
wide *adv.* widely
wiȝt *n.* weight

wil(e)we *n.* willow; marshmallow (*Althaea officinalis* L., → **2420**)
wil(l *v.* want (*used generally as an auxiliary to mark the future tense*)
wilde *a.* wild, not cultivated
wylde hempe *n.* hemp agrimony (*Eupatorium cannabinum* L., → **2495**)
wilde malowe *n.* marshmallow (*Althaea officinialis* L., → **849**)
wilde rewe *n.* fumewort (*Corydalis solida* (L.) Clairv., → **681**)
wylde sanagrene *n.* black cumin (*Nigella sativa* L., → **2538**)
wilde sauge *n.* ?wood sage (*Teucrium scorodonia* L., → **133**)
wilde spurge *n.* sun spurge (*Euphorbia helioscopia* L., → **2332**)
wylde tansy *a.* silverweed (*Potentilla anserina* L., → **2501**)
wilde tyme *a.* wild thyme (*Thymus serpyllum* L., → **1631**)
wilde worte *n.* ?wild clary (*Salvia verbenaca* L., → **1616**)
will *n.* will
wynde *n.* wind; air in the digestive tract
wyn(e *n.*[1] wine
wyne *n.*[2] vine (*Vitis vinifera* L.)
wynter *n.* year
wirchinge *a.* therapeutic
wise *a.* wise
wit(t *n.* wit, intelligence; mind, sense
with *prep.* with, in addition to; next to; by means of; by (*in passive constructions*)
with(e)-oute(n *prep.* without
with-hold* *v.* retain, hold back
wythi, -e *n.* willow (*Salix* L. spp., → **2511**)
wiþ-in *prep.* within
with-in(ne *adv.* within; (in the) inside
with-inforþ *adv.* inside
with-oute *adv.* (in the) outside
withwynde *n.* woodbine (*Lonicera*

periclymenum L., → **2484**)
wlake *a.* lukewarm
wlatynge *n.* nausea
wode* *n.* wood, forest
wode *a.* insane; rabid
wodebynd(e *n.* woodbine (*Lonicera periclymenum* L., → **2484**)
wodebroune *n.* bugle (*Ajuga reptans* L., → **919**)
wode-merche *n.* ?wood sage (*Teucrium scorodonia* L., → **133**)
wod(e)roff(e *n.* sweet woodruff (*Galium odoratum* (L.) Scop., → **2341**)
wodesoure *n.* wood sorrel (*Oxalis acetosella* L., → **2469**)
wolde *n.* asarabacca (*Asarum europaeum* L., → **2379**)
wolfe-ys þistill *n.* ?black chameleon (*Cardopatium corymbosum* (L.) Pers., → **2490**)
woll → **olde**
woll(e *n.* wool
wolshele *n.* scarlet pimpernel (*Anagallis arvensis* L., → **1859**)

woman *n.* woman
womb(e, -me *n.* intestine; womb
wonder *adv.* extremely, very
wondyrly *adv.* extremely, very
wone* *v.* be accustomed
worcher *n.* remedy, sth. which does good to health
word* *n.* word
worme *n.* snake; maggot; parasite, helminth; vermin
wormesede *n.* hog's fennel (*Peucedanum officinale* L., → **2186**)
worste → **evil(l**
worte *n.* decoction of malted grain
worthi, -e *a.* worthy, valuable
wote → **wete**
wound *n.* wound
wound *v.* wound
wrap* *v.* wrap
wrynge *v.* squeeze
write* *v.* write

INDEX OF PROPER NAMES

Diascardias Pedacius Dioscorides → **1682**
Galean, -lyen Claudius Galen → **189**, **355**, **1582**, **1677**, **2241**
Herforde est Hereford **2548**
Inde India **1539**
Ypocras Hippocrates → **83**, **385**, **1112**, **2398**
Johannes Lelamour John Lelamour **2547**
Saynt Johann Baptista Saint John the Baptist **651**
Macer Macer Floridus **214**, **2544**, → **2546**
Place(u)s Matthaeus Platearius → **1428**, **2295**
Perys Mithridates → **1962**
Palydius Rutilius Taurus Aemilianus Palladius → **1980**
Plenius Pliny the Elder → **171**, **178**, **182**, **323**, **374**, **800**, **826**, **982**, **1169**, **1290**, **1343**, **1369**, **1586**, **2398**, **2417**, **2442**

Appendix A. Botanical names

Binomen	ME Name	PDE Name	Latin Heading
Achillea millefolium	myllefoly, yarowe	yarrow	——
Aeonium arboreum	souredok	tree houseleek	acedula
Agrimonia eupatoria	agrymony, ambros(e, hyndale, wilde sauge, wode-merche	agrimony	agrimonia
Ajuga reptans	browne bugill, hart-worte, hertwort, silfe-hele, [wodebroune]	bugle	bigula, fraxinus
Alliaria petiolata	cardiake, cilsper	garlic mustard	cardiaca
Allium cepa	beatis, oynown[e]is	onion	/beata/
Allium porrum	lekys	leek	——
Allium sativum	garlek	garlic	alium domesticum
Althaea officinalis	wylwe, holyhok, wilde malowe	marshmallow	——
Ammi majus	ameos	bishopsweed	ameos
Anacyclus pyrethrum	pelletir	pellitory of Spain	piretum domesticum
Anagallis arvensis	kennyng-worte, pympirnell, [wa]yworte, wolshele	scarlet pimpernel	ippia maior
Anchusa arvensis	borage, longe de [be]ffe, oxetonge	alkanet	borago, lingua bouis
Anethum graveolens	annete, annys, dyll	dill	anisum, anetum
Angelica archangelica	erbe moyntayne, herba Plenius	garden angelica	/herba Plenius/
Anthemis cotula	dogfynell, houndfynell, maythen	stinking camomile	amarusca
Anthemis ssp.	camamyll	camomiles	camamilla
Anthriscus sylvestris	cheruell, kerwell, serfoyle	wild chervil	/apium risus, apium siluaticum/
Apium graveolens	(h)ache	wild celery	——
Aristolochia spp.	astrologie, medewort, rede mader	birthworts	/aristologia/
Aristolochia clematitis	hertwort, silfehale, [wodebroune]	birthwort	fraxinus

BINOMEN	ME NAME	PDE NAME	LATIN HEADING
Artemisia abrotanum	sowtheryne-wode	southernwood	abrotanum
Artemisia absinthium	wermode	wormwood	——
Artemisia maritima	lavandyr coton	sea wormwood	——
Artemisia vulgaris	mogwort	mugwort	arthemesia
Arum maculatum	herbe yue, hertishorne, ive	cuckoo's pint	ostragium
Asarum europaeum	wolde	asarabacca	——
Asphodelus aestivus	affodill	summer asphodel	centum capita
Asphodelus sp.	woderofe	asphodels	hastula regia
Asplenium scolopendrium	cerelonge, hertistonge	hart's tongue fern	lingua cerui
Asplenium trichomanes	maydenhere	maidenhair spleenwort	capilli Veneris
Aster amellus	lvnary	Italian starwort	[astericon]
Atropa bella-donna	dowechs, doworte, lesior, more morell	deadly nightshade	s[o]latrum
Bellis perennis	bon-worte, brisewort, daysye	daisy	consolida minor
Berula erecta	bellyre	narrow-leaved water-parsnip	birula
Borago officinalis	borage,bvgill, longe de [be]ffe, oxetonge	borage	bigula, borago, lingua bouis
Brassica nigra	mostarde	black mustard	——
Brassica oleracea	caule	cabbage	caulus domesticus
Calamintha ssp.	calamynte	calamints	calament
Calendula officinalis	marygoldye, rodewort	pot marigold	solsequium
Capsella bursa-pastoris	herdys purse, sanguynary, stanche, totheworte	shepherd's purse	bursa pastoris
Cardopatium corymbosum	wolfe-ys þistill	black chameleon	camelion
Carlina gummifera	wolfe-ys þistill	pine thistle	camelion
Carum carvi	carwey	caraway	caruium
Centaurea calcitrapa	kalketrap	caltrops	spica celtica
Centaurea centaurium	more centory	greater centaury	——
Centaurea nigra	more centory	greater centaury	——
Centaurium erythraea	fethirfoy, hersgall, lasse centory	common centaury	/febrefuga/
Chelidonium majus	more celedony	greater celandine	——
Chenopodium bonus-henricus	mercury, papwort, smere-worte	allgood	mercurialis
Cichorium intybus	marygoldye, rodewort	chicory	solsequium
Clinopodium nepeta	catt-mynte, nepis, nepte ryall	lesser calamint	nepta, rapa domestica

Lelamour Herbal

BINOMEN	ME NAME	PDE NAME	LATIN HEADING
Commiphora gileadensis	balme	balsam-tree	balsamum
Conium maculatum	erbe benet, hemloke	hemlock	[cicuta], herba benedicta
Conopodium majus	[e]arthnote	pignut	ciclaminum
Coriandrum sativum	coryandyr	coriander	coriandrum
Corydalis solida	fvmyter, wilde rewe	fumewort	fumus terre
Crocus sativus	safur	saffron	crocus
Cuminum cyminum	comyn	cumin	cummin
Cuscuta epilinum	dodyr	dodder	linum
Cuscuta epithymum	tyme	thyme dodder	epetimum
Cyclamen hederifolium	[e]arthnote	sow-bread	ciclaminum
Cynoglossum officinale	houndystonge	hound's-tongue	lingua canis
Cyperus longus	galynga	English galingale	galanga
Cytisus scoparius	brome	common broom	genestula
Daphne laureola	lawreoll	spurge laurel	———
Daucus carota	birdis-neste, dauke, pasnepe, pastyrnepe	wild carrot	daucus asininus, pastita domestica
Delphinium staphisagria	[stafisagre]	stavesacre	[stafisagria]
Dioscorea communis	godhishond, Seynt Mary seall	black bryony	sigilum Sancte Marie
Dracunculus vulgaris	addyrworte, dragancia femall, dragans, sepentary	dragons	dragancia (femina)
Drimia maritima	oy[n]one gresse	sea onion	———
Ecballium elaterium	spurge	squirting cucumber	elactuericum
Eruca vesicaria	costmaryn, sky[r]white	rocket	/eruca/
Eryngium maritimum	kalketrap	caltrops	spica celtica
Erysimum × cheiri	vyolett	wallflower	viola alba
Eupatorium cannabinum	donnetyl, holy rope, wylde hempe	hemp agrimony	canabaria
Euphorbia helioscopia	tvtymallys, wilde spurge	sun spurge	anabulla
Euphrasia spp.	eufrase	eyebrights	eufrasia
Filago germanica	chauuede, horeworte, wey-hor	cudweed	———
Filago pyramidata	chauuede, horeworte, wey-hor	cottonrose	———
Filipendula vulgaris	dropwort, filipendula	dropwort	filipendula
Foeniculum vulgare	finell	fennel	feniculum
Fragaria vesca	strawbery	wild strawberry	fragra
Galium aparine	aron, clyuer, hayreff	cleavers	rubia minor
Galium boreale	croswort	Northern bedstraw	herba cruciaca
Galium odoratum	erbe Waltir, woderofe	sweet woodruff	hastula regia, herba Waltery

Binomen	ME Name	PDE Name	Latin Heading
Galium palustre	croswort	common marsh-straw	herba cruciaca
Gentiana amarella	gencyan	gentian	genciana
Geranium columbinum	coluyr-fote	long stalked cranesbill	pes columbe
Geranium robertianum	erbe Robert	herb Robert	herba Roberti
Geranium sanguineum	maworte	bloody cranesbill	spicarius
Geum urbanum	avance, garofull, hare-fote	wood avens	gariofilum, sana munda
Glechoma hederacea	heyhofe	ground ivy	edera terrestris
Glycyrrhiza glabra	lycorys	licorise	liquericia
Gymnocarpium dryopteris	polypody, oke-verne	oak-fern	filex campestris, polipodium
Hedera helix	ivy	ivy	edera nigra
Helleborus niger	clofe-tonge, elebyr, longwort, pedelyon, piletir of Spayne, walworte	black hellebore	/eleborus/
Helminthotheca echioides	endyue, horse-þistill	bristly ox-tongue	endiuia
Hyoscyamus spp.	henbane	henbanes	——
Hypericum androsaemum	pa[r]k-levis, tutesayne	tutsan	agnus castus
Hypericum perforatum	erbe Johann, more centuary	St. John's wort	fuga demonum
Hyssopus officinalis	isope	hyssop	isopus
Inula britannica	polycary	British yellowhead	policaria
Inula elenium	elenacampana, horshele	elecampane	/elenacampana/
Iris × germanica	flour delice	German flag	iris
Iris × germanica florentina	safe	Florentine iris	irios
Iris pseudacorus	gladoyne	gladdon	gladiolus
Jacobaea vulgaris	fly-fo, ragworte	ragwort	——
Juniperus sabina	sawyn	savin	——
Knautia arvensis	scabyeus	field scabious	scabiosa
Lactuca sativa	letuse	lettuce	lacctuca
Lavandula angustifolia	lauandyr	English lavender	lauandula
Leonurus cardiaca	cardiake, cilsper	motherwort	cardiaca
Lepidium latifolium	ditander	pepperwort	diptanum
Lepidium sativum	crasse	garden cress	——
Levisticum officinale	cowslope, lovache	lovage	/herba Petri/
Lilium candidum	lylly	lily	—
Linum usitatissimum	flax, lyne	flax	linum
Lithospermum officinale	gromyll	common gromwell	granum solis
Lolium temulentum	kokkyll, wylde sanagrene	darnel	lollium

Lelamour Herbal

Binomen	ME Name	PDE Name	Latin Heading
Lonicera periclymenum	cheuyrfoyle, serfoyle, withwynde, wodebynd	woodbine	caprifolium, apium siluaticum
Lupinus albus	lvpyne	lupin	lupinus fabe
Malva sylvestris	hokkys, maloys	common mallow	malua minor
Mandragora spp.	mandrake	mandrakes	mandragora
Marchantia polymorpha	levirwort	liverwort	epatica
Marrubium vulgare	horehounde, howndbene, morall	white horehound	marubium
Matthiola incana	vyolett	gilliflower	viola alba
Medicago spp.	hony-sokyll, melilote, þre-levid-grasse	burclovers	—
Melilotus spp.	hony-sokyll, melilote, þre-levid-grasse	melilots	—
Melissa officinalis	medewort	common balm	—
Mentha aquatica	horsmynte, medemynt, water-mynte	water-mint	balsa[m]ita
Mentha spp.	mynte	mints	—
Mentha longifolia	white mynte	horsemint	menta romana
Mentha pulegium	pulyoll	pennyroyal	—
Myristica fragrans	notemyge	nutmeg	nux muscata
Nasturtium officinale	watyr-cars	watercress	nasturcium aquaticum
Nigella sativa	kokkyll, wylde sanagrene	black cumin	lollium
Ocimum spp.	basilicon	basils	basilica
Ononis spinosa procumbens	kammok	restharrow	resta bouis
Orchis mascula	ȝekesterris, s[t]andilgose, s[t]andylwelkys	early purple orchid	saturion maior
Origanum dictamnus	ditander, hilwort, pulyoll monten, wilde tyme	dittany of Crete	/diptanum/
Origanum majorana	magiron	sweet marjoram	magirona
Origanum vulgare	broþer-worte, origanum, pygele	wild marjoram	/origanum/
Osmunda regalis	osm(o)unde	royal fern	filex campestris, osmunda
Oxalis acetosella	cokkowe-brede, sorell de boys, stokwort, wodesoure	wood sorrel	alleluya
Paeonia officinalis	pyany	peony	—
Pallenis spinosa	erbe Christofyr male	spiny starwort	herba Christofer
Papaver spp.	chessboll, papy	poppies	papauer

Binomen	ME Name	PDE Name	Latin Heading
Parietaria judaica	hem[er]worte, lithwort, paratory	pellitory-of-the-wall	paratorum
Pastinaca sativa	birdis-neste, dauke, pasnepe, pastyrnepe	parsnip	daucus asininus, pasti[nac]a domestica
Persicaria hydropiper	arsmeche, cvlrage	water-pepper	persicaria
Persicaria maculosa	arsmeche, cvlrage	willow-weed	persicaria
Petroselinum crispum	persely	parsley	petrocillium
Peucedanum officinale	swynes-fenyll, wormesede	hog's fennel	feniculus porci[n]us
Pilosella officinarum	mowsere	mouse-ear hawkweed	auricula muris
Pimpinella anisum	comyn	anise	cummin
Pimpinella saxifraga	saxfrage	burnet saxifrage	saxifragia
Plantago coronopus	(herbe) yue, hertishorne	buck-horn's plantain	ostragium
Plantago indica	polycary(a)	fleawort	policaria, p[s]ilium
Plantago lanceolata	launcell, rybwort	ribwort	lanceolata
Plantago major	playnteyn, waybrede	waybread	arnoglossa
Polygonatum multiflorum	godhishond, Seynt Mary seall	Solomon's seal	sigilum Sancte Marie
Polygonum aviculare	gasar, knotwort, sparowe-tonge, stryle, swynes-carsse	knotgrass	centinodium, mirtus
Polypodium vulgare	euere-verre[n]e	common polypody	filex campestris
Portulaca oleracea	coltisfote, diuee, fole-fote, helow, horshoue, horshoo, portulake	purslane	pes pulli (agrestis), portulaca
Potentilla anserina	gose gresse, whityn more, wylde tansy	silverweed	iacea alba
Potentilla erecta	turmentile	common tormentil	tana[s]etum
Potentilla reptans	quynfoyly, synkefoly	cinquefoil	quinque folium
Primula elatior	cowslope	oxlip	herba Petri
Primula vulgaris	prymerose	primrose	ligustrum
Ranunculus bulbosus	lode-worte, ram-ys-fote	bulbous buttercup	pes arietis
Ranunculus ficaria	lasse celedony	lesser celandine	———
Ranunculus flammula	las[se] sper-wort	lesser spearwort	f[l]amula minor
Ranunculus lingua	launcell, spereworte, sper-hede	greater spearwort	f[l]amula maior
Ranunculus sardous	clofe-tonge, pedelyon	hairy buttercup	eleborus
Raphanus raphanistrum	white pepir	white charlock	rapistrum domesticum

BINOMEN	ME NAME	PDE NAME	LATIN HEADING
Raphanus sativus	radich	radish	rappan[us]
Reseda luteola	wolde	weld	——
Rhinanthus spp.	germandir	rattles	——
Rosa spp.	rosse	roses	——
Rosmarinus officinalis	rose-mary	rosemary	——
Rubia tinctorum	madyr, warance	madder	rubia maior
Rumex acetosa	souredok	common sorrel	acedula
Rumex spp.	dokkys	docks	lappa
Ruscus aculeatus	gasar, knotwort	butcher's broom	mirtus
Ruta graveolens	rewe	rue	——
Salix spp.	wylwe, wythi	willows	/salix/
Salvia officinalis	sagge	sage	——
Salvia verbenaca	oculus Christi, scabwort, wilde worte	wild clary	oculus Christi
Sambucus ebulus	(herbe) yue, hertishorne, walworte	danewort	/ostragium/
Sambucus nigra	walworte	elder	——
Sanguisorba spp.	bornete	burnets	burneta
Saponaria officinalis	ostricium, savygill	soapwort	/ostricium/
Satureja spp.	savory	savories	——
Scorzoneroides autumnalis	morre y-bitt	autumnal hawkbit	morsus diaboli
Sedum acre	stonecrop	common stonecrop	crassula minor
Sedum telephium	orpyn	orpine	crassula maior
Sempervivum tectorum	full, houseleke, jubarbe	houseleek	Barba Jouis, sacrefolium
Senecio vulgaris	gryniswelly, growndswelow, swython	common groundsel	——
Sinapis alba	white pepir	white mustard	rapistrum domesticum
Sisymbrium officinale	verveyn	hedge mustard	——
Smyrnium olusatrum	alixsandir, stannmarche	horse parsley	alexandrum
Solanum nigrum	houndbery, morell, nyght-shade, pety morell	black nightshade	/morella medica/
Sonchus oleraceus	sowe-þistill	common sowthistle	labium Veneris
Stachys betonica	betayne	betony	betayne
Stellaria holostea	pygele	greater stitchwort	——
Succisa pratensis	scabyeus	devil's-bit scabious	scabiosa
Symphytum officinale	confery	comfrey	consolida maior
Tanacetum parthenium	fethirfoy, hersgall	feverfew	febrefuga
Tanacetum vulgare	tansy	tansy	tanacetum

Binomen	ME Name	PDE Name	Latin Heading
Taraxacum spp.	dent de lyon	dandelions	dens leonis
Teucrium chamaedrys	colombyne, germandir	wall germander	——
Teucrium scorodonia	ambros(e, hyndale, wilde sauge, wodemerche	wood sage	euperatorium
Thymus serpyllum	hilwort, pulyoll monten, wilde tyme	wild thyme	——
Thymus vulgaris	tyme	garden thyme	epetimum
Trifolium spp.	hony-sokyll, melilote, þre-levid-grasse	clovers	——
Trigonella foenum-graecum	fenygreke	fenugreek	fenigre[c]um
Tussilago farfara	coltisfote, diuee, folefote, horshoue	coltsfoot	pes pulli agrestis
Urtica spp.	nettyll	nettles	vrtica
Valeriana celtica	kalketrap	Celtic spikenard	spica celtica
Veratrum album	elebyr, longwort, piletir of Spayne, walworte	white hellebore	/eleborus/
Verbascum thapsus	moleyne, taperwort	great mullein	——
Verbena officinalis	colombyne, verveyn	vervein	——
Veronica beccabunga	brokleuys	brooklime	fabaria
Viola odorata	vyolett	sweet violet	viola alba
Viscum album	arbuste, mistilte	mistletoe	osmunda
Vitex agnus-castus	pa[r]k-levis, tutesayne	chaste tree	agnus castus

Appendix B. Medical virtues

abortifacient (to cause abortion): 305, 340, 346, 434, 593, 987, 1229, 1283, 1390, 1396, 1534, 1576, 1654, 1806, 2047, 2060, 2083, 2102, 2317, 2362, 2388, 2414
acoustic (to improve hearing): 545, 1234, 2273, 2415
acrepalous (against drunkenness): 454, 2520
adipsic (to relieve thirst): 1251, 1891, 2032
alexipharmic (against poison, including bites from poisonous snakes): 4, 42, 70, 129, 174, 217, 306, 318, 395, 412, 484, 507, 535, 551, 695, 718, 729, 760, 810, 952, 1127, 1304, 1332, 1407, 1433, 1512, 1555, 1610, 1661, 1725, 1742, 1781, 1812, 1827, 1862, 1943, 1962, 2084, 2101, 2115, 2192, 2212, 2252, 2270, 2289, 2327, 2368, 2437, 2446, 2487
analgesic (pain-killer): 3, 184, 226, 236, 298, 303, 527, 726, 748, 1404, 1486, 1715, 1726, 1772, 1782, 1793, 1926, 2098, 2242
anamnestic (to improve memory): 209, 1184
anaphrodisiac (to quell sexual desire): 401, 483, 882, 1501, 1948, 2154, 2278, 2293, 2516
antacid (against heartburn, i.e., burning sensation in the stomach): 4, 704, 1659, 1970
antephialtic (against nightmares): 2002
anthelminthic (against worms in the womb or bowels): 126, 356, 396, 416, 448, 780, 989, 995, 1195, 1198, 1279, 1319, 1457, 1513, 1564, 1669, 1767, 2127, 2187, 2270, 2283, 2357
anthemoptyic (against spitting blood): 151, 170, 1114, 1749, 1876, 2243
anthydropic (against dropsy): 151, 170, 256, 349, 770, 990, 1198, 1383, 1609, 1638, 1744, 1802, 2295, 2396, 2413
antiabortive (against miscarriage): 48
antiacne (against black spots in the skin): 1740, 2429
antialopecic (against baldness and hair loss): 304, 1496, 1602, 1990, 2041
antiaphthic (against canker, i.e. wounds in the mouth): 993, 1562, 1598, 1746, 1791, 1794, 1925, 1973, 2140, 2162, 2347, 2434
antiarthritic (against illnesses of the joints, particularly arthritis and gout): 47, 257, 445, 519, 1911, 1953, 2030
antiasthmatic (against asthma): 452
anticallus (against corns in the feet): 197, 1596, 2475
anticancerous (against cancer): 46, 424, 549, 639, 857, 888, 1082, 1090, 1483, 1731, 1938, 2007, 2485
anticaries (against rotting of the teeth): 73, 1996
anticatarrhal (against catarrh, flux from the head): 225, 1845, 2370
anticaustic (against corrosion of the skin): 2264
anticephalalgic (against headache): 119, 272, 380, 576, 773, 1011, 1373, 1434, 1465, 1776, 1826, 1844, 1957, 1977, 2240, 2267, 2305, 2321, 2442
anticholecystic (against disorders in the gall-bladder): 1676, 1803, 2427
anticholeric (against excess of bile): 206, 219, 290, 295, 1185, 1621, 1901
anticolic (against colic, i.e., pain in the bowels): 59, 370, 928, 1164, 1405, 2142
anticontusive (against bruises): 491, 527, 764, 1556, 2368
anticteric (against jaundice): 175, 221, 235, 331, 372, 612, 772, 1382, 1393, 1514, 1559, 1676, 1796, 2069, 2079, 2105, 2366, 2382, 2432
antidiaphoretic (against excessive sweating): 2018

antidiarrheic (against diarrhea): 6, 359, 436, 568, 594, 925, 1110, 1704, 1712, 1901, 1971
antidinic (against vertigo): 1068, 2064, 2143
antidysenteric (against dysentery): 80, 202, 483, 568, 887, 978, 1027, 1379, 1428, 1601, 1674, 1732, 1739, 1779, 1787, 1872, 2025, 2269, 2310, 2330, 2348, 2426
antiemetic (against vomit): 273, 417, 703, 1659, 1723, 2055, 2106, 2264
antiemmenagogue (against the emission of woman menses): 363, 756, 1753, 2122, 2513
antiephelic (against freckles): 200, 1606, 1666
antiepilectic (against epilepsia): 75, 279, 466, 1262, 1350, 1464, 1492, 1678, 1745, 1836, 2396, 2521
antiepistactic (against nosebleed): 495, 1114, 1380, 2249
antigingivitic (against disorders of the gum): 590, 1665, 1752
antigonorrheic (against the accidental effusion of semen): 1221
antihalitosic (against bad breath): 488, 791, 809, 1546, 1603, 2543
antihematuric (against pissing blood): 148, 1854
antihemorrhoidal (against hemorrhoids): 115, 859, 1395, 1446, 1524, 1604, 1630, 2454
antihepatitic (against swollen liver): 1336
antiherpetic (against herpes, erysipelas, eczema, scabs, tetters etc.): 334, 360, 603.690, 719, 877, 953, 1375, 1426, 1577, 1708, 1748, 1960, 1970, 2209, 2342
anti-inflammatory (against swelling): 161, 248, 292, 299, 357, 429, 442, 527, 688, 764, 909, 925, 931, 941, 1000, 1009, 1041, 1092, 1204, 1218, 1347, 1433, 1440, 1628, 1666, 1726, 1743, 1758, 1768, 1802, 1863, 1893, 1931, 1954, 1968, 2003, 2014, 2213, 2246, 2285, 2349, 2373, 2424, 2460
antilethargic (against lethargy): 1350, 2052, 2299, 2321
antilumbalgic (against lumbago): 1347, 1491, 1810, 2144, 2239
antimalarial (against tertian fever, i.e. malaria): 612, 1309, 1761, 1817
antimanic (against madness): 626, 1745, 2026, 2395, 2407
antimastitic (against swelling of the breasts): 642, 879
antimelancholic (against melancholy): 1887, 2163, 2396
antimetrorrhagic (against metrorrhagia, i.e. flux of woman's menses): 1373, 1684, 1704, 1712, 1971
antinephritic (against nephritis): 596, 701
antineuropathic (against problems of the nerves): 2120
antiodontalgic (against toothache): 303, 331, 567, 800, 897, 910, 1001, 1237, 1369, 1566, 1598, 1752, 1821, 1977, 2417, 2486
antiotalgic (against earache): 44, 153, 775, 944, 1003, 1373, 1523, 1561, 1592, 1716, 1748, 1958
antiparalytic (against palsy): 77, 1173, 1657, 1690, 1822, 1839, 2113, 2409
antipernius (against chilblains): 53, 2481
antipestilential (against pestilence): 626, 782
antiphtheiriac (against lice): 65, 310, 1178
antiphthisic (against phthisis): 937, 996, 1334, 1750, 1817, 2038, 2043, 2087
antipleuritic (against pleuresy): 1950
antipleurodynic (against stitch in the side): 75, 627, 808, 897, 942, 1569, 2087

antipodagric (against podagra): 75, 276, 427, 445, 643, 671, 753, 851, 883, 1485, 1665, 1717, 1773, 1782, 1793, 2266, 2346, 2408
antipruritic (against itching): 564, 1373, 1403, 1557, 1669, 2089, 2120, 2233, 2339
antipyrotic (against burns on the skin): 743, 1039, 1637, 1741, 1977, 2253, 2430, 2519
antirabic (against rabies): 1481, 1742, 1781
antiraucedo (against hoarseness of the voice): 452, 777, 995
antisciatic (against sciatica): 309, 338, 595, 900, 1095, 1188, 1335, 1528, 2278
antiscrofulous (against scrofula): 1353
antiseptic (to cleanse wounds): 129, 634, 941, 1737, 2059, 2420, 2508
antisingultus (against hiccups): 109, 274, 401, 1517
antispasmodic (against spasms: shaking of members, cramp in the stomach, etc.): 717, 729, 945, 958, 1412, 2101
antispermatorrheic (against effusion of semen): 882
antitenesmus (against tenesmus, i.e. the feeling that one needs to pass stool despite an empty colon): 778
antitonsillitic (against tonsillitis, quinsy, etc.): 859, 1475
antitumoral (against tumours): 524, 612, 1729
antitussive (against cough): 5, 50, 155, 166, 312, 315, 347, 411, 594, 598, 727, 775, 807, 903, 926, 931, 947, 996, 1125, 1249, 1334, 1478, 1557, 1575, 1670, 1706, 1712, 1816, 1949, 2018, 2087, 2099, 2525
antiulcerous (against ulcers, botches, whelks, etc.): 1765, 1804, 2266, 2458, 2486
antiuvulitic (against staphyledema, i.e. swollen uvula): 450, 456, 1494, 1560
antiverrucous (against warts): 2516
aphrodisiac (to arouse sexual desire): 300, 321, 554, 695, 793, 847, 1734, 1886, 2056, 2131
apophlegmatic (to help discharge excessive phlegm from the head): 451, 1230, 1327, 1333, 2389
calefacient (to give heat): 119, 128, 352, 717, 867, 1507, 1522, 1998, 2147
cardiac (against disorders of the heart): 206, 219, 290, 295, 577, 686, 1185, 1814, 2362
carminative (to expel wind in the bowels): 81, 108, 127, 370, 410, 480, 503, 563, 678, 791, 853, 867, 999, 1083, 1164, 1547, 1800, 1950, 2050, 2197, 2320, 2358, 2398, 2542
caustic (causing a burning sensation): 1328, 2264
cephalgic (to cure disorders of the head): 2520
cholagogue (to expel bile): 746, 1239, 1638, 2358
conceptive (to help pregnancy): 1387, 1430
consolidative (to join together broken bones, cut veins or sinews, etc.): 142, 262, 317, 495, 526, 719, 1044, 1100, 1132, 1246, 1276, 2449, 2529
contraceptive (against pregnancy): 1325, 1948
corroborant (to strengthen): 1400, 2000
corrosive (causing a burning sensation): 390
cosmetic (to obtain a healthy skin colour): 8, 192, 316, 482, 1024, 1161, 1236, 1278, 1393, 1557, 1587, 1848, 1990, 2041, 2062, 2091,
demonifuge (to exorcize demons): 78
deoppilant (to open obstructions): 80, 143, 226, 233, 295, 505, 537, 611, 686,

743, 1166, 1212, 1272, 1287, 1623, 1845, 1944, 1975, 2294

desiccant (to dry the excess of humidity): 1484

detergent (to clean): 371, 379, 399, 547, 690, 1201, 1272, 1313, 1537, 2504

diaphoretic (to increase sweat): 388, 1495, 1505, 1568

dietetic (to lose weight): 1026

diuretic (to pass water): 19, 107, 150, 235, 314, 368, 419, 481, 505, 592, 691, 701, 787, 810, 1084, 1166, 1329, 1398, 1472, 1491, 1564, 1573, 1670, 1829, 1839, 2047, 2122, 2316, 2358, 2380

eloquent (to help speak): 866, 1497, 1594, 1692, 1846, 2533

emetic (to produce vomit): 1150, 1225, 1608, 2229, 2382, 2394

emmenagogue (to help the emission of woman's menses): 117, 175, 340, 348, 368, 391, 414, 434, 505, 572, 702, 756, 1118, 1143, 1148, 1166, 1329, 1388, 1528, 1573, 1596, 1655, 1674, 1801, 1806, 1948, 2047, 2060, 2083, 2317, 2358, 2380, 2414, 2539

emollient (to soften): 895, 954, 981, 1296, 1927

encephalic (to cure disorders of the brain): 688, 1545

epistactic (to produce nosebleed): 1380

eupeptic (to help digestion): 116, 178, 269, 290, 295, 314, 416, 481, 503, 508, 791, 845, 1459, 1563, 1620, 1809

exfoliant (to remove dead skin): 2474

exhilarant (to cause laughter or happiness): 78, 212, 217, 288, 1190, 1993, 2433, 2436, 2446

exorcist (to expel devils and ghosts): 650, 1402

expectorant (to expel mucus from the breast): 50, 311, 729, 1658, 2049, 2100, 2122, 2211, 2319

febrifuge (against fever): 8, 34, 75, 168, 268, 277, 361, 389, 558, 716, 952, 1211, 1245, 1309, 1411, 1438, 1466, 1507, 1761, 1770, 1823, 1838, 1869, 1952, 1973, 2124, 2178, 2191, 2284, 2408, 2448, 2497

fertilizer (to make the land more productive): 2020

galactogenous (to produce milk): 6, 16, 116, 202, 433, 700, 1088, 1210, 1831, 2540

galactogogue (to secrete milk): 1321

galactophygus (to stop the production of milk): 879

hematogenous (to form blood): 1210, 1816

hematogogue (to draw blood): 1299, 1488, 2488

hemostatic (to stop bleeding): 972, 1116, 1488, 1740, 1792, 1958, 2085, 2302, 2310, 2344, 2512, 2528

hepatic (to cure disorders of the liver): 128, 143, 678, 805, 989, 1083, 1243, 1275, 1548, 1572, 1722, 1803, 2082, 2215, 2303, 2362

herpetofuge (to expel snakes from some place): 178, 306, 403, 576, 761, 1515, 1827, 2009, 2029, 2036, 2124

hysteric (against disorders of the uterus): 756, 1391, 1480, 2121, 2381

indurant (to harden sinews, skin, etc.): 320, 671, 797

laxative (to help pass stools): 167, 232, 436, 743, 999, 1022, 1050, 1127, 1135, 1297, 1493, 1587

leprostatic (against leprosy): 392, 440, 689, 1087, 1236, 1353, 1513, 1577, 1235, 2397, 2416

lithontriptic (to break the stone): 128, 261, 368, 572, 592, 678, 691, 786, 1016, 1303, 1329, 1398, 1470, 1573, 1629, 1677, 1815, 2113, 2159, 2163, 2203, 2244, 2287, 2315, 2448, 2467

maturative (to make swellings ripe): 933, 1036, 1293, 1295, 2116, 2179, 2485

mazolytic (to help the expulsion of the placenta): 71, 274, 766, 940, 1655, 1772, 1806, 2426

mucolytic (to make mucus less thick or sticky): 2087

muscicide (to kill flies): 1234, 2392

nephretic (to cure disorders of the kidneys): 117, 128, 447, 747, 770, 793, 901, 1722, 1756, 1774, 1803, 2121

ophthalmic (to cure disorders of the eyes): 3, 46, 153, 159, 199, 203, 292, 299, 315, 329, 351, 378, 433, 508, 514, 552, 620, 695, 756, 874, 944, 979, 988, 1084, 1233, 1316, 1333, 1346, 1369, 1450, 1605, 1618, 1650, 1652, 1751, 1864, 1875, 1979, 2108, 2129, 2182, 2199, 2266, 2328, 2368, 2390, 2411, 2523

orectic (to build up an appetite): 692, 1268, 1603, 2022

oxen (to cure them from illnesses): 660, 2280

oxytocic (to speed childbirth): 732, 869, 940, 1086

panacea (to cure everything): 1987

phlegmagogue (to expel phlegm): 173, 791, 999, 1125, 1239, 1621, 1834, 2358, 2411

poultry (to make it fatter): 973

preservative (to keep food fresh): 2011

prognostic (to know the outcome of an illness): 1413, 1474, 2439

prophylactic (to avoid illnesses): 961, 1273, 1866, 2045, 2493

psychostimulant (to help mental health and acumen): 1329, 1545

pulmonic (to cure disorders of the lungs): 208, 598, 770, 990, 995, 1186, 1950

purgative (to cleanse through the womb or bowels): 135, 341, 576, 866, 899, 1150, 1226, 1329, 1632, 2047, 2054, 2217

refrigerant (to lessen heat): 200, 614, 644, 883, 980, 1040, 1209, 1890, 2032, 2526

regenerative (to create new skin or flesh): 462, 1484, 2509

reinvigorant (to regain strength): 2005

rejuvenatory (to look young): 707, 2005

relaxant (to soften muscles, sinews, tendons, etc.): 119, 281, 2424

resolvent (to dissolve gatherings): 753, 1088, 2540

rodenticide (to kill mice, rats, and other rodents): 1232, 1857, 2391

soporific (to induce sleep): 184, 193, 201, 291, 1215, 1216, 1219, 1419, 1700, 1703, 1705, 1712, 1715, 1716, 1718, 2107, 2375

spasmolytic (to relieve spasm): 89, 145

splanchnic (to cure disorders of the viscera): 10, 162, 373, 397, 414, 1409, 1810, 2444

splenetic (to cure disorders of the spleen): 64, 75, 308, 348, 377, 571, 678, 805, 989, 995, 1336, 1485, 1572, 1668, 1673, 1722, 1731, 1830, 2184, 2303, 2367

sternutatory (to sneeze): 197, 295, 1230, 1266, 1580, 1595

stomachal (to cure disorders of the stomach): 35, 116, 155, 192, 401, 436, 686, 715, 805, 845, 865, 950, 1083, 1267, 1275, 1318, 1409, 1535, 1542, 1620, 1627, 1817, 1885, 1948, 2106, 2215, 2343, 2350

thoracic (good for the chest): 747, 2120

tonic (to restore the general well-being): 184, 980, 988, 1567, 1663, 1687

trichogenous (promoting the growth of hair): 413, 441, 463, 2118, 2209

vermifuge (to expel parasitic worms from the body): 301, 332, 696, 910, 1201, 1316, 1458, 1460, 1532, 1996

vesical (to cure disorders of the urinary bladder): 983, 1756, 1774

vulnerary (to cure wounds): 36, 61, 73, 111, 137, 144, 157, 224, 337, 350, 351, 405, 423, 475, 549, 634, 638, 720, 797, 841, 888, 914, 920, 1082, 1090, 1132, 1133, 1145, 1167, 1181, 1245, 1273, 1310, 1481, 1551, 1633, 1737, 1778, 1784, 1864, 1896, 1938, 2059, 2183, 2198, 2312, 2420, 2434, 2508

Late Middle English Texts

General Editors:
Antonio Miranda-García, University of Málaga (amiranda@uma.es)
& Santiago González, University of Oviedo (sigonzalez@uniovi.es)

This series is conceived to facilitate the edition of unpublished scientific treatises written in Late Middle English (late 13th century to the very early 16th century) as well as the publication of monographs dealing with their transmission, palaeographical and dialectal features, and/or their lexical, syntactic and pragmatic characteristics. The second aspect of the series seeks to favour studies specializing in linguistic variation or any of the multi-faceted aspects of the Middle English language even from a diachronic perspective.

The Late Middle English Texts series is directed towards a wide scholarly readership that includes Textual Edition, Textual Criticism and Transmission – especially on electronic and digital formats both as standalone and online –, Ecdotics, History of Science, History of the English Language and Linguistics, Late Medieval Studies, History of Cultural Artifacts and Librarianship. The chronological scope we contemplate will range approximately from the mid 1200's to the early 1500's, and will include both manuscripts, incunabula and early prints that have come down to us in English, with the occasional excursion into analogues in other languages. Editions will include codicological and language studies that will enhance the relevance of the text within the cultural transmission European framework.

The series includes both scholarly and academic editions and monograph studies with a specialised and comprehensive focus. Thematic and teaching textual anthologies will also be considered for the series. We do not aim primarily at publishing collected papers from conferences, symposia, meetings and other reunions, unless the occasion had a very relevant topic and was strongly coherent and specialised in its discussions.

Each publication is subject to a rigorous blind double peer-review system that involves at least five readers from five different institutions (Universities or Research Institutes).

1   Antonio Miranda-García & Santiago González Fernández-Corugedo
    Benvenutus Grassus' On the well-proven art of the eye
    Practica oculorum & De probatissima arte oculorum
    524 pages / 2011 / 978-3-0343-0698-0

2   Javier Calle-Martín & Antonio Miranda-García
    The Middle English Version of *De viribus herbarum*
    (GUL MS Hunter 497, ff. 1r-92r)
    258 pages / 2012 / 978-3-0343-0697-3

3   Laura Esteban-Segura
        System of Physic
        (GUL MS Hunter 509, ff. 1r-167v)
        A Compendium of Mediaeval Medicine
        Including the Middle English Gilbertus Anglicus
        461 pages / 2012 / 978-3-0343-0077-3

4   Forthcoming

5   Javier Calle-Martín and Miguel Ángel Castaño-Gil.
        A Late Middle English Remedy-book (MS Wellcome 542, ff. 1r-20v)
        A Scholarly Edition
        183 pages / 2013 / 978-3-0343-1369-8

6   David Moreno Olalla
        Lelamour Herbal
        An Annotated Critical Edition of MS Sloane 5, ff. 13r-57r
        510 pages / 2018 / 978-3-0343-3155-5